A-Z of Neurological Practice

Second Edition

Erratum to:

A-Z of Neurological Practice

A.J. Larner et al., *A-Z of Neurological Practice*,
© Springer-Verlag London Limited 2011

The Preface to the second edition, in the references, the first name Larner A.J., changed to Lerner A.J.

Preface to the Second Edition

References

1. Lerner AJ. Diagnostic Criteria in Neurology. Totawa, NJ: Humana Press; 2006.
2. Larner AJ. A Dictionary of Neurological Signs. 3rd ed. New York: Springer; 2011.
3. Larner AJ. Neuropsychological Neurology: The Neurocognitive Impairments of Neurological Disorders. Cambridge, UK: Cambridge University Press; 2008.

The online version of the original chapter can be found at DOI: 10.1007/978-1-84882-994-7

Andrew J. Larner • Alasdair J. Coles
Neil J. Scolding • Roger A. Barker

A-Z of Neurological Practice

A Guide to Clinical Neurology

Second Edition

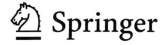 Springer

Authors
Dr. Andrew J. Larner, MA, MD,
MRCP(UK), DHMSA
Consultant Neurologist
Walton Centre for Neurology and
Neurosurgery, Liverpool, UK

Dr. Alasdair J. Coles, PhD, FRCP
Lecturer in Neurology
Addenbrooke's Hospital
Cambridge, UK

Prof. Neil J. Scolding, PhD, FRCP
Burden Professor of Clinical
Neurosciences, Institute of Clinical
Neurosciences
Bristol, UK

Dr. Roger A. Barker, BA, MBBS,
MRCP, PhD
Reader in Clinical Neuroscience
Addenbrooke's Hospital
Cambridge, UK

ISBN: 978-1-84882-993-0   e-ISBN: 978-1-84882-994-7
DOI: 10.1007/978-1-84882-994-7
Springer Dordrecht Heidelberg London New York

A catalogue record for this book is available from the British Library

Preface to the Second Edition

As with the first publication, the aim of this new, slimmer edition is to present information about neurological disorders in a structured and succinct way, following a "trickle down" principle: beginning with overviews and then moving on to specific disease categories. The latter address clinical features (i.e., information accessed by history-taking and physical examination), investigations, differential diagnosis, treatment, and prognosis. In this new edition, diagnostic criteria have been referenced where appropriate, but not included, both for fear of making the book too unwieldy and because this has already been done elsewhere.[1] Neurological signs are omitted and neuropsychology is not discussed in detail, since both these undertakings have been presented elsewhere.[2,3] Cross-references to the Online Mendelian Inheritance in Man (OMIM) database have been given where relevant.

George Orwell pointed out ("Why I write," 1946) that "writing a book is a horrible, exhausting struggle, like a long bout of some painful illness." It has sometimes seemed so with this book, but we hope that Orwell's other dictum, that "every book is a failure," does not prove entirely true and that our readers find something of use in these pages. We thank Manika Power at Springer for taking the book on, and for her unstinting encouragement in bringing it to fruition.

References

1. Larner AJ. Diagnostic Criteria in Neurology. Totawa, NJ: Humana Press; 2006.
2. Larner AJ. A Dictionary of Neurological Signs. 3rd ed. New York: Springer; 2011.
3. Larner AJ. Neuropsychological Neurology: The Neurocognitive Impairments of Neurological Disorders. Cambridge, UK: Cambridge University Press; 2008.

A

Abetalipoproteinemia [OMIM#200100]

Bassen–Kornzweig syndrome

Bassen and Kornzweig first described the association of a progressive ataxic syndrome with fat malabsorption, atypical retinitis pigmentosa, and acanthocytosis with a lack of serum betalipoproteins in two siblings of consanguineous parents in the 1950s. Abetalipoproteinemia is a rare autosomal recessive condition characterized by the defective assembly and secretion of apolipoprotein-B-containing lipoproteins, which are required for secretion of plasma lipoproteins that contain apolipoprotein B. In consequence, there are very low plasma concentrations of cholesterol and triglyceride, and of fat-soluble vitamins, especially vitamin E, which produces the clinical features of peripheral neuropathy, retinitis pigmentosa, and cerebellar degeneration. The condition is caused by mutations in the gene coding for microsomal triglyceride transfer protein (MTP) on chromosome 4q22-24, a protein required for the assembly of lipoproteins which contain apolipoprotein B. A related condition, hypobetalipoproteinemia, is inherited in an autosomal dominant fashion, with a defect in the apolipoprotein-B gene in some cases, and in the homozygous state may be indistinguishable from abetalipoproteinemia.

Clinical features

- Malabsorption: steatorrhea, with failure to thrive in children.
- Retinal degeneration: usually before the age of 10 years, with impaired night vision (nyctalopia) initially, and progressive retinitis pigmentosa; vitamin A deficiency may be significant. However, visual impairment is seldom severe.
- Peripheral neuropathy: a sensorimotor neuropathy with areflexia is often the presenting feature and is usually present by 10–30 years of age; vitamin E deficiency may be significant.
- Ataxic syndrome: with dysarthria, nystagmus, and head titubation. It results from a combination of peripheral neuropathy, spinocerebellar tract degeneration, and direct cerebellar damage (i.e., sensory and cerebellar ataxia); vitamin E deficiency may be significant.

A.J. Larner et al., *A-Z of Neurological Practice*,
DOI: 10.1007/978-1-84882-994-7_1,
© Springer-Verlag London Limited 2011

- Dorsal column sensory loss and extensor plantar responses.
- Ophthalmoplegia in later stages.
- Skeletal abnormalities: pes cavus, scoliosis; may be secondary to the peripheral neuropathy.
- Subdural, retroperitoneal hemorrhages; excessive blood loss during surgery (vitamin K deficiency may be significant).
- No autonomic abnormalities, but cardiac involvement with cardiomegaly is found in the late stages of the disease.

Investigation

Blood: low ESR; often a mild hemolytic anemia; acanthocytosis on blood film (which must be fresh to exclude false negatives), usually 50% or more of the red blood cells showing acanthocytic morphology; and low levels of apolipoprotein B (as demonstrated with immunoelectrophoresis), with very low plasma levels of chylomicrons, very low-, intermediate-, and low-density lipoproteins (VLDL, IDL, LDL). The plasma levels of cholesterol and triglycerides are very low, in the region of 1–2 and 0–1 mmol/L, respectively. The concentrations of fat-soluble vitamins, especially vitamin E, are also low. Neuroimaging (CT/MRI) shows no specific abnormalities. CSF is usually normal. Neurophysiology (EMG/NCS) shows peripheral sensorimotor neuropathy (axonal, demyelinating, or mixed); SSEPs may show abnormal posterior column function; VERs may be consistent with optic neuropathy; ERG may be consistent with retinal degeneration. Malabsorption tests may be required; jejunal biopsy reveals normal villi but the intestinal mucosal cells are vacuolated due to the presence of fat droplets that accumulate within them as they cannot be taken up by the chylomicrons.

Differential diagnosis

- *Friedreich's ataxia*
- Vitamin E deficiency secondary to other malabsorption syndromes (e.g., *coeliac disease*, cystic fibrosis)
- Isolated vitamin E deficiency (*ataxia with vitamin E deficiency* [AVED])

Treatment and prognosis

Treatment of the malabsorption syndrome is achieved by substitution and restriction of fat intake (i.e., low fat diet and medium chain triglycerides). Many of the neurological complications can be prevented by oral administration of vitamin E (1–10 g/day). Replacement of other fat-soluble vitamins (vitamins A, D, and K) is required. Untreated patients are usually unable to stand or walk by the time they reach adolescence and rarely survive beyond the age of 40 years.

References

Hardie RJ. Acanthocytosis and neurological impairment – a review. Q J Med. 1989; 71:291–306
Rowland LP, Pedley TA. Abetalipoproteinemia. In: Rowland LP, ed. Merritt's Textbook of Neurology. 9th ed. Baltimore, MD: Williams & Wilkins; 1995:594–596
Vongsuvanh R, Hooper AJ, Coakley JC, et al. Novel mutations in abetalipoproteinaemia and homozygous familial hypobetalipoproteinaemia. J Inherit Metab Dis. 2007;30:990

Abscess: overview

An abscess is a focal suppurative process, which may occur within or adjacent to nervous tissue, with resultant neurological features as well as systemic disturbance (pyrexia) from infection.

* Cerebral abscess:
  - Focal suppuration within brain parenchyma may present with the symptoms and signs of a space-occupying lesion: headache, focal signs, impaired level of consciousness, and epileptic seizures. Fever is not universally present, so its absence should not rule out the diagnosis. Predisposing causes include penetrating head trauma, hematogenous spread (e.g., infective *endocarditis*), and immunosuppression (e.g., *HIV/AIDS*), but the most common cause is contiguous spread of infection, for example in the ear, paranasal sinuses, or teeth. Pulmonary fistulae in *hereditary hemorrhagic telangiectasia* (Osler–Weber–Rendu syndrome) predispose to cerebral abscesses. Fungal infections may also result in cerebral abscess formation (aspergillosis, blastomycosis, coccidioidomycosis, mucormycosis), as may filamentous bacteria (actinomycosis).
* Spinal cord abscess:
  - Abscess within the spinal cord is extremely rare; symptoms and signs are indistinguishable from epidural abscess.
* Epidural or extradural abscess:
  - These are located between dura and bone; they may be spinal or, less often, cranial.
    o Spinal: Spread of infection is from vertebral osteomyelitis or retroperitoneal, mediastinal, or paraspinal infection. Severe back +/– radicular pain; compressive spinal cord syndrome (myelopathy +/– radiculopathy) may develop (thoracic > lumbar > cervical), often with systemic features of infection. Bloods may show leucocytosis, elevated ESR. Plain radiographs may show narrowing of disc spaces and/or lytic changes but MRI is investigation of choice for visualization of abscess. CSF, which should

only be done if MR imaging shows there is spinal block, reveals raised white count (typically <100 cells/µl), raised protein, and normal glucose. Treatment is with surgical decompression with appropriate antibiotic cover: Staphylococcus aureus is the most common organism, but others include streptococci, enterobacteria, Mycobacterium tuberculosis, and various fungi and parasites. Prognosis is good if surgical intervention is early; delayed diagnosis is associated with a poor prognosis.

- o Cranial: Almost always associated with an overlying osteomyelitis or local paranasal sinus infection. The features and management are similar to those of *subdural empyaema*. CSF may show pleocytosis (20–100 cells/µL) with normal glucose and protein. Treatment is with antibiotics; *Staphylococcus aureus* is the most commonly identified organism. Surgery has a place if there is significant mass effect or if an organism cannot be identified from peripheral cultures.

- Subdural abscess/empyaema:
  - These are located between dura and arachnoid. Spinal subdural abscess is clinically indistinguishable from epidural abscess.

References

Calfee DP, Wispelwey B. Brain abscess. Semin Neurol. 2000;20:353–360
Infection in Neurosurgery Working Party of the British Society for Antimicrobial Chemotherapy. The rational use of antibiotics in the treatment of brain abscess. Br J Neurosurg 2000;14:525–530
Pradilla G, Ardila GP, Hsu W, Rigamonti D. Epidural abscesses of the CNS. Lancet Neurol. 2009;8:292–300

Acanthamoeba

Acanthamoeba is one of the free-living amoebae, which, like *Naegleria*, may cause sporadic (primary amoebic) meningoencephalitis, spreading hematogenously from a cutaneous (skin ulcer) or pulmonary source, particularly in immunocompromised (e.g., *HIV/AIDS*, transplantation) patients. CSF shows pleocytosis; organisms are never cultured from CSF. Bacterial, fungal, and tuberculous meningitides could be considered in the differential diagnosis. Treatment with pentamidine is recommended and single cerebral *abscess* may be surgically removed. Mortality is very high.

Reference

Grunnert ML, Cannon GH, Kushner JP. Fulminant amebic meningoencephalitis due to *Acanthamoeba*. Neurology. 1981;31:174–177

Aceruloplasminemia [OMIM#604290]

This rare, recessively inherited disorder, in which ceruloplasmin is absent from the plasma, is clinically similar to *Wilson's disease*, individuals presenting with cerebellar ataxia, dementia, and involuntary movements, although copper metabolism is normal. Diabetes mellitus may also be present. Iron deposition in the basal ganglia is thought to be the cause. Similar cases with raised serum ferritin (ceruloplasmin deficiency with hemosiderosis) are also reported from Japan. Oral iron chelation has been reported to improve symptoms.

References

Logan JL, Harveyson KB, Wisdom GB, Hughes AE, Archbold GPR. Hereditary caeruloplasmin deficiency, dementia and diabetes mellitus. Q J Med. 1994; 87:663–670

Skidmore FM, Drago V, Foster P, et al. Aceruloplasminaemia with progressive atrophy without brain iron overload: treatment with oral chelation. J Neurol Neurosurg Psychiatry. 2008;79:467–470

Achondroplasia [OMIM#100800]

Chondrodystrophy

Achondroplasia is the most common form of bone dysplasia, inherited as an autosomal dominant condition, with an incidence of 1:25,000. Failure of normal endochondral bone formation, as a consequence of mutations in the fibroblast growth factor 3 gene, results in diminished vertebral body height and short stature. Such changes may be exacerbated with age due to further flattening and wedging of vertebral bodies, disc prolapse, and osteophyte formation. In 20–50% of cases, there are neurological complications, including the following:

Skull base compression with *hydrocephalus, syringomyelia,* +/– lower cranial nerve palsies, with myelopathy.

Spinal cord/root compression: can be anywhere, but typically in the cervicomedullary region (*foramen magnum syndrome*, causing progressive paraparesis or quadriparesis) or the cauda equina.

Respiratory disturbances, including *obstructive sleep apnea–hypopnea syndrome.*

Surgery for cord or root compression is often difficult due to the extent of the stenosis but seems to be most successful when done in young patients. However, in some cases decompression is ineffective and the stenosis continues to progress and is ultimately fatal.

Reference

Gordon N. The neurological complications of achondroplasia. Brain Dev. 2000;22:3–7

Acromegaly

Pituitary disease, resulting in excessive secretion of growth hormone (hyper-somatotropism) in adults, leads to acromegaly (*cf.* gigantism in children). This is a cause of secondary *diabetes mellitus*, so untreated acromegalics are at risk of all the potential neurological complications of diabetes. In addition, recognized neurological features of acromegaly include:

- Headache
- Acroparesthesia
- Visual disturbance (bitemporal hemianopia)
- Proximal myopathy (acromegalic myopathy; arthropathic > myopathic?)
- Thickening of the peripheral nerves +/– peripheral neuropathy (distal paresthesia, weakness, and areflexia, slowed nerve conduction velocities, soft tissue compression, nerve stretching?)
- *Carpal tunnel syndrome*
- Central sleep apnea syndrome

The myopathy may be accompanied by a raised creatine kinase, with myopathic features on EMG and muscle biopsy, variation in fiber size, type 2 fiber atrophy, and nonspecific increase in glycogen and lipofuscin on electron microscopy.

References

Khaleeli AA, Levy RD, Edwards RH, et al. The neuromuscular features of acromegaly: a clinical and pathological study. J Neurol Neurosurg Psychiatry. 1984;47:1009–1015
Woo CC. Neurological features of acromegaly: a review and report of two cases. J Manipulative Physiol Ther. 1988;11:314–321

Actinomycosis

Actinomycosis is caused by various Gram-positive anaerobic or microaerophilic rods (filamentous bacteria) of the genus Actinomyces. The most common clinical manifestation is "lumpy jaw," cervicofacial abscess formation. Infection may spread to the brain by direct extension or hematogenous spread to cause cerebral *abscess*(es) and/or acute or chronic nonspecific *meningitis*. Organisms are seldom identified from the CSF, but culture from extraneural sites may be possible. Yellow exudates from cutaneous abscesses contain "sulfur granules." Actinomycosis resembles *nocardiosis* as both may be a consequence of prolonged nonspecific immunosuppression; actinomycosis may occur, however, in immunocompetent patients.

Reference

Jacobson JR, Cloward RB. Actinomycosis of the central nervous system: a case of meningitis with recovery. JAMA. 1948;137:769–771

Action myoclonus–renal failure syndrome (AMRF) [OMIM#254900]

Action myoclonus–renal failure syndrome is characterized by tremor, action myoclonus, cerebellar signs, epilepsy, and renal failure, with onset in teenage or the early twenties. It was initially reported in several French-Canadian kindreds in Quebec and presumed to be an autosomal recessive disorder. The neurological features do not seem to be related to renal failure per se in this condition, which is thought to result from an inherited metabolic defect.

Clinical features

- Tremor of fingers, hands: onset age 17–18 years
- Proteinuria: onset age 17–18
- Action myoclonus: onset age 19–23; most disabling symptom
- Renal failure: onset age 20–22
- Cerebellar signs, ataxia, dysarthria: onset age 21–23; not severe
- Epilepsy (infrequent generalized seizures): onset age 21–23
- +/– Mild axonal degenerative neuropathy
- No extrapyramidal, pyramidal signs. Intelligence probably normal

Investigation

Neuroimaging shows nonspecific cerebral or cerebellar atrophy. EEG may show spike wave complexes, slowing, and photoparoxysmal discharges. Brain pathology shows pigment granules in astrocytes. Renal biopsy shows a nonspecific nephritis.

Differential diagnosis

Other causes of hereditary myoclonus, epilepsy, cerebellar syndrome, for example, sialidosis type I, neuronal ceroid lipofuscinosis (*Kuf's disease*), *neurodegeneration with brain iron accumulation*.

Treatment and prognosis

Symptomatic treatment of myoclonus and epilepsy; renal dialysis +/− transplantation (no recurrence in transplanted organ).

References

Badhwar A, Berkovic SF, Dowling JP, et al. Action myoclonus-renal failure syndrome: characterization of a unique cerebro-renal disorder. Brain. 2004;127:2173–2182
Berkovic SF, Dibbens LM, Oshlack A, et al. Array-based gene discovery with three unrelated subjects shows SCARB2/LIMP-2 deficiency causes myoclonus epilepsy and glomerulosclerosis. Am J Hum Genet. 2008;82:673–684

Acute disseminated encephalomyelitis (ADEM)

Acute hemorrhagic leukoencephalitis, acute necrotizing hemorrhagic encephalomyelitis, acute postinfectious encephalomyelitis (APEM), Hurst's disease

Acute disseminated encephalomyelitis (ADEM) is a monophasic illness characterized by a meningitic and encephalomyelitic syndrome, usually following an infective illness or vaccination, with evidence of widespread demyelination within the CNS. In its less fulminant form, it may be difficult to distinguish from the first episode of *multiple sclerosis (MS)*: because abnormalities in CSF, evoked potentials and MRI are similar in both conditions, continued follow-up may be the only way to make the distinction. ADEM typically occurs in children and young adults, is uncommon, and has a significant morbidity and mortality. Treatment with high-dose parenteral steroids is often tried, but is of unproven benefit.

Clinical features

- ADEM is a clinical syndrome: there are currently no accepted diagnostic criteria.
- Preceding infection: measles, rubella, chickenpox; rarely mumps, influenza, *Mycoplasma pneumoniae*.
- Preceding vaccination: rabies, smallpox, rarely tetanus antitoxin.
- Prodromal phase: fever, malaise, myalgia.
- Rapid onset (hours, days) of:
  - Focal or multifocal signs and symptoms of white matter lesions: e.g., optic neuritis (may be bilateral), ataxia, and paraparesis (*transverse myelitis*) with varying degrees of bladder and bowel involvement.

- Focal cortical deficits (e.g., dysphasia, seizures, and hemiparesis) are more common in ADEM than in episodes of multiple sclerosis.
- Encephalopathy, ranging from confusion and somnolence to fits, stupor, and coma, may be seen in adults, but is more commonly seen in children.
- Meningism with headache, fever, and neck stiffness is classically associated with hemorrhagic ADEM.

Investigation

Blood: usually unhelpful, but leukocytosis is not uncommon, especially in cases of acute necrotizing hemorrhagic encephalomyelitis, when there is also an elevated ESR. Neuroimaging: MRI demonstrates multifocal white matter lesions that are often more symmetric in their distribution, than those found in MS. As with MS the lesions enhance and persist, but in contrast with MS no new lesions develop beyond the time the disease typically evolves, which rarely extends beyond 2 weeks. New symptoms or signs, or new MRI lesions, appearing after 4 weeks from the start of the episode should be considered a second episode and raise the possibility of multiple sclerosis. Hence, interval scanning may help differentiate ADEM from MS. CSF usually shows increased protein and cells (lymphocytes) with a normal glucose concentration. This is most florid with the acute necrotizing hemorrhagic encephalomyelitis variant (which has all the same causes as the regular form of ADEM, although Mycoplasma is especially relevant) when there may be associated red blood cells in the CSF. Oligoclonal bands may be found, but usually do not persist; persistent oligoclonal bands are more suggestive of MS. Neurophysiology: evoked potentials and EEG may be abnormal, depending on extent and distribution of lesions. Pathology is rarely available. Perivascular inflammation with lymphocytes and mononuclear cells may be seen, with edema and microglial activation, and disseminated foci of demyelination throughout the brain and spinal cord centered on small- and medium-sized veins (peripheral nervous system spared). In its most severe form (acute hemorrhagic leukoencephalitis, Hurst's disease), there is necrosis of small blood vessels and brain tissue around the vessels; these lesions may coalesce and lead to almost complete hemorrhagic necrosis of whole hemispheres.

Differential diagnosis

The major differential diagnosis is between ADEM and the first episode of MS. Other conditions that may enter the differential diagnosis include:

- Multiple emboli
- Viral encephalitis
- Granulomatous disease (e.g., *neurosarcoidosis*)
- *Vasculitis*

Treatment and prognosis

Nearly 10–30% mortality rate; in the fulminant hemorrhagic form, death may occur in a few days. About 5% make a complete recovery, usually beginning within weeks. Recurrence may occur: multiphasic disseminated encephalomyelitis (MDEM). No treatment has been critically evaluated in ADEM, but there is some anecdotal evidence of benefit with intravenous methylprednisolone and plasmapharesis, with less compelling evidence for intravenous immunoglobulin. The development of more purified vaccines has greatly reduced the incidence of ADEM as a postvaccinial disorder. Rate of reclassification of ADEM as MS varies, but a recent large retrospective survey found that 35% of affected adults were reclassified as MS in 1 year.

References

De Seze J, Debouverie M, Zephir H, et al. Acute fulminant demyelinating disease: a descriptive study of 60 patients. Arch Neurol. 2007;64:1426–1432

Höllinger P, Sturzenegger M, Mathis J, Schroth G, Hess CW. Acute disseminated encephalomyelitis in adults: a reappraisal of clinical, CSF, EEG, and MRI findings. J Neurol. 2002;249:320–329

John L, Khaleeli AA, Larner AJ. Acute disseminated encephalomyelitis: a riddle wrapped in a mystery inside an enigma. Int J Clin Pract. 2003;57:235–237

Weinshenker B, O'Brien P, Petterson T, et al. A randomized trial of plasma exchange in acute central nervous system inflammatory demyelinating disease. Ann Neurol. 1999;46:878–886

Adrenoleukodystrophy (X-ALD) [OMIM#300100]

Adrenomyeloneuropathy (AMN), Siemerling–Creutzfeldt disease

X-linked adrenoleukodystrophy (X-ALD), the most common of the peroxisomal disorders, is characterized by a variable clinical phenotype, even within families, the spectrum of disease varying from an aggressive cerebral form of progressive demyelination with deafness, blindness, dementia, spasticity, as well as adrenal insufficiency, to an adult presentation (including carrier females) with a spastic paraparesis and a mild distal polyneuropathy, termed adrenomyeloneuropathy (AMN). X-ALD is due to mutations in a gene encoding a peroxisomal membrane protein ("ALD protein") that belongs to the ATP-binding cassette (ABC) protein family. This leads to accumulation of very long chain fatty acids (VLCFA) that characterizes the disease.

Clinical features

Heterogeneity of expression is very common in X-ALD, including within families. It affects approximately 1:25,000 males.

- Childhood cerebral presentation: age of onset <10 years:
  - Progressive personality change and intellectual decline, leading to dementia.
  - Gait abnormalities that evolve into a spastic quadriparesis.
  - Development of hearing and visual impairments at a later stage, leading to deafness and blindness.
  - Epileptic seizures rare.
  - Adrenal insufficiency (hypotension, skin pigmentation) found in >90% of cases but to varying degrees, some clinically overt, some biochemical only. In 70–80% of cases, the neurological deficits precede the adrenal insufficiency.
  - Pathology is more inflammatory than in other varieties of leukodystrophy.
- Adolescent cerebral presentation: 10–21 years:
  - Same as for childhood presentation but with a slower or "stuttering" onset. Motor involvement and cortical blindness may be absent.
- Adrenomyeloneuropathy (AMN): age 28 ± 9 years:
  - Progressive spastic paraparesis
  - Mild distal polyneuropathy
  - Adrenal insufficiency
  - Hypogonadism
  - Perhaps 45% develop later cerebral involvement, including neuropsychiatric disturbances, typically schizophreniform psychosis; dementia occurs late and is slowly progressive.
- Adult cerebral: age >21 years:
  - Rapidly progressive cerebral disease, as in childhood form, without preceding AMN; dementia may be a presenting feature (rare).
- Addison's disease only; no neurological features.
- Asymptomatic: genetic abnormality only, without endocrine or neurological features.
- Female heterozygotes:
  - Twenty percent have an AMN-like illness of variable severity (mild spastic paraparesis to wheelchair bound); 1–3% develop dementia, behavioral disturbance, or visual failure.

Investigation

Blood electrolytes, ACTH, and cortisol may demonstrate adrenal insufficiency. Very long chain fatty acids (VLCFA) are raised in serum, white cells, or cultured fibroblasts (in particular, the C26:C22 ratio). Neurogenetic testing reveals mutations in an ATP-binding-cassette transporter gene; over 500 have been described. Neuroimaging: brain CT/MRI shows extensive white matter demyelination, predominantly parieto-occipital, with incomplete sparing of U-fibers; contrast enhancement at the advancing margin of demyelination is characteristic and may be predominantly posterior or anterior in distribution. MR spectroscopy shows reduced *N*-acetyl aspartate, increased choline. CSF may show nonspecific raised protein and increased cell counts. Neurophysiology (EMG/NCS) may show a demyelinating neuropathy.

Differential diagnosis

Other *leukodystrophies*, especially *metachromatic leukodystrophy*, in adults. In adults, other conditions to consider include

- *Hereditary spastic paraplegia (HSP)*
- *Subacute combined degeneration of the cord*
- *Multiple sclerosis*
- CIDP with central demyelination

Treatment and prognosis

Adrenal replacement therapy for adrenal insufficiency. Symptomatic treatments of spasticity.
    Treatment of ALD per se:

- Dietary: Lorenzo's oil (a mixture of glycerol trioleate acid and trierucic acid in 4:1 ratio) normalizes plasma VLCFA, and if given early to asymptomatic boys, it reduces the risk of developing MRI abnormalities; its use may therefore be appropriate in asymptomatic boys with no MRI changes.
- Bone marrow transplantation: of no use in rapidly advancing disease, but may have a place in early disease to arrest, stabilize, and maybe even reverse early cerebral disease as measured by MR imaging and neuropsychology; no current indication in asymptomatic patients.
- Immunosuppressive therapy has no proven place.
- Gene therapy remains a hope.

Nearly two thirds of ALD patients escape the most severe phenotype.

References

Moser HW, Raymond GV, Dubey P. Adrenoleukodystrophy: new approaches to a neurodegenerative disease. JAMA. 2005;294:3131–3134
Moser HW, Raymond GV, Lu SE, et al. Follow-up of 89 asymptomatic patients with adrenoleukodystrophy treated with Lorenzo's oil. Arch Neurol. 2005;62:1073–1080
X-linked Adrenoleukodystrophy Database, www.x-ald/nl

Albers–Schönberg disease

Osteopetrosis

A condition characterized by increased bone density throughout the skeleton, which may occasionally lead to cranial nerve palsies or *hydrocephalus*.

Alcohol and the nervous system: overview

Alcohol can have many effects on the central and peripheral nervous system. The pleasurable short-term effects are familiar to most people. However, adverse effects of alcohol consumption are common and may be classified as acute or chronic in nature. This distinction relates to the amount of and the period of time over which alcohol has been consumed. Many of the chronic complications of alcoholism are due to a combination of the toxic effects of alcohol coupled with the nutritional deficiencies commonly coexisting with excessive alcohol consumption (e.g., thiamine deficiency), along with some as yet unidentified genetic predisposition. Alcohol does not act at specific receptors but does appear to selectively stimulate chloride ion flux through the GABA/Barbiturate/Benzodiazepine receptor, with a particular anatomical preference for the brain stem.

Damage to the nervous system may possibly result from

- Direct toxic effects
- Oxidation to glutaraldehyde
- Nonoxidative metabolism to fatty-acid ethyl esters
- Malnutrition

Alcohol-induced pathology differs in different sites:

- Muscle: muscle fiber damage and myopathy, including an acute necrotizing myopathy (*rhabdomyolysis*) after an alcoholic binge
- Peripheral nerve/optic nerve: axonal loss (peripheral neuropathy; optic atrophy)
- Cerebellum: Purkinje cell loss, especially in anterior/superior vermis
- Cerebral hemispheres: cortical atrophy and possibly cholinergic deafferentation of cortex
- Brain stem: symmetrical pallor and hemorrhage around the third/fourth ventricles, aqueduct, and in the mammillary bodies and medial thalamus (*Wernicke–Korsakoff syndrome*)

Clinical features

Not everyone who consumes excessive quantities of alcohol develops neurological complications. It is unclear why only certain individuals do, and why they should develop some of the neurological complications but not others.

- Alcohol intoxication:
  - Dependent on the plasma level of alcohol, although chronic consumption of alcohol leads to tolerance:
  - >5.4 mmol/L; mild intoxication: altered mood (usually excitement); impaired cognition and incoordination
  - >21.7 mmol/L; vestibular and cerebellar signs, autonomic dysfunction with hypotension and hypothermia, stupor, and eventually coma as the plasma level rises
  - >108.5 mmol/L; usually results in death from respiratory depression
  - In addition, heavy alcohol consumption over short periods of time may result in episodes of amnesia that cannot be accounted for by either a global depression of consciousness or coincident disorders, such as epileptic seizures.
- Alcohol withdrawal state:
  - Nausea, vomiting, perceptual difficulties, tremor, visual hallucinations, fits, delirium tremens (DTs). This latter condition is a severe confusional state that is usually seen within the first 4 days of stopping drinking alcohol, and usually lasts for 1–3 days. It consists of profound agitation, with insomnia, visual hallucinations and delusions, tremor, and autonomic hyperactivity. There may be associated hypophosphatemia.
- Nutritional deficiencies of the nervous system secondary to alcoholism:
  - Wernicke–Korsakoff syndrome (WKS): Wernicke's acute encephalopathy with (or without) ophthalmoplegia and ataxia precedes a chronic Korsakoff's syndrome, which is characterized by a profound anterograde and retrograde memory deficit, which may (or, more often, may not) be associated with confabulation. Thiamine deficiency is thought to be causative.
  - Pellagra.
  - Peripheral neuropathy: a painful axonal sensorimotor polyneuropathy.
  - Optic neuropathy (so-called tobacco– alcohol amblyopia): often occurs in association with heavy smoking. It presents with a painless bilateral visual loss that develops over weeks.
- Conditions of uncertain pathogenesis associated with excessive alcohol consumption:
  - Cerebellar degeneration: M > F, usually in association with peripheral neuropathy. It predominantly involves the rostral vermis, developing over weeks to years, and typically presents with walking difficulties secondary to truncal ataxia. Nystagmus, dysarthria, and intention tremor are uncommon. There may be some recovery on stopping the alcohol.
  - *Marchiafava–Bignami syndrome*: characterized by stupor, coma, fits, dementia, and emotional lability. Pathologically, there is demyelination,

predominantly of the corpus callosum. Said to affect, predominantly, drinkers of Italian Chianti, M > F.
- *Central pontine and extrapontine myelinolysis (CPEPM)*: often correlated with rapid electrolyte changes associated with alcoholic liver disease. It typically presents with a rapidly progressive flaccid quadriparesis, with brain stem signs and bulbar failure.
- Alcoholic myopathy and cardiomyopathy.
- Alcoholic dementia (the differential diagnosis of cognitive decline in alcoholic patients includes traumatic subdural hematomas, which must actually be excluded, because they are potentially reversible).
- Cerebral atrophy.
- Fetal alcohol syndrome (FAS):
  - Occurs in ~6% of alcoholic females. There is aberrant fetal neuronal and glial migration, with cerebellar dysplasia. Affected babies are microcephalic and have pre- and postnatal growth retardation, facial dysmorphology, neurological deficits, and other systemic abnormalities.
- Neurological disorders associated with alcoholic liver disease:
  - Hepatic encephalopathy.
  - Chronic hepatocerebral degeneration, or "non-Wilsonian hepatocerebral degeneration".
- Neurological disorders sometimes responsive to alcohol:
  - *Essential tremor*.
  - Alcohol-responsive *myoclonus–dystonia syndrome* (DYT11): autosomal dominant, starts early in life with combination of dystonia and myoclonic jerks; alcohol in small amounts affects dystonia to some extent but has a dramatic effect on the myoclonic jerks.

Treatment and prognosis

Specific treatment depends on the particular syndrome, but general recommendations include

- Stop alcohol consumption in the context of an alcohol detoxification program.
- Treat with high-dose thiamine, initially intravenously, then orally.
- Replace any other vitamin deficiencies, normalize any electrolyte abnormalities (e.g., hyponatremia, hypophosphatemia) slowly.
- Check for any other treatable conditions (e.g., subdural hematoma).

Reference

McIntosh C, Chick J. Alcohol and the nervous system. J Neurol Neurosurg Psychiatry. 2004;75(Suppl III):iii16–iii21

Alexander's disease [OMIM#203450]

This rare disorder, classified with the *leukodystrophies* and first described in 1949, is typically a childhood condition characterized by megalencephaly, progressive neurological deterioration, and pathological findings of diffuse Rosenthal fiber formation. It has very rarely been described in adults. Autosomal dominant mutations in the gene encoding glial fibrillary acidic protein (GFAP) on chromosome 17 have been associated with the condition.

Clinical features

- Infantile group: from birth to early childhood
  - Psychomotor retardation with failure to thrive.
  - Epileptic seizures.
  - Quadriparesis.
  - Megalencephaly: progressive head enlargement is a major (but not consistent) feature.
- Juvenile group: age 7–14 years
  - Progressive bulbar/pseudobulbar symptoms.
  - Spasticity.
  - Epileptic seizures and cognitive decline are less common.
- Adult group: age 20–60
  - Similar to juvenile group.
  - Occasionally present with a course resembling *multiple sclerosis*.
  - Occasionally asymptomatic.

Investigation

Neuroimaging (CT/MRI) shows extensive white matter demyelination; large head in infants, may also have evidence of hydrocephalus; CSF usually normal; nonspecific protein elevation. Neurophysiology (EEG) may show some epileptiform features. Neurogenetic testing for mutations in the GFAP gene is diagnostic. This may supersede the need for brain biopsy: the pathological focus is in the white matter, with demyelination and morphological abnormalities in astrocytes, with the pathological hallmark of diffuse accumulation of Rosenthal fibers. These represent a gliotic reaction in which astrocytes appear to have been converted into hyalinized eosinophilic bodies. While not unique to Alexander's disease, Rosenthal fibers are characteristic of it, especially in the subependymal, subpial, and perivascular regions, more so in frontal white matter areas than occipitally. The later the onset of disease, the less severe is the demyelination.

Differential diagnosis

Other leukodystrophies, especially Canavan's disease.

Enlarged head:

- Hydrocephalus (in juvenile cases)
- Canavan's disease
- Glutaric aciduria type I
- Gangliosidoses
- *Metachromatic leukodystrophy*
- L-*2-hydroxyglutaric acidemia*

Treatment and prognosis

No specific treatment. Symptomatic measures for epilepsy, spasticity. The younger the onset, the worse the prognosis: survival in the infantile group is ~2.5 years; in the juvenile group, it is ~8 years.

References

Brenner M, Johnson AB, Boespflug-Tanguy O, et al. Mutations in GFAP, encoding glial fibrillary acidic protein, are associated with Alexander disease. Nat Genet. 2001;27:117–120
Jacob J, Robertson NJ, Hilton DA. The clinicopathological spectrum of Rosenthal fibre encephalopathy and Alexander's disease: a case report and review of the literature. J Neurol Neurosurg Psychiatry 2003;74:807–810

Altitude illness

Acute Mountain Sickness, Chronic Mountain Sickness, Monge disease

High altitude environments (i.e., greater than 5,300 ft) are characterized by a lower atmospheric partial pressure of oxygen and hence the risk of hypoxia in humans. All travelers to high altitude will experience varying degrees of acute mountain sickness (AMS), but only in a small percentage does this become life-threatening with acute pulmonary and/or cerebral edema. This most often occurs with rapid ascent to over 12,000 ft in unacclimatized individuals.

Clinical features

- Acute mountain sickness (AMS):
  - Headache, insomnia, anorexia, nausea and dizziness; a syndrome of burning feet and burning hands is also described.
  - More serious manifestations: vomiting, dyspnea, muscle weakness, oliguria, peripheral edema and retinal hemorrhages; the latter may progress to visual

failure. In addition, the patient may develop ataxia, abnormal behavior, drowsiness, and hallucinations, which may progress to coma and death from severe pulmonary and cerebral edema.
- Cerebral edema may first manifest with slight mental impairments or change in behavior, accompanied by headache, nausea, vomiting, and hallucinations, sometimes with epileptic seizures and ataxia, which may progress to coma and death.
- Prolonged exposure to high altitude has been reported to cause some mild impairment of neurobehavioral function, especially memory.
- Chronic mountain sickness (Monge disease):
  - Pulmonary hypertension, cor pulmonale, and secondary polycythemia induced by hypoxia and the systemic effects of long-term habitation at high altitudes.
  - Neurological features may occur, such as mental slowness, fatigue, nocturnal headache, and sometimes papilledema.

Treatment and prognosis

- Prevention:
  - Slow ascent with acclimization at around 6,000–8,000 ft.
  - Increased fluid intake; avoidance of alcohol.
  - Conditioning exercise before departure, especially if over 35 years old.
  - High carbohydrate, low fat, low salt diet.
  - Carbonic anhydrase inhibitors (acetazolamide or faster acting methazolamide), dexamethasone, and nifedipine have been shown to have a prophylactic role in AMS.
- Treatment:
  - In established cases, treatment is with supplemental oxygen, descent to lower altitude, and rest; dexamethasone is indicated in cases of cerebral edema.

References

Barry PW, Pollard AJ. Altitude illness. BMJ. 2003;326:915–919
Basnyat B, Murdoch DR. High-altitude illness. Lancet. 2003;361:1967–1974
Wilson MH, Newman S, Imray CH. The cerebral effects of ascent to high altitudes. Lancet Neurol. 2009;8:175–191

Alzheimer's disease (AD)

Dementia of the Alzheimer type (DAT)

Alzheimer's disease (AD) is a common neurodegenerative disease, first described by Alois Alzheimer in 1906. It characteristically affects the elderly population and usually presents with episodic memory difficulties. Sporadic and familial cases are reported, the latter tending to occur earlier. As the disease progresses, there is increasing difficulty with memory, language, and orientation, leading to global impairment of cognitive faculties within 5–10 years from symptom onset. Death is usually from secondary causes such as bronchopneumonia. The neuropathological accompaniments of intellectual decline are

- Neurofibrillary tangles composed ultrastructurally of paired helical filaments, composed largely of the microtubule associated protein tau
- Plaques composed largely of amyloid protein, with various morphologies
- Dystrophic neurites containing paired helical filaments: surrounding some plaques, and in the cortical neuropil (neuropil threads, cortical neuritic dystrophy)
- Synaptic and neuronal loss

Abnormal cellular processing and subsequent aggregation of certain proteins may be the key pathophysiological process. The amyloid (cascade) hypothesis remains the most favored explanation of disease pathogenesis, largely because many of the genetic mutations identified as deterministic for AD (in the genes encoding amyloid precursor protein [OMIM#104300], presenilin 1 [OMIM#607822] and presenilin 2 [OMIM#606889]) lead to increased cellular production of the long variant (42–43 amino acids) of amyloid β-peptide (Aβ42) from its precursor molecule, amyloid precursor protein (APP). Apolipoprotein E (ApoE) genotype is a risk factor for the development of AD, the ε4/ε4 genotype carrying the greatest risk, although this is neither necessary nor sufficient for the development of AD. Extracellular amyloid brain burden is not sufficient to cause disease; disruption of intraneuronal cytoskeletal integrity leading to formation of neurofibrillary tangles and dystrophic neurites, with synapse loss and neuronal death, is also required for the development of dementia. Neurofibrillary pathology follows a predictable pattern of spread from transentorhinal cortex to neocortex. Gross atrophy of the cerebral cortex with extensive gliosis and neuronal cell loss, associated with atrophy of the cholinergic forebrain nuclei including the basal nucleus of Meynert, and cholinergic insufficiency is the end result.

Clinical features

- Cognitive deficits: impairment of episodic memory is the most common presenting symptom, with relative preservation of working memory/sustained attention. It is advisable to obtain a history from other family members or carers, to help ascertain the nature, extent, and duration of the problems. The patient often makes light of difficulties or attempts to explain them away. Isolated amnesia, insufficient to fulfill diagnostic criteria for AD, may be labeled as mild cognitive impairment (MCI), a condition that may progress to AD.

- Cognitive deficits progress to involve other domains, e.g.,:
  - Language difficulties, including word finding and comprehension problems.
  - Visuospatial dysfunction: occasionally a presenting feature (*posterior cortical atrophy*, visual variant AD).
  - Dysexecutive syndrome.
- Impaired activities of daily living (ADL): initially operational (shopping, cooking, finances), but latterly basic (dressing, toileting, feeding).
- Behavioral features: depression may be common in the early stages, and it is sometimes difficult to differentiate cognitive deficits due to depression and dementia. Agitation, wandering, and psychosis may also occur. These are the features which most often lead to breakdown of care at home and necessitate institutionalization.
- Neurological features: there are no specific signs. Some patients develop extrapyramidal signs, but these are usually mild. Myoclonus and epileptic seizures may occur, with increasing frequency as the disease progresses and probably more common in familial than sporadic disease. A variant with spastic paraparesis associated with certain presenilin-1 gene mutations is described.

Clinical variants of AD that have been described include:

- Posterior cortical atrophy (PCA): patients present with progressive visual agnosia but with relative preservation of memory; may be associated with depression.
- Lewy body variant (LBV) of AD: this name has been applied to those patients with *dementia with Lewy bodies* (*DLB*), with additional pathology sufficient to meet standard pathological criteria for AD; this condition may be distinguished from "diffuse Lewy body disease" (DLBD), which lacks concomitant AD pathology.
- A frontal variant of AD (rare).
- *Mild cognitive impairment* (*MCI*) may in some instances be prodromal AD, especially the amnestic type of MCI.

Various forms of Familial AD (FAD) have been identified, and in certain cases deterministic genetic mutations identified:

- Mutations in the amyloid precursor protein (APP) gene on chromosome 21: rare families (ca. 25 worldwide) in which dominant mutations show complete penetrance by the age of 60, with most cases presenting from 30 to 60 years of age. (One of the amyloid angiopathies, hereditary cerebral hemorrhage with angiopathy, Dutch type [HCHWAD], also results from mutation within the APP gene.)
- Mutations in the presenilin-1 (PS-1) gene on chromosome 14, and in the presenilin-2 gene on chromosome 1: PS-1 mutations are the most common identified cause of FAD, over 170 different mutations are recorded. Mutations usually result in disease with the same age of onset within,

but not necessarily between, families; there are occasional cases of incomplete penetrance. These observations suggest a role for other genetic or epigenetic factors (but not ApoE). PS-1 FAD generally presents earlier and runs a more rapid course than sporadic cases of AD. In addition, myoclonus and epileptic seizures are more prominent than in sporadic AD.

- In trisomy 21 (*Down syndrome*), AD neuropathology usually develops before the age of 40 due to a gene dosage effect of APP.
- Polymorphisms in the gene encoding apolipoprotein E (ApoE) on chromosome 19 influence the risk of developing both sporadic and some familial AD (e.g., APP mutation families) in a dose-dependent manner; possession of two ApoE ε4 alleles increases risk by about eightfold; however, this is neither necessary nor sufficient for the development of AD. In contrast the ε2 allele may offer some protection against developing AD.

Other families have been described that do not map to any of the above loci.

Investigation

Blood: usually all normal; should assay thyroid function, calcium, vitamin B_{12}, syphilis serology to identify potentially treatable causes of dementia (extremely rare). Neuropsychology is often helpful in defining the nature and extent of cognitive deficits. Earliest changes are typically in episodic memory, although some patients present with visuospatial problems. Difficulties in language and executive function also emerge with time. Often a global pattern of cognitive impairment is evident by the time of the patient's presentation. Islands of preserved ability may remain (e.g., reading, but without comprehension). Neuroimaging: Structural imaging (CT/MRI) may show cortical atrophy, but this may overlap with that seen in normal ageing. Longitudinal study of volumetric indices (e.g., hippocampal volume) may be helpful in showing progressive atrophy, but determining hippocampal volume on one-off standard clinical service MRI scans is rarely reliable. Functional imaging (SPECT/PET) changes may demonstrate hypoperfusion/hypometabolism in the parietotemporal regions. Magnetic resonance spectroscopy may show reductions in neuronal markers (*N*-acetyl-aspartate). CSF: regular indices are usually normal, but assay of tau protein (raised) and Aβ (lower) may be useful in diagnosis. Neurophysiology: EEG shows nonspecific changes only, such as slowing of background alpha rhythm; this may be helpful in distinction from *frontotemporal lobar degeneration*, where EEG remains largely normal. Pathological change remains the "gold standard" for diagnosis, but this is seldom present antemortem. Neurogenetic testing: for early onset AD with a family history suggestive of autosomal dominant transmission (= at least three affected individuals in at least two generations), searching for mutations in APP, PS-1, and PS-2 may be worthwhile.

Differential diagnosis

- Normal aging
- *Mild cognitive impairment*
- Depression
- *Delirium*
- The differential diagnosis of *dementia* per se is broad; mixed pathology (AD + vascular change) is also common. *Vascular cognitive impairment, vascular dementia*

Treatment and prognosis

Support and information for patients and families. Cholinesterase inhibitors, whose aim is to potentiate the central cholinergic network, are licensed for the symptomatic treatment of mild-to-moderate AD. Memantine, an antagonist at NMDA receptors, may also have a therapeutic effect. Behavioral features may require behavioral therapy and pharmacotherapy, although the latter may be associated with increased cerebrovascular mortality. Disease-modifying drugs are not yet available, but research into agents influencing amyloidogenesis and tau aggregation are ongoing. Institutionalization may eventually be necessary, often because of behavioral features or incontinence; early intervention may avoid the need for institutionalization. The disease is progressive and the median survival time from diagnosis to death is around 7–10 years.

Diagnostic criteria

Dubois B, Feldman HH, Jacova C, et al. Research criteria for the diagnosis of Alzheimer's disease: revising the NINCDS-ADRDA criteria. Lancet Neurol. 2007;6:734–746
McKhann G, Drachman D, Folstein M, et al. Clinical diagnosis of Alzheimer's disease. Report of the NINCDS-ADRDA work group under the auspices of the Department of Health and Human Service Task forces on Alzheimer's disease. Neurology. 1984;34:939–944

References

Alzheimer Disease and Frontotemporal Dementia Mutation Database, www.molgen.ua.ac.be/Admutations
Larner AJ. Alzheimer's disease. In: Cappa SF, Abutalebi J, Démonet JF, Fletcher PC, Garrard P, eds. Cognitive Neurology: A Clinical Textbook. Oxford: Oxford University Press; 2008:199–227

Larner AJ, Doran M. Genotype-phenotype relationships of presenilin-1 mutations in Alzheimer's disease: an update. J Alzheimers Dis. 2009;17:259–265
Perry G, Avila J, Kinoshita J, Smith MA, eds. Alzheimer's Disease: A Century of Scientific and Clinical Research. Amsterdam, The Netherlands: IOS Press; 2006

Aminoacidopathies: overview

Aminoacidopathies are rare autosomal recessive, inborn errors of metabolism, in which amino acid synthesis or transport is affected. These disorders do not impair growth, maturation, or development in utero, but may present in the early months of life with neurological features, which may be episodic or chronically progressive, such as encephalopathy. Examples of some of the more common aminoacidopathies with neurological features are given here.

- Phenylketonuria (PKU): phenylalanine hydroxlase deficiency.
    - Developmental delay, +/– vomiting from around 2 months; permanent deficits thereafter if untreated. Musty odor. Can be screened for at birth.
- Tyrosinemia: Type I (hepatorenal tyrosinemia): fumaryl-acetoacetate hydrolase deficiency.
    - Neonatal liver failure; cabbage-like odor. Chronic form with hepatic disease and Fanconi syndrome. Episodic porphyric complications.
- Tyrosinemia: Type II (oculocutaneous tyrosinemia, Richner–Hanhart disease): tyrosine amino-transferase deficiency.
    - Corneal, plantar, and palmar erosions. Variable neurological involvement with mental retardation and motor delay.
- Tyrosinemia: Type III (Benign transient neonatal tyrosinemia): 4-hydroxy-phenylpyruvate bisoxygenase/dioxygenase deficiency.
- *Homocystinuria*: cystathionine β-synthase deficiency.
    - May present in adulthood with marfanoid habitus, cerebral thromboembolic disease, +/– psychiatric and extrapyramidal features with mental retardation.
- Hartnup's disease: neutral amino acid (e.g., tryptophan) transport defect in kidney and gut with consequent deficiency of niacinamide and a clinical syndrome presenting in childhood, reminiscent of *pellagra* (skin rash), with progressive ataxia, +/– optic atrophy, dystonia, pyramidal signs, tremor, and delirium. The urine contains large amounts of neutral, monamino-monocarboxylic amino acids, which are decreased in plasma. Many subjects with aminoaciduria are asymptomatic (Hartnup's disorder). Treatment is with oral nicotinamide, with or without a high protein diet.
- Maple Syrup Urine disease (MSUD): catabolic disorders of branched chain amino acids.
    - Wide range in severity of defects and of clinical presentation: neonatal encephalopathy, later onset fulminant encephalopathy with mental retardation; episodic encephalopathy in early childhood; ataxia, mental retardation, failure to thrive common; maple syrup odor.

- Nonketotic hyperglycinaemia (glycine encephalopathy): defect in glycine cleavage system.
  - Severe neonatal encephalopathy, myoclonus and apnea, leading to death. Less severe enzyme deficits present with mental retardation, spasticity, and myoclonic fits.
- Histidinemia: histidase deficiency.
  - Association with epileptic seizures, mental retardation, attention deficits, tremor, ataxia, and other neurological deficits may be fortuitous rather than causal; many "normals" may be shown to have histidinemia.
- Lysine intolerance: defect in dibasic amino acid transport mechanism in kidney and gut.
  - Feeding difficulties with growth failure, osteoporosis, bone marrow depression and hepatomegaly. Developmental delay with episodic encephalopathy. Mental retardation, psychoses, epileptic seizures.
- Cystinosis: intralysosomal accumulation of the amino acid cystine in kidney, cornea, thyroid, and brain.
  - Proximal tubulopathy: De Toni–Debre–Fanconi syndrome, characterized by hyperphosphaturia, hyperaminoaciduria, and glucosuria; polyuria and proteinuria; may lead to rickets. Ocular damage: corneal cystine crystals, retinopathy. Neuropsychological deficits. Distal vacuolar myopathy also described. May present in adulthood.

Investigation

As a general rule, biochemical diagnosis is usually straightforward due to the accumulation of metabolites proximal to the enzyme defect, which, being water-soluble, may be detected in plasma and urine.

References

Charnas LR, Luciano CA, Dalakas M, et al. Distal vacuolar myopathy in nephropathic cystinosis. Ann Neurol. 1994;35:181–188

Evans OB, Parker CC, Haas RH, Naidu S, Moser HW, Bock H-GO. Inborn errors of metabolism of the nervous system. In: Bradley WG, Daroff RB, Fenichel GM, Marsden CD, eds. Neurology in Clinical Practice. 3rd ed. Boston, MA: Butterwoth-Heinemann; 2000:1595–1664

Gascon GG, Ozand PT. Aminoacidopathies and organic acidopathies, mitochondrial enzyme defects, and other metabolic errors. In: Goetz CG, ed. Textbook of Clinical Neurology. 2nd ed. Philadelphia, PA: W.B. Saunders; 2003:629–664

Holme E, Lindstedt S. Diagnosis and management of tyrosinemia type I. Curr Opin Pediatr. 1995;7:726–732

Menkes JH. Disorders of amino acid metabolism. In: Rowland LP, ed. Merritt's Textbook of Neurology. 9th ed. Baltimore, MD: Williams & Wilkins; 1995:538–546

Amoebic infection: overview

Amoebae (*Entamoeba histolytica*) may rarely invade the brain (amoebiasis) producing abscesses, especially in the frontal lobes or basal ganglia. A combination of surgery and antibiotics (metronidazole) may be required, but mortality is very high.

Free-living amoebae of the species *Naegleria* or *Acanthamoeba* may cause acute or granulomatous meningoencephalitis. Amoebic trophozoites may be identified in CSF or in skin nodules. Purulent CSF (raised white cell count, mostly polymorphs, raised protein, low glucose, often hemorrhagic) with negative Gram stain may stimulate a search for amoebae. Treatment is with intravenous and intrathecal amphotericin or miconazole. Though rare, the mortality of these conditions is very high.

Amyloid diseases: overview

Amyloid is the name given to predominantly extracellular fibrillar material composed primarily of protein, in the form of insoluble β-pleated sheets, the origin of which varies with the type of amyloidosis and disease state. Amyloid deposits are best visualized using the dye Congo red: light microscopy shows amyloid deposits to be pink or red in color, but under polarized light the Congo red-stained amyloid demonstrates an apple-green birefringence. Antibodies against the specific protein component of amyloid (e.g., amyloid β-peptide) allow its visualization by immunohistochemistry. Around 20 different proteins have been defined as causing amyloid deposition. These deposits may occur in a number of different organs in a number of different diseases, some of which include, or are exclusive to, the nervous system.

Amyloidosis may be classified in various ways (e.g., systemic vs localized), but probably the division into acquired and hereditary causes, based on the pathogenetic protein, is most useful:

- Acquired:
  - *Primary systemic amyloidosis*: amyloid (AL: amyloid light chain) is derived from immunoglobulin light chains associated with aberrant expansion of B-cell clones (e.g., multiple myeloma).
  - Secondary amyloidosis, Reactive amyloidosis: amyloid (AA: amyloid fibril protein) is derived from serum amyloid associated protein (SAA), normally secondary to chronic inflammatory conditions (e.g., bronchiectasis, rheumatoid arthritis).
  - β-Microglobulin amyloidosis: associated with renal dialysis. Rarely associated with neurological complications.
- Hereditary:
  - A-Bri, A-Dan: *familial British dementia (FBD)* and *familial Danish dementia (FDD)*, respectively.

- Amyloid β-peptide: some forms of *intracerebral hemorrhage* (*cerebral amyloid angiopathy*), *Alzheimer's disease.*
- Apolipoproteins AI, AII: non-neuropathic.
- Cystatin: some forms of intracerebral hemorrhage (cerebral amyloid angiopathy).
- Fibrinogen: non-neuropathic.
- *Gelsolin amyloidosis*: cranial neuropathy, corneal dystrophy.
- Lysozyme: non-neuropathic.
- Transthyretin: *familial amyloid polyneuropathy.*

Reference

Gibbs SDJ, Hawkins PN. Biochemical basis of the amyloid diseases. Br J Hosp Med. 2010;71:70–75

Andersen–Tawil syndrome [OMIM#170390]

This is a rare disorder characterized by the following triad:

- *Periodic paralysis* (hyperkalemic or hypokalemic).
- Malignant ventricular arrhythmia; this may postdate the periodic paralysis by many years; there may be a prolonged QT interval on ECG (hence, may be classified with *long QT syndromes*, as LQT7).
- Craniofacial dysmorphism: may be subtle.

Mutations in the voltage-independent skeletal muscle potassium channel gene (KCNJ2) have been found in this condition; hence, it is a *channelopathy*.

References

Davies NP, Imbrici P, Fialho D, et al. Andersen-Tawil syndrome: new potassium channel mutations and possible phenotypic variation. Neurology. 2005;65:1083–1089
Tawil R, Ptacek LJ, Pavlakis SG, et al. Andersen's syndrome: potassium sensitive periodic paralysis, ventricular ectopy, and dysmorphic features. Ann Neurol. 1994;35:326–330

Aneurysm: overview

Intracranial aneuryms may be classified in various ways:

- Morphology: helpful in defining different natural history
  - Saccular
  - Fusiform

- Dissecting: small dissecting (Charcot–Bouchard) aneurysms or microaneurysms arise from the small perforating arteries of the brain, possibly as a consequence of vessel wall weakening from lipohyalinosis and often in the context of *hypertension*. They may be implicated in hypertensive *intracerebral hemorrhage*, affecting the basal ganglia, thalamus, pons, and subcortical white matter.
- Size:
  - <3 mm, 3–6 mm, 7–10 mm, 11–25 mm, >25 mm (giant)
- Location:
  - Anterior, posterior circulation, specific vessels, especially at arterial branch points

In addition, there are a number of disorders, some hereditary, which may be associated with aneurysms:

- *Arteriovenous malformations*
- *Dural arteriovenous fistula*, spinal arteriovenous malformations
- Cardiac myxoma (tumor metastasis)
- *Sickle-cell disease*
- *Superficial siderosis of the nervous system*
- Head trauma
- Mycotic aneurysms, most often with infective endocarditis
- Cocaine abuse
- *Coarctation of the aorta*
- Hereditary:
  - *Ehlers–Danlos syndrome* type IV
  - *Pseudoxanthoma elasticum*
  - Infantile *fibromuscular dysplasia*
  - *Neurofibromatosis*
  - α_1-Antitrypsin deficiency
  - *Hereditary hemorrhagic telangiectasia* (Osler–Weber–Rendu syndrome)
  - Autosomal dominant polycystic kidney disease

Clinical features

Most cerebral aneurysms are asymptomatic and do not rupture. Symptomatic features other than *subarachnoid hemorrhage*, if present, depend on aneurysm location and may be acute ischemia, headache, epileptic seizures, cranial neuropathy; or chronic headache, visual loss, pyramidal tract dysfunction, and facial pain due to mass effect.

Investigation

Many aneurysms are discovered incidentally, when cranial imaging is undertaken for some other purpose. If aneurysms are being specifically sought, then some form of angiography is required; catheter angiography has been the gold standard although it carries a definite morbidity; other options include CT angiography, magnetic resonance angiography (MRA), and digital subtraction angiography (DSA).

Treatment and prognosis

Screening for aneurysms should probably be confined to family members when two or more first degree relatives have had a subarachnoid hemorrhage. Therapeutic interventions include surveillance (small aneurysms, <10 mm diameter, have a very low rupture rate, and hence the risks of intervention probably outweigh any potential benefits), endovascular coiling, or open surgery (clipping). Long-term follow-up suggests a slightly increased risk of rebleeding in coiled as opposed to clipped aneurysms, but the risk of death was significantly lower at 5 years in the coiled group.

Reference

Molyneux AJ, Kerr RS, Birks J, et al. Risk of recurrent subarachnoid haemorrhage, death, or dependence and standardised mortality ratios after clipping or coiling of an intracranial aneurysm in the International Subarachnoid Aneurysm Trial (ISAT): long-term follow-up. Lancet Neurol. 2009;8:427–433

Angelman syndrome [OMIM#105830]

Happy puppet syndrome

Angelman syndrome is a neurogenetic disorder linked to chromosome 15, and is of great biological interest as it demonstrates the phenomenon of imprinting. Approximately 70% of cases result from de novo maternal deletions involving chromosome 15q11.2-q13, whereas the same deletions of paternal origin result in Prader–Willi syndrome. Approximately 2% of cases result from paternal uniparental disomy of 15q11.2-q13; maternal disomy causes Prader–Willi syndrome. Some of the remaining cases are caused by mutations in the gene encoding ubiquitin-protein ligase E3A gene (UBE3A).

Clinical features

- Developmental delay; microcephaly, virtually absent speech, feeding difficulties
- Mental retardation: mild to severe; +/– autism

- Happy demeanor (constant), unprovoked laughter (may not be prominent)
- Movement disorder: ambulation age 5–6 years, distinctive gait with jerky ataxia and lower extremity hypertonia (the "happy puppet")
- Seizure disorder: tonic, atonic > tonic–clonic epileptic attacks
- Moderate dysmorphism: prognathism

Investigation

Neurogenetic testing: for 15q11-q13 deletion of maternal orgin. EEG is often suggestive of diagnosis: runs of slow 3 Hz waves, especially posteriorly, often notched +/– spikes. Neuroimaging (CT/MRI) unremarkable.

Differential diagnosis

Behavioral features are fairly characteristic; may be mistaken for Rett's syndrome in girls, or ataxic *cerebral palsy*.

Treatment and prognosis

No specific treatment; symptomatic therapy for epileptic seizures (ethosuximide, topiramate). Although long-term survival is reported, prognosis is generally poor.

References

Angelman H. "Puppet" children: a report on three cases. Dev Med Child Neurol. 1965;7:681–688
Dan B. Angelman Syndrome (Clinics in developmental medicine No. 177). London: Mac Keith Press; 2008

Angiostrongyliasis

Infection with the rat lungworm *Angiostrongylus cantonensis*, following ingestion of snails, slugs, or undercooked prawns, may cause an eosinophilic meningitis or meningoencephalitis; cranial nerve palsies, epileptic seizures, and coma may also be features. The absence of focal features on structural brain imaging helps to distinguish this condition from *neurocysticercosis* and *gnathostomiasis*. CSF pressure is elevated and the white cell count is raised with a high percentage of eosinophils. Larvae may be found in the CSF or seen in the eye on ophthalmoscopy or slit-lamp examination. Because of possible toxicity of larvicidal agents, supportive treatment only may be appropriate in patients who are improving since the disease is often self-limiting.

Reference

Jones M, Mohanraj R, Shaunak S. Eosinophilic meningitis due to Angiostrongylus Cantonensis: first reported case in the UK. Adv Clin Neurosci Rehabil. 2007; 6(6):20–21

Ankylosing spondylitis

Marie-Strümpel disease, Von Bechterew's disease

Ankylosing spondylitis (AS) is a chronic spondyloarthropathy caused by an autoimmune-mediated process directed against a cartilage proteoglycan. It is strongly associated with the HLA antigen B27. It affects particularly Europeans, men more than women (prevalence 1–3:1,000), with onset in the second and third decades of life. Characteristically, the sacroiliac joints and lumbosacral spine are affected initially, with symptoms of early morning pain and stiffness. Extra-articular manifestations include uveitis, aortic regurgitation, pulmonary fibrosis, and amyloidosis, as well as neurological features. The latter include a cauda equina syndrome, radiculopathy, myelopathy, and spinal stenosis. Spinal fracture may also lead to neurological complications. Treatment is designed to reduce inflammation; in some cases surgery may be necessary.

Clinical features

- Neurological features:
  - *Cauda equina syndrome* (CES): The clinical picture is like that for other cauda equina syndromes, but sensory and sphincter abnormalities tend to be more common than motor weakness. CES is rare, yet it is the most common neurological complication of ankylosing spondylitis.
  - Radiculopathy involving the lumbosacral roots.
  - Myelopathy is rare in this condition and is usually due to a secondary complication, such as meningeal fibrosis, *atlanto–axial dislocation* (more commonly seen with *rheumatoid arthritis*), spinal fracture +/– an epidural hematoma +/– cord concussion (especially in the cervical region, in response to minor trauma, as there is marked osteoporosis in this condition).
  - Lumbar *spinal stenosis*.

- Systemic features: chronic back pain, which is often insidious at onset, worse in the morning and made better by exercise (*cf.* osteoarthritis). Pain often radiates to the groin and thighs and with time is associated with a limitation of movement.
- Nonarticular, non-neurological manifestations: include Reiter's syndrome, psoriasis, inflammatory diseases of the bowel, uveitis, pulmonary fibrosis, aortic regurgitation, and amyloidosis.

Investigation

Blood often reveals a nonspecific inflammatory response with raised ESR, raised acute phase proteins, and mild normochromic normocytic anemia. Rheumatoid factor and other autoantibodies are negative, but 90% of patients are HLA B27 positive. Imaging: spinal radiographs demonstrate bony bridging of the vertebral bodies to produce the so-called bamboo spine. Plain radiographs of the sacroiliac joints reveal sacroilitis, which evolves to obliteration of the joint. MRI of the spine, and/or myelography, often reveals dorsal arachnoid diverticulae. In addition, there may be evidence of radicular involvement, meningeal thickening, enlargement of the thecal sac, and dilatation of the lumbosacral nerve root sleeves. There is usually little or no meningeal enhancement with gadolinium. CSF may show a raised protein. Neurophysiology (EMG/NCS) may reveal a radiculopathy.

Differential diagnosis

The lack of spinal movement may also occur in acute painful conditions such as *intervertebral disc prolapse*. The loss of lordosis may occur in *rigid spine syndrome*, extrapyramidal disorders, especially *progressive supranuclear palsy*; and *stiffness* as in stiff man/person syndrome may lead to lower back symptoms.

Treatment and prognosis

Ankylosing spondylitis is poorly responsive to immunotherapies; steroids are unhelpful, but there may be a role for the anti-TNFα biologicals such as etanercept and infliximab. Joint pain and stiffness may be treated symptomatically with non-steroidal anti-inflammatory medications (e.g., indomethacin) and physiotherapy. Surgical intervention may be required in some patients with either the cauda equina syndrome or myelopathy. In cases of symptomatic atlanto-axial dislocation surgical intervention is mandatory. Steroids are without benefit in CES.

References

Ahn NU, Ahn UM, Nallamshetty L, et al. Cauda equina syndrome in ankylosing spondylitis (the CES-AS syndrome): meta-analysis of outcome after medical and surgical treatments. J Spinal Disord. 2001;14:427–433
Matthews WB. The neurological complications of ankylosing spondylitis. J Neurol Sci. 1968;6:561–573

Anterior choroidal artery infarction

Stroke following occlusion of the anterior choroidal artery, most usually a branch of the internal carotid artery before its terminal bifurcation into the anterior and middle cerebral arteries, produces inconsistent deficits, including

- Contralateral hemiparesis and hemisensory deficit (proprioception often spared).
- +/– Impaired language (aphasia), visuospatial function (including spatial neglect).
- +/– Visual field defect, typically homonymous horizontal sectoranopia (lateral geniculate nucleus involvement).

In situ thrombosis of the artery seems more common than embolism from proximal sources. Many have *lacunar syndromes* despite the absence of lacunar infarction.

References

Palomeras E, Fossas P, Cano AT, Sanz P, Floriach M. Anterior choroidal artery infarction: a clinical, etiologic and prognostic study. Acta Neurol Scand. 2008;118:42–47
Rousseaux M, Cabaret M, Serafi R, Kozlowski O. An evaluation of cognitive disorders after anterior choroidal artery infarction. J Neurol. 2008;255:1405–1410

Anterior interosseous neuropathy

Kiloh–Nevin syndrome

The anterior interosseous nerve is a purely motor branch of the median nerve, arising distal to pronator teres and lying anterior to the interosseous membrane. It innervates the flexor digitorum profundus I and II, flexor pollicis longus, and pronator quadratus muscles. Selective palsy of the anterior interosseous nerve is a rare restricted form of *median neuropathy*, with a characteristic clinical picture of subacute weakness in the hand, with or without pain. Weakness of the terminal phalanx of the index finger causes the "pinch sign" or "okay sign," inability to form a small circle by pinching the thumb and index finger together, and the "straight thumb sign" is evident when making a fist. There is no sensory involvement. Diagnosis may be confirmed by electrophysiological studies showing abnormalities confined to the three muscles innervated by the anterior interosseous nerve. Local trauma, fractures, *neuralgic amyotrophy*, mononeuritis multiplex, or compression by a fibrous band between the two heads of pronator teres are the most common causes. Partial median nerve palsies located proximally (e.g., supracondylar region) may also produce a picture resembling anterior interosseous neuropathy (= pseudo-anterior interosseous neuropathy) because fibers destined for the anterior interosseous nerve are located posteriorly in the median nerve and prone to selective injury in the supracondylar region (e.g., following fracture or compression by ligament of Struthers).

Reference

Goulding PJ, Schady W. Favourable outcome in non-trauamtic anterior interosseous nerve lesions. J Neurol. 1993;240:83–86

Anterior spinal artery syndrome (ASAS)

Beck syndrome

Anterior spinal artery syndrome (ASAS) is perhaps the most common of the *spinal cord vascular diseases*. The normal blood supply of the spinal cord is from paired posterior spinal arteries supplying the posterior third of the cord, and from a single anterior spinal artery formed by branches from both vertebral arteries, "reinforced" at thoracic levels by segmental arteries such as the artery of Adamkiewicz (arteria radicularis magna). Thus, the anterior two-thirds of the cord is relatively vulnerable to ischemia and infarction, particularly at middle to lower thoracic levels. Many cases of anterior spinal artery syndrome remain idiopathic, although recognized causes include aortic surgery (for resection of thoracic or thoracolumbar aortic aneurysms), occlusion (e.g., systemic atherosclerosis, embolus from aortic aneurysm), systemic hypotension, and, much less commonly, inflammatory vessel disease, arachnoiditis, vasculopathies, or thrombophilic syndromes. The symptoms and signs in cases related to surgery may be masked by epidural analgesia. Fibrocartilaginous embolism of the spinal cord is a rare cause of anterior spinal artery syndrome, in which fibrocartilaginous emboli are found in the vascular bed; there may be a preceding history of minor trauma or Valsalva maneuver.

Clinical features

- Paraparesis, paraplegia: initially flaccid with reflex loss, evolving to spasticity, hyperreflexia, and extensor plantar responses
- Sensory level with impaired spinothalamic modalities (pain, temperature) below the level, preserved dorsal column modalities (e.g., proprioception)
- Sphincters: bladder and bowel paralysis usual

Investigation

The clinical picture is often diagnostic. Neuroimaging with spinal cord MRI may show ischemic lesions and exclude other structural causes of myelopathy.

Treatment and prognosis

No specific treatment, other than in embolic cases where anticoagulation or antiplatelet agents may be used. Risk factors for vascular disease merit treatment in their own right. Recovery is extremely variable, dependent probably on the extent and duration of impaired cord perfusion: one series reported <20% of survivors to be fully ambulatory, with >20% in-hospital mortality and worse prognosis with increasing patient age. Neurorehabilitation to maximize potential is indicated.

Reference

De la Barrera S, Barca-Buyo A, Montoto-Marqués A, et al. Spinal cord infarction: prognosis and recovery in a series of 36 patients. Spinal Cord. 2001;39:520–525.

Anthrax

Anthrax is a zoonotic infection with the sporulating Gram-positive bacillus *Bacillus anthracis*, usually a disease of herbivores, acquired from contact with spores in the soil. Exposure to infected animals is one cause of human disease. The possible use of this bacterium as an agent of bioterrorism, because it is relatively easy to weaponize, has led to increased awareness of its possible effects.

Clinical features

- Main forms of disease are respiratory, cutaneous, and gastrointestinal.
- Inhalational anthrax rapidly progresses to septicemia, shock, and respiratory failure, with a high mortality despite intensive care.

- Cutaneous anthrax is less likely to produce septicemia and is common in some parts of the tropics.
- A pyogenic *meningitis* occurs in less than 5% of cases, the clinical features of which are identical to other causes of pyogenic meningitis. A primary site of infection such as a pustule or pulmonary syndrome should be evident in anthrax meningitis.

Investigation

CXR may show widened mediastinum, hilar lymphadenopathy. CT/MRI brain may show subarachnoid hemorrhage. CSF is inflammatory, may also be hemorrhagic; Gram-positive rods on Gram stain.

Differential diagnosis

Other causes of bacterial meningitis; once Gram-positive rods are seen in CSF, differential diagnosis includes Listeria.

Treatment and prognosis

Antibiotic regime, initially intravenous, for example, ciprofloxacin, doxycycline, imipenem. Role of dexamethasone is unclear. Oropharyngeal edema may necessitate intubation. Mortality may be high despite appropriate treatment. Cutaneous anthrax may respond to penicillin alone.

References

Beeching NJ, Dance DAB, Miller ARO, Spencer RC. Biological warfare and bioterrorism. BMJ. 2002;324:336–339
Meselson M, Guillemin J, Hugh-Jones M, et al. The Sverdlovsk anthrax outbreak of 1979. Science. 1994;266:1202–1207

Antiphospholipid syndrome (APS)

Hughes syndrome

Antiphospholipid antibodies may be

- Primary: not associated with an underlying connective tissue disease
- Secondary: to systemic lupus erythematosus or other connective tissue disorder

These antibodies are definitely associated with a tendency to venous or arterial thromboses and, as such, the antiphospholipid syndrome includes cerebrovascular

events (venous thrombosis, TIA, or completed stroke) and their secondary consequences (e.g., focal epilepsy). There is strong anecdotal evidence also that chorea
can be seen in patients with these antibodies, in the absence of basal ganglia
infarcts, especially in association with oral contraceptive use. However, the association of this syndrome with some non-ischemic neurological manifestations is
controversial: in particular, there is little evidence for the claim that these antibodies cause an illness that mimics multiple sclerosis, which is treatable by
anticoagulation.

Clinical features

- Neurological:
  - *Transient ischemic attack*, ischemic *stroke*, retinal artery occlusion (all
    these may be associated with *migraine*)
  - *Transverse myelitis*, multiple sclerosis-like syndrome
  - Epileptic seizures
  - Headaches, *migraine*
  - Cognitive impairment, *dementia*
  - Chorea
  - Acute inflammatory neuropathy (*Guillain–Barré syndrome*), periph-
    eral neuropathy
- Limb deep venous thrombosis; retinal, renal, and hepatic venous
  thrombosis
- Myocardial infarction, peripheral vascular disease
- Pregnancy failure
- Livedo reticularis (*Sneddon syndrome*: may also occur without antiphos-
  pholipid antibodies)
- Thrombocytopenia
- Mitral valve vegetations

In catastrophic APS, rapidly progressive microvascular thrombosis leads to
multiorgan failure.

Investigation

- Repeated assays for IgG and IgM anticardiolipin antibodies: these assays
  are notoriously fluctuant, so only high concentrations of antibodies sustained over at least 6 weeks should be regarded as significant.
- Prothrombotic screen to look for lupus anticoagulant.

Differential diagnosis

Other causes of venous or arterial vascular disease.

Treatment and prognosis

- General: Modification of cardiovascular risk factors.
- Specific: The presence of anticardiolipin antibodies alone is not an indication for treatment. In patients with these antibodies who have had venous or arterial thromboses, secondary prevention is indicated, although there is no class 1 evidence to discriminate between the efficacy of anticoagulation or antiplatelet therapy. Immunotherapy has been suggested, but no randomized trials have yet been undertaken. In catastrophic APS, plasma exchange is recommended.

References

Cohen D, Berger SP, Steup-Beekman GM, Bloemenkamp KWM, Bajmea IM. Diagnosis and management of the antiphospholipid syndrome. BMJ. 2010; 340:1125–1132
Keswani SC, Chauhan N. Antiphospholipid syndrome. J R Soc Med. 2002;94:336–342
Rodrigues CE, Carvalho JF, Shoenfeld Y. Neurological manifestations of antiphospholipid syndrome. Eur J Clin Investig. 2010;40:350–359

Anton–Babinski syndrome

Anton–Babinski syndrome refers to unilateral asomatognosia, the inability to recognize a paralyzed (usually left) limb as one's own, with left hemiparesis. In addition, there may be anosognosia (denial or unawareness of neurological deficits, left sensory extinction), left homonymous hemianopia, and left visual neglect. This usually follows a destructive lesion (commonly, infarction) of the right (nondominant) superior parietal lobule, but is also recorded with nonconvulsive status epilepticus.

Reference

Thomas P, Giraud K, Alchaar H, Chatel M. Ictal asomatognosia with hemiparesis. Neurology. 1998;51:280–282

Arachnoid cyst

Arachnoid *cysts* are cystic areas bounded by arachnoid membranes; they may occur above or below the tentorium but the most common site is in the middle cranial fossa. They are congenital (developmental) in origin, secondary to arachnoid maldevelopment, with trapping of arachnoid membrane, often with a one-way valve which communicates with the ventricular CSF system. Arachnoid cysts are often noted as incidental findings on CT or MRI scanning, but rarely cause symptoms themselves. They can occasionally be symptomatic when they enlarge sufficiently to compress neighboring structures, and they are associated with a slightly increased risk of subdural hematoma.

Clinical features

- Usually asymptomatic, incidental findings on structural brain imaging.
- Headache: may occur with a large cyst in the posterior fossa.
- *Subdural hematoma.*
- Local compressive symptoms, especially when they originate in the posterior fossa.
- In children they may cause macrocrania.
- Occasionally, arachnoid cysts may be found in the suprasellar region; they present in childhood with bobbing and nodding of the head, the "bobble head doll syndrome."
- Occasionally, arachnoid cysts have been implicated in cognitive decline, *syringomyelia.*

Investigation

Neuroimaging (CT/MRI) reveals the cyst, most commonly at the anterior pole of the temporal lobe.

Differential diagnosis

If local compression occurs, the differential diagnosis is that of a space-occupying lesion.

Treatment and prognosis

They are usually found by chance on neuroimaging; patient reassurance as to their nonmalignant, nonprogressive nature may be required. If there are focal neurological effects, then surgical intervention may be required.

Arachnoiditis

Chronic adhesive arachnoiditis, Idiopathic progressive ascending adhesive arachnoiditis, Meningitis circumscripta spinalis

Arachnoiditis literally means inflammation of the arachnoid, but in clinical practice the term is used to refer to meningeal scarring (fibrosis) as a consequence of injury or inflammation. There may be subsequent obliteration of the subarachnoid space, adhesions between the cord and dura, and occasionally the development of calcification and ossification (arachnoiditis ossificans). These changes may lead to cord compression. Clumping and adhesion of spinal roots (+/− arachnoid cyst development) may cause further compression. Blood vessel involvement may lead to ischemia with myelomalacia and cavitations in the cord, which may coalesce to form syringomyelia. The initiating injury may take various forms, including a prolapsed disc, spinal surgery, or the presence of foreign material in the subarachnoid space such as blood, infection, intrathecal drugs and, in the past, radiological contrast dyes used in myelography (particularly Myodil). The advent of modern improved contrast dyes, MR spinal imaging, better surgical techniques and treatment of spinal infection has meant that arachnoiditis has become much less common. Diagnosis and treatment of this condition is difficult.

Clinical features

- Usually occurs between the ages of 40 and 60 years; M > F. There is often a long latent period between insult and symptom onset, of up to 25 years. Many cases are asymptomatic.
- Spinal root involvement: low back pain that worsens with exercise, with lumbosacral radiculopathy that is usually recurrent and bilateral, often causing a *cauda equina syndrome.*
- Spinal cord compression and ischemia: this is now relatively rare, but patients used to present with thoracic cord involvement and paraparesis/paraplegia.
- Presentation with *syringomyelia* may still occur.
- An *anterior spinal artery syndrome* of cord infarction secondary to fibrosis and vessel involvement may occur.
- Idiopathic progressive ascending adhesive arachnoiditis: a rare condition that usually leads to death after 5–10 years. It presents with a painful progressive cauda equina syndrome, which then progresses to involve the conus and spinal cord in an ascending fashion. Clinically, there is a painful ascending severe paraplegia with sensory loss, muscle wasting, and weakness, leading to upper motor neurone features, and autonomic dysfunction.

Investigation

Neuroimaging with MRI may demonstrate adherent roots +/− thickening of the meninges, with little or no enhancement following gadolinium. CSF may reveal a mildly elevated protein and occasional pleocytosis. Neurophysiology (EMG/NCS) may reveal radiculopathy.

Differential diagnosis

- Tumor
- Malignant meningitis

Arachnoiditis may contribute to the neurological complications in *ankylosing spondylitis*.

Treatment and prognosis

The treatment of arachnoiditis is difficult and controversial. Optimum treatment is probably conservative with analgesics; anti-neuropathic pain agents such as carbamazepine, pregabalin, gabapentin, tricyclic antidepressants, and TENS; anti-inflammatory agents are usually not helpful. Surgical intervention is usually ineffective. Patients often have significant morbidity, although rarely die from their condition unless there is significant cord involvement.

References

Caplan LR, Noronha AB, Amico LL. Syringomyelia and arachnoiditis. J Neurol Neurosurg Psychiatry. 1990;53:106–113
Jellinek E. Myodil arachnoiditis: iatrogenic and forensic illness. Pract Neurol. 2002;2:237–239

Arbovirus disease: overview

Arboviruses are RNA viruses which are probably the most common cause of encephalitis worldwide, different types occurring in different geographical areas. The name derives from the fact that they are arthropod-borne: many have life cycles involving transmission by mosquitoes. Examples include

- Flaviviruses:
  - Dengue
  - St. Louis encephalitis virus
  - *Japanese encephalitis* virus
  - Murray Valley encephalitis virus (Australian X disease)
  - Tick-borne encephalitis virus
  - Louping ill
  - West Nile virus
- Bunyaviruses:
  - Rift Valley Fever virus
- Alphaviruses:
  - Eastern equine encephalitis virus
  - Western equine encephalitis virus

Argyrophilic grain disease (AGD)

Braak disease

Argyrophilic grain disease (AGD) is characterized morphologically on the basis of abundant neuropathological grains, consisting of abnormally phosphorylated tau protein, mainly in the CA1 subfield of the cornu ammonis, entorhinal, and transentorhinal cortices, amygdala, and hypothalamic lateral tuberal nucleus. Neurofibrillary tangles are also present in entorhinal and limbic areas, but are less prominent than in symptomatic *Alzheimer's disease* (*AD*). Oligodendroglial tau filamentous inclusions (coiled bodies) are also seen. Immunohistochemistry suggests that AGD is a 4R *tauopathy* and, hence, akin to *progressive supranuclear palsy* and *corticobasal degeneration*. Clinically, argyrophilic grain disease is a dementing disorder but with more prominent behavioral features and less prominent memory problems than in AD. Hence, some authors consider it distinct from AD.

Reference

Ferrer I, Santpere G, van Leeuwen FW. Argyrophilic grain disease. Brain. 2008;131:1416–1432

Arteriovenous malformations (AVMs)

Arteriovenous malformations (AVMs) of the CNS are formed from the abnormal development of blood vessels. Their classification is based on morphology and the location of the nidus or fistula. The key feature is arteriovenous shunting of blood, a *sine qua non* that excludes other intracranial vascular malformations such as *cavernomas*. AVMs vary in size, from a few millimeters to several centimeters, and in location. The most common presenting features are hemorrhage and *epilepsy*.

Clinical features

- The most common presentation of AVMs is with hemorrhage: primary *intracerebral hemorrhage* (*ICH*) > *subarachnoid hemorrhage* > intraventricular hemorrhage. AVMs may account for 1–2% of all strokes, and perhaps 4% in young adults; 9% of subarachnoid hemorrhages (SAH); and about 4% of all ICH, but possibly one-third of ICH, in young adults.

- The second most common presentation is with epileptic seizures, although AVMs are not a common cause of first presentations with unprovoked seizures (1%).
- Many AVMs are asymptomatic at the time of detection, for example, in patients undergoing brain imaging for some other reason.
- Progressive neurological deficit can occur with large or strategically placed AVMs (e.g., myelopathy with spinal AVM).
- In rare instances, *hydrocephalus* can develop if the vein of Galen is involved with the AVM. However, a more common cause for hydrocephalus is basal meningeal fibrosis secondary to subarachnoid hemorrhage.
- Headache, particularly persistently unilateral migraine, was once thought to be a common presentation; in fact, only 0.3% of patients with headache without focal neurological signs harbor an AVM; for migraineurs, the figure is 0.07%.
- Retinal and cutaneous vascular malformations may be found in patients with AVMs of the CNS and they may be in communication with the centrally placed vascular abnormality.

Investigation

Neuroimaging: CT with contrast will visualize most AVMs but MRI is more reliable. Although MRA can demonstrate some of the anatomy of AVMs, catheter angiography still remains the investigation of choice to define the origin and extent of arterial supply, and the venous drainage, of AVMs. CSF may confirm subarachnoid hemorrhage.

Differential diagnosis

Other causes of intracranial hemorrhage, focal epileptic seizures, progressive myelopathy.

Treatment and prognosis

Studies of the natural history of AVMs suggest an annual risk of first-ever hemorrhage of about 1%, but this does vary with location (greater with deep brain location) and drainage (greater with exclusively deep venous drainage). However, rebleed rates are higher, particularly in the first 6–12 months. The annual risk of developing *de novo* seizures is around 1%, with good prospects for control with antiepileptic medications. The long-term crude annual fatality rate is approximately 1–1.5%; 50–70% of deaths are due to hemorrhage.

A number of treatment modalities have evolved, the three main options being surgical excision, stereotactic radiotherapy, and endovascular embolization; there are no randomized controlled or comparative trials. It is not clear if treatment of unruptured AVMs is worthwhile.

References

Al-Shahi Salman R, Mast H, Stapf C. Unruptured arteriovenous malformations of the brain. Adv Clin Neurosci Rehabil. 2007;6(6):6–7
Choi JH, Mohr JP. Brain arteriovenous malformations in adults. Lancet Neurol. 2005;4:299–308
Friedlander RM. Clinical practice. Arteriovenous malformations of the brain. N Engl J Med. 2007;356:2704–2712
Spetzler RF, Martin NA. A proposed grading system for arteriovenous malformations. J Neurosurg. 1986;65:476–483
Wedderburn CJ, van Beijnum J, Bhattacharya JJ, et al. Outcome after interventional or conservative management of unruptured brain arteriovenous malformations: a prospective, population-based cohort study. Lancet Neurol. 2008;7:223–230

Aseptic meningitis: overview

Aseptic meningitis may be defined as a syndrome of clinical meningism with an inflammatory cerebrospinal fluid (leukocytosis) but with no organism identified (e.g., by Gram stain, Ziehl–Nielsen stain, culture, polymerase chain reaction). The differential diagnosis is broad:

- Partially treated bacterial *meningitis*
- Viral meningitis or meningoencephalitis
- *Tuberculous meningitis*
- Fungal meningitis
- Other bacterial/protozoal infections: brucellosis, leptospirosis, malaria
- Parameningeal infection: epidural/subdural abscess/empyema
- Chemical meningitis: blood (*subarachnoid hemorrhage*), myelographic agents
- *Endocarditis*
- Malignant meningitis: carcinoma, lymphoma, leukemia
- Venous sinus thrombosis
- Autoimmune disorders: *vasculitis*, *Behçet's disease*, *Sjögren's syndrome*
- *Neurosarcoidosis*
- Mollaret's (recurrent) meningitis: *dermoid, epidermoid*
- Chronic (benign) lymphocytic meningitis
- Idiosyncratic drug reaction (intravenous immunoglobulin, NSAIDs)

Aspergillosis

This fungal infection (*Aspergillus fumigatus*) may present as a chronic sinusitis with skull base osteomyelitis, with involvement of cranial nerves adjacent to infected bone. Clinical manifestations include brain *abscess* and granuloma, *meningitis*, meningomyelitis, *aneurysm*, and stroke-like syndromes from *vasculitis* or disseminated infection. Immunocompromised individuals are particularly vulnerable, for example, following organ transplantation. Diagnosis is by culture of the organism, or identification on biopsy specimens; there are no reliable serodiagnostic markers. CSF may show pleocytosis and elevated protein, but normal glucose, an important point in the differential diagnosis from *tuberculosis*. Treatment is with amphotericin +/– 5-flucytosine or voricanozole. Outcome is poor, even in immunocompetent patients.

References

Marr KA, Patterson T, Denning D. Aspergillosis. Pathogenesis, clinical manifestations and therapy. Infect Dis Clin North Am. 2002;16:875–894
Narayan SK, Kumar K, Swaminathan RP, Roopeshkumar VR, Bhavna B. Isoalted cerebral aspergilloma in a young immunocompetent patient. Pract Neurol. 2009;9:166–168

Astrocytoma

Astrocytomas are CNS *tumors* of neuroectodermal origin, which fall within the rubric of *glioma*, most cells containing glial fibrillary acidic protein (GFAP). Histologically, several types are described (fibrillary, pilocytic, protoplasmic, gemistocytic, pleomorphic xanthoastrocytomas), but the histological features do not correlate well with prognosis.

Ataxia telangiectasia (AT) [OMIM#208900]

Louis–Bar disease, Louis–Bar syndrome

Ataxia telangiectasia is a rare autosomal recessive condition in which there is defective DNA repair as a consequence of mutations in the ATM gene on chromosome 11, which results in a progressive ataxia, with loss of cerebellar Purkinje cells (possibly due to a failure to protect cells from oxidative stress). ATM is a protein kinase with critical signaling roles in the cellular response to ionizing radiation. Immunological deficiency leads to susceptibility to pyogenic infection and tumor development. AT may be regarded as a chromosome instability syndrome (along with Fanconi's anemia, Bloom syndrome, Nijmegen breakage syndrome, and AT-like disorder). Patients usually present before the age of 10 years with a progressive motor disorder and a characteristic oculomotor apraxia. At a later stage, they develop telangiectasia.

Clinical features

- Initial development is usually normal, problems becoming apparent when the child learns to walk. Ataxia of gait typically develops between the ages of 12 to 18 months; by age 10 years patients are usually unable to walk. The initial presentation may be complicated by athetosis with occasional myoclonic jerks.
- Progressive dystonia of the fingers may emerge with development.
- Oculomotor apraxia: an impairment of voluntary ocular motility, such that to move the eyes an abrupt head thrust may be required. Disordered smooth pursuit and limitation of upgaze may also occur.
- Dysarthria and drooling due to the cerebellar and extrapyramidal involvement.
- A peripheral polyneuropathy with distal muscular atrophy may be seen in adult patients, as may involvement of spinal cord dorsal columns with loss of proprioception.
- Recurrent infections, especially sinopulmonary, are a major feature. Children tend to be small and underweight. Bronchopulmonary infections may progress to bronchiectasis and atrophy of the secondary lymphoid organs.
- Cutaneous features: telangiectasia develop after the ataxia (3–6 years), and are seen on the conjunctiva and skin (ears, exposed parts of the neck, nose, and cheek in a butterfly pattern, flexor creases of forearm). Hypertrichosis and infrequent grey hairs are also a feature.
- About 10–15% of patients develop malignancy in early adulthood, usually T-cell tumors. Many other tumor types have also been reported in AT.
- Significant neuropsychological impairments are unusual; mild mental retardation may occur.

Investigation

Blood: standard blood tests are normal, but there is usually a raised α-feto-protein (90%), and hypogammaglobulinemia (80%); selective deficiency of the IgG2 subclass is characteristic. Neuroimaging (CT/MRI) shows cerebellar atrophy with relative sparing of cerebral cortex. CSF is normal. Neurophysiology (EMG/NCS) may show a peripheral polyneuropathy. Neurogenetic testing may show one of numerous mutations identified in the *ATM* gene at chromosome 11q22.23. Cultured fibroblasts have increased radiosensitivity due to faulty repair of DNA. Pathology: striking loss of cerebellar Purkinje cells and degenerative changes in dentate and inferior olivary nucleus; loss of myelinated fibers in the dorsal columns, spinocerebellar tracts, and peripheral nerves; degenerative changes in the dorsal roots, with cell loss in the sympathetic ganglia and some anterior horn cell loss.

Differential diagnosis

Young onset cerebellar syndromes. The differential diagnosis for the eye movement disorder includes Cogan's congenital oculomotor apraxia (see *Cogan syndrome (2)*), *Niemann–Pick disease* type C, and *Gaucher's disease*.

Treatment and prognosis

There is no specific treatment. Infections should be treated; postural drainage for bronchiectasis. The disease is relentlessly progressive; survival into adulthood is rare. The usual cause of death is intercurrent bronchopulmonary infection or neoplasia, usually during the second decade of life. Routine surveillance for leukemia/lymphoma is recommended.

References

Spacey SD, Gatti RA, Bebb G. The molecular basis and clinical management of ataxia telangiectasia. Can J Neurol Sci. 2000;27:184–191
Verhagen MM, Abdo WF, Willemsen MA, et al. Clinical spectrum of ataxia-telangiectasia in adulthood. Neurology. 2009;73:430–437

Ataxia with isolated vitamin E deficiency (AVED) [OMIM#277460]

Ataxia with isolated vitamin E deficiency (AVED) is a rare autosomal recessive disorder with deficiency of vitamin E, but without evidence of fat malabsorption and with normal lipoproteins (*cf. abetalipoproteinemia*). Clinically, the features are of progressive cerebellar ataxia, proprioceptive sensory loss (axonal peripheral neuropathy), tendon areflexia, extensor plantar responses, dysarthria, *scoliosis*, pes cavus, with or without a cardiomyopathy. The features are thus identical to *Friedreich's ataxia*, emphasizing the importance of measuring vitamin E levels in any progressive ataxia. The mutant gene for AVED has been mapped to chromosome 8q and encodes alpha-tocopherol transfer protein (TTPA) which incorporates tocopherol into very low density lipoproteins. The condition may be treated with vitamin E supplements, but clinical efficacy is uncertain.

Acquired vitamin E deficiency, for example associated with prolonged fat malabsorption, may be associated with similar neurological features (cerebellar ataxia, spinal cord syndrome, peripheral neuropathy).

References

Mariotti C, Gellera C, Rimoldi M, et al. Ataxia with isolated vitamin E deficiency: neurological phenotype, clinical follow-up and novel mutations in TTPA gene in Italian families. Neurol Sci. 2004;25:130–137
Ouahchi K, Arita M, Kayden H, et al. Ataxia with isolated vitamin E deficiency is caused by mutations in the alpha-tocopherol transfer protein. Nat Genet. 1995;9:141–145

Ataxia with oculomotor apraxia (AOA)

Two forms of ataxia with oculomotor apraxia (AOA) are characterized:

- AOA1 [OMIM#208920]:
  - Autosomal recessive cerebellar ataxia associated with oculomotor apraxia
  - Hypoalbuminemia, hypercholesterolemia
  - Axonal sensorimotor neuropathy
  - Choreiform movements (often at onset, but transient)
  - Cerebellar atrophy on MRI
  - Age range at onset 2–18 years
  - Results from mutations in the aprataxin gene
- AOA2 [OMIM#606002], also known as autosomal recessive spinocerebellar atrophy 1 (SCAR1):
  - Autosomal recessive cerebellar ataxia associated with (occasional) oculomotor apraxia
  - Peripheral (motor) neuropathy
  - Pyramidal signs
  - Head tremor
  - Dystonia
  - Strabismus
  - Chorea
  - Raised serum α-fetoprotein level
  - Cerebellar atrophy on MRI
  - Results from mutations in the senataxin gene

The differential diagnosis includes *ataxia telangiectasia* (AT) and *Friedreich's ataxia* (FA).

References

Anheim M, Monga B, Fleury M, et al. Ataxia with oculomotor apraxia type 2: clinical, biological and genotype/phenotype correlation study of a cohort of 90 patients. Brain. 2009;132:2688–2698
Le Ber I, Moreira MC, Rivaud-Péchoux S, et al. Cerebellar ataxia with oculomotor apraxia type 1: clinical and genetic studies. Brain. 2003;126:2761–2772

Atlantoaxial dislocation, subluxation

Dislocation or subluxation of the atlantoaxial articulation often results from failure of the stabilizing function of the odontoid peg of C2. This may occur in

- Cervical trauma
- Congenital malformation
- *Rheumatoid arthritis*
- *Down syndrome*
- *Ankylosing spondylitis*
- Foramen magnum lesions
- *Grisel syndrome*
- Morquio's disease

The resulting cord compression results in myelopathy or medullary compression, sometimes even in sudden death.

Atypical facial pain

Atypical facial pain is the name given to a syndrome of poorly localized unilateral or bilateral *facial pain*, often over the cheek or nose, lasting weeks or years, provoked by stress or fatigue, largely unresponsive to typical analgesics, without abnormal neurological signs, and for which no structural cause is found. Anxiety, depression, and other bodily pains are often associated factors. Diagnostic criteria are lacking (some consider it a diagnosis of exclusion), which makes epidemiological surveys difficult, but it is generally agreed to be more common in women, occurring usually in the fourth to sixth decades. Treatment is with a tricyclic antidepressants such as amitriptyline or nor-triptyline, which may need to be continued for up to 2 years.

Reference

Elrasheed AA, Worthington HV, Arivaratnam S, Duxbury AJ. Opinions of UK specialists about terminology, diagnosis, and treatment of atypical facial pain: a survey. Br J Oral Maxillofac Surg. 2004;42:566–571

Atypical pneumonias: overview

The term "atypical pneumonia" has been used to describe pneumonia, which, in contrast to typical pneumonia, is characterized by a relatively gradual onset, dry cough, shortness of breath, and prominent extrapulmonary symptoms, including headache, encephalopathy, myalgia, fatigue, nausea, vomiting, and diarrhea. Agents considered to be causes of atypical pneumonia include

- *Mycoplasma pneumoniae*
- *Chlamydia psittaci* (*psittacosis*)
- *Coxiella burnetti* (*Q fever*)
- *Legionella pneumophila* (*Legionnaires' disease*)
- *Francisella tularensis* (tularemia)
- *Histoplasma capsulatum*
- *Coccidiodes immitis*

as well as others, such as Influenza A virus. These agents may account for up to one-third of pneumonias, for which reason it has been suggested that the term "atypical" be dropped.

These conditions may be accompanied by neurological features.

Autonomic failure: overview

The autonomic nervous system (ANS) is composed of two major components: the sympathetic and parasympathetic nervous systems. They have a common origin from the hypothalamus and are involved with the homeostatic mechanisms maintaining cardiovascular stability as well as providing the neural input to visceral structures. There is a close functional relationship with the endocrine system that is similarly largely controlled from the hypothalamus. Disorders of the ANS may be due either to central or peripheral damage, disease, or interference from pharmacological agents.

Causes of autonomic failure include:

- Central causes:
  - *Primary autonomic failure* (*PAF*)
  - *Multiple system atrophy* (*MSA*)
  - Idiopathic *Parkinson's disease* (PD)
  - Structural lesions involving the hypothalamus and brain stem in the region of the fourth ventricle, spinal cord lesions
- Peripheral causes:
  - *Diabetes mellitus*
  - Amyloidosis
  - Alcohol
  - *Guillain–Barré syndrome*
  - Connective tissue disorders (especially *Sjögren's syndrome*)
  - *Lambert–Eaton myasthenic syndrome* (*LEMS*)
  - *Porphyria*
  - *Fabry's disease*
  - *Tangier disease*

- Vitamin B$_{12}$ deficiency states (rare)
- *Hereditary sensory and autonomic neuropathies* (*HSAN*)
- Infections: *botulism*, neurosyphilis, *HIV*, Chagas' disease
- Paraneoplastic syndrome (usually in association with ANNA 1 antibodies, or antibodies against the ganglionic nicotinic ACh receptor)
- Renal failure
- Dopamine-β-hydroxylase deficiency
- Drug effects:
  - Antihypertensive agents that block the sympathetic network (e.g., α-adrenoceptor, ganglion blockers)
  - Antidepressant drugs: tricyclic antidepressants, monoamine oxidase inhibitors
  - Major tranquilizers: phenothiazines, barbiturates (possibly central action)

Clinical features

- Postural hypotension/orthostatic hypotension/orthostatism: may present as *syncope* or presyncope, often precipitated by standing, exertion, or meals.
- Sexual impotence in males.
- Urinary symptoms: frequency and nocturia.
- Bowel symptoms: either nocturnal diarrhea or constipation. In the latter case, the patient may present with gastroparesis, recurrent vomiting, or intestinal pseudo-obstruction.
- Heat intolerance: associated with loss of sweating.
- Poor tolerance of bright lights, easily dazzled with difficulty accommodating.

Investigation

- Bedside testing:
  - Pupillary responses to light.
  - Postural blood pressure readings: a drop of >30/15 mmHg is significant if the patient is not fluid depleted.
  - Heart rate response to standing: should consist of an increase in rate between 10–30 beats/min.
  - Sweat test using quinizarin powder: should be positive when body temperature is raised by 1°C using space and electric blankets.
  - Valsalva maneuver with ECG monitoring: should demonstrate an increase in heart rate and there should be variation in heart rate with respiration.

- Laboratory testing:
  - Baroreflex sensitivity with changes in posture using a tilt table: on tilting, the normal response is a rise in blood pressure and a drop in heart rate. The test is normally done at 45° and 90° tilts.
  - Cardiovascular response to liquid meal: in normal individuals there is no significant change in heart rate or blood pressure, but in cases of autonomic failure blood pressure often drops after the meal due to failed compensation for increased splanchnic bed blood flow.
  - Bladder function: cystometrography.
  - Gastrointestinal motility: may be measured most simply using a barium meal.
  - Pupillary testing: rarely performed, but one of the few tests that can reliably distinguish central, sympathetic, or parasympathetic lesions. Responses are recorded at 15 min intervals for up to an hour after instillation of the eyedrops:

	Normal response	Peripheral sympathetic lesion	Central sympathetic lesion	Parasympathetic lesion
REST	–	Small pupil	Small pupil	Large pupil
4% Cocaine (prevents catecholamine uptake)	Dilatation (mydriasis)	Remains small	Slight dilatation	No effect, remains dilated
0.1% Adrenaline (acts on supersensitive adrenergic receptors)	No effect	Dilates	Small effect with dilatation	No effect
1% Hydroxy-amphetamine (stimulates catecholamine release)	Dilates	No response	Dilates	No effect
2.5% Meta-choline/0.125% Pilocarpine (acts on muscarinic receptors)	Constricts	?Further constriction	?Further constriction	Constriction (miosis)

Treatment and prognosis

Autonomic failure is difficult to treat effectively, but a number of symptomatic measures often help, at least initially. It is imperative to stop any medication that may be contributing to the symptomatology; for example, levodopa in MSA may exacerbate the autonomic failure without producing any significant anti-Parkinsonian action.

- Postural hypotension:
  - Head-up bed tilt of about 15° at night: resets the renin-angiotensin system.
  - Non-steroidal anti-inflammatory drugs (e.g., indomethacin): causes some fluid retention.
  - Desmopressin nasal spray: causes fluid retention and also helps with nocturnal urinary frequency, a common symptom in autonomic failure.
  - Fludrocortisone: causes fluid retention.
  - Ephedrine: causes vasoconstriction and some increase in cardiac output.
  - Midodrine.
  - "Marmite."
- Impotence:
  - Papaveretum injections into corpora cavernosa.
  - Sildenafil (Viagra).
- Urinary frequency/retention:
  - Oxybutynin, desmopressin spray for urinary frequency.
  - Intermittent self-catheterization in the event of urinary retention or large residual urinary volumes.
- Bowel immotility:
  - Cisapride and/or maxolon can increase gastrointestinal motility.

Overall prognosis is dependent on the cause. In PAF and MSA autonomic failure tends to worsen and often leads to death. If the cause of autonomic failure is transient (drugs, structural lesions, GBS and some of the infective and metabolic causes) prognosis is better.

References

Low PA, Bennaroch E, eds. Clinical Autonomic Disorders. 3rd ed. Philadelphia, PA: Lippincott Williams & Wilkins; 2008
Mathias CJ, Bannister R, eds. Autonomic Failure. A Textbook of Clinical Disorders of the Autonomic Nervous System. 4th ed. Oxford: Oxford University Press; 1999
Mathias CJ. Autonomic diseases: management. J Neurol Neurosurg Psychiatry. 2003;74(Suppl III):iii42–iii47

Autosomal dominant cerebellar ataxia (ADCA): overview

A clinical phenotypic classification of autosomal dominant cerebellar ataxias (ADCA) was proposed by Harding, as follows:

- ADCA type I:
  - Ataxia with ophthalmoplegia, optic atrophy, dementia, or extrapyramidal features, including Machado–Joseph disease (SCA3)

- ADCA type II:
  - Ataxia with pigmentary maculopathy, with or without ophthalmoplegia or extrapyramidal features
- ADCA type III:
  - "Pure" ataxia

ADCA type IV, cerebellar ataxia with myoclonus and deafness, probably represents *mitochondrial disease*, possibly including May–White syndrome, and so is probably obsolete.

To these categories of autosomal dominant cerebellar ataxia may be added:

- Autosomal dominant cerebellar ataxia with sensory neuropathy (Biemond's ataxia; SCA4): sensory symptoms affect the face and limbs in this rapidly progressive condition (unlike ADCA I-III).
- *Dentatorubral-pallidoluysian atrophy (DRPLA)*.
- *Episodic ataxias* with autosomal dominant inheritance.

Harding's phenotypic classification has been superseded to some extent by genotypic classification of the *spinocerebellar ataxias (SCA)* based on the discovery of genetic loci and specific genes responsible for the various syndromes: around 30 loci have now been described. Locus heterogeneity or phenotypic convergence has been demonstrated as ADCA type I may be a result of mutations in SCA1, 2, 3, and 4, and ADCA type III may be associated with SCA 5, 6, and 11. Several of the SCAs are *trinucleotide repeat diseases*, as is DRPLA. The episodic ataxias have been found to result from mutations in ion channel genes (*channelopathies*). Increased understanding of these conditions suggests that a pathogenetic classification may succeed Harding's phenotypic classification.

References

De Michele G, Coppola G, Cocozza S, Filla A. A pathogenetic classification of hereditary ataxias: is the time ripe? J Neurol. 2004; 251:913–922
Harding AE. The Hereditary Ataxias and Related Disorders. Edinburgh, UK: Churchill Livingstone; 1984

Autosomal dominant nocturnal frontal lobe epilepsy (ADNFLE) [OMIM#600513, #605375]

Autosomal dominant nocturnal frontal lobe epilepsy (ADNFLE) is a rare *epilepsy* syndrome, sometimes resulting from mutations in ligand-gated nicotinic acetylcholine receptor channels (i.e., a *channelopathy*).

Clinical features

- Nocturnal seizures, occurring in clusters, onset in childhood, with persistence to adult life; seizures characterized by vocalization, thrashing, stiffening, sometimes with preserved consciousness. May look bizarre and be mistaken for non-epileptic attacks.
- Normal clinical examination.
- Positive family history (although penetrance incomplete).

Investigation

EEG may show bifrontal epileptiform discharges. Neuroimaging normal. Neurogenetic testing may show mutations in either of two neuronal nicotinic acetylcholine receptor subunits, α_4 and β_2. Other genetic linkages have been described.

Differential diagnosis

Parasomnia; dyskinesia.

Treatment and prognosis

Carbamazepine monotherapy is often effective.

Reference

Combi R, Dalpra L, Tenchini ML, Ferini-Strambi L. Autosomal dominant frontal lobe epilepsy – a critical overview. J Neurol. 2004;251:923–934

B

Balò's concentric sclerosis

Encephalitis periaxialis concentrica

Balò's concentric sclerosis is a rare form of demyelinating disease, characterized by concentric alternating bands of myelin destruction and preservation within the cerebral hemispheres. Originally a pathological diagnosis, this appearance has also been documented antemortem using MRI: lesions show a hypointense center and intermediate rings, which enhance with gadolinium, and hyperintense inner and outer rings. Lesions that have this appearance microscopically occur in typical *multiple sclerosis* ("type 3" lesions). Occasionally, patients present with a monophasic or relapsing–remitting syndrome of epileptic seizures or cortical deficits and, on imaging, are found to have a single, or a few large Balò's-type lesions; it is not clear whether this is an unusual form of multiple sclerosis or a distinct disorder. There is no consensus on the treatment for such patients.

References

Balò J. Encephalitis periaxialis concentrica. Arch Neurol Psychiatry. 1928;19:242–264
Kastrup O, Stude P, Limmroth V. Balò's concentric sclerosis. Evolution of active demyelination demonstrated by serial contrast-enhanced MRI. J Neurol. 2002;249:811–815

Barth syndrome

Barth's X-linked cardiomyopathy and neutropenia syndrome

Barth syndrome is an X-linked mitochondrial disease that presents with dilated cardiomyopathy, proximal myopathy, short stature, and increased susceptibility to infection in boys. Cyclic neutropenia and 3-methylglutaconic aciduria are also features. Barth syndrome is associated with mutations in the tafazzin (TAZ) gene at Xq28, resulting in cardiolipin deficiency and abnormal mitochondria.

Reference

Bione S, D'Adano P, Maestrini E, et al. A novel X-linked gene, G4.5, is responsible for Barth syndrome. Nat Genet. 1996;12:385–389

Bartonellosis

Bartonella (*Rochalimaea*) *henselae* is the major cause of cat scratch disease, a febrile illness with lymphadenopathy most often occurring in children after a cat scratch (earlier studies had suggested that *Afipia felis* was the cause). It also causes bacillary angiomatosis, a multisystem disorder characterized by proliferation of small blood vessels, seen primarily in patients with acquired immunodeficiency syndrome. Neurological manifestations have been reported in both, including:

* Encephalopathy/encephalitis
* Myelitis
* Radiculitis
* Cerebellar ataxia
* Compressive neuropathy
* Neuroretinitis, optic neuritis, papillitis

The organism may be identified by culture, PCR, and serology. Various antibiotics (ciprofloxacin, gentamicin, erythromycin, cotrimoxazole) have been reported of benefit in cat scratch disease, but not bacillary angiomatosis.

In South America, *Bartonella bacilliformis* causes a febrile illness variously known as Oroya fever, verruga peruana, and Carrion's disease, the organism transmitted by the bite of sandflies. Invasion of the CNS may cause meningoencephalitis, myelitis, or venous thrombosis. The differential diagnosis includes *malaria*. First-line treatment is with chloramphenicol, although penicillin, tetracycline, and cotrimoxazole may be used.

Reference

Marra CM. Neurologic complications of Bartonella henselae infection. Curr Opin Neurol. 1995;8:164–169

Basal ganglia calcification: overview

Deposition of calcium within the basal ganglia was increasingly noted following the advent of CT brain scanning, occurring in a variety of neurological diseases and as an incidental finding in a significant proportion (0.5–1.0%) of neurologically normal individuals. Calcification of other CNS structures, including cortex (especially the occipital lobe), white matter, and cerebellum, may also be present (e.g., occipital lobe in *coeliac disease*, amygdala in *Urbach–Wiethe disease*). The calcification occurs in the walls of capillaries, arteries, small veins, and perivascular spaces, and may be associated with neuronal degeneration and gliosis.

The most commonly recognized associations of basal ganglia calcification include:

- Hypoparathyroidism, pseudohypoparathyroidism
- Mitochondrial cytopathy, for example, MELAS
- Idiopathic familial syndrome (*Fahr's disease*)
- Sporadic ("physiological"; no disorder of calcium metabolism)

Basal ganglia calcification has also been reported in

- *Wilson's disease*
- Birth anoxia
- Cockayne's syndrome
- *Carbon monoxide poisoning*
- Lead poisoning
- *Tuberous sclerosis*
- *HIV/AIDS*
- Radiation therapy
- Methotrexate therapy
- *Down syndrome*
- Aicardi–Goutières syndrome
- *Neurobrucellosis*
- *Systemic lupus erythematosus*

Dependent upon the clinical phenotype, further investigation of these conditions may be required. At the minimum, assessment of calcium status should be undertaken (blood calcium and phosphate +/ parathormone level).

References

Fénelon G, Gray F, Paillard F, et al. A prospective study of patients with CT detected pallidal calcifications. J Neurol Neurosurg Psychiatry. 1993;56:622–625
Koller WC, Cochran JW, Kláwans HL. Calcification of the basal ganglia: computerized tomography and clinical correlation. Neurology. 1979;29:328–333

Basedow's paraplegia

A paraplegia-like weakness occurring in the context of severe hyperthyroidism, with flaccid weakness, absent reflexes, minimal or no sensory disturbance and without sphincter disturbance, was described in the nineteenth century by various authors including Charcot. It is possible that this reflected coincident postinfective polyneuropathy or *Guillain–Barré syndrome* (GBS). However, cases of acute asymmetric mixed axonal and demyelinating senso-rimotor neuropathy in the context of acute hyperthyroidism, with mitochon-drial and cytoskeletal tissue changes compatible with thyrotoxicosis in the absence of GBS type changes, have been reported. Weakness and thyrotoxi-cosis are also rarely seen as part of the syndrome of thyrotoxic hypokalemic *periodic paralysis* in males of Asian or Latin American descent.

Reference

Pandit L, Shankar SK, Gayathri N, Pandit A. Acute thyrotoxic neuropathy – Basedow's paraplegia revisited. J Neurol Sci. 1998;155:211–214

Becker muscular dystrophy (BMD) [OMIM#300376]

This condition is allelic with *Duchenne muscular dystrophy;* hence, it is a dys-trophinopathy, with the same distribution of muscle wasting and weakness, but more benign: onset is around 12 years, and death does not occur until the fourth or fifth decade, sometimes even later. There may be associated mental impairment.

References

Bushby KM, Gardner-Medwin D. The clinical, genetic and dystrophin characteristics of Becker muscular dystrophy. I. Natural history. J Neurol. 1993;240:98–104 [Erratum Journal of Neurology. 1993; 240:453]
Emery AEH. The muscular dystrophies. Lancet. 2002;359:687–695
Sinnreich M. Dystrophinopathies. In: Karpati G, Hilton-Jones D, Bushby K, Griggs RC, eds. Disorders of Voluntary Muscle. 8th ed. Cambridge: Cambridge University Press; 2010:205–229

Behçet's disease

Behçet's disease is a chronic, multisystem, inflammatory disorder, named after the Turkish dermatologist Hulusi Behçet who formally described the condition in 1937 (although it was possibly described in the fifth century BCE in the Hippocratic corpus). It is found throughout the world, but is more common in Japan and the Mediterranean countries. Women are more commonly affected (F:M = 2–5:1), with presentation around 20–40 years of age. The disease can present in diverse ways (to dermatologists, chest physicians, ophthalmologists, neurologists) although the cardinal features are mucocutaneous ulceration, uveitis, skin lesions, and thrombotic events.

An International Study Group has suggested the following diagnostic criteria for Behçet's disease:

- Recurrent oral ulceration (sine qua non) in combination with two or more of the following:
- Recurrent genital ulceration
- Eye lesions
- Skin lesions or a positive pathergy test

However, Behçet's disease can occasionally present with isolated neurological features; the diagnosis may then rely on biopsy. Management often requires long-term immunosuppressive therapy.

Clinical features

- Recurrent oral aphthous ulceration (at least three times in a 12-month period).
- Recurrent genital aphthous ulceration.
- Ophthalmic lesions: anterior or posterior uveitis; retinal vasculitis; cells in vitreous humor in asymptomatic individuals.
- Skin lesions: erythema nodosum; pseudofolliculitis; papulopustular lesions; acneiform nodules.
- Joint involvement: recurrent seronegative arthritis, often involves individual large joints, is subacute, self-limiting, and nondeforming.
- Intestinal involvement: ulcerative hemorrhagic lesions of stomach, intestine, and anus that may be indistinguishable from ulcerative colitis.
- Vascular complications: include thrombophlebitis, deep venous thrombosis, *venous sinus thrombosis*, hepatic vein occlusion, and, rarely, arterial occlusions.
  - Neurological features (rarely seen together):
  - Parenchymal: inflammatory mass lesions are seen, especially in the brain stem or diencephalon.
  - Lymphocytic meningitis, occasionally with encephalopathy (epileptic seizures and reduced level of awareness).
  - Cerebral *venous sinus thrombosis* with raised intracranial pressure.
  - Peripheral nerve involvement is rare (polyneuropathy, mononeuropathy multiplex).

Investigation

Blood is usually nonspecific. There is often an inflammatory response with raised ESR and CRP with raised α-gammaglobulin and leukocytosis. Consider HLA testing (more common in those positive for HLA B51). Neuroimaging: MRI may reveal large space-occupying enhancing lesions that often involve the brain stem, +/− basal ganglia. Scattered nonspecific white matter lesions may be seen and are usually asymptomatic. MR angiography may reveal a thrombosed sagittal sinus. CSF may be normal; however, there may be raised intracranial pressure in the context of dural sinus thrombosis. With parenchymal CNS disease, hypercellular CSF (neutrophils, lymphocytes) is found in 60%, occasionally with positive oligoclonal bands. Ophthalmological assessment using a slit lamp may be helpful in defining ocular involvement. Dermatological and gastroenterological assessments as appropriate. Brain biopsy: if diagnosis suspected and not established by any other means.

Differential diagnosis

- Neurological disorders:
  - Multiple sclerosis
  - Cerebral vasculitis
  - Neurosarcoidosis
  - Vogt–Koyanagi–Harada syndrome
- Systemic disorders:
  - Reiter's disease
  - Stevens–Johnson syndrome
  - *Systemic lupus erythematosus*
  - Crohn's disease/ulcerative colitis
  - *Ankylosing spondylitis*
  - *Sweet's syndrome*

Treatment and prognosis

- Disease course varies:
  - Relapsing–remitting (40%)
  - Secondary progressive (30%)
  - Primary progressive (10%)
  - Silent neurological involvement (20%)
- Local therapy:
  - Oral ulcers can be treated with topical tetracycline or interferon-α.
  - Genital ulcers can be treated with topical steroids.
  - Uveitis can be treated with mydriatics and topical steroids.
- Systemic therapy for parenchymal disease:
  - Various immunosuppressive treatments have been tried, either singly or in combination. None have been submitted to a randomized controlled trial:
  - Corticosteroids (1 mg/kg/day initially, then a maintenance dose of 5–10 mg/day)
  - Azathioprine 2.5 mg/kg/day

- Chlorambucil 6–8 mg/day
- Cyclophosphamide, orally or via pulsed iv infusions
- Ciclosporin 5–10 mg/kg/day for 3 months (although there are anecdotal reports that ciclosporin may exacerbate neurological Behçet's)
- Colchicine 1 mg/day for 2–24 months
- Other therapies that have been tried include plasma exchange, thalidomide, and dapsone.
- Thrombotic events: warfarin may be indicated.
- Non-steroidal anti-inflammatory drugs may be used for arthritis.
- The prognosis is highly variable. It is worse with parenchymal neurological involvement, raised CSF cell count or protein, brain stem + involvement, primary or secondary progressive course, and relapse during tapering of steroid therapy.

Diagnostic criteria

International Study Group for Behçet's disease. Criteria for the diagnosis of Behçet's disease. Lancet. 1990;335:1078–1080.

Reference

Al-Araji A, Kidd DP. Neuro-Behçet's disease: epidemiology, clinical characteristics, and management. Lancet Neurol. 2009;8:192–204

Behr syndrome

Behr complicated optic atrophy, Optic atrophy-ataxia syndrome

Behr syndrome, first described in 1909, is an autosomal recessive disease characterized by

- Optic atrophy, nystagmus
- Spinocerebellar degeneration: spasticity and cerebellar ataxia
- +/– Learning disability
- +/– Peripheral neuropathy (sensory axonal)
- +/– Deafness
- +/– Tremor

Autosomal dominant inheritance has also been described. Onset is in infancy and the condition is slowly progressive.

Behr syndrome may be classifed as an early onset ataxia with optic atrophy, and may need to be differentiated from *Friedreich's ataxia, leukodystrophies, mitochondrial disease*, neuronal ceroid lipofuscinosis, and Wolfram syndrome. Alternatively it may be classified within the *hereditary spastic paraplegia* rubric.

3-Methylglutaconic aciduria may be noted in Behr syndrome, suggesting that it may result from enzyme deficiency or mitochondrial disorder.

Reference

Felicio AC, Godeiro-Junior C, Alberto LG, et al. Familial Behr syndrome-like pheno-type with autosomal dominant inheritance. Parkinsonism Relat Disord. 2008; 14:370–372

Bell's palsy

Bell's palsy is the most common cause of a lower motor neurone facial (VII cranial nerve) palsy. The eponym is reserved for idiopathic facial nerve palsy as there are many recognized symptomatic causes for facial palsy. Bell's palsy is speculated to have a viral etiology. Men and women are affected equally. The majority of patients require no investigation and make a full and complete spontaneous recovery. A minority (15%) fails to make a full recovery, and, in some cases, the regenerating nerve forms aberrant connections with symptomatic consequences, for example, crocodile tears.

Clinical features

- Onset is usually with pain in or behind the ear on the side that becomes affected, followed by a lower motor neurone VII nerve palsy of varying severity.
- Unilateral facial weakness evolves over hours, reaching a maximum within 2–3 days of symptom onset.
- Symptoms of numbness of the face on the ipsilateral side are almost invariable, possibly due to altered sensory return caused by subcutaneous muscle flaccidity; there is usually no objective evidence of sensory loss.
- Ipsilateral impairment of taste (ageusia, hypogeusia) and hyperacusis may be features, and have localizing value. Lesions within the facial canal proximal to the meatal segment cause both hyperacusis and ageusia; lesions in the facial canal between the nerve to stapedius and the chorda tympani cause ageusia but no hyperacusis; lesions distal to the branching off of the chorda tympani cause neither ageusia nor hyperacusis (i.e., facial motor paralysis only).
- Idiopathic facial nerve palsy can be recurrent but this is rare and has a distinct differential diagnosis, as does a bilateral onset of facial weakness.

Investigation

Generally, no investigations are required. Blood, imaging, and CSF are normal unless facial weakness is symptomatic. Neurophysiology (EMG/NCS) may show relative inexcitability of the facial nerve: if <10% of the normal side within 14 days of onset, it suggests that recovery will be incomplete.

Differential diagnosis

Other causes of an isolated lower motor neurone facial nerve palsy include:

• Geniculate herpes zoster (Ramsay Hunt syndrome)
• Diabetes mellitus
• *Neuroborreliosis* (Lyme disease, Bannwarth's disease)
• *Neurosarcoidosis*
• Leukemic infiltration, lymphoma
• HIV seroconversion
• Neoplastic compression (e.g., cerebellopontine angle tumor; rare)
• Entrapment: *Paget's disease*, hyperostosis cranialis interna
• Facial nerve neuroma
• *Idiopathic intracranial hypertension* (rare false localizing sign)

Recurrent lower motor neurone facial nerve palsy should prompt consideration of

• Diabetes mellitus
• Neuroborreliosis
• Neurosarcoidosis
• Leukemia, lymphoma
• *Melkersson–Rosenthal syndrome*

Facial weakness may also result from disease of muscle (e.g., *facioscapulohumeral dystrophy*, *dystrophia myotonica*, *mitochondrial disease*) and of the neuromuscular junction (*myasthenia gravis*). Upper motor neurone lesions may cause facial weakness, distinguished clinically by sparing of frontalis, which may be unilateral (e.g., hemisphere infarct +/– hemiparesis, lacunar infarct, space-occupying lesions: intrinsic tumor, metastasis, abscess) or bilateral (motor neurone disease, diffuse cerebrovascular disease, pontine infarct).

Treatment and prognosis

There is now robust evidence to support a role for steroids (prednisolone) early in the treatment of Bell's palsy, with associated better outcome at 3 and 9 months. Meta-analyses find no evidence to support the use of antiviral agents (aciclovir) alone, but disagree as to whether they do confer additional benefit in combination with steroids. Facial nerve decompressive surgery has been advocated in some cases.

If eye closure is incomplete, eye protection with artificial tears may be required, and antibiotics for any exposure conjunctivitis. Tarsorrhapy may be required if recovery is insufficient to achieve eye closure.

Poorer prognosis is associated with older patient age (over 40 years) and if no recovery is seen within 4 weeks of onset. Aberrant nerve regeneration may occur, leading to autonomic synkineses such as involuntary tearing of the eye on the affected side with eating (crocodile tears, Bogorad's syndrome) and gustatory sweating (Frey's syndrome). Synkinesis of the facial musculature with chewing may also occur: jaw opening leads to eye closure, jaw winking, on the involved side (Marin–Amat syndrome). *Hemifacial spasm* sometimes appears after Bell's palsy, and there is also a report of blepharospasm following Bell's palsy.

References

De Almeida JR, Al Khabori M, Guyatt GH, et al. Combined corticosteroid and antiviral treatment for Bell palsy: a systematic review and meta-analysis. JAMA. 2009;302:985–993

Quant EC, Jeste SS, Muni RH, Cape AV, Bhussar MK, Peleq AY. The benefits of steroids versus steroids plus antivirals for treatment of Bell's palsy: a meta-analysis. BMJ. 2009;339:b3354

Sullivan FM, Swan IR, Donnan PT, et al. Early treatment with prednisolone or acyclovir in Bell's palsy. N Engl J Med. 2007;357:1598–1607

Belly dancer's dyskinesia

Belly dancer's dyskinesia is the name given to a focal involuntary movement disorder characterized by undulating rhythmical movement of the anterior abdominal wall causing circular rotatory umbilical motion. Most cases follow a laparotomy; there is disagreement amongst the authorities as to whether or not cases may be related to neuroleptic use. Pain may also be present. The movements have no associated neurological lesion in the spinal cord. Treatment with botulinum toxin injections and pallidal deep brain stimulation has been reported.

Reference

Iliceto G, Thompson PD, Day BL, et al. Diaphragmatic flutter, the moving umbilicus syndrome and "belly dancers' dyskinesia." Mov Disord. 1990;5:15–22

Benign epilepsy syndromes: overview

A number of epilepsy syndromes of childhood have an extremely good prognosis, with spontaneous seizure cessation with increasing age and, hence, may be described as benign. These include

- Absence seizures ("petit mal")
- Rolandic epilepsy, benign epilepsy with centrotemporal spikes
- Panayiotopoulos syndrome (benign occipital epilepsy)
- Gastaut's occipital epilepsy
- Benign partial epilepsies:
  - With affective symptoms
  - With extreme somatosensory evoked potentials
  - With frontal spikes
- Benign infantile seizures: familial, nonfamilial (Watanabe–Vigevano syndrome)
- Benign myoclonic epilepsy of infancy
- Benign familial myoclonus
- Benign neonatal seizures: familial, nonfamilial
- Benign neonatal convulsions ("fifth day fits")

The syndrome of benign familial neonatal convulsions is an autosomal dominant condition, shown to be a channelopathy, affecting voltage-gated potassium channels, M-type subunit (mutations in genes KCNQ2 and KCNQ3; OMIM#121200 and #121201, respectively).

Nonepileptic movement disorders may need to be differentiated from some of these syndromes, for example, benign neonatal sleep myoclonus and benign nonepileptic myoclonus of infancy ("shuddering attacks").

Reference

Panayiotopoulos CP. A Clinical Guide to Epileptic Syndromes and Their Treatment: Based on the ILAE Classifications and Practice Parameter Guidelines. 2nd ed. London: Springer; 2007:285–318

Benign hereditary chorea (BHC) [OMIM#118700]

This autosomal dominant condition with childhood onset is characterized by chorea, which is nonprogressive or only slowly progressive; the first symptom may be delayed walking. There is no dementia, PET brain scans are normal and there is no overt pathological change (cf. *Huntington's disease*). There is genetic heterogeneity: some families have mutations in the thyroid transcription factor (TITF-1) gene on chromosome 14. Abnormalities in thyroid and lung have been identified in the clinical spectrum since identification of the gene.

References

Kleiner-Fisman G, Lang AE. Benign hereditary chorea revisited: a journey to understanding. Mov Disord. 2007;22:2297–2305
Kleiner-Fisman G, Rogaeva E, Halliday W, et al. Benign hereditary chorea: clinical,
genetic and pathological findings. Ann Neurol. 2003;54:244–247

Benign paroxysmal positional vertigo (BPPV)

Benign paroxysmal positional vertigo (BPPV) is a common disorder resulting from damage to the peripheral vestibular apparatus. It is often idiopathic
in origin, but, in a significant number of cases, it is associated with a preceding
history of head trauma or vestibular neur(on)itis, presumbaly of viral origin.
The condition is characterized by paroxysmal positional vertigo and nystagmus, which is normally induced by certain movements of the head such as
lying down or rolling over in bed at night. In all cases, there is a disruption of
flow of endolymph in the semicircular canals, most usually the posterior but
occasionally the horizontal. There are two theories of pathogenesis: *cupulo-
lithiasis* suggests that detached otoconia (calcium carbonate crystals) from
the utricle become adherent to the cupula of the posterior semicircular canal,
rendering it a gravity sensitive organ; whereas *canalithiasis* refers to debris,
including possibly degenerating otoconia, which becomes free-floating in the
endolymph and disturbs the endolymph when the head is moved, stimulating
the ampulla. The latter is the more compelling explanation for the clinical
phenomenology. Moreover, it is readily treatable by manipulation to reposition the debris (Epley maneuver).

Clinical features

- Paroxysms of vertigo with nausea and gait ataxia, and occasionally vomiting; induced by turning the head into certain positions, especially lying
  down and rolling over in bed or bending forward. The attacks last for a few
  minutes at most.
- There may be a secondary anxiety disorder.
- Attacks may be induced on clinical examination using the Dix–Hallpike
  (or Nylen–Barany) maneuver. Prior to performing this, the patient should
  be warned that an attack may be induced, and if it is severe, prophylactic
  prochlorperazine may be given. The patient must be told to keep his or her
  eyes open during the maneuver despite the vertigo:
  - The patient sits on the side of the examination couch.
  - Examiner turns the patient's head through 45° to right or left, then tips
    the patient back in this position so that the head lies 30° below the hori-
    zontal (i.e., hanging over the end of the couch).

- The eyes are observed in this position for at least 30 s. In a positive test, torsional nystagmus with the upper pole of the eye beating toward the ground will be observed.
- It must be remembered that there will be a delay before the nystagmus emerges; it rapidly fatigues.
- The test is done in both directions (i.e., right and left head turning).

Investigation

The positional maneuver (Dix–Hallpike, Nylen–Barany) is diagnostic when positive. Blood, neuroimaging, CSF, and other tests are necessary only when there is doubt about the diagnosis, and/or a central cause for vertigo is considered possible. (A central vestibular lesion may cause a "false-positive" Hallpike, where the nystagmus is distinguished from that of BPPV by being of rapid onset and not fatigable.)

Differential diagnosis

- Vestibular neur(on)itis
- Labyrinthine concussion
- Ménière's disease, vestibular-only form
- Posterior fossa (cerebellum, brain stem) disease: vascular, demyelinating, neoplastic
- Vertebrobasilar insufficiency (the labyrinthine artery arises from the vertebrobasilar system)
- Panic attacks

Treatment and prognosis

The condition is often self-limiting, with the majority of attacks passing off within 10 weeks. However, there is a tendency to recurrence. The mainstay of therapy is manipulation to reposition the displaced otolith crystals or otoconia, of which the most successful is the Epley maneuver:

- The patient may need prophylactic prochlorperazine as the procedure begins with a Dix–Hallpike maneuver.
- The patient's head is tipped to the side that is affected, provoking vertigo and nystagmus.
- The head is then turned through 90° while the body remains in the supine position.
- The head and body are then rotated so that the head is facing down; this may provoke further brief vertigo.

- The patient is then brought to the seated position, with the head still turned toward the shoulder.
- The patient's head is then recentered and the head tipped forward (chin down) by about 20°.

The patient should keep his or her head in the upright position as much as possible in the first 48 h after the procedure. About 80% of patients gain improvement after the first session, and this figure rises to 98% after a second session a week later.

Habituating exercises, such as the Brandt–Daroff exercises, may be undertaken if the patient cannot tolerate the Epley maneuver. Drug treatment is usually ineffective, and surgical elimination of posterior semicircular canal function is rarely needed.

References

Bronstein AM, Lempert T. Dizziness: A Practical Approach to Diagnosis and Management. Cambridge: Cambridge University Press; 2007:132–145 [includes videos]
Epley JM. The canalith repositioning procedure: for treatment of benign paroxysmal positional vertigo. Otolaryngol Head Neck Surg. 1992;107:399–404
Furman JM, Cass SP. Benign paroxysmal positional vertigo. N Engl J Med. 1999;341:1590–1596

Beriberi

Beriberi is a condition that affects the heart and peripheral nervous system, and is due to thiamine or vitamin B1 deficiency. When the disease predominantly affects the heart, the patient presents with congestive cardiac failure, or "wet beriberi," whereas when the disease involves the peripheral nerves, the patient presents with a painful peripheral neuropathy or "dry beriberi." In its pure form it is relatively rare, but thiamine deficiency is not uncommonly found to be an etiological agent in the neuropathies associated with malnutrition and chronic alcoholism.

Clinical features

- Insidious onset, usually over weeks, of pain (ache, cramp-like, burning), paresthesia and weakness, more apparent distally and especially in the legs, where it may be associated with skin changes (glossy, atrophic, hairless).
- On examination, there is usually a predominantly motor neuropathy, affecting especially the lower limbs and which may be so severe as to prevent walking; there is symmetrical distal sensory impairment, with hyperesthesia and allodynia. Tendon jerks are usually lost early.

- Sensory loss is very variable in terms of which modalities are lost and which spared. There is often hyperhidrosis of the hands and feet. Bulbar and respiratory muscle involvement is rare (cf. *Guillain–Barré syndrome*).
- In addition to the neurological features, there may be evidence of malnutrition, alcoholism, and congestive cardiac failure.

Investigation

Blood: FBC may show anemia, liver function tests may be abnormal, low vitamin B_{12}, folate, pyruvate (often raised in thiamine deficiency), and reduced RBC transketolase (must be measured before thiamine repletion). Imaging: CXR may reveal features of congestive cardiac failure. Neuroimaging (CT/MRI) is usually normal, unless there is concurrent disease associated with the thiamine deficiency (e.g., *Wernicke–Korsakoff syndrome*). CSF is usually normal, with occasionally slightly raised protein. Neurophysiology (EMG/NCS) shows evidence of an axonal neuropathy, with denervation on needle EMG. Pathologically, there is axonal degeneration with secondary demyelination, involving the largest and most distal myelinated fibers; degeneration may extend to the anterior and posterior roots, anterior horn cells, dorsal root ganglia, and dorsal columns. In the early stages of the disease, the neuropathy may be curable with vitamin supplementation.

Differential diagnosis

Other painful neuropathies:

- Guillain–Barré syndrome (acute motor axonal neuropathy)
- Diabetes mellitus
- Critical illness polyneuropathy
- Vasculitis (pain as each nerve is infarcted)
- Porphyria
- Infection: neuroborreliosis (Lyme disease), diphtheria, poliomyelitis
- Paraneoplastic syndromes
- Heavy metal poisoning
- Fabry's disease
- HIV/AIDS
- Cryoglobulinemia

Treatment and prognosis

The mainstay of treatment is thiamine replacement, at a dose of 50–100 mg/day, as soon as the diagnosis is considered. In the short term, aspirin, non-steroidal anti-inflammatory medications, and tricyclic antidepressants may be needed to control the pain. Physiotherapy is required, especially as atrophy and weakness may develop due to disuse, secondary to the pain. The majority of patients start to improve in days, but in the more severe cases, especially with cardiac involvement, improvement may take months and is incomplete.

Reference

Murphy C, Bangash IH, Varma A. Dry beriberi mimicking the Guillain-Barré syndrome. Pract Neurol. 2009;9:221–224

Bethlem myopathy [OMIM#158810]

Early-onset limb-girdle myopathy with contractures

A rare autosomal dominant muscle disease, with onset from infancy to adolescence, with proximal lower limb weakness, and slow progression; most patients remain ambulant. Contractures of interphalangeal joints, elbows, and ankles are common. There is no facial or cardiac involvement (cf. *Emery–Dreifuss muscular dystrophy*). Creatine kinase may be normal or slightly elevated, EMG is myopathic, and muscle biopsy is nonspecific. Mutations in the genes encoding the three peptide chains of collagen VI (COL6A1, A2, A3 genes), an extracellular matrix protein, have been detected in this condition and also in *Ullrich congenital muscular dystrophy*.

References

Jobsis GJ, Boers JM, Barth PG, de Visser M. Behtlem myopathy: a slowly progressive congenital muscular dystrophy with contractures. Brain. 1999;122:649–655
Jobsis GJ, Keizers H, Vreijling JP, et al. Type VI collagen mutations in Bethelm myopathy, an autosomal dominant myopathy with contractures. Nat Genet. 1996;14:113–115

Bickerstaff's brainstem encephalitis (BBE)

Bickerstaff's brain stem encephalitis is a syndrome of acute ophthalmoplegia and cerebellar ataxia, which is clinically very similar to *Miller Fisher syndrome*, with which it may form a clinical spectrum It is preceded by infection and is probably due to autoimmune attack on brain stem structures; anti-GQ1b ganglioside autoantibodies, as found in Miller Fisher syndrome, are found in most, but not all, cases, and are the unifying feature of the "anti-GQ1b syndrome." At its most severe, ventilatory support may be required, but overall prognosis for recovery is extremely good.

Clinical features

- Prodrome: general malaise +/− myalgia
- Evolution of brain stem signs (downward):
  - Drowsiness, but easily rousable (not always present)
  - Mild headache, occasional vomiting
  - Acute ophthalmoplegia (downgaze spared), +/− diplopia, ptosis, fixed dilated pupils
  - Motor trigeminal (V) involvement
  - Lower motor neurone facial (VII) nerve involvement
  - Cerebellar ataxia (especially trunk)
  - Bulbar weakness
  - Limb power normal; reflexes brisk to absent; plantars may be extensor
- Maximum disability in 5–30 days
- Great improvement thereafter; may be complicated by Parkinsonism for 2 weeks, but eventual total recovery

Clustering of cases has been noted on occasion.

Investigation

Blood: Anti-GQ1b antiganglioside autoantibodies. Serological screening for recognized antecedent infections (herpes simplex virus, Epstein–Barr virus, cytomegalovirus, varicella zoster, *Campylobacter jejuni* enteritis). Neuroimaging (MRI) may show brain stem lesions, anywhere from midbrain to medulla. CSF may show pleocytosis, raised protein; may be normal.

Differential diagnosis

- Miller Fisher syndrome
- Brain stem inflammatory disease: *multiple sclerosis*, *Behçet's disease*
- Unusual presentation of *herpes simplex encephalitis*
- Direct brain stem infection with Listeria or Legionella (when there may be an accompanying peripheral neuropathy)

Treatment and prognosis

Relapses are not recorded. If the patient is appropriately supported through the acute phase, total recovery occurs. Uncontrolled studies suggest that plasma exchange and IVIg may be of benefit.

References

Bickerstaff ER. Brain stem encephalitis (Bickerstaff encephalitis). In: Vinken PJ, Bruyn GW, eds. Handbook of Clinical Neurology: Infections of the Nervous System Part II. Vol 34. Amsterdam, The Netherlands: North Holland; 1978: 605–609
Chataway SJS, Larner AJ, Kapoor R. Anti-GQ1b antibody status, magnetic resonance imaging, and the nosology of Bickerstaff's brainstem encephalitis. Eur J Neur. 2001;8:355–357
Ito M, Kuwabara S, Odaka M, et al. Bickerstaff's brainstem encephalitis and Fisher syndrome form a continuous spectrum: clinical analysis of 581 cases. J Neurol. 2008;255:674–682

Bing–Neel syndrome

Bing–Neel syndrome refers to malignant infiltration of the CNS by lympho-plasmacytic cells in Waldenström's macroglobulinemia, which may be either "tumoral" or "diffuse." The former is more common and presents with focal neurological deficits and/or seizures, whilst the latter manifests as nonfocal cognitive and psychiatric change or depression of consciousness. Diffuse disease may be due to leptomeningeal infiltration or to slowing of the cerebral circulation secondary to blood hyperviscosity. The latter may also cause episodic visual disturbances through slowing of the retinal circulation.

Reference

Mackenney J. A possible case of diffuse Bing-Neel syndrome in Waldenström's macroglobulinaemia. Adv Clin Neurosci Rehabil. 2009;9(2 Suppl):14–15

Binswanger's disease

Subcortical arteriosclerotic encephalopathy (SAE)

Binswanger in 1894 described a vascular disorder consisting of a subcortical obliteration of small arteries and arterioles, often in association with systemic *hypertension*, leading to pathological periventricular demyelination and clinical *dementia*. The condition was judged to be relatively rare until the advent of neuroimaging, when neuroradiological evidence of white matter disease led to increased use of this diagnostic category. However, such white matter changes, now sometimes labeled leukoaraiosis, are relatively common in the elderly both without and with dementia (which may be of Alzheimer type or vascular in origin). The term Binswanger's disease is probably best reserved for pathological changes, modern reports of which are relatively few, and suggest hypertensive small artery disease as the pathological substrate. Such cases might be better incorporated under the rubric of subcortical ischemic vascular disease.

Clinical features

- The classic history is of stepwise deterioration, with episodes of acute deterioration from lacunar syndromes, and periods of stability and occasionally even improvement. However, a considerable proportion of patients present with steadily progressive neurological deficits.
- Abnormal gait: wide-based, shuffling; due to a combination of pyramidal and, particularly, extrapyramidal dysfunction.
- Urinary incontinence.
- Mood changes including apathy, inertia, abulia.
- Pseudobulbar palsy.
- *Vascular dementia, vascular cognitive impairment*: typically frontal subcortical pattern of deficits.
- +/– Focal cerebrovascular deficits.
- +/– Epileptic seizures.
- Immobility.

Investigation

Blood is usually normal; need to exclude hypercholesterolemia, thrombophilia. Neuroimaging: CT/MRI show an ischemic periventricular leukoencephalopathy, often with sparing of subcortical U-fibers; patchy periventricular white matter changes (leukoaraiosis), with lacunar infarcts in the basal ganglia +/– brain atrophy, ventricular dilatation. Carotid angiography shows no significant extra- or intracranial abnormality. CSF is usually normal. Neuropsychology: subcortical-frontal executive dysfunction is prominent. Investigation for other hypertensive end-organ damage, for example, echocardiogram and renal ultrasound, may be indicated.

Differential diagnosis

Other causes of leukoaraiosis:

- Hypertensive small vessel disease (*lacunar syndromes*)
- Multi-infarct dementia
- Vascular syndromes including *CADASIL* and *cerebral amyloid angiopathy*
- Cerebral *vasculitis*

- *Normal pressure hydrocephalus*
- Inflammatory CNS disease including *neurosarcoidosis, Behçet's disease, multiple sclerosis*

Treatment and prognosis

Reduce the risk of further vascular events: control blood pressure, hypercholesterolemia; low-dose aspirin. The disease usually progresses, regardless of blood pressure control, with mean survival between 5 and 10 years.

References

Bennett DA, Wilson RS, Gilley DW, Fox JH. Clinical diagnosis of Binswanger's disease. J Neurol Neurosurg Psychiatry. 1990;53:961–965
Caplan LR. Binswanger's disease revisited. Neurology. 1995;45:626–633
Fisher CM. Binswanger's encephalopathy: a review. J Neurol. 1989;236:65–79

Blastomycosis

Blastomycosis is a fungal infection that causes a self-limiting respiratory illness, but which may occasionally cause chronic nonspecific *meningitis* or intracranial *abscess*, more often in immunocompromised individuals. The organism, *Blastomyces dermatitidis*, is seldom identified from the CSF; culture from extraneural sites may be possible. Treatment is with intravenous amphotericin, followed by itraconazole.

Blue rubber bleb naevus syndrome

Blue rubber bleb naevus syndrome is a rare viscero- cutaneous hemangiomatosis, in which bluish rubbery naevi occur on the skin and also in the lungs, liver, skeletal muscle, and, rarely, the CNS. Neurological presentations include focal seizures and cerebellar syndrome. MR imaging shows high signal intensity lesions on T_2-weighted scans. Hemorrhage and calcification may also be observed. Surgical ablation is possible, but conservative management is often adequate. The differential diagnosis encompasses *hereditary hemorrhagic telangiectasia*.

References

Fernandes C, Silva A, Coelho A, Campos M, Pontes F. Blue rubber bleb naevus: case report and literature review. Eur J Gastroenterol Hepatol. 1999;11:455–457
Wills AJ, Marsden CD, eds. Fifty Neurological Cases from the National Hospital. London: Martin Dunitz; 1999:133–135 [Case 41]

Botulism

Botulism is an extremely rare condition resulting from infection with the Gram-positive anaerobic bacillus *Clostridium botulinum*, which produces a polypeptide exotoxin that exerts neurological effects. Botulinum toxin (Btx) blocks synaptic transmission at the neuromuscular junction (and indeed has been used as a therapeutic agent for dystonic movement disorders and spasticity). Specifically, holotoxin comprises heavy (H) and light (L) chains joined by a disulphide bond; a sequence at the carboxyl end of the heavy (H_C) chain binds with high affinity to a specific presynaptic neuronal surface receptor at cholinergic synapses, allowing toxin to cross the plasma membrane via receptor-mediated endocytosis. From the endosome, toxin enters the cell cytoplasm via a pH-dependent conformational change mediated by the amino end of the heavy chain (H_N). Reduction of the disulphide bond releases the L chain, the toxic moiety, which is an endopeptidase that selectively cleaves proteins essential for the recognition and docking of neurotransmitter-containing vesicles with the plasma membrane (e.g., synaptobrevin or vesicle-associated membrane protein [VAMP], syntaxin, SNAP-25). This prevents the quantal release of acetylcholine (ACh) and, hence, clinical features (autonomic dysfunction, muscle paralysis) appear 12–36 h after toxin ingestion. Bacterial contamination of foodstuffs is the most common cause of botulism, but it may also occur in wounds and as an infantile infection. In the Western world, the most common cause of wound bolutism is contamination of the deliberate injection of illicit drugs into the skin ("skin-popping"). The clinical presentation is with autonomic failure and muscle paralysis. Treatment is supportive; recovery may be prolonged and incomplete.

Three clinical variants are recognized:

- Infantile botulism: infants between 2 weeks and 11 months of age are susceptible to intestinal colonization by *C. botulinum*, leading to flaccid paralysis, cranial nerve signs, and autonomic signs.
- Foodborne botulism: causes an afebrile descending paralysis with autonomic and cranial nerve signs.
- Wound botulism: conditions predisposing to this are similar to those encountered in tetanus.

Clinical features

- In infantile and foodborne botulism, first symptoms after toxin ingestion (12–36 h) are anorexia, nausea, vomiting, and diarrhea (gastroenteritis); not a feature of wound botulism.
- Parasympathetic features generally precede muscle weakness: blurred vision and diplopia with an ophthalmoplegia, ptosis, and large unreactive pupils, and concurrent bulbar failure.
- Descending flaccid paralysis, and signs of autonomic failure (bradycardia, postural hypotension, dry mouth) then occur.

- Sensory and cognitive functions are normal.
- In foodborne botulism, there may be a history of other people with similar symptoms, or of home canning or bottling of foods (spores can survive for long periods of time and germinate in anaerobic conditions of increased alkalinity with a rise in temperature).
- Intravenous drug use is a risk factor for the development of wound botulism.

Investigation

Bloods: usually normal; may be able to assay for the toxin in blood. Neuroimaging: usually normal. CSF: usually normal. Neurophysiology: EMG/ NCS is the key investigation, showing decreased amplitude of the evoked compound muscle action potentials and, characteristically, an incremental response on rapid repetitive nerve stimulation but a decrement with slow repetitive nerve stimulation. Nerve conduction studies reveal normal conduction velocities (i.e., no neuropathy).

Differential diagnosis

- *Myasthenia gravis* (bulbar weakness)
- *Miller Fisher syndrome* variant of Guillain–Barré syndrome
- *Bickerstaff's brain stem encephalitis*
- *Diphtheria*
- *Poliomyelitis*
- *Brain stem vascular syndromes*

Treatment and prognosis

Treatment is supportive, with respiratory monitoring and, if necessary, ventilation in the intensive care unit. Prolonged parenteral feeding may be required due to autonomic involvement of the gut. Antibiotic treatment may be given but aminoglycosides should be avoided since they can potentiate neuromuscular blockade. In the early stages, trivalent equine antitoxin is recommended (after intradermal hypersensitivity testing). The recovery phase may be prolonged, up to years, and is often incomplete. Botulism is a notifiable disease.

References

Critchley EMR, Mitchell JD. Human botulism. Br J Hosp Med. 1990;43:290–292
Shapiro RL, Hatheway C, Swerdlow DL. Botulism in the United States: a clinical and epidemiologic review. Ann Intern Med. 1998;129:221–228
Wenham TN. Botulism: a rare complication of injecting drug use. Emerg Med J. 2008;25:55–56

Boucher–Neuhauser syndrome

A syndrome comprising the triad of

- *Spinocerebellar ataxia*
- Hypogonadotropic hypogonadism
- Choroidal dystrophy

Movement disorders have also been described.

References

Limber ER, Bresnick EH, Lebovitz RM, et al. Spinocerebellar ataxia, hypogonadotropic hypogonadism and choroidal dystrophy (Boucher-Neuhauser syndrome). Am J Med Genet. 1989;33:409–414

Ling H, Unnwongse K, Bhidayasiri R. Complex movement disorders in a sporadic Boucher-Neuhauser syndrome: phenotypic manifestations beyond the triad. Mov Disord. 2009;24:2304–2306

Brachial plexopathy: overview

The brachial plexus is a collection of nerves, taking their origin from the C5 to T1 anterior and posterior nerve roots, which is located in the region from the lateral aspect of the neck to the axilla, just superior to the apex of the lung. The brachial plexus gives rise to all the nerves of the upper limb. It may be selectively involved in disease processes, and is subject to traumatic injury (e.g., motorbike injuries). Recovery is dependent on the etiology and extent of the insult.

Recognized causes of brachial plexopathy include

- Trauma:
  - Upper plexus: C5-6 roots and upper trunk (*Erb–Duchenne palsy*)
  - Lower plexus: C8-T1 roots and lower trunk (*Klumpke palsy*)
- Inflammatory:
  - *Neuralgic amyotrophy*, also known as acute brachial neuropathy/plexitis, brachial neuritis, Parsonage Turner syndrome
- Neoplastic:
  - Upper plexus:
    - Primary: neurofibroma, schwannoma, neurogenic sarcoma/fibrosarcoma (rare)
    - Secondary: metastatic disease from lung, breast
  - Lower plexus:
    - Primary: *Pancoast syndrome* (lung apex tumor).
    - Secondary: metastatic disease from lung, breast

- Postirradiation (especially radiotherapy to axillary nodes in breast cancer treatment)
- Inherited: *hereditary neuropathy with liability to pressure palsies (HNLPP)*, hereditary neuralgic amyotrophy
- Structural: *thoracic outlet syndrome*
- Drug abuse: heroin (causing an inflammatory brachial or sacral plexopathy)

Clinical features

- Upper limb sensory and/or motor dysfunction (depressed or absent tendon reflexes) in the territory of more than one cervical root or peripheral nerve (i.e., not explicable as single root or nerve lesion).
- Pain may be a feature (striking in neuralgic amyotrophy, tumor infiltration) or may be absent (postirradiation).
- Historical features may suggest etiology:
  - Trauma, for example, caused by motorbike accidents, obstetric trauma, gunshot wounds, carrying heavy rucksack, electrical injury
  - Previous tumor, radiation
  - Drug abuse
  - Individual or family history of previous entrapment neuropathies (HNLPP)

A particularly difficult situation occurs when women previously treated for breast cancer, including radiation therapy of axillary nodes, present with a brachial plexopathy, the differential lying between neoplastic infiltration and postirradiation change. Clues to correct diagnosis include

- Pain: typically absent in postirradiation change; may be major clinical symptom in neoplastic infiltration.
- Lower plexus more likely to be involved in postirradiation change (upper plexus relatively protected by other anatomical structures).
- Neurophysiology: myokymia typical of postirradiation change.

Investigation

Neuroimaging: MRI scanning of the cervical cord and plexus for focal lesions, swelling. Apical views on a chest X-ray, +/– high-resolution CT scan through chest, lung apices, and plexus. Neurophysiology: EMG/NCS is usually critical in distinguishing plexus lesions from cervical radiculopathies if this cannot be done clinically. A reduced sensory action potential implies the lesion is postganglionic and therefore not a *radiculopathy*. The distribution and size of reduction of SAPs and CMAPs helps localize the site of the lesion within the plexus, as does the pattern of denervation on EMG sampling. In particular, denervation in the cervical paraspinal muscles implies a root lesion, since the plexus does not innervate these muscles. Myokymia is seen in postradiation plexopathy and not in neoplastic plexopathies. SSEPs from the upper limb can help localize site of lesion, in terms of plexus versus cervical roots. CSF is usually normal; may be nonspecific elevation of protein. Axon reflex test: scratching the skin with 1% histamine or intradermal injection will normally induce a wheal and vasodilatory response. If there is a postganglionic lesion, this reaction is lost. This test may be used for localization of the level of the lesion by applying it to different dermatomes.

Differential diagnosis

- Cervical radiculopathies
- Multiple mononeuropathies
- *Motor neurone disease*
- Neurogenic thoracic outlet syndrome
- Focal upper limb chronic inflammatory demyelinating polyneuropathy
- Rotator cuff injuries
- Acute poliomyelitis

Treatment and prognosis

Of cause, where identified. Inflammatory lesions may be treated with steroids. Traumatic injury may sometimes be amenable to microsurgical repair.

References

Harris W. The Morphology of the Brachial Plexus. Oxford: Oxford University Press; 1939
Russell JW, Windebank AJ. Brachial and lumbar neuropathies. In: McLeod JG. ed. Inflammatory Neuropathies. London: Baillière Tindall; 1994:173–191

Brain death

Brain death is the permanent cessation of all brain function, both cerebral cortex and brain stem. Brain stem death is the permanent cessation of all brain stem function. Patients are unconscious, apneic, and have lost all brain stem reflexes. These are clinical diagnoses. Because individuals suffering brain or brain stem death are potential donors of organs for transplantation, the necessity to establish such diagnoses definitively has become of increased importance. This remains an area of ethical dispute.

The diagnosis of brain stem death should not normally be considered until at least 6 h have elapsed from the onset of *coma*, or 24 h if coma was secondary to anoxia and/or a cardiac arrest. The diagnosis requires a number of criteria to be fulfilled by two independent medical doctors, one of whom should be a neurologist. It is normally convenient for one to do the testing and the other to witness, or the testing can be done sequentially. Either way, the tests should be repeated after a "short period of time." Respiratory disconnection is usually supervised by an anesthetist and witnessed by the assessors.

The cause of the irreversible brain damage needs to be established, and the reasons why it is irremediable. The time of onset of coma needs to be known.

Clinical features

Criteria vary in different countries.

- Preconditions:
  1. Could primary hypothermia, drugs, or metabolic-endocrine abnormalities be contributing significantly to the apneic coma? (Where appropriate, plasma and urine should be checked for drugs, as well as for plasma pH, glucose, sodium, and calcium.)
  2. Have any neuromuscular blocking drugs been administered during the preceding 12 h?
  3. Is the rectal temperature over 35°C? If not, warm the patient up and reassess.

Only if all the preconditions have been met can the examination be undertaken.

- Examination:

All questions must be answered in the negative for the diagnosis to be made.

1. In some but not all countries, Doll's eye (oculocephalic) movements: is there any contraversive conjugate deviation of the eyes when the head is gently and fully rotated to either side (i.e., doll's eye movements intact)?
2. Do the pupils react to light?
3. Is there any response to corneal stimulation on either side?
4. Do the eyes deviate when either ear is irrigated with 50 mL of ice cold water for 30 s (i.e., oculovestibular reflexes intact)? Check whether the tympanic membranes are intact first.
5. Is there a gag reflex?
6. Is there a cough reflex following bronchial stimulation by a suction catheter?
7. Is there any motor response within the cranial nerve distribution to a painful stimulus?
8. Is there any spontaneous ventilation? If not, then preoxygenate the patient for 10 min with 100% oxygen and record arterial blood gases (ABG). The $PaCO_2$ must exceed 5.3 kPa before disconnection from the ventilator. Disconnect the

patient from the ventilator and give oxygen at 6 L/min via a suction catheter in the trachea and wait for 10 min before repeating the ABG: the $PaCO_2$ must exceed 6.65 kPa at the end of the disconnection period. Is there any spontaneous respiratory movement?

Investigation

As mentioned, this is a clinical diagnosis, but it would be unusual to declare brain death in the absence of abnormalities on cranial imaging. It has been suggested that investigations such as the EEG, transcranial Doppler ultrasonography, or brain SPECT or PET imaging might be helpful in establishing the diagnosis, but these have not been incorporated in accepted diagnostic criteria in the UK.

Differential diagnosis

- Possibly reversible brain dysfunction, as a consequence of drug/toxin ingestion or hypothermia, must be considered.
- *Locked-in syndrome.*

Treatment and prognosis

The diagnosis implies that there is no hope of recovery.

References

Academy of Medical Royal Colleges. A Code of Practice for the Diagnosis and Confirmation of Death. London: Academy of Medical Royal Colleges; 2008

Heran MK, Heran NS, Shemie SD. A review of ancillary tests in evaluating brain death. Can J Neurol Sci. 2008;35:409–419

O'Brien MD. Criteria for diagnosing brain stem death. BMJ. 1990;301:108–109

Pallis C, Harley DH. ABC of Brainstem Death. 2nd ed. London: BMJ; 1996

The Quality Standards Subcommittee of the American Academy of Neurology. Practice parameters for determining brain death in adults (summary statement). Neurology. 1995;45:1012–1014

Brain stem vascular syndromes: overview

Numerous eponymous brain stem vascular syndromes have been described, characterized on the basis of the particular combination of neurological signs, and encompassing cranial nerve palsies, cerebellar signs, and long tract signs.

However, such splitting is not helpful in management as this depends on etiology (these syndromes may occur with pathologies other than cerebro-vascular disease), irrespective of the precise clinical picture.

Brain stem vascular syndromes include:

Midbrain: these often result from occlusion of a penetrating branch of the posterior cerebral artery to the midbrain, less commonly to basilar artery involvement.

- Weber's syndrome: ipsilateral oculomotor (fascicular) nerve palsy with pupil involvement (parasympathetic fibers); and contralateral hemiplegia including the face, due to involvement of corticospinal and corticobulbar fibers in the cerebral peduncle
- Benedikt's syndrome: ipsilateral oculomotor nerve palsy and contralateral involuntary movements (tremor, chorea, athetosis, due to red nucleus involvement), +/− contralateral hemiparesis
- Chiray–Foix–Nicolesco syndrome: almost identical to Benedikt's syndrome, but with additional contralateral sensory disturbances
- Claude's syndrome: ipsilateral oculomotor nerve palsy and contralateral cerebellar ataxia, asynergy, dysdiadochokinesis, due to a lesion in the region of the brachium conjunctivum
- Nothnagel's syndrome (ophthalmoplegia-ataxia syndrome): ipsilateral oculomotor nerve palsy and contralateral cerebellar ataxia +/− trochlear nerve palsy, +/− sensory loss, +/− nystagmus
- *Top of the basilar syndrome* (rostral basilar artery syndrome): visual, oculomotor, and behavioral features without prominent motor or sensory features

Pons:

- Millard–Gubler syndrome: ipsilateral lateral rectus (VI) and facial (lower motor neurone VII) palsies, with contralateral hemiplegia sparing the face
- Raymond syndrome (alternating abducens hemiplegia): lateral rectus paralysis (involvement of abducens [VI] cranial nerve fascicles), with contralateral hemiplegia sparing the face (pyramidal tract involvement), due to a ventral medial pontine lesion
- Raymond–Céstan syndrome: ipsilateral cerebellar ataxia, contralateral hypoesthesia to all modalities (medial lemniscus and spinothalamic tract involvement), +/− contralateral hemiparesis (ventral extension involving corticospinal tract), due to a rostral lesion of the dorsal pons
- Foville syndrome: ipsilateral gaze paresis (looking away from the lesion), ipsilateral lower motor neurone VII nerve palsy with contralateral hemiplegia, due to dorsolateral pontine involvement usually from infarction in the territory of the anterior inferior cerebellar artery
- Marie–Foix syndrome: ipsilateral cerebellar ataxia, contralateral hemiparesis, +/− contralateral hypoesthesia (pain and temperature)
- *Gasperini syndrome*: ipsilateral VI and VII

- *Locked-in syndrome* (de-efferented state): with bilateral ventral pontine lesions

Medulla: often associated with vertebral artery occlusion/dissection

- Déjerine's anterior bulbar syndrome (medial medullary syndrome): ipsilateral tongue paresis with atrophy and fibrillation (hypoglossal (XII) nerve involvement), contralateral hemiparesis sparing the face (due to involvement of the pyramid), contralateral hemisensory loss for position and vibration sensation (involvement of the medial lemniscus) +/− neuro-ophthalmological signs: upbeat nystagmus. Medial medullary infarcts classified by MRI appearances may sometimes be associated with pure hemiparesis ("incomplete syndrome"). Bilateral medial medullary infarction causes quadriparesis, bilateral sensory loss, dysphagia, dysarthria, and dysphonia. Medial and lateral medullary infarction produce the hemimedullary syndrome of Babinski–Nageotte.
- Wallenberg's syndrome (lateral medullary syndrome): ipsilateral facial hypoesthesia for pain and temperature (trigeminal spinal nucleus and tract involvement); nausea, vomiting, vertigo, oscillopsia (vestibular nuclei); ipsilateral Horner's syndrome +/− ipsilateral hypohidrosis of the body (descending sympathetic tract involvement); contralateral hypoalgesia, thermoanesthesia (spinothalamic tract involvement); ipsilateral ataxia of limbs (involvement of olivocerebellar/spinocerebellar fibers, inferior cerebellum); palatal, pharyngeal, and vocal cord paralysis leading to dysphagia, dysphonia, impaired gag reflex; +/− eye movement disorders, including nystagmus, abnormalities of ocular alignment (skew deviation, ocular tilt reaction, environmental tilt), smooth pursuit and gaze holding, and saccades; +/− hiccup; +/− tinnitus, hearing loss, facial weakness. This clinical syndrome may also occur in association with demyelination, neoplasm, hematoma, and trauma.
- Céstan syndrome (Céstan–Chenais syndrome, medial medullary tegmentum syndrome): ipsilateral vocal cord and palatal paralysis, ipsilateral Horner's syndrome, contralateral hemiplegia, contralateral hemianesthesia for proprioception and discriminative touch (medial lemniscus involvement) with sparing of pain and temperature (spinothalamic) sensation. This syndrome may be characterized as equivalent to Wallenberg's lateral medullary syndrome without the ipsilateral ataxia, but with additional contralateral hemiparesis, and hence, a rare variant of lateral medullary syndrome ("Wallenberg plus").
- Avellis syndrome (palatopharyngeal paralysis of Avellis): soft palate and vocal cord paralysis with contralateral hemianesthesia for pain and temperature, with or without a Horner's syndrome, with spared laryngeal function (lesion involves tegmentum of the medulla with the Xth cranial nerve, cephalad portion of nucleus ambiguus, the spinothalamic tract, and sometimes descending pupillary sympathetic fibers).

- Babinski–Nageotte syndrome (hemibulbar syndrome, medullary tegmental paralysis): contralateral hemiplegia and sensory loss in the limbs and trunk, ipsilateral hemiataxia and facial sensory loss, dysarthria, dysphonia, and dysphagia but no tongue (XII) involvement (cf. medial mdullary syndrome), = variant of lateral medullary syndrome with additional contralateral hemiparesis ("Wallenberg plus").
- Reinhold's syndrome, hemimedullary syndrome = lateral + medial medullary syndrome.
- Opalski's (submedullary) syndrome: lateral medullary (Wallenberg) syndrome with ipsilateral hemiplegia: lesion below the decussation of the pyramids (cf. Babinski–Nageotte syndrome).

References

Bogousslavsky J, Maeder P, Regli F, Meuli R. Pure midbrain infarction: clinical syndromes, MRI, and etiologic patterns. Neurology. 1994;44:2032–2040

De Freitas GR, Moll J, Araujo AQC. The Babinski-Nageotte syndrome. Neurology. 2001;56:1604

Gan R, Noronha A. The medullary vascular syndromes revisited. J Neurol. 1995;242: 195–202

Krasnianski M, Neudecker S, Schluter A, Zierz S. Babinski-Nageotte syndrome and hemimedullary (Reinhold's) syndrome are clinically and morphologically distinct conditions. J Neurol. 2003;250:938–942

Kumral E, Afsar N, Kirbas D, Balkir K, Özdemirkiran T. Spectrum of medial medullary infarction: clinical and magnetic resonance findings. J Neurol. 2002;249:85–93

Liu GT, Crenner CW, Logigian EL, et al. Midbrain syndromes of Benedikt, Claude and Nothnagel: setting the record straight. Neurology. 1992;42:1820–1822

Montaner J, Alvarez-Sabín J. Opalski's syndrome. J Neurol Neurosurg Psychiatry. 1999;67:688–689

Sacco RL, Freddo L, Bello JA, Odel JG, Onesti ST, Mohr JP. Wallenberg's lateral medullary syndrome. Clinical-magnetic resonance imaging correlations. Arch Neurol. 1993;50:609–614

Silverman IE, Lui GT, Galetta SL. The crossed paralyses. The original brain-stem syndromes of Millard-Gubler, Foville, Weber and Raymond-Cestan. Arch Neurol. 1995;52:635–638

Takizawa S, Shinohara Y. Magnetic resonance imaging in Avellis' syndrome. J Neurol Neurosurg Psychiatry. 1996;61:17

Brody disease [OMIM#601003]

Brody disease is a rare disorder of childhood characterized by poor relaxation of muscles after exercise, initially in the limbs, then in the face and trunk. Mild muscle atrophy and weakness may develop. Despite the clinical resemblance to myotonia, EMG shows no myotonic discharges; hence, this is a pseudomyotonia syndrome. It results from abnormalities of the fast-twitch skeletal muscle sarcoplasmic reticulum Ca²⁺ ATPase, and some cases with recessive inheritance have mutations in the ATP2A1 gene encoding the sarcoplasmic/endoplasmic reticulum Ca²⁺ ATPase (SERCA1) protein.

References

Odermatt A, Taschner PE, Scherer SW, et al. Mutations in the gene encoding SERCA1, the fast-twitch skeletal muscle sarcoplasmic reticulum Ca²⁺ ATPase, are associated with Brody disease. *Nat Genet.* 1996;14:191–194
Vattemi G, Gualandi F, Oosterhof A, et al. Brody disease: insights into biochemical features of SERCA1 and identification of a novel mutation. *J Neuropathol Exp Neurol.* 2010;69:246–252

Brown's syndrome

Superior oblique tendon sheath syndrome

Brown's syndrome is restriction of active and passive elevation of the eye in adduction (i.e., compromised superior oblique muscle action), resulting in intermittent vertical diplopia. There may be an associated pulling sensation or clicking noise in the orbit; there may be focal pain at the corner of the orbit. This is due to a restriction of free movement through the trochlea pulley mechanism. The condition may be congenital or acquired, the recognized causes including trauma and inflammation (e.g., collagen vascular diseases such as *Sjögren's syndrome*). The previous name of "superior oblique tendon sheath syndrome" is not justified, since surgery to the sheath seldom produced clinical benefit. Spontaneous resolution may occur or treatment of the underlying cause (e.g., inflammation) may be required. Superior oblique tenotomy with or without ipsilateral inferior oblique recession may be appropriate in congenital cases.

Reference

Wilson ME, Eustis HS, Parks MM. Brown's syndrome. *Surv Ophthalmol.* 1989;34:153–172

Brown–Vialetto–van Laere syndrome

Pontobulbar palsy with deafness

This is a rare, fatal, brain stem degeneration occurring in childhood, with early and prominent sensorineural hearing deficit. There is involvement of all muscles supplied by cranial nerves below the fifth (bulbar *spinal muscular atrophy*). Spinal motor neurones and the pyramidal tract may also be affected. The condition is probably recessive.

Reference

Sathasivam S. Brown-Vialetto-Van Laere syndrome. Orphanet J Rare Dis. 2008;3:9

Burning mouth syndrome

Glossodynia, Glossopyrosis

Burning mouth syndrome is a sensation of oral burning, pain of the tongue and mucosa, usually bilateral, and of unknown etiology. There is no associated erythema, tongue weakness, or alterations in taste. There may also be jaw pain, taste changes, painful teeth, headache, and neck and shoulder pain. There is an association with anxiety and depression. It is more common in women, and in the middle-aged and elderly. Systemic and local features that might cause oral pain, such as vitamin B_{12} deficiency, sicca syndrome, ill-fitting dentures, and oral candidiasis should be excluded. The pain is thought to be neuropathic and may respond to medications effective for neuropathic pain, such as topical capsaicin, antidepressants, gabapentin.

Reference

Grushka M, Ching V, Epstein J. Burning mouth syndrome. In: Hummel T, Welge-Lussen A, eds. Taste and Smell. An Update. Basel, Switzerland: Karger; 2006:278–287

C

CADASIL

Cerebral autosomal dominant arteriopathy with subcortical infarcts and leukoencephalopathy, Chronic familial vascular encephalopathy, Hereditary multi-infarct dementia

Cerebral autosomal dominant arteriopathy with subcortical infarcts and leukoencephalopathy (CADASIL) is a genetic vasculopathy resulting from mutations within the gene encoding the notch3 protein. The mechanisms by which mutations lead to disease are not currently understood. An autosomal recessive variant (CARASIL) has also been described, often associated with alopecia and degenerative disease in the lumbar spine and knees.

Clinical features

- Ischemic stroke, often recurrent, subcortical (*lacunar syndromes*).
- Migraine with aura: often adult onset.
- Psychiatric disturbance: apathy, mood disorder.
- Dementia, of "subcortical" type (late).
- Pseudobulbar palsy (late).
- Acute encephalopathy: "CADASIL coma"; self-limiting, may be recurrent.
- There is marked variability in disease course and phenotype.
- Family history: there may be family members with "multiple sclerosis" or "Alzhemier's," which may represent incorrectly diagnosed CADASIL.

Investigation

Neuroimaging (MRI) shows confluent high signal in periventricular and deep white matter, plus focal areas of lacunar infarction and basal ganglia lesions. Anterior temporal pole and external capsule high signal lesions may point to diagnosis. Skin biopsy shows granular osmiophilic material, an abnormal protein deposit, adjacent to basement membrane of smooth muscle cells of arterioles in the dermis; this is highly specific but sensitivity may be only around 50%. Neurogenetic testing shows *notch3* mutations, especially in exons 3, 4, 11, 19. Brain biopsy has largely been superseded by neurogenetic testing and skin biopsy.

Differential diagnosis

Other causes of vascular dementia, although risk factors for stroke are often absent in CADASIL.

Treatment and prognosis

No specific treatment currently known. Aspirin or other antiplatelet agents may be used; the place of warfarin remains uncertain. Acetazolamide has been reported of benefit for migraine. Although there is evidence of a cholinergic deficit in CADASIL brain, a trial of cholinesterase inhibitor for the dementia of CADASIL was negative.

References

Chabriat H, Joutal A, Dichgans M, Tournier-Lasserve E, Bousser MG. CADASIL. Lancet Neurol. 2009;8:643–653

Schon F, Martin RJ, Prevett M, Clough C, Enevoldson TP, Markus HS. "CADASIL coma": an underdiagnosed acute encephalopathy. J Neurol Neurosurg Psychiatry. 2003;74:249–252

Valenti R, Poggesi A, Pescini F, Inzitari D, Pantoni L. Psychiatric disturbances in CADASIL: a brief review. Acta Neurol Scand. 2008;118:291–295

Caisson disease

Decompression sickness

Caisson disease or decompression sickness results from too rapid an ascent from a deep underwater dive, leading to the production of nitrogen bubbles within the circulation ("the bends"). These primarily affect the spinal vessels (especially posteriorly), characteristically in the upper thoracic region, producing myelopathic symptoms. Occasionally, cerebral involvement is seen. Treatment is immediate hyperbaric oxygen therapy.

References

Dick AP, Massey EW. Neurological presentations of decompression sickness and air embolism in sport divers. Neurology. 1985;35:667–671

Hallenbeck JM, Bove AA, Elliott DH. Mechanisms underlying spinal cord damage in decompression sickness. Neurology. 1975;25:308–316

Camptocormia

Bent spine syndrome, Souques disease

Camptocormia is abnormal flexion of the trunk and neck that appears when standing or walking and disappears in the supine position. It was first described as a "war neurosis": it was believed to be a psychiatric disorder occurring in men facing armed conflict. Subsequently, it has been realized that reducible lumbar kyphosis may also result from neurological disorders, including muscle disease (paravertebral myopathy, *nemaline myopathy*), *Parkinson's disease*, *dystonia*, and, possibly, as a paraneoplastic phenomenon. Cases with associated lenticular (putaminal) lesions have also been described. Camptocormia may be related in some instances to *dropped head syndrome*. Treatment in PD with botulinum toxin has been reported, and also sometimes with surgery.

References

Jankovic J. Camptocormia, head drop and other bent spine syndromes: heterogeneous etiology and pathogenesis of parkinsonian deformities. Mov Disord. 2010;25:527–528

Tiple D, Fabbrini G, Colosimo C, et al. Camptocormia in Parkinson disease: an epidemiological and clinical study. J Neurol Neurosurg Psychiatry. 2009;80:145–148

Umapathi T, Chaudhry V, Cornblath D, et al. Head drop and camptocormia. J Neurol Neurosurg Psychiatry. 2002;72:1–7

Camptodactyly

Isolated crooked little fingers, Streblomicrodactyly

Camptodactyly ("bent finger") is angulation at the proximal interphalangeal joint of the little finger, either as part of a dysmorphic syndrome or in isolation, the latter either as a sporadic or a familial condition. Inheritance in the latter is probably autosomal dominant with variable penetrance. It is seen incidentally in neurological outpatients more frequently than *ulnar neuropathy* with which it may be confused.

Clinical features

- Nontraumatic, painless, flexion deformity at the proximal interphalangeal joint of the little finger. Other fingers, and occasionally toes (especially the second), may also be affected.
- No sensory or motor signs (cf. ulnar neuropathy).
- A noninflammatory arthropathy may coexist with the flexion deformity.

Investigation

None required.

Differential diagnosis

- Trauma to little finger
- Ulnar neuropathy causing claw hand (*main en griffe*)
- Dupuytren's contracture
- Scleroderma
- Focal dystonia or neuromyotonia
- Diabetic cheiroarthropathy

Treatment and prognosis

Various surgical approaches have been suggested, but there are no trial data. There is little functional compromise as a result of the deformity, which is nonprogressive.

Reference

Larner AJ. Camptodactyly in a neurology outpatient clinic. Int J Clin Pract. 2001;55: 592–595

Candidiasis

Moniliasis

Systemic infection with the fungus *Candida* may occur in the context of immunosuppression (including diabetes mellitus), burns, and total parenteral nutrition, affecting the brain as microabscesses, noncaseating granulomata, meningitis, meningoencephalitis, and ependymitis. CSF shows pleocytosis but the organism is rarely identified by culture; extraneural sites (blood, urine, skin) are usually more helpful. Systemic infection carries a grave prognosis, even with intravenous amphotericin treatment.

CANOMAD

CANOMAD is a rare sensory neuropathy; the name is an acronym denoting the key features, *viz.*:

- *C*hronic *a*taxic *n*europathy
- *O*phthalmoplegia

- Ig*M* paraprotein
- Cold *a*gglutinins
- *D*isialosyl antibodies

Clinically there is a chronic neuropathy causing sensory ataxia and areflexia, but with preserved motor function in the limbs. Ocular and bulbar weakness may be fixed or relapsing–remitting. EMG/NCS and nerve biopsy reveal both axonal and demyelinating features. The anti-disialosyl antibodies react with an epitope common to the gangliosides GD1b, GD3, GT1b, and GQ1b. It may be considered a persistent form of the acute *Miller Fisher syndrome*. A partial response to IVIg or rituximab may be observed.

Reference

Willison HJ, O'Leary CP, Veitch J, et al. The clinical and laboratory features of chronic sensory ataxic neuropathy with anti-disialosyl IgM antibodies. Brain. 2001; 124:1968–1977

Capsular warning syndrome

Donnan syndrome

The capsular warning syndrome is a syndrome characterized by a cluster of stereotyped *transient ischemic attacks* (TIAs), typically causing weakness of the whole of one side of the body without cognitive or language deficit (hence, a pure motor lacunar TIA), followed within hours to days usually by a lacunar infarct of the internal capsule, but sometimes associated with pontine lesions. The syndrome is presumed to reflect intermittent and then complete closure of a single lenticulostriate or other perforating artery. As in other *lacunar syndromes*, a proximal arterial or cardiac cause is unlikely.

Reference

Donnan GA, O'Malley HM, Quang L, Hurley S, Bladin PF. The capsular warning syndrome: pathogenesis and clinical features. Neurology. 1993;43:957–962

Carbon monoxide poisoning

The neurotoxic effects of carbon monoxide (CO) were first investigated by Claude Bernard in the nineteenth century. Acute CO poisoning causes depression of CNS function which may be fatal. Various symptoms may occur, including headache, dizziness, weakness, nausea, impaired concentration, shortness of breath, and visual changes; loss of consciousness is unusual.

The diagnosis may be established by measuring carboxyhemoglobin level in venous blood. Treatment is by removal of the patient from the CO source, and administration of normobaric or hyperbaric oxygen until the carboxyhemoglobin level returns to normal.

Some patients with carbon monoxide poisoning develop a delayed encephalopathy with motor and/or cognitive deficits, a few days to weeks after recovering from the acute poisoning, or without history of acute poisoning. Motor features are usually extrapyramidal and dystonic, including a progressive akinetic-mute syndrome or a delayed *parkinsonian syndrome*, although pyramidal signs may be seen. There may be additional personality changes (sometimes psychosis), and cognitive deficits such as impaired executive function, slowed mental processing, and impaired visuospatial function; deficits may be very focal (e.g., visual agnosia). MR imaging may show white matter changes in periventricular or centrum semiovale, although these are less common in unselected patients than cognitive sequelae; MR changes may also be seen in caudate nucleus, globus pallidus, cerebellum, or hippocampus.

Chronic exposure to low-level carbon monoxide, such as occurs with faulty gas appliances, may cause a syndrome of headache and cognitive symptoms.

Patients typically improve with time, but may be left with permanent neurological and/or neuropsychological sequelae.

References

Ernst A, Zibrak JD. Carbon monoxide poisoning. N Engl J Med. 1998;339:1603–1608
Larner AJ. Delayed motor and visual complications after attempted suicide. Lancet. 2005;366:1826
Parkinson RB, Hopkins RO, Cleavinger HB, et al. White matter hyperintensities and neuropsychological outcome following carbon monoxide poisoning. Neurology. 2002;58:1525–1532
Weaver LK, Hopkins RO, Chan KJ, et al. Hyperbaric oxygen for acute carbon monoxide poisoning. N Engl J Med. 2002;347:1057–1067

Carnitine palmit(o)yltransferase (CPT) deficiency

DiMauro syndrome

Carnitine palmit(o)yltransferase (CPT) is an enzyme involved in the transport of fatty acid across the mitochondrial membrane: from outside to inside (CPT I) and unhooking carnitine once the complex is inside (CPT II), hence one of the *fatty acid oxidation disorders (FAOD)*. Two types of deficiency are recognized; both are defects of acylcarnitine synthesis-translocation. CPT II deficiency is the more commonly encountered.

Clinical features

- Type I (CPT I): presents in neonatal period with hepatomegaly and severe hepatocellular dysfunction (hypoglycemia), encephalopathy, hyperammonemia, metabolic acidosis, and hypotonia.
- Type II (CPT II): may present in neonatal period as for CPT I; also presents in young adults with a history of episodic muscle stiffness, pain, tenderness, and weakness, induced by exercise, cold, fasting, or intercurrent infection. Accompanying myoglobinuria may precipitate acute renal failure. No "second wind phenomenon" (cf. *McArdle's disease*). A chronic myopathy is also described.

Investigation

Type I: plasma carnitine concentration often elevated, acylcarnitines unremarkable; CPT I deficiency demonstrated in fibroblasts or white cells.
Type II (CPT II): Bloods: plasma carnitine concentration elevated; creatine kinase elevated during attacks; raised triglycerides. Muscle biopsy: lipid accumulation (not all cases). CPT II deficiency demonstrated in fibroblasts or white cells. Neurogenetics: mutations in CPT II gene have been identified.

Differential diagnosis

- Type I: carnitine deficiency
- Type II (CPT II): glutaric aciduria type II (GAII); McArdle's disease (myophosphorylase deficiency)

Treatment and prognosis

Neonatal: protective therapy: avoid fasting, frequent feeding to avoid mobilizing fatty acids; dietary supplementation with medium chain triglycerides. Adult CPT II: avoid strenuous exercise, avoid muscle pain, or exercise when fasted. In cases of *rhabdomyolysis*, forced alkaline diuresis may be helpful.

References

DiMauro S, Melis-DiMauro PM. Muscle carnitine palmityltransferase deficiency and myoglobinuria. Science. 1973;182:929–931
Hug G, Bove KE, Soukup S. Lethal neonatal multiorgan deficiency of carnitine palmitoyltransferase II. N Engl J Med. 1991;325:1862–1864

Carotid artery disease: overview

The carotid artery is vulnerable to occlusive (stenotic) atheromatous disease, particularly at the bifurcation of the common carotid artery and in the proximal internal carotid artery, which may lead to embolic cerebrovascular disease. The extent of narrowing and the presence or absence of symptomatic consequences are the most important determinants of treatment. Carotid artery *dissection*, usually following trauma, is also a cause of embolic disease. Aneurysmal disease and fistula formation are less common diseases of the carotid arteries.

Clinical features

- Stenosis, asymptomatic: mild narrowing is common in the elderly, associated with hypertension, hypercholesterolemia; a bruit may be present due to turbulent flow but is not an indication for investigation/treatment per se.
- Stenosis, symptomatic: may be associated with *transient ischemic attacks* (*TIA*), either ocular or hemispheric, from emboli breaking off the ulcerated surface of atheromatous plaque, or, less commonly, hemodynamic (e.g., *limb shaking* attacks); total occlusion in childhood may lead to collateral vessel formation at the base of the brain with resultant risk of cerebral hemorrhage (*moyamoya*). Cognitive disorder as a consequence of occlusive disease is also possible.
- Dissection: unilateral facial pain, often periorbital, +/– Horner's syndrome +/– hemispheric infarct with "stuttering" onset +/– lower cranial nerve palsies. May be history of trauma to neck; other associations of carotid dissection include *fibromuscular dysplasia, Ehlers–Danlos syndrome* (type IV), *Marfan's syndrome, pseudoxanthoma elasticum.*
- Aneurysm: trauma, surgery, irradiation, fibromuscular dysplasia, may lead to internal carotid artery aneurysm formation, which may be a source of brain embolism; intracranial aneurysms more likely to rupture and bleed (subarachnoid hemorrhage).
- Fistula: in neck, may follow trauma, especially penetrating (e.g., gunshot, stabbing); in cavernous sinus either spontaneously or following trauma, as a *carotid-cavernous fistula* (*CCF*).

Investigation

- Imaging of carotid artery: options are Doppler ultrasound, magnetic resonance angiography, CT angiography, and catheter angiography. First two are usually adequate for detecting accurately the degree of stenosis; catheter angiography has higher morbidity.
- Specific investigations for possible underlying vasculopathy (fibromuscular dysplasia, Ehlers–Danlos syndrome) may be required.
- Risk factors for atherosclerosis.

Differential diagnosis

Stenosis, symptomatic: consider emboli from other sources, for example, cardiac, aortic arch. Also encompasses differential diagnosis of TIA, for example, migraine.

Treatment and prognosis

- Stenosis, asymptomatic: mainstay of management has been no specific treatment, but control of modifiable risk factors (hypertension, hypercholesterolemia, smoking); results from the Asymptomatic Carotid Surgery Trial suggest that early surgery is associated with a reduced risk of subsequent stroke and death, provided cardiovascular status is sufficiently good (major cause of postoperative deaths).
- Stenosis, symptomatic: if stenosis <70%, antiplatelet agents recommended (aspirin, dipyridamole, clopidogrel, ticlopidine); if TIAs continue despite these, formal anticoagulation with warfarin may be considered. Stenosis >70% probably merits carotid endarterectomy, but decision must also take into account cardiovascular status (most common cause of morbidity and mortality). Stenting is associated with a higher restenosis rate than surgery. Control of vascular risk factors.
- Dissection: anticoagulation with warfarin usually recommended (notwithstanding the current absence of randomized controlled trials).
- Aneurysm: if a source of embolism, may require medical/surgical intervention.

References

Halliday A, Mansfield A, Marro J, et al. Prevention of disabling and fatal strokes by successful carotid endarterectomy in patients without recent neurological symptoms: randomised controlled trial. Lancet. 2004;363:1491-1502 [Erratum: Lancet 2004;364: 416]
Rothwell PM. Endarterectomy for symptomatic and asymptomatic carotid stenosis. Neurol Clin. 2008;26:1079–1097

Carotid-cavernous fistula (CCF)

This common type of *dural arteriovenous fistula* links the internal carotid artery with a portion of the cavernous sinus. They may occur spontaneously (especially in postmenopausal women) or following trauma, rupture of an intracavernous carotid aneurysm, or in association with connective tissue disorders such as *Ehlers–Danlos syndrome*. Classification may be into direct (high-flow) or indirect (low-flow) types, although more sophisticated classification schemes exist (e.g., Barrow).

Clinical features

- Injected sclera, chemosis, proptosis (may be pulsatile)
- Ophthalmoplegia, diplopia
- Pain
- Ocular bruit
- +/– Visual loss

Investigation

Brain imaging may show a mass in the cavernous sinus. The shunt may be visualized by transcranial Doppler ultrasonography, but to define the anatomy precisely, and as a possible prelude to treatment, catheter angiography is required.

Differential diagnosis

Other causes of painful ophthalmoplegia.

Treatment and prognosis

Embolization via a catheter may be possible, dependent upon the precise anatomy. Occlusion by intermittent pressure on the carotid artery is also an option. Carotid-cavernous fistulae rarely cause *subarachnoid hemorrhage* when they occur spontaneously; those due to trauma are more likely to cause intracerebral bleeding. A significant number of carotid-cavernous fistulae thrombose spontaneously. All treatments are designed to prevent progression and hemorrhage, and will do nothing for the physical appearance of the proptosed eye.

Reference

Barrow DL, Spector RH, Braun IF, et al. Classification and treatment of spontaneous carotid-cavernous sinus fistulas. J Neurosurg. 1985;62:248–256

Carpal tunnel syndrome (CTS)

Putnam's acroparesthesia

Compression of the median nerve in the carpal tunnel by the transverse carpal ligament (flexor retinaculum) is probably the most common *entrapment neuropathy*, commoner in women, often between the ages of 40–60 years. Although a number of clinical tests have been described for carpal tunnel syndrome (CTS), electrophysiological testing is still the gold standard for diagnosis.

Recognized associations include

- Rheumatoid arthritis
- Acromegaly
- Hypothyroidism
- Uremia, dialysis
- Amyloidosis
- Pregnancy
- *Hereditary neuropathy with liability to pressure palsies*

Most instances occur in otherwise healthy people.

Clinical features

- Pain: classically involving the thumb, index, middle, and radial half of ring finger, but on occasion reported to involve all digits; may extend to the whole hand and, in some cases, also up the forearm, occasionally even to the shoulder. Often causes nocturnal waking, when patients may shake or "flick" their hands ("to get the circulation going again") or get up and walk about to relieve symptoms.
- Sensory disturbance: hypoesthesia generally confined to median nerve distribution in the hand, but anomalous findings may be encountered.
- Motor wasting and/or weakness affecting the median innervated muscles of the thenar eminence may occur.
- Symptoms often bilateral.

A number of clinical tests have been described which aim to provoke the typical symptoms of tingling (Tinel's "sign of formication") in the cutaneous distribution of the damaged nerve ("peripheral reference"). These include:

- Tinel's sign: tapping over transverse carpal ligament, for example, with a tendon hammer (sensitivity 60–67%; specificity 59–77%)
- Phalen's sign: prolonged forced wrist flexion (as in carrying heavy shopping bags)
- Carpal tunnel compression test: application of moderate pressure over the transverse carpal ligament (sensitivity 52.5%; specificity 61.8%)
- Pressure provocative test: pressure cuff + direct median nerve pressure (sensitivity 54.5%; specificity 68.4%)
- "Flick test": clinical history of relieving symptoms by flicking or shaking hands (occurs with same frequency in cases with and without EMG confirmation)

Investigation

Bloods: thyroid function tests, rheumatoid factor, may be assayed if clinical features suggest relevant underlying diagnosis. Neurophysiology (EMG/ NCS) is the gold standard for the diagnosis of carpal tunnel syndrome: decreased amplitude and prolonged median motor and sensory latencies; EMG shows denervation abnormalities in advanced cases.

Differential diagnosis

Sensory polyneuropathy, radiculopathy, hyperventilation.

Treatment and prognosis

There are a number of options, including splinting of the wrist, analgesia, steroid injections, hand therapy, ultrasound, and surgical decompression. A recent randomized controlled trial has suggested that surgery is the more efficacious in terms of overall outcome than hand therapy and ultrasound, but patients in both groups improved.

References

Hi ACF, Wong S, Griffith J. Carpal tunnel syndrome. Pract Neurol. 2005;5:210–217
Jarvik JG, Comstock BA, Kliot M, et al. Surgery versus non-surgical therapy for carpal tunnel syndrome: a randomised parallel-group trial. Lancet. 2009;374:1074–1081
Rosenbaum RB, Ochoa JL. Carpal Tunnel Syndrome and Other Disorders of the Median Nerve. 2nd ed. Boston, MA: Butterworth-Heinemann; 2002

Cauda equina syndrome and conus medullaris syndrome: overview

The conus medullaris is the most distal part of the spinal cord, adjacent to the vertebral body of L1 in most adults, and the cauda equina ("the horse's tail") is the sheaf of nerve roots which lies below it, the roots running distally to the intervertebral foramina of the lower lumbar, sacral, and coccygeal vertebrae. Local pathology may involve both structures or, less likely, affect them individually. Although this anatomical distinction may be attempted on clinical grounds, it is often difficult and of little practical value.

Recognized causes of cauda equina and conus medullaris syndromes include

- Central disc herniation. If acute, this is a neurosurgical emergency.
- Tumor: primary (e.g., ependymoma, meningioma, schwannoma); metastasis.
- Hematoma.

- Abscess.
- Lumbosacral fractures.
- Inflammation (e.g., cauda equina syndrome in *neurosarcoidosis*; rare).
- *Ankylosing spondylitis* (cauda equina syndrome in association with dorsal arachnoid diverticula: rare).

Clinical features

- Motor:
  - Wasting: glutei, posterior thigh, anterolateral leg and foot muscles; more evident in cauda equina lesions
  - Fasciculations: if conus involved
  - Weakness of legs: flaccid paralysis in cauda equina syndrome; hip flexor weakness said to be relatively specific for conus lesion
  - Reflex loss or diminution, especially ankle jerk
- Sensory:
  - Pain: lumbar region, thighs, buttocks, perineum, legs (may be symmetric or asymmetric); may be worse in recumbent position and increased by Valsalva maneuver
  - Sensory loss: so-called saddle anesthesia (sacral dermatomes), dorsal aspect of thigh; more asymmetric in cauda equina syndromes. Sensory deficits may extend to trunk in conus lesion, and position sense may be affected (cf. cauda equina syndrome).
- Sphincter:
  - Sphincter disturbance: incomplete: impaired initiation of micturition, loss of bladder sensation; complete: retention/overflow; bladder symptoms said to occur earlier in conus lesions; constipation
  - Impotence: impaired erection, ejaculation

Disease confined to the conus medullaris is said to produce early sphincter involvement, late pain, and symmetrical sensory involvement, whereas pure cauda equina lesions are said to produce early pain, late sphincter involvement, and asymmetric sensory deficits.

Investigation

Imaging: MRI is the modality of choice, for example, for disc disease, tumors, inflammation. Neurophysiology (EMG/NCS) may help to determine whether roots are affected. CSF may show nonspecific raised protein.

Differential diagnosis

Polyneuropathy, multiple radiculopathy, lumbar *spinal stenosis*.

Treatment and prognosis

Dependent on cause; discs, tumors, hematomas, abscesses may be surgically resected or aspirated; inflammatory disease may require steroids; the cauda equina syndrome of ankylosing spondylitis may be stabilized by lumboperitoneal shunting. Recovery is said to be more likely with lesions of the conus than the cauda equina.

References

Gleave JR, Macfarlane R. Cauda equina syndrome: what is the relationship between timing of surgery and outcome? Br J Neurosurg. 2002;16:325–328
Lavy C, James A, Wilson-MacDonald J, Fairbank J. Cauda equina syndrome. BMJ. 2009;338:881–884
Swash M, Katifi HA. The conus medullaris and cauda equina syndromes. J Neurol Neurosurg Psychiatry. 1996;61:216–217

Cavernoma, cavernous hemagioma [OMIM#116860]

Cavernoma, or cavernous hemagioma, is a type of *vascular malformation*, characterized by thin walled vascular spaces, lacking a shunt, and hence not *arteriovenous malformations* (*AVMs*). More often supratentorial than infratentorial, they may be single or multiple ("cavernomatosis"), sporadic or familial. Mutations in three genes have to date been shown to cause cavernous hemangiomas: CCM1 (Krit1 gene on chromosome 7q21-q22); CCM2 (CCM2/malcavernin gene); and CCM3 (PDCD10 gene).

Although cavernomas are readily identified by MR imaging, cerebral angiography is usually negative because of the absence of AV shunting. They may present as space-occupying lesions, with epileptic seizures, or with hemorrhage; sometimes with relapsing–remitting symptoms which may be confused with *multiple sclerosis*, especially if located in the brainstem. Many are asymptomatic and found by chance when the brain is imaged for other reasons.

Treatment is either symptomatic (e.g., antiepileptic medication) with neuroradiological surveillance, or surgical.

References

Moran NF, Fish DR, Kitchen N, Shorvon S, Kendall BE, Stevens JM. Supratentorial cavernous haemangiomas and epilepsy: a review of the literature and case series. J Neurol Neurosurg Psychiatry. 1999;66:561–568
Revencu N, Vikkula M. Cerebral cavernous malformations: new molecular and clinical insights. J Med Genet. 2006;43:716–721

Cavernous sinus disease

Cavernous sinus syndrome

The cavernous sinus lies behind the eye and lateral to the pituitary gland. It contains the internal carotid artery, the nerves that innervate the extraocular muscles, and the first two divisions of the trigeminal nerve. A number of disease processes may affect the cavernous sinus and present with a progressive ophthalmoplegia with or without involvement of the first and second divisions of the trigeminal nerve. A cavernous sinus syndrome may result from

- Granulomatous inflammatory conditions: *neurosarcoidosis*; idiopathic inflammation (so-called *Tolosa–Hunt syndrome*).
- Aneurysms of the internal carotid artery.
- Thrombophlebitis and thrombosis: cavernous sinus thrombosis may be a consequence of sepsis, associated with infections of the orbit, paranasal sinuses and teeth, usually resulting in bilateral signs and symptoms.
- *Carotid-cavernous fistula* (*CCF*).
- Metastatic disease: especially from the nasopharynx.
- Tumor: *meningioma, glioma.*
- *Mucormycosis* (especially in context of diabetes mellitus).

The advent of MRI has greatly improved the visualization of the cavernous sinus and diagnosis of conditions involving it.

Clinical features

- Diplopia: due to involvement of III, IV, or VI cranial nerves; isolated palsies or any combination of nerves can be involved. The sixth cranial nerve lies adjacent to the carotid artery in the cavernous sinus and so an aneurysm may present with an isolated sixth nerve palsy.
- Sensory loss: with a depressed corneal reflex. If the lesion is far back in the cavernous sinus then the second division of the trigeminal nerve can be involved; a lesion in the posterior part of the cavernous sinus may present with a sixth nerve palsy and a Horner's syndrome, as a branch of the sympathetic chain briefly links up with the abducens nerve in the posterior part of the cavernous sinus (= *Parkinson's syndrome*). If the lesion is toward the orbital apex or superior orbital fissure, only the first part of the trigeminal nerve is involved and optic nerve involvement is more likely.
- Proptosis: may occur in any of the conditions involving the cavernous sinus. In the case of carotid-cavernous fistula, the exophthalmos is often pulsatile and associated with an ocular bruit.
- Pain: located retro-orbitally is common, especially with metastatic and granulomatous conditions involving the cavernous sinus.

- Reduced visual acuity: may occur on occasion, due to compression of the optic nerve at the apex of the cavernous sinus, or in the case of carotid-cavernous fistula due to ischemia.
- Chemosis and injected conjunctival vessels: may be found in cases of carotid-cavernous fistula.

In the case of a cavernous sinus thrombosis, the signs may be bilateral and often develop acutely in the context of local infection in the orbit, paranasal sinuses, or teeth. The patient is usually systemically unwell with prominent retro-orbital pain with chemosis, proptosis, orbital congestion with a variable ophthalmoplegia and sensory loss over the forehead. There is often ocular edema or optic nerve compression which can lead to blindness, which may also occur secondary to occlusion of the ophthalmic artery.

Investigation

Bloods may include FBC, ESR, CRP, serum ACE. Imaging may include CXR (?sarcoid; neoplasm), brain MRI +/- gadolinium, CT to ascertain if any bone erosion, MRA or angiogram to localize any aneurysm/fistula. This may need to be repeated as the lesions can sometimes be occult. CSF is usually normal. Other investigations may need to be considered, for example, for sarcoidosis, ENT opinion for exclusion of a nasopharyngeal carcinoma.

Differential diagnosis

- Orbital disease:
  - Thyroid eye disease
  - Orbital pseudotumor (*Tolosa–Hunt syndrome*)
  - Metastatic orbital disease
  - Primary tumors of the eye (e.g., melanoma)
  - Sarcoidosis within the orbit

A similar clinical picture may occur with lesions at the orbital apex or the superior orbital fissure; the term Foix–Jefferson syndrome has been used to describe a combination of III, IV, V, and VI cranial nerve palsies with exophthalmos and eyelid edema associated with tumor, aneurysm, or thrombosis of the cavernous sinus.

Treatment and prognosis

Dependent on cause. Granulomatous disease normally responds dramatically to steroids (e.g., prednisolone initially at a dose of 80 mg/day). Long-term follow-up is recommended and some patients may require long-term treatment with steroids. Tumors, whether primary or secondary, are usually inoperable. The treatment of choice is, therefore, chemo- or radiotherapy. Aneurysms of the carotid artery in the cavernous sinus do not cause subarachnoid hemorrhage. If they are saccular they can be embolized, if fusiform then the only option is occlusion of the ipsilateral carotid artery. Often the treatment of choice is observation.

Reference

Bone I, Hadley DM. Syndromes of the orbital fissure, cavernous sinus, cerebello-pontine angle, and skull base. J Neurol Neurosurg Psychiatry. 2005;76(Suppl III):iii29–iii38

Cayman disease

Cayman cerebellar ataxia

Cayman disease is an autosomal recessive cerebellar ataxia, confined to one area of Grand Cayman in the Cayman Islands, first described in 1978. It is characterized by psychomotor retardation, nonprogressive ataxia, nystagmus, intention tremor, and hypotonia, without retinal changes or optokinetic nystagmus. Linkage to chromosome 19p13.3 was established, leading to the characterization of mutations in a neuronal protein named caytaxin.

References

Bomar JM, Benke PJ, Slattery EL, et al. Mutations in a novel gene encoding a CRAL-TRIO domain cause human Cayman ataxia and ataxia/dystonia in the jittery mouse. Nat Genet. 2003;35:264–269 [Erratum: Nat Genet. 2005;37:555]
Nystuen A, Benke PJ, Merren J, Stone EM, Sheffield VC. A cerebellar ataxia locus identified by DNA pooling to search for linkage disequilibrium in an isolated population from the Cayman Islands. Hum Mol Genet. 1996;5:525–531

Central core disease [OMIM#117000]

This rare autosomal dominant myopathy was the first congenital myopathy to be described. Infants present in the neonatal period with hypotonia, areflexia, delayed motor milestones, proximal limb and facial weakness. Associated features include pes cavus, short stature, kyphoscoliosis, and dislocation of the hips. The condition is usually nonprogressive. Adult presentation with muscle cramps or limb girdle weakness may occur, or the condition may remain asymptomatic. Susceptibility to anesthesia-related *malignant hyperthermia* occurs in one-third of patients. Creatine kinase is usually normal but may be mildly elevated. Neurophysiology shows nonspecific myopathic change. Muscle histology reveals densely packed and disorganized myofibrils ("cores") in the center of most type 1 muscle fibers, seen as central pallor with stains for mitochondrial enzymes. Central core disease may be associated with mutations in the gene (*RYR*1) on chromosome 19q13.1 encoding the ryanodine receptor of the sarcoplasmic membrane; hence, this may be classified as one of the *channelopathies*. The malignant hyperthermia phenotype is also associated with mutations in this gene, and some forms of *multi-minicore disease* are allelic. There is no specific treatment.

References

Jungbluth H, Lillis S, Zhou H, et al. Late-onset axial myopathy with cores due to a novel heterozygous dominant mutation in the skeletal muscle ryanodine receptor (RYR1) gene. Neuromuscul Disord. 2009;19:344–347
Zhang Y, Chen HS, Khanna VK, et al. A mutation in the human ryanodine receptor gene associated with central core disease. Nat Genet. 1993;5:46–50

Central pontine and extrapontine myelinolysis (CPEPM)

Osmotic demyelination syndrome

This disorder is characterized by the destruction, usually symmetrical, of myelin sheaths in the basal pons, sometimes extending beyond the pons (hence "pontine myelinolysis" may be a misnomer). Reported cases are most often, but not exclusively, associated with hyponatremia and its rapid correction with intravenous fluids. Other recognized associations include chronic alcoholism and undernutrition, dehydration associated with vomiting (e.g., pregnancy) and diarrhea, diuretic therapy, postoperative overhydration, compulsive water drinking (dipsomania), organ (especially liver) transplantation, and following severe burns. A feature common to many of these situations is change in plasma osmolality, leading to the notion that CPEPM may represent an "osmotic demyelination syndrome." Why the myelin of the neurones and the white matter tracts of the pons should be particularly susceptible to such changes has not been clearly explained. Neuronal death may be apoptotic.

Clinical features

May affect pyramidal, extrapyramidal, and cerebellar pathways and lower cranial nerves:

- Most commonly presents as a severe quadriparesis.
- Behavioral changes.

- Eye movement disorders.
- Bulbar/pseudobulbar palsy.
- Locked-in syndrome.
- Seizures.
- Coma.
- Delayed onset movement disorders.
- Some cases are asymptomatic being discovered only at autopsy.

Investigation

Bloods: review changes in serum sodium, +/– osmolality. Neuroimaging (MRI) demonstrates signal changes in the pons and elsewhere in the brain stem, cerebellum, basal ganglia, which are indicative of demyelination. Neurophysiology (BSAEP) may demonstrate prolonged latencies consistent with pontine lesions. Pathology shows demyelination, often symmetrical in pons.

Differential diagnosis

Inflammatory demyelination is unlikely to be confused with CPEPM from the context, likewise *brain stem vascular syndromes* secondary to basilar artery occlusion.

Treatment and prognosis

Prevention is the best treatment; hence judicious (= slow) correction of hyponatremia is advisable, although the precise rate remains debatable (ca. 12 mmol/L/day). For those with malnutrition and/or alcoholism, vitamin supplemetation (e.g., thiamine) is appropriate. Once the damage is done, only symptomatic treatment is available.

References

Adams RD, Victor M, Mancall EL. Central pontine myelinolysis: a hitherto undescribed disease occurring in alcoholic and malnourished patients. Arch Neurol Psychiatry. 1959;81:154–172

Ashrafian H, Davey P. A review of the causes of central pontine myelinolysis: yet another apoptotic illness? Eur J Neurol. 2001;8: 103–109

Martin RJ. Central pontine and extrapontine myelinolysis: the osmotic demyelination syndromes. J Neurol Neurosurg Psychiatry. 2004;75 (supplIII):iii22–iii28

Pearce JM. Central pontine myelinolysis. Eur Neurol. 2009;61:59–62

Sterns RH, Riggs JE, Schochet SS. Osmotic demyelination syndrome following correction of hyponatraemia. N Engl J Med. 1986;314:1535–1542

Cerebellar disease: overview

The cerebellum, located in the posterior fossa behind the brain stem and below the tentorial membrane, is part of the motor system. Its organization may best be thought of in terms of three systems:

- Vestibulo- or archeocerebellum: involved in balance and eye movement control
- Spino- or paleocerebellum: primarily involved with the control of axial movement and posture
- Ponto- or neocerebellum: coordinates limb movements
  - Recognized causes of cerebellar syndromes are many, but they may be broadly separated into hereditary and acquired.
- Inherited: of the hereditary degenerative disorders, recessive conditions tend to present early (before age 20 years) whereas late onset (after age 20 years) is more suggestive of an autosomal dominant disorder:

Autosomal dominant:

- Clinically classified as *autosomal dominant cerebellar ataxia (ADCA)* types I, II, and III; now increasingly reclassified on the basis of underlying genetic mutations as *spinocerebellar ataxias (SCA)*
- *Episodic ataxias*: *channelopathies* involving potassium (type 1) and calcium (type 2) channels
- *Huntington's disease (HD)*
- *Dentatorubral-pallidoluysian atrophy (DRPLA)*
- Inherited *prion diseases*, especially *Gerstmann–Sträussler–Scheinker (GSS) disease.*

Autosomal recessive:

- Friedreich's ataxia (FA)
- Ataxia with isolated vitamin E deficiency (AVED)
- Ataxia telangiectasia (AT)
- Ataxia with oculomotor apraxia (AOA)
- Charlevoix–Saguenay syndrome (autosomal recessive spastic ataxia of Charlevoix–Saguenay, ARSACS)
- Refsum's disease
- Other inherited metabolic disorders associated with progressive ataxia:
  - *Abetalipoproteinemia* (Bassen–Kornzweig disease)
  - *Behr's syndrome*
  - *Cerebrotendinous xanthomatosis (CTX)*
  - Cockayne's syndrome
  - GM2 gangliosidosis: adult onset (partial hexosaminidase A deficiency)
  - Gillespie's syndrome
  - Hartnup's disease

- Joubert syndrome
- Marinesco–Sjögren syndrome
- *Mitochondrial disease*
- *Neuronal ceroid lipofuscinoses (NCL)*
- *Niemann–Pick disease* (NPD) type B ("non-neuropathic")
- Paine syndrome
- Pontocerebellar hypoplasia
- Sialidosis
- Sjögren–Larsson syndrome
- *Unverricht–Lundborg disease*
- Urea cycle enzyme defects (UCED)
- *Wilson's disease*
- Xeroderma pigmentosa (XP)

Pathogenetic mechanisms are starting to be defined, including impaired defence from oxidative stress (e.g., FA, AVED, Abetalipoproteinemia), impaired DNA repair (e.g., AT, Cockayne's syndrome, XP), and impaired metabolic homeostasis.

- Acquired:
  - Vascular:
    - Cerebellar infarction: 40% posterior inferior cerebellar artery (PICA) territory; 5% anterior inferior cerebellar artery (AICA) territory; 35% superior cerebellar artery (SCA) territory; and 20% watershed infarcts.
    - Cerebellar hemorrhage: patient may present with an acute cerebellar syndrome +/– *hydrocephalus* secondary to brainstem compression and/or tonsillar herniation. There may also be brainstem signs. Urgent imaging is required; with tonsillar herniation, urgent neurosurgical intervention may be necessary in the form of posterior fossa decompression or shunt.
    - *Superficial siderosis.*
  - Infective:
    - Viral infection: For example, EBV and varicella (especially in children), congenital rubella syndrome.
    - Bacterial: direct spread from middle ear disease or mastoiditis, with possible abscess formation, in which case the patient is usually unwell and toxic with severe headache.
    - Parasitic: *neurocysticercosis.*
    - Prion disease: *Creutzfeldt–Jakob disease* (sporadic, iatrogenic), *kuru.*
  - Inflammatory:
    - *Multiple sclerosis*: often with other signs of disseminated CNS lesions
    - Other CNS inflammatory conditions: especially *Behçet's disease*; *neurosarcoidosis, vasculitis*
    - Miller Fisher variant of Guillain–Barré syndrome
    - *Bickerstaff's brainstem encephalitis*

- Metabolic/Endocrine:
  o Gluten ataxia (with or without gluten-sensitive enteropathy = *coeliac disease*)
  o Vitamin E deficiency (isolated deficiency, acquired with gastrointestinal disease)
  o *Wernicke–Korsakoff syndrome*
  o Hypothyroidism (rare)
- Neoplasia:
  o Primary CNS tumor: including hemangioblastoma, medulloblastoma, glioma, ependymoma, vestibular schwannoma, meningioma
  o Secondary metastatic tumors: lung, breast, kidney, thyroid, gastrointestinal, melanoma
  o *Paraneoplastic syndromes* of cerebellar degeneration: especially with breast and gynecological tumors
- Drug/Toxin induced:
  o *Alcohol*: acute (reversible), chronic (truncal ataxia +/– peripheral neuropathy)
  o Antiepileptic drugs (phenytoin, carbamazepine)
  o *Chemotherapy* (e.g., 5-fluorouracil, cytosine arabinoside)
  o Toluene (glue sniffing)
  o Thallium poisoning (rare)
- Degenerative:
  o Multiple system atrophy (MSA): MSA-C
  o Idiopathic late onset cerebellar ataxia (ILOCA) – diagnosis of exclusion

Clinical features

- Ataxia: if the vermal structures are involved there is truncal ataxia with little or no limb, speech, or eye involvement. The patient walks with a wide-based, staggering gait. With severe vermal/paravermal damage, there may be an inability to stand or sit. If lateral cerebellar structures are involved there is ipsilateral limb ataxia, manifest as inaccurate reaching for targets. (NB Ataxia per se may result from disorders in sensory and optic, as well as cerebellar, pathways.)
- Decomposition of movement (asynergia): a loss of smooth fluid movement in the performance of skilled tasks, leading to clumsiness or jerkiness.
- Dysmetria or pastpointing: errors may be made in reaching for targets. Tremor may become more evident as the target is approached (intention tremor).
- Dysdiadochokinesis: clumsiness in performing rapid alternating movements, for example, supination/pronation of the forearm.

- Dysarthria: speech may be slurred and broken up, often referred to as scanning dysarthria. This is associated with damage in the region of the paravermal zone of the rostral cerebellum. In some cases of severe acute bilateral cerebellar damage, particularly in children, there maybe muteness that can last for months (cerebellar mutism).
- Nystagmus; eye movment abnormalities: various eye movement abnormalities have been described with cerebellar disease, many of which are also seen with brainstem lesions. These include gaze-evoked nystagmus (nystagmus directed toward the side of the lesion, cf. vestibular nystagmus), ocular dysmetria, and opsoclonus.
- Hypotonia: reduced muscular tone in ipsilateral limbs, +/– reduced tendon jerks, may be seen with acute cerebellar lesions. The hypotonia is more evident in arm than leg, and proximal more than distal. It may result from reduced cerebellar outflow to the muscle spindle. (Hypertonia is often seen in cerebellar lesions due to involvement of adjacent brainstem and the descending motor pathways.)

A number of clinical cerebellar syndromes are recognized, related to cerebellar anatomy:

- Rostral vermis syndrome (anterior lobe): wide-based stance and gait; little limb ataxia, hypotonia, nystagmus, dysarthria (e.g., alcoholic cerebellar degeneration).
- Caudal vermis syndrome (flocculonodular and posterior lobe): axial dysequilibrium, staggering gait, no limb ataxia, sometimes nystagmus (e.g., medulloblastoma in children).
- Cerebellar hemispheric syndrome: ipsilateral limb ataxia, dysarthria.
- Pancerebellar syndrome: combination of all the above, with bilateral signs in trunk, limbs, and axial musculature.

Investigation

Investigation scheme for an ataxic individual will be tailored to the specific situation but may involve:
- Neuroimaging (CT/MRI): for atrophy, structural lesion, inflammatory change.
- CSF: especially if inflammatory cause suspected, for example, for oligoclonal bands.
- Neurogenetic testing as appropriate. Testing for SCA6 should be considered in late-onset ataxia even without a family history.

References

Giunti P, Wood NW. The inherited ataxias. Adv Clin Neurosci Rehabil. 2007;7(5):18–21
Klockgether T, ed. Handbook of Ataxia Disorders. New York: Marcel Dekker; 2000

Klockgether T. Sporadic ataxia with adult onset: classification and diagnostic criteria. Lancet Neurol. 2010;9:94–104
Manto MU, Pandolfo M, eds. The Cerebellum and Its Disorders. Cambridge: Cambridge University Press; 2002

Cerebellopontine angle syndrome

Extra-axial mass lesions at the cerebellopontine angle, abutting the internal auditory meatus, produce a typical constellation of neurological signs ipsilaterally:

- Depression of the corneal reflex (V; early)
- Lower motor neurone facial (VII) weakness
- Sensorineural hearing loss (VIII)
- Hemiataxia

The most common cause of this syndrome is a *vestibular schwannoma* (acoustic neuroma) but it may also occur with a *meningioma, dermoid, epidermoid* (cholesteatoma), or *chordoma*. Metastases are rare.

References

Baloh RW, Konrad HR, Dirks D, et al. Cerebellar-pontine angle tumors. Arch Neurol. 1976;33:507–512
Bone I, Hadley DM. Syndromes of the orbital fissure, cavernous sinus, cerebellopontine angle, and skull base. J Neurol Neurosurg Psychiatry. 2005;76(Suppl III):iii29–iii38
Cross J, Coles A. Anatomy primer: the cerebello-pontine angle. Adv Clin Neurosci Rehabil. 2002;2(3):16–17

Cerebral amyloid angiopathy (CAA)

Congophilic angiopathy, Dyshoric angiopathy

Cerebral amyloid angiopathy (CAA) is used to refer to conditions characterized by the deposition of amyloid within cerebral blood vessels, and may be regarded as an organ-specific form of amyloidosis. In many cases, the protein is predominantly amyloid β-peptide, but other proteins may also be responsible for CAA, such as cystatin c in the Icelandic form of hereditary cerebral hemorrhage with amyloidosis (HCHWA-I). There may sometimes be concurrent inflammatory changes. CAA may be sporadic or familial.

CAA may be observed in

- *Alzheimer's disease*
- *Down syndrome*

- *Dementia pugilistica*
- *Familial British dementia, familial Danish dementia*
- Postirradiation
- Normal elderly
- Hereditary cerebral hemorrhage with amyloidosis – Dutch type (HCHWA-D) [OMIM#605714]
- Hereditary cerebral hemorrhage with amyloidosis – Icelandic type (HCHWA-I) [OMIM#105150]

Clinical features

- May be asymptomatic
- Recurrent *intracerebral hemorrhage* in a lobar pattern: headache, nausea, vomiting, focal neurological deficit +/– impaired consciousness
- Cognitive impairment, dementia
- Transient neurological symptoms: transient ischemic events, focal seizures, myoclonus
- +/– Positive family history

Investigation

Definitive diagnosis relies on the examination of brain tissue, but this is seldom available: brain biopsies may be taken at the time of evacuation of cerebral hemorrhages, if this is clinically indicated. Neurogenetic testing for HCHWA-D (APP gene) and HCHWA-I (cystatin c gene) if appropriate. Neuroimaging (MRI, especially with a diffusion gradient sequence) reveals new and old hemorrhages predominantly involving the subcortical white matter.

Differential diagnosis

- Primary *intracerebral hemorrhage*, for example, from hypertension, excessive anticoagulation (INR > 3.0), blood dyscrasias
- Head trauma
- *Vascular malformations*
- *Vasculitis*
- CNS tumor, metastases

Treatment and prognosis

No specific treatment. Surgical evacuation of lobar hemorrhages may be indicated on occasion. In HCHWA-D, there is a 50% mortality rate at presentation with a cerebral hemorrhage; gradual development of dementia syndrome occurs with repeated hemorrhage, and cognitive decline has been noted in some patients even in the absence of hemorrhage.

References

Chung KK, Anderson NE, Hutchinson D, Synek B, Barber PA. Cerebral amyloid angiopathy associatd inflammation (CAA-I): three case reports and a review. J Neurol Neurosurg Psychiatry. 2011;82:20–26

Plant GT, Ghiso J, Holton JL, Frangione B, Revesz T. Familial and sporadic cerebral amyloid angiopathies associated with dementia and the BRI dementias. In: Esiri M, Lee VMY, Trojanowski JQ, eds. The Neuropathology of Dementia. 2nd ed. Cambridge: Cambridge University Press; 2004;330–352

Cerebral palsy (CP)

Cerebral palsy (CP) denotes a variety of persisting and evolving disorders of movement and motor function caused by nonprogressive brain lesions. CP is a common (1–2 per 1,000 births) cause of persisting neurological disability. In the majority of cases, the cause is unknown, with less than 15% of cases following perinatal complications. Although relatively underinvestigated in the past, thorough evaluation is now recommended; many cases labeled as "CP" may have another disorder. A trial of levodopa to try to identify cases of *dopa-responsive dystonia* is recommended by some authorities.

Clinical features

CP may be classified according to

- Topography: tetraplegic, hemiplegic, diplegic (Little's disease)
- Clinical features: spastic, dystonic, dyskinetic, hypotonic, ataxic

However, these labels should not be used as a substitute for thorough investigation of potential underlying causes.

Investigation

No specific investigation is diagnostic, but some may be helpful, for example, MR imaging of the brain may show a vascular insult in hemiplegic CP. Investigations may be used principally to establish alternate diagnosis (see below), for example, MRI brain, blood/urine analysis for aminoacids, urine organic acid analysis, white blood cell enzymes.

Differential diagnosis

CP needs to be differentiated from a developmental coordination disorder (clumsy child, "developmental dyspraxia") and global developmental delay. Other conditions need to be considered in specific situations:

- In the absence of a history of perinatal insult
- A positive family history of "cerebral palsy"
- Developmental regression
- Presence of oculomotor abnormalities, ataxia, muscle atrophy, sensory loss, involuntary movements

Conditions which may be confused with CP may be listed according to the clinical features:

- With apparent or real muscle weakness:
  - Duchenne/Becker muscular dystrophy
  - Infantile neuroaxonal dystrophy
  - Mitochondrial cytopathy
- With predominant diplegia/tetrapelgia:
  - Adrenoleukodystrophy/adrenomyeloneuropathy (X-ALD/AMN)
  - Arginase deficiency
  - Metachromatic leukodystrophy (MLD)
  - Hereditary spastic paraplegia (HSP)
  - Holocarboxylase synthetase deficiency
- With significant dystonia/involuntary movements:
  - Dopa-responsive dystonia (DRD)
  - Glutaric aciduria type I
  - Pyruvate dehydrogenase complex deficiency
  - Lesch–Nyhan disease
  - Rett's syndrome
  - Juvenile neuronal ceroid lipofuscinosis
  - Pelizaeus–Merzbacher disease (PMD)
  - 3-Methylglutaconic aciduria
  - 3-Methylcrotonyl CoA carboxylase deficiency
- With significant ataxia:
  - Ataxia telangiectasia (AT)
  - Angelman syndrome
  - Chronic/adult GM1 gangliosidosis
  - Mitochondrial cytopathy (especially *NARP syndrome*, 8993 mutation)
  - Niemann–Pick disease type C
  - Pontocerebellar atrophy/hypoplasia
  - Posterior fossa tumor
  - X-linked spinocerebellar ataxia
- With significant bulbar/oromotor dysfunction:
  - Worster–Drought syndrome (perisylvian, opercular, Foix–Chavany–Marie syndrome)

Treatment and prognosis

Treatment is of underlying cause if identified. The most important treatable cause is dopa-responsive dystonia which responds to small doses of levodopa.

Symptomatic treatment is indicated for spasticity, including physiotherapy. Orthopedic interventions are generally unhelpful.

Late adult deterioration is seen in many cases for reasons that are often unclear, but investigation to exclude treatable complications secondary to the cerebral palsy is recommeneded, such as accelerated cervical spine degenerative disease.

References

Gupta R, Appleton RE. Cerebral palsy: not always what it seems. Arch Dis Child. 2001;85:356–360

Lin J-P. The cerebral palsies: a physiological approach. J Neurol Neurosurg Psychiatry. 2003;74 (suppl I):i23–i29

Panteliadis CP, Strassburg H-M, eds. Cerebral Palsy. Principles and Management. Stuttgart, Germany: Thieme; 2004

Cerebral salt wasting (CSW) syndrome

Natriuresis with consequent hyponatremia is a recognized complication of *subarachnoid hemorrhage*, space-occupying lesions (or following neurosurgery for these conditions), and, occasionally, *meningitis* or *encephalitis*. Clinically, it may be mistaken for the *syndrome of inappropriate antidiuretic hormone secretion (SIADH)*, since hyponatremia is common to both. The distinction is important since the management is different. In CSW, hyponatremia results from natriuresis resulting in renal sodium and water loss with reduced intravascular volume, whereas in sIADH renal conservation of water results in dilutional hyponatremia. Hence, the appropriate management of CSW is intravenous saline (under central venous presure guidance) with intravenous hydrocortisone or fludrocortisone, the mineralocorticoid effects of which reduce renal sodium loss.

Variable	CSW	sIADH
Serum sodium	↓	↓
Weight	↓	↑
Central venous pressure (CVP)	↓	↑ or N
Orthostatic hypotension	+	-
Serum osmolality	↑ or N	↓

Variable	CSW	sIADH
Serum uric acid	N	↓
Plasma urea	N or ↑	↓ or N
Packed cell volume (PCV)	↑	↓ or N
Urine sodium	↑↑	↑
Urine volume	↑↑	↓ or N

Reference

Harrigan MR. Cerebral salt wasting syndrome: a review. Neurosurgery. 1996;38:152–160

Cerebrotendinous xanthomatosis (CTX) [OMIM#213700]

Cholestanolosis

Cerebrotendinous xanthomatosis (CTX) is a rare autosomal recessive lipid storage disorder in which there is impaired bile acid synthesis due to various mutations in the gene encoding the mitochondrial enzyme 27-sterol hydroxylase (CYP27) on the distal portion of chromosome 2p. The enzyme deficiency causes an absence of chenodeoxycholic acid in the bile with consequent elevated cholestanol in the plasma and other tissues (e.g., neurones, tendons, and lungs). The condition may present in late childhood with bilateral cataracts and diarrhea, followed by an ataxic syndrome, spasticity, dementia, peripheral neuropathy, and tendon xanthomata. It is a progressive disorder; early treatment with chenodeoxycholic acid can be effective.

Clinical features

- Juvenile bilateral cataracts (97%)
- Diarrhea (50%)
- Tendon xanthomata, especially Achilles' tendon (visible or palpable; 41%)
- Pyramidal signs: spasticity (81%)
- Cerebellar ataxia (56%)
- Dementia, around the age of 20 years (66%)
- Peripheral neuropathy (31%)
- Osteoporosis secondary to abnormal vitamin D metabolism
- Premature atherosclerosis

Investigation

Bloods: raised serum cholestanol; low to normal cholesterol. Urine: elevated bile alcohols. Neuroimaging (CT/MRI) shows global cerebral atrophy and parenchymal demyelination (CTX may be classified with the *leukodystrophies*). CSF is usually normal. Neurophysiology (EMG/NCS) may show peripheral neuropathy; evoked potentials may show delayed central conduction; EEG may show diffuse slowing. Neurogenetic testing may show mutations in the 27-sterol hydroxylase gene.

Treatment and prognosis

Treatment with chenodeoxycholic acid (750 mg/day) can be effective if early diagnosis is made.

References

Moghadasian MH, Salen G, Frohlich JJ, Scudamore CH. Cerebrotendinous xanthomatosis: a rare disease with diverse manifestations. Arch Neurol. 2002;59:527–529
Verrips A, Hoefsloot LH, Steenbergen GCH, et al. Clinical and molecular genetic characteristics of patients with cerebrotendinous xanthomatosis. Brain. 2000;123:908–919

Cervical cord and root disease: overview

Cervical myelopathy, Cervical radiculopathy

The cervical spine consists of seven vertebrae, C1 to C7, and the cervical spinal cord provides eight sets of cervical nerves, each arising above the corresponding numbered vertebra with the exception of C8 which emerges between the C7 and T1 vertebrae. The cervical nerves provide motor innervation for the muscles in the upper limb, the shoulder, and upper chest and back, and sensory innervation of the upper limb, shoulder, neck, and back of the head. Damage to the nerve roots (cervical radiculopathy) causes wasting and weakness in the upper limb musculature often with pain and sensory loss, and is most commonly due to degenerative cervical spine disease: hypertrophic facet joint osteophytes, degenerative ligaments, and bulging/herniation of intervertebral discs. In such cases there is often narrowing of the cervical canal which may lead to compression of the spinal cord (cervical myelopathy) causing spastic paraparesis, triparesis, or quadriparesis, depending on the level of the compression. A similar clinical picture may be produced by other pathologies, including inflammation, tumors, trauma, and anterior horn cell disease. The advent of MR imaging has greatly improved the ability to visualize adequately this part of the neuraxis and hence diagnostic precision.

Causes of cervical myelopathy +/– radiculopathy include

- Extradural:
  - Degenerative disease of cervical spine (cervical spondylotic myelopathy)
  - Vertebral collapse, for example, secondary to metastatic disease, *tuberculosis*
  - Traumatic vertebral fracture/dislocation
  - Craniocervical junction anomalies: platybasia, basilar invagination, odontoid peg abnormalities, *ankylosing spondylitis*, *Paget's disease*, *rheumatoid arthritis*
- Intradural, extramedullary:
  - Meningioma
  - Neurofibroma
  - Epidural *abscess*
- Intramedullary:
  - Tumor: glioma, ependymoma, hemangioblastoma
  - Vascular lesions: anterior spinal artery occlusion, spinal AVMs, Caisson disease
  - *Syringomyelia*: may be associated craniovertebral anomaly, spinal tumor
  - Inflammation: *multiple sclerosis, neuromyelitis optica, acute disseminated encephalomyelitis, neurosarcoidosis, systemic lupus erythematosus, vasculitis*; parainfectious (e.g., mycoplasma)
  - *Subacute combined degeneration of the cord* (vitamin B_{12} deficiency, *copper deficiency-associated myeloneuropathy*)
  - *HIV/AIDS* vacuolar myelopathy
  - Postradiation myelopathy
  - Spinal cord abscess (rare)
  - Lightning or electrical injuries (rare)
  - Nutritional (e.g., *lathyrism* from a bean-rich diet)

Clinical features

- Myelopathy:
  - History:
    ○ Pain may or may not be a feature
    ○ Complaint of limb weakness; legs giving way, dragging, tripping
    ○ May be sphincter involvement, especially if intramedullary lesion
  - Examination:
    ○ Upper motor neurone signs: spasticity, pyramidal pattern of weakness (flexors > extensors), hyperreflexia, Babinski sign
    ○ Minor sensory signs: when present involve joint position sense and vibration perception (i.e., dorsal column); occasionally a Brown–Séquard syndrome
    ○ May have radicular signs in one or both upper limbs

- Radiculopathy:
  - History:
    - ○ Dermatomal pain
    - ○ Paroxysmal pain, increased by coughing, sneezing, straining at stool
  - Examination:
    - ○ Paresis appropriate to root(s) involved
    - ○ Reflex loss appropriate to root(s) involved
- Specific roots:
  - C1: motor only; minor weakness of head flexion, extension
  - C2: posterior scalp sensory change, +/– minor weakness of head flexion, extension
  - C3: sensory disturbance lower occiput, angle of jaw, upper neck; "red ear syndrome"; weakness of scalene and levator scapulae muscles, +/– diaphragm
  - C4: sensory signs on lower neck; weakness of scalene, levator scapulae and rhomboid muscles, +/– diaphragm
  - C5: neck, shoulder, upper anterior arm pain; weakness of levator scapulae, rhomboid, serratus anterior, supraspinatus, infraspinatus, deltoid, biceps, brachioradialis muscles, +/– (rarely) diaphragm; biceps and supinator reflexes may be depressed
  - C6: pain in lateral arm, dorsal forearm, first and second digits; weakness of serratus anterior, biceps, pronator teres, flexor carpi radialis, brachioradialis, extensor carpi radialis longus and brevis muscles; biceps and supinator reflexes may be depressed; inverted reflex may be seen if concurrent cord compression at C5-C6
  - C7: pain in dorsal forearm; sensory change in third and fourth digits; weakness of serratus anterior, pectoralis major, latissimus dorsi, biceps, pronator teres, flexor carpi radialis, triceps, extensor carpi radialis longus and brevis muscles, extensor digitorum; triceps reflex may be depressed
  - C8: pain in medial arm and forearm; sensory signs on medial forearm and hand, and fifth digit; weakness of flexor digitorum superficialis, flexor pollicis longus, flexor digitorum profundus, pronator quadratus, small hand muscles; finger flexor reflex may be depressed; +/– ipsilateral Horner's syndrome
  - [T1: sensory signs on medial arm; weakness of small hand muscles; finger flexor reflex may be depressed; +/– ipsilateral Horner's syndrome.]
- Specific levels:
  - C3-C4 central cord syndrome: "Numb and clumsy hands" syndrome
  - Often follows hyperextension neck injury, in elderly patients; ischemia, syringomyelia
  - No obvious wasting but increased tone and hyperreflexia in upper limbs
  - Loss of joint position sense and light touch in upper limbs
  - Numbness in fingertips and palms, +/– pain in shoulder girdle.
  - Loss of vibration perception in lower limbs

Investigation

Bloods: may include FBC, ESR, vitamin B_{12}, autoantibody profile, serum ACE.

Neuroimaging: MRI is imaging technique of choice for cervical spine; occasionally a myelogram is required if a dural AVM is suspected but not seen with MRI.

Neurophysiology: EMG/NCS to exclude peripheral neuropathy or widespread anterior horn cell disease; to define level of radiculopathy, the sites of greatest denervation are:

- C5 radiculopathy: spinati, deltoid, biceps, brachioradialis.
- C6 radiculopathy: 50% are similar to C5 radiculopathy with additional involvement of pronator teres; the other 50% are identical to the findings in a C7 radiculopathy.
- C7 radiculopathy: pronator teres, flexor carpi radialis, triceps.
- C8 radiculopathy: first dorsal interosseous, abductor digiti minimi, abductor pollicis brevis, flexor pollicis longus.

CSF may be required to exclude an inflammatory or malignant process. Occasionally evoked potentials and central motor conduction times are useful in diagnosing demyelinating CNS disease and upper motor neurone involvement.

Differential diagnosis

Other causes of arm pain, weakness, sensory disturbance, for example, *brachial plexopathy* (such as neuralgic amyotrophy).

Treatment and prognosis

Dependent on the cause of the cervical cord syndrome. In the case of spondylotic cervical radiculomyelopathy, conservative management is normally the first line of treatment (collar, physical therapy). However, surgery may become necessary when there is a progressive impairment of function with no remission. Best results are expected with only a single level of compression diagnosed clinically with appropriate neuroradiological correlate. Multiple compressive lesions may be approached surgically, but pose greater problems. The aim of surgery is to prevent progression rather than reverse the neurological deficits. However, in a significant number of cases there is some neurological improvement postoperatively. The surgical approach may be either posterior, with laminectomy and foraminotomy, or anterior (Cloward's procedure) with laminectomy and osteophyte-posterior ligament removal. The latter approach gives a better decompression and has a complication rate of between 2% and 8%. Comparative studies suggest that discectomy, collar, or physical therapy, all give similar outcomes at 12-month follow-up.

Reference

Malcolm GP. Surgical disorders of the cervical spine: presentation and management of common disorders. J Neurol Neurosurg Psychiatry. 2002;73(Suppl I):i34–i41

Cervical dystonia

Nuchal dystonia, Spasmodic torticollis, Wryneck

Cervical dystonia is a focal *dystonia* which is usually idiopathic but may follow neck or head trauma, and occasionally has been associated with brainstem and basal ganglia lesions. It typically presents between the ages of 30–50 years and there is a female preponderance. In about one-third of patients, dystonia spreads to other sites (e.g., face, arm) as a segmental dystonia and in another third the disease spontaneously remits, usually in the first 5 years of the illness, although this is often transient.

Clinical features

- The head is twisted around one or several planes of the neck, often with an element of jerking +/– "no-no" head tremor and shoulder elevation, due to involuntary contraction of neck muscles, most usually sternocleidomastoid, trapezius, and splenius capitis, although other muscles can be involved in more complex cases, such as levator scapulae.
- Patients sometimes discover that the dystonic movements may be overcome by a "sensory trick" or *geste antagoniste* such as placing a finger lightly on the face or back of the neck.
- There may be associated dystonic features elsewhere, as in a cranial segmental dystonia such as *Meige's syndrome*. Cervical dystonia is also a feature of *Grisel syndrome*.
- Severity of cervical dystonia may be graded using the Tsui severity scale.

Investigation

Diagnosis is clinical and generally no specific are investigations required.

Differential diagnosis

Unlikely to be mistaken; acute dystonic reactions may produce a similar picture.

Treatment and prognosis

Treatment is with botulinum toxin, giving relief in ca. 80% of cases, although repeated injections, usually every 3 months, are required indefinitely.

Other treatments that have been tried include ventral rhizotomy of upper cervical roots and section of the spinal accessory nerve with denervation of the sternocleidomastoid. Bilateral thalamotomy has been tried but surgical treatment has no benefit over botulinum toxin injections, and may be associated with significant side effects. Uncontrolled movements may result in premature degenerative disease of the cervical spine which may become clinically apparent, for example, compressive myelopathy/radiculopathy from disc disease.

References

Costa J, Borges A, Espirito-Santo C, et al. Botulinum toxin type A versus botulinum toxin type B for cervical dystonia. Cochrane Database Syst Rev. 2005;25;(1):CD004314
Sheean G. Cervical dystonia: unresolved issues and future challenges. Neurol Clin. 2008;26(Suppl 1):66–76
Tsui JK, Eisen A, Stoesl AJ, Calne S, Calne DB. Double blind study of botuilinum toxin in spasmodic torticollis. Lancet. 1986;2:245–24

Channelopathies: overview

Channelopathy is the generic name applied to a wide variety of neurological diseases caused by dysfunction of ion channels in excitable membranes. Many of these are due to inherited mutations of genes encoding ion channels in muscle, neurones, and glia. Acquired channelopathies, of autoimmune and transcriptional pathogenesis, may also occur. The channelopathies may be classified as

- Muscle channelopathies:
  - Voltage-gated channels:
    - Sodium channels:
      - Hyperkalemic periodic paralysis
      - Hypokalemic periodic paralysis (rare)
      - Paramyotonia congenita
      - Potassium-aggravated myotonia (PAM)
    - Potassium channels:
      - Hypokalemic periodic paralysis
      - Andersen–Tawil syndrome
    - Calcium channels:
      - Hypokalemic periodic paralysis (common)
      - Malignant hyperthermia
      - Central core disease

- o Chloride channels:
  - Myotonia congenita (Becker, Thomsen types)
- o Ligand-gated channels:
  - Nicotinic Acetylcholine receptors: congenital myasthenic syndromes
- Neuronal channelopathies:
  - Voltage-gated channels:
    - o Sodium channels:
      - Generalized epilepsy with febrile seizures plus (GEFS+)
      - Severe myoclonic epilepsy of infancy
    - o Potassium channels:
      - Episodic ataxia type 1
      - Benign familial neonatal convulsions
    - o Calcium channels:
      - Familial hemiplegic migraine (FHM)
      - Spinocerebellar ataxia type 6 (SCA6)
      - Episodic ataxia type 2
    - o Ligand-gated channels:
      - Nicotinic acetylcholine receptors: Autosomal dominant nocturnal frontal lobe epilepsy (ADNFLE)
      - Glycine receptors: Familial hyperekplexia
      - GABA receptors: Generalized epilepsy with febrile seizures plus
- Glial channelopathies:
  - Gap junction proteins: Charcot–Marie–Tooth disease CMTX or CMT1X.

Several of the inherited *long QT syndromes* are also channelopathies.

References

Fontaine B, Hanna MG. Muscle ion channelopathies and related disorders. In: Karpati G, Hilton-Jones D, Bushby K, Griggs RC, eds. Disorders of Voluntary Muscle. 8th ed. Cambridge: Cambridge University Press; 2010:409–426
Rose MR, Griggs RC, eds. Channelopathies of the Nervous System. Boston, MA: Butterworth-Heinemann; 2001

Charcot–Marie–Tooth (CMT) disease

Charcot and Marie, and independently, Tooth, in 1886 described hereditary peripheral neuropathy with a peroneal muscular atrophy phenotype: distal weakness and atrophy, distal sensory loss, areflexia, and foot deformity (pes cavus). The heterogeneity of this group of conditions soon became apparent, falling within the rubric of *hereditary motor and sensory neuropathy (HMSN)* in the classification of hereditary neuropathies proposed by Dyck and Lambert in 1968. The observation that nerve conduction velocities might be low or normal, implying demyelinating and axonal variants, respectively, led to the division into HMSN I (or CMT I) and HMSN II (or CMT II). The definition of the genetic basis of some of these inherited neuropathies has forced a revision of classification.

Currently, the following varieties fall within the rubric of Charcot–Marie–Tooth disease:

- CMT 1: Autosomal dominant, hypertrophic demyelinating neuropathy:
  - CMT1A: duplications or point mutations in peripheral myelin protein 22 (PMP22) gene on chromosome 17p11.2-p12; constitutes 60–90% of CMT1
  - CMT1B: mutations in myelin protein zero (MPZ or P_0) gene on chromosome 1q22; includes *Roussy–Lévy syndrome*
  - CMT1C: linked to chromosome 16p13.1-p12.3, SIMPLE/LITAF gene
  - CMT1D: due to mutations in early growth response element 2 (EGR2) gene on chromosome 10q21.1-q22.1
  - CMT1F: early onset, +/– tremor and cerebellar ataxia, due to mutations in NEFL gene on chromosome 8p21
- CMTX: X-linked dominant:
  - CMTX1: mutations in gap junction protein beta-1 (GJB1) gene, also known as Connexin 32, at chromosome Xq13.1; 7–12% of CMT, males more severely affected than females, no male-to-male transmission, may have central nervous system demyelination as well
- CMTX: X-linked recessive:
  - CMTX2: linked to chromosome Xq22.2
  - CMTX3: linked to chromosome Xq26.3-q27.1
  - CMTX4: linked to chromosome Xq24.q26.1
  - CMTX5: linked to chromosome Xq22.3, PRPS1 gene
- CMT 2: Autosomal dominant, axonal neuropathy:
  - CMT2A: mutations in mitofusin 2 (MFN2) gene on chromosome 1p36.2; up to 20% of CMT2
  - CMT2B: mutations in RAB7 gene on chromosome 3q21
  - CMT2C: linked to chromosome 12q23-q24
  - CMT2D: mutations in GARS gene on chromosome 7p15
  - CMT2E: mutations in neurofilament light chain (NEFL) gene on chromosome 8p21
  - CMT2F: mutations in HSPB1 (HSP27) gene on chromosome 7q
  - CMT2G: linked to chromosome 12q12–13.3
  - CMT2I/2J: mutations in myelin protein zero (MPZ or P_0) gene (hence, allelic with CMT1B); 5% of autosomal dominant CMT2
  - CMT2K: mutations in GDAP1 gene on chromosome 8q13-q21.1
  - CMT2L: mutations in HSPB8 (HSP22) gene on chromosome 12q24
- CMT 2: Autosomal recessive, axonal neuropathy:
  - CMT2B1: mutations in LMNA gene on chromosome 1q21.2 (hence, allelic with *Emery–Dreifuss muscular dystrophy*, *limb girdle muscular dystrophy* type 1B, *progeria*)
  - CMT2B2: mutations in MED25 gene on chromosome 19q13.3
  - CMT2H/K: mutations in GDAP1 gene on chromosome 8q13-q21.1

- CMT4: Autosomal recessive, demyelinating neuropathy:
  - CMT4A: mutations in GDAP1 gene on chromosome 8q13-q21.1
  - CMT4B1: mutations in myotubularin-related protein 2 (MTMR2) gene on chromosome 11q22
  - CMT4B2: mutations in SBF2/MTMR13 gene on chromosome 11p15
  - CMT4C: mutations in KIAA1985 gene on chromosome 5q32
  - CMT4D: mutations in N-myc-downstream regulated gene 1 (NDRG1) on chromosome 8q24.3
  - CMT4E: mutations in early growth response element 2 (EGR2) gene (hence allelic with CMT1D)
  - CMT4F: mutations in periaxin (PRX) gene on chromosome 19q13.1-q13.2
  - CMT4G: linked to chromosome 10q23.2
  - CMT4H: mutations in FGD4 gene on chromosome 12p11.21-q13.11
  - CMT4J: mutations in FIG4 gene on chromosome 6q21
- Dominant intermediate CMT (DI-CMT): conduction velocities intermediate between those of CMT 1 and CMT 2:
  - DI-CMTA: linked to chromosome 10q24.1-q25.1
  - DI-CMTB: mutations in DNM2 gene on chromosome 19p12-p13.2
  - DI-CMTC: mutations in YARS gene on chromosome 1p34-p35
  - DI-CMTD: mutations in myelin protein zero (MPZ or P_0) gene on chromosome 1q22

Of these, the most common are CMT-1A, CMT-1B, CMTX1, and CMT2A.

Clinical features

In addition to distal sensory and motor findings, there may be additional clinical features such as deafness, learning disability, scoliosis, diaphragm weakness, tremor, and cerebellar ataxia which may give clues to specific CMT type and guide genetic testing, as does crucially the inheritance pattern gleaned from family history.

Investigation

Neurophysiology: EMG/NCS: motor conduction velocities allow assignment to CMT1, CMT2, or DI-CMT groups. Neurogenetic testing guided by inheritance pattern, neurophysiological findings, and phenotype.

Differential diagnosis

Other demyelinating or axonal neuropathy, or a distal myopathy, but the clinical phenotype with positive family history is unlikely to lead to confusion.

Treatment and prognosis

No specific drug therapy. Mainstay of management is rehabilitation, orthotics, supportive and symptomatic treatment, occasionally surgery for skeletal/foot deformities. Variable prognosis according to subclassification.

References

Pareyson D, Marchesi C. Diagnosis, natural history, and management of Charcot-Marie-Tooth disease. Lancet Neurology. 2009;8:654–667

Reilly MM. Sorting out the inherited neuropathies. Pract Neurol. 2007;7:93–105

Charlevoix–Saguenay syndrome [OMIM#270550]

ARSACS

An autosomal recessive disorder of childhood, initially reported from Quebec, Canada, characterized by a slowly progressive pyramidal syndrome, dysarthria, cerebellar ataxia, abnormal eye movements (vertical pursuit), sphincter involvement, mitral incompetence, and motor neuropathy, linked to chromosome 13q11–12 with mutations in the SACS gene (homozygous and compound heterozygous). It may be classified as a "complicated" *hereditary spastic paraplegia* or as an early-onset autosomal recessive cerebellar ataxia with retained reflexes (autosomal recessive spastic ataxia of Charlevoix–Saguenay, ARSACS). Initially thought to be a rare condition confined to Quebec, it is now known to occur worldwide.

Reference

Vermeer S, Meijer RP, Pijl BJ, et al. ARSACS in the Dutch population: a frequent cause of early-onset cerebellar ataxia. Neurogenetics. 2008;9:207–214

Cheiralgia paresthetica

Handcuff neuropathy

Cheiralgia paresthetica describes paresthesia and pain in the distribution of the superficial dorsal sensory branch of the radial nerve (radial side of the thumb, dorsoradial side of hand). Ulnar flexion of the hyperpronated forearm may exacerbate the pain. It is a sensory mononeuropathy of the superficial ramus of the radial nerve which may result from pressure trauma to the nerve from handcuffs or tight wristbands (hence an *entrapment neuropathy*) and is usually self-limiting. It has also been recorded with diabetes mellitus.

Reference

Massey EW, Pleet AB. Handcuffs and cheiralgia paresthetica. Neurology. 1978; 28:1312–1313

Cheiro-oral syndrome

Restricted acral sensory syndrome

Cheiro-oral syndrome is an abnormal sensory syndrome involving the perioral region, sometimes bilaterally, and the ipsilateral palm, sometimes only certain digits ("pseudoradicular"), +/– ipsilateral foot. Most commonly this reflects thalamic pathology (VPN), usually stroke, but may also occur with lesions of the corona radiata and sensory cortex, the latter especially if there is an isolated pseudoradicular syndrome.

References

Chen WH. Cheiro-oral syndrome: a clinical analysis and review of the literature. Yonsei Med J. 2009;50:777–783
Kim JS. Restricted acral sensory syndrome following minor stroke: further observations with special reference to differential severity of symptoms among individual digits. Stroke. 1994;25:2497–2502

Chemotherapy-induced neurological disorders

Drug therapies given to inhibit or destroy neoplastic cells are nonspecific in their effects and may adversely affect normal neuronal function in brain, spinal cord, and the peripheral nervous system, transiently or permanently. Neurotoxicity is more likely with high-dose therapy, combined therapies, and intrathecal drug administration. Some of the more common adverse effects are listed here, along with the drugs most often culpable.

Clinical features

- Encephalopathy: acute, subacute, chronic, with focal signs, seizures, cognitive deficit, coma: methotrexate, cytosine arabinoside, 5-fluorouracil, intra-arterial nitrosoureas, ifosfamide, L-asparaginase
- Chemical meningitis: intrathecal drugs, for example, methotrexate, cytosine arabinoside

- Cerebellar syndrome: cytosine arabinoside, 5-fluorouracil
- Peripheral neuropathy: vinca alkaloids, taxanes, cis-platinum, procarbazine, etoposide
- Ototoxicity: cis-platinum
- Ocular toxicity: intra-arterial nitrosoureas, tamoxifen
- Syndrome of inappropriate ADH secretion: vincristine, cis-platinum

Investigation

Usually the clinical picture is clearly related to drug use, but investigations to exclude other diagnostic possibilities, especially opportunistic infection or recurrence of the original tumor, may be appropriate.

Differential diagnosis

Metastatic disease, opportunistic infection, metabolic derangement, other drug toxicities.

Treatment and prognosis

Therapeutic options are often limited. Drug withdrawal may be appropriate if acute toxicity occurs. Some toxicities reverse spontaneously, others do not.

References

Keime-Guibert F, Napolitano M, Delattre JY. Neurological complications of radiotherapy and chemotherapy. J Neurol. 1998;245:695–708

Paleologos NA. Complications of chemotherapy. In: Biller J, ed. Iatrogenic Neurology. Boston, MA: Butterworth-Heinemann; 1998; 439–459

Quasthoff S, Hartung HP. Chemotherapy-induced peripheral neuropathy. J Neurol. 2002;249:9–17

Chiari malformations

Arnold–Chiari malformations

Chiari in the 1890s described a number of congenital anomalies at the base of the brain, which have become known as Chiari (or Arnold–Chiari) malformations. They are characterized by descent of the cerebellar tonsils and parts of the brainstem into the cervical canal, often with associated *hydrocephalus*. Two types of Chiari malformation are recognized: type I without, and type II with, an associated myelomeningocoele and other signs of dysraphism. Diagnosis has become easier with the advent of MRI. Management by surgery is controversial and complex. Several hypotheses have been advanced to explain the mechanism whereby hindbrain anomalies cause associated hydrocephalus and *syringomyelia* and syringobulbia, with the hope that this will inform surgical approaches. The issues are not entirely resolved. Descent of the brainstem and cerebellum into the cervical canal occludes the foramen magnum; in addition there may be narrowing of the cerebral aqueduct, and obstruction to the outflow of CSF from the foramina of Luschka and Magendie. A piston-type mechanism may then lead to hydrocephalus and syrinx formation. There may be associated developmental abnormalities such as cervical myelomeningocoele, polymicrogyria, and a low termination of the spinal cord.

Clinical features

* Type I Chiari malformation: not associated with meningocoele or other signs of dysraphism
  – Symptoms and signs usually develop in adolescence or adult life.
  – Symptom onset may be sudden, especially after neck manipulation (especially extension).
  – A significant number of patients have an anatomically short ("bull") neck.
  – Raised intracranial pressure.
  – Progressive cerebellar ataxia.
  – Syringomyelia
    Lower cranial nerve palsies +/– long tract signs and sensory loss due to spinal cord compression +/– cerebellar ataxia.
  – Downbeat nystagmus.
  – Cough headache (hindbrain headache).
* Type II Chiari malformation: associated with meningocoele
  – Symptoms usually develop early in life, often in the neonatal period.
  – Progressive hydrocephalus.
  – Progressive lower cranial nerve abnormalities (VI to XII).
  – Signs as for type I anomaly.

Investigation

MRI is the diagnostic investigation. CSF is not usually required but raised protein and pressure.

Differential diagnosis

Type I: multiple sclerosis, high cervical tumor, skull base tumor, magnum involvement.
Type II: other causes of hydrocephalus, spina bifida, brainstem

Treatment and prognosis

The optimal management of Chiari malformations remains uncertain. If the clinical picture in type I is stable, then conservative management may be most appropriate. If the signs and disability are progressing, surgical intervention may be indicated, for example, upper cervical laminectomy and foramen magnum decompression. Associated syringomyelia may merit treatment in its own right.

References

Anson JA, Benzel EC, Awad IA, eds. Syringomyelia and the Chiari Malformations. Park Ridge, IL: American Association of Neurological Surgeons; 1997
Arnett B. Arnold-Chiari malformation. Arch Neurol. 2003;60:898–900
Hadley DM. The Chiari malformations. J Neurol Neurosurg Psychiatry. 2002;72 (Suppl II):ii38–ii40
Pillay PK, Awad IA, Little JR, Hahn JF. Symptomatic Chiari malformation in adults: a new classification based on magnetic resonance imaging with clinical and prognostic significance. Neurosurgery. 1991;28:639–645

Cholesteatoma

Cholesteatoma (*epidermoid*) of the ear is a skin cyst within the middle ear space that behaves like a localized tumor. It may be congenital or acquired; the fact that the incidence of cholesteatoma has not fallen since the introduction of antibiotic therapy for middle ear infection suggests that most are congenital, like epidermoids elsewhere. Cholesteatoma predisposes to repeated acute middle ear infections and mastoid infections and is usually found in the presence of chronic otitis media. It may also erode bone in the vestibular labyrinth which may lead to a perilymphatic fistula causing vertigo, sensorineural deafness, and facial nerve palsy. Central extension may cause *meningitis*, venous sinus thrombosis, or dural abscess.

On clinical grounds alone, it may not be possible to differentiate chronic otitis media from cholesteatoma; this requires debridement of the external ear and otological examination.

Cholesteatoma may invade the cerebellopontine angle from the middle ear, mimicking a *vestibular schwannoma* or other cause of a *cerebellopontine angle syndrome*. Clinical signs reported with cholesteatomas also include *Gradenigo's syndrome* and spontaneous periodic hypothermia. Glomus jugulare tumors also enter the differential diagnosis.

If a "Bell's palsy" continues to progress after 72 h, the possibility that it is caused by a cholesteatoma should be considered and imaging arranged urgently.

Surgical approach to cholesteatoma necessitates tumor excision and exteriorizing the skin cyst.

Cholesterol embolization syndrome

In patients with widespread atheroma, cholesterol emboli may enter the circulation spontaneously or, more commonly, as a consequence of instrumentation, and possibly anticoagulant or thrombolytic therapy. Cholesterol emboli occlude the microcirculation causing a syndrome of malaise, fever, renal failure, abdominal pain, skin petechiae, confusion, and even peripheral gangrene. Blood tests show anemia, thrombocytopenia, leukocytosis, eosinophilia, and raised ESR. The differential diagnosis includes infective endocarditis and systemic vasculitis.

References

Fine MJ, Kapoor W, Falanga V. Cholesterol crystal embolisation: a review of 221 cases in the English literature. Angiology. 1987;38:769–784
Van Jaarsveld BC, Bartelink AK, Erkelens DW. Cholesterol crystal embolisation. Neth J Med. 1991;38:86–92.

Chordoma

Chordomas are rare tumors that originate from the remnant of the notochord. They are found most commonly either at the level of the clivus, sellar, or parasellar region, or sacrococcygeal region, but may also cause a *cerebellopontine angle syndrome*. Tumors are locally invasive, have a tendency to recur, and potential to metastasize. They present most often in the 30–50-year age group. Cerebral lesions typically cause diplopia and other cranial nerve palsies with headache, sacrococcygeal lesions cause lower back pain with a *cauda equina syndrome and conus medullaris syndrome*.

Neuroimaging (MRI) shows a circumscribed, extrinsic lesion, often with heterogeneous signal intensity. Biopsy may be required for definitive diagnosis, the characteristic microscopic feature being the presence of physaliphorous cells. Other mass lesions enter the differential diagnosis (meningioma, neurofibroma, and carcinoma of the local tissue), as do inflammatory disorders such as Wegener's granulomatosis. Clival lesions may be difficult to access surgically. Although full removal may be possible, there is a tendency to recurrence. Chordomas are largely refractory to both radio- and chemotherapy, although some centers report improved survival with surgery + radiotherapy; proton beam therapy may be helpful. A 5-year survival of around 60% is quoted.

References

Cohen-Gadol AA, Al-Mefty O. Skull base tumors. In: Bernstein M, Berger MS, eds. Neuro-oncology. The Essentials. 2nd ed.. New York: Thieme; 2008:320–333
Watkins L, Khudados ES, Kaleoglu M, et al. Skull base chordomas: a review of 38 cases, 1958–1988. Br J Neurosurg. 1993;7:241–248

Choriocarcinoma

Choriocarcinoma is a *germ cell tumor* characterized by differentiation into trophoblastic tissue which is highly vascular and prone to hemorrhage. It may occur as a metastatic *pineal tumor*, or in the cauda equina or spinal canal, often after a molar pregnancy or abortion. Presentation may be with epileptic seizures, hemorrhages, or gradually progressive deficits. It is associated with increased CSF levels of β-human chorionic gonadotrophin. The management may involve chemotherapy, radiotherapy, and surgery.

Reference

Ilancheran A, Ratnam SS, Baratham G. Metastatic cerebral choriocarcinoma with primary neurological presentation. Gynecol Oncol. 1988;29:361–364

Choroid plexus papilloma

Choroid plexus papilloma is a rare tumor which may cause headache with *hydrocephalus* and raised intracranial pressure due to excessive CSF secretion, or may remain asymptomatic. It may occur in the context of *incontinentia pigmenti*.

Chronic inflammatory demyelinating polyradiculoneuropathy (CIDP)

Chronic inflammatory demyelinating polyradiculoneuropathy (CIDP) is an acquired peripheral sensorimotor *neuropathy* of presumed immunological pathogenesis. Although its presentation and course is heterogeneous, CIDP may be clinically distinguished – by definition – from *Guillain–Barré syndrome* (GBS) by its progressive worsening over a period of at least 8 weeks. Key features are electrophysiological (and pathological) evidence of demyelination and elevated CSF protein concentration. CIDP is often responsive to immunosuppressive therapy.

Clinical features

- Variable course: usually progressive, subacute monophasic, and occasionally relapsing–remitting. Unlike GBS the neurological deficits are still developing 8 weeks after disease onset and often continue to evolve over months or years.
- Symmetrical demyelinating sensorimotor polyradiculoneuropathy: involves distal and proximal musculature, although the distal weakness is usually more prominent. The degree of weakness is usually much greater than muscle atrophy, and deep tendon reflexes are depressed or absent. About 65% of

cases have sensory loss, paresthesiae or pain in the limbs, with occasional involvement of the trunk. Pure sensory variants have been described.

- The nerves may be thickened and palpable; rarely cord compression from hypertrophied nerve roots has been described.
- Occasionally patients have cranial nerve or autonomic involvement; presentation with subacute progressive sensory ataxia may occur.
- Focal forms of the disease are described, for example, with involvement of only one limb; *ophthalmoplegic migraine* may be a focal variant of demyelinating neuropathy.
- In some patients there is evidence of concurrent central demyelination.
- Conditions occasionally associated with CIDP include:
  - Hereditary motor and sensory neuropathy (HMSN)
  - Lymphoma/carcinoma
  - Monoclonal gammopathy of uncertain significance (MGUS)
  - Collagen vascular disorders

Investigation

Bloods: serum electrophoresis and quantitation of immunoglobulins should be performed to exclude *paraproteinemic demyelinating neuropathy (PDN)*; raised anti-ganglioside antibodies (anti-GM1) may be found, although this is more typical of *multifocal motor neuropathy* with conduction block (MMN). Neuroimaging: on spinal MRI thickened nerve roots may be seen, which may narrow the spinal canal and cause cord compression if very large; on brain MRI (not routinely indicated) periventricular white matter lesions, similar to those seen in *multiple sclerosis*, are sometimes seen, and may cause clinical manifestations, but this is very rare. CSF protein is typically raised to between 0.9 and 2.5 g/L; there are usually no cells, normal glucose ratio, and no oligoclonal bands. However, patients with central demyelination may have oligoclonal bands. Neurophysiology: EMG/NCS electrophysiological criteria for a diagnosis of CIDP include:

- Reduced motor conduction velocities, <75% of lower limit of normal (i.e., demyelinating neuropathy)
- Prolonged distal motor latencies, >140% of normal
- Conduction block and/or temporal dispersion of compound muscle action potential
- Increased F wave latency, >120% of normal

Although CIDP is usually clinically symmetrical, there are often electrophysiological differences between limbs, which, like conduction block, are not seen in the hereditary demyelinating neuropathies. Nerve biopsy (not routinely indicated) shows features of multifocal demyelination, principally proximal, and remyelination with onion bulb formation +/– a mononuclear cell (macrophage and lymphocyte) infiltration.

Differential diagnosis

- Guillain–Barré syndrome: it is extremely rare (<5%) to have recurrent GBS with complete recovery between attacks. Furthermore, GBS does not progress after 6 weeks by definition, although the patient may still be severely debilitated at this and later stages.
- Hereditary motor and sensory neuropathy (HMSN) type I: a symmetrical neuropathy with a long history; pes cavus frequent; CSF protein is normal. (However, a handful of cases of HMSNI patients have been described with inflammatory demyelination on nerve biopsy, suggesting superimposed CIDP.)
- Paraproteinemic demyelinating neuropathy.
- Paraneoplastic polyneuropathies, including the *POEMS syndrome*.
- Metabolic neuropathies.
- Polyradiculoneuropathy associated with *HIV* and *neuroborreliosis* (Lyme disease).
- Vasculitic neuropathy, including the very rare non-systemic "isolated" vasculitic neuropathy.

Treatment and prognosis

In mild cases there may be no need to treat. In those disabled by their condition or continuing to progress, the mainstay of treatment is immunosuppression. Most patients with CIDP respond to 8 weeks of steroid therapy, starting with high doses (cf. MMN, often does not respond and may actually get worse). Intravenous immunoglobulin (IVIg: 0.4 g/kg/day for 5 days; or 1 g/kg/day for 2 days) has good evidence as first-line therapy for both short- and long-term use, usually needing to be repeated at intervals. Plasma exchange (PEx) is equally effective as IVIg. Evidence for other immunosuppressants and immunomodulatory treatment (interferons, azathioprine, methotrexate, ciclosporin, cyclophosphamide) is weaker. Antibodies such as rituximab and etanercept may sometimes succeed where other treatments have failed. The majority of patients with CIDP respond to therapy and remain ambulant and employed. Only a minority fail to respond and become wheelchair-bound.

References

Hughes RAC, Bouche P, Cornblath DR, et al. European Federation of Neurological Societies/Peripheral Nerve Society guideline on management of chronic inflammatory demyelinating polyradiculoneuropathy: report of a joint task force of the European Federation of Neurological Societies and the Peripheral Nerve Society. Eur J Neurol. 2006;13:326–332

Krishnan A, Lecky B, Sathasivam S. Immune therapy in chronic inflammatory demyelinating polyneuropathy. Adv Clin Neurosci Rehabil. 2008;8(3):10–12

Overell JR, Willison HJ. Chronic inflammatory demyelinating polyradiculoneuropathy: classification and treatment options. Pract Neurol. 2006;6:102–110

Sander HW, Latov N. Research criteria for defining patients with CIDP. Neurology. 2003;60:8–15

Vallat JM, Sommer C, Magy L. Chronic inflammatory demyelinating polyradiculoneuropathy: diagnostic and therapeutic challenges for a treatable condition. Lancet Neurol. 2010;9:402–412

Chronic progressive external ophthalmoplegia (CPEO)

Chronic progressive external ophthalmoplegia (CPEO) is one of the classical phenotypes of *mitochondrial disease*. Sporadic and familial cases are recognized; the latter may be autosomal dominant or recessive. The phenotype may result from a number of mutations, including multiple deletions (sporadic) of mitochondrial DNA (mtDNA), single base pair mutations of mitochondrial DNA (e.g., mtDNA bp 3243, 4977), mitochondrial tRNA mutations, and defects in nuclear genes encoding mitochondrial proteins: POLG1 (encodes mtDNA polymerase), C10ORF2 (encodes the mitochondrial helicase Twinkle), and ANT1 (encodes adenine nucleotide translocase). In CPEO, the mutated mtDNA is confined to muscle, unlike the situation in Pearson's syndrome and *Kearns–Sayre syndrome* (*KSS*) wherein mutated mtDNA is found in a wide variety of tissues.

Clinical features

CPEO is perhaps more loosely defined than KSS, consisting clinically of

- Slowly progressive paresis of eye musculature
- Bilateral ptosis
- +/− Cardiac conduction defects
- +/− Proximal muscle weakness, fatigue (especially in later stages)
- +/− Pigmentary retinopathy
- +/− Sensory ataxic neuropathy

Onset is usually in the third or fourth decade, but may be as late as the fifth or sixth decade. Hence, it shares many features in common with the definition of KSS but with later onset.

Investigation

Ophthalmology consultation for fundus photography, ERG. Muscle biopsy: COX negative fibers, ragged red fibers on Gomori trichrome stain.

Neurogenetics: muscle mtDNA deletions or point mutations may be found; or nuclear DNA mutations.

Differential diagnosis

- Ocular myasthenia.
- Thyroid ophthalmopathy.
- Ocular abnormalities may be similar to those of progressive supranuclear palsy, but additional features should rule this out.

Treatment and prognosis

No specific treatment, although coenzyme Q10 and carnitine may be used. Supportive treatment as appropriate, for example, treatment of diabetes mellitus, cardiac pacemaker.

Reference

Caballero PE, Candela MS, Alvarez CI, Tejerina AA. Chronic progressive ophthalmoplegia: a report of 6 cases and a review of the literature. Neurologist. 2007; 13:33–36

Chronic relapsing inflammatory optic neuropathy (CRION)

Chronic relapsing inflammatory optic neuropathy (CRION) describes a rare syndrome of subacute, painful visual loss, often bilaterally sequential, in which the degree of visual loss is usually more severe than in other causes of demyelinating optic neuropathy. The condition is exquisitely corticosteroid-responsive, but quickly relapses once steroids are weaned, often requiring long-term immunosuppression. VERs show prolonged latency but preserved amplitude, and ERG shows reduced amplitude of the N95 peak, indicating that this is a purely optic nerve disease. CSF is normal. Superficially, CRION resembles the granulomatous optic neuropathy of *neurosarcoidosis*, but with prolonged follow-up patients do not develop signs of widespread disease. Some patients have been found to have antibodies to aquaporin-4, suggesting that this disorder may fall within the spectrum of *neuromyelitis optica (NMO)*.

References

Kidd D, Burton B, Plant GT, Hughes EM. Chronic relapsing inflammatory optic neuropathy (CRION). Brain. 2003;126:276–284
Matthews LAE, Baig F, Palace J, Turner MR. The borderland of neuromyelitis optica. Pract Neurol. 2009;9:335–340

Churg–Strauss syndrome

Churg–Strauss syndrome is a systemic *vasculitis* involving the peripheral nerve and characterized by asthma and peripheral eosinophilia. The clinical features include:

- Neurological: acute painful mononeuritis multiplex most common, but distal symmetric polyneuropathy, radiculopathy, ischemic optic neuropathy/visual loss, and bilateral trigeminal neuropathy have also been recorded; cerebrovascular disease is rare but does occur.
- Pulmonary: asthma, allergic rhinitis.
- Cutaneous: erythema multiforme, leukocytoclastic vasculitis.
- Cardiac.

In a typical case, biopsy of peripheral nerve is not necessary. High-dose corticosteroids usually lead to rapid control of disease, but recurrence within 2 years is high, so steroids should be maintained (with steroid-sparing agents) for that time. Severe cases may require IVIG and/or cyclophosphamide.

Diagnostic criteria

Masi AT, Hunder GG, Lie JT, et al. The American College of Rheumatology 1990 criteria for the classification of Churg-Strauss syndrome (allergic granulomatosis and angiitis). Arthritis Rheum. 1990;33:1094–1100

References

Sehgal M, Swanson JW, DeRemee RA, Colby TV. Neurologic manifestations of Churg-Strauss syndrome. Mayo Clin Proc. 1995;70:337–341
Wolf J, Bergner R, Mutallib S, Buggle F, Grau AJ. Neurologic complications of Churg-Strauss syndrome – a prospective monocentric study. Eur J Neurol. 2010;17:582–588

Ciguatera

This is a form of marine food poisoning, common in the tropics, following consumption of reef fish (barracuda, grouper, red snapper) which are transvectors for dinoflagellates which produce the toxins ciguatoxin, maitotoxin, and scaritoxin. These act by activating sodium and calcium ion channels in excitable membranes; hence, this may be regarded as an acquired *channelopathy*. Initial gastrointestinal features are followed within hours of eating reef fish by paresthesiae (limbs, oral cavity, trunk, genitalia), headache, myalgia, and occasionally ataxia and limb weakness. Cardiovascular effects may also occur. Neurophysiology shows slowing of sensory and motor nerve conduction velocities. Supportive care is indicated, with eventual recovery. Mannitol has been found helpful although the mechanism is unclear. Chronic pain may be a sequela.

Reference

Pearn J. Neurology of ciguatera. J Neurol, Neurosurg Psychiatry. 2001;70:4–8

Cluster headache (CH)

Erythroprosopalgia, Harris's syndrome, Horton's headache, Horton's neuralgia, Migrainous neuralgia

Cluster headache (CH) is an episodic stereotypic *headache* of extreme severity, classified with the *trigeminal autonomic cephalalgias* (*TAC*), occurring more often in men than women (3.5–7:1). Headache is strictly unilateral and associated with cranial autonomic features. Onset is most commonly in the third or fourth decade of life although it may begin at any age. Circannual and circadian periodicity of the headaches is typical. CH typically responds to a number of drugs; hence, correct diagnosis is important.

Clinical features

• Cluster attack:
Orbital/temporal pain of abrupt onset and cessation, strictly unilateral, of extreme severity, lasting minutes to hours, usually 45–180 min. Frequency of attacks ranges from 8/day to 1 every second day; attacks may occur at identical times each day, often at night. During an attack, cranial autonomic features are present: lacrimation, nasal congestion, rhinorrhea, forehead/facial sweating, miosis and ptosis (partial Horner's syndrome), eyelid edema, conjunctival injection. These features are transient, with the possible exception of the partial Horner's syndrome. Occasionally, there may be migrainous phenomena such as nausea, vomiting, photophobia, and phonophonia. Sufferers are often restless and irritable during an attack, preferring to move about (cf. *migraine*); the pain may be so severe that they will bang their head against a wall for relief.
Recognized precipitants: alcohol (usually within an hour; cf. migraine, several hours), nitroglycerine, exercise, elevated environmental temperature.
There is usually no family history (cf. migraine). CH may be associated with a higher incidence of peptic ulceration.

- Cluster bout:
  Episodic cluster headache (80–90%): recurrent bouts lasting more than a week and separated by remissions of more than 2 weeks.
  Chronic cluster headache (10–20%): no remissions within 1 year, or remissions less than 2 weeks.

Investigation

History, and examination during the attack, is diagnostic. Bloods are usually normal, as is structural neuroimaging. PET may show focal hypothalamic activity.

Differential diagnosis

- Migraine
- Other trigeminal autonomic cephalalgias: paroxysmal hemicranias, SUNCT syndrome
- Hypnic headache
- Trigeminal neuralgia
- Carotid dissection; Raeder's paratrigeminal syndrome
- Granulomatous disease of the cavernous sinus ("Tolosa-Hunt syndrome")
- Glaucoma
- Giant cell arteritis
- Dental disease (not too unusual for teeth to be removed in CH patients)

Treatment and prognosis

- Acute treatment:
  - Avoid triggers (alcohol, vasodilator drugs).
    - Sumatriptan 6 mg subcutaneously (bd if necessary), or intranasal triptans; oral triptans act too slowly.
  - Intranasal triptan (sumatriptan, zolmitriptan).
  - Oxygen 100% at flow rate 9–12 L/min for 15 min (requires special mask).
  - Intranasal lignocaine 20–60 mg: adjunct, rarely adequate alone.
- Prophylactic treatment:
  - Short term (episodic cluster headache):
    - Prednisolone: short intensive courses, 2–3 weeks in tapering doses, for example, 60 mg/day for 5 days, taper dose by 10 mg every 3 days (often associated with relapse)
    - Naratriptan, eletripan bd
    - Greater occipital nerve injection

– Long term (prolonged episodic cluster headache, chronic cluster headache):
  ○ Verapamil = drug of choice; 240–960 mg daily with baseline ECG and monitoring for PR interval prolongation
  ○ Lithium: 300 mg bd, titrated (following *British National Formulary*) to serum lithium concentration in upper part of therapeutic range; monitoring blood tests for renal and thyroid function required
  ○ Methysergide: 4–10 mg/day (~ 60% improve); monitor for retroperitoneal fibrosis; require drug holiday every 6 months
  ○ Topiramate
  ○ Gabapentin
  ○ Melatonin

References

Cohen AS, Goadsby PJ. Prevention and treatment of cluster headache. Prog Neurol Psychiatry. 2009;13(3):9-10, 12–14, 16
May A, Leone M, Afra J, et al. EFNS guidelines on the treatment of cluster headache and other trigeminal-autonomic cephalalgias. Eur J Neurol. 2006;13:1066–1077

Coarctation of the aorta

Neurological complications of coarctation of the aorta, which may be congenital or acquired (e.g., following childhood irradiation, or in *Takayasu's disease*), are variable, and include:

* Ruptured intracerebral aneurysm/*subarachnoid hemorrhage*: may be related or coincidental.
* Headache (secondary to proximal hypertension?): may be related or coincidental.
* Spinal cord ischemia/infarction, possibly as a consequence of a steal phenomenon: this may result in neurogenic intermittent claudication.
* Spinal cord compression: from enlarged collateral vessels; may also cause spinal subarachnoid hemorrhage.
* Episodic loss of consciousness: syncope? seizures?
* Left recurrent laryngeal nerve palsy: compression by aneurysmal dilatation proximal to coarctation.

Reference

LeBlanc FE, Charrette EP, Dobell AR, Branch CL. Neurological complications of aortic coarctation. Can Med Assoc J. 1968;99:299–303

Cobb syndrome

Cutaneomeningospinal angiomatosis

In this sporadic neurocutaneous syndrome, a dural angioma is associated with a cutaneous angioma in the corresponding dermatome. The former may behave as an extradural mass lesion, compressing the spinal cord or roots.

Reference

Clark MT, Brooks EL, Chong WS, Pappas C, Fahey M. Cobb syndrome: a case report and systematic review of the literature. Pediatr Neurol. 2008;39:423–425

Cocaine

Neurological consequences of cocaine use include stroke (a significant cause in young adults), epileptic seizures, encephalopathy, and acute headache. These are probably due to cocaine's vasoconstrictor (sympathomimetic) action causing a spastic vasculopathy; more rarely, it induces an inflammatory *vasculitis* of the CNS, prompting speculation on the value of steroid treatment for some of these conditions. Psychiatric effects ranging from mania and delusions to depression (following drug withdrawal) are also recognized. A handful of case reports suggest that "chasing the dragon" with either cocaine or heroin may lead to a toxic central nervous system demyelinating syndrome, with radiological similarities to ADEM, but clinically more severe and without inflammation pathologically.

The use of "crack" cocaine, the free base, produces high blood levels almost instantaneously after smoking and increases the likelihood of toxicity. The only treatment is abstinence.

References

Enevoldson TP. Recreational drugs and their neurological consequences. J Neurol, Neurosurg Psychiatry. 2004;75 (Suppl III): iii9–iii15
Rowbotham MC, Lowenstein DH. Neurologic consequences of cocaine use. Annu Rev Med. 1990;41:417–422

Coccidioidomycosis

This is a fungal infection, due to the soil fungus *Coccidioides immitis*, common in the south-western USA that presents with an influenza-like illness with pulmonary infiltrates and is usually self-limiting. Occasionally, disease becomes disseminated, and *meningitis* may be a feature, with papilledema and sixth nerve palsy, and CSF findings similar to tuberculous meningitis. The organism is hard to culture from CSF but may be identified in lung, lymph node, and skin lesions. The differential diagnosis also encompasses other fungal causes of meningitis (histoplasmosis, *blastomycosis*) and actinomycosis. Treatment is with intravenous amphotericin, often required for months, and CSF drainage if *hydrocephalus* occurs, despite which the condition may be fatal.

Coeliac disease

Gluten ataxia, Gluten-sensitive enteropathy

Coeliac disease may be associated in about 10% of cases with a variety of neurological abnormalities which cannot be otherwise explained, including:

- Epilepsy
- Migraine
- Cerebellar syndrome
- Spinocerebellar ataxia
- Peripheral neuropathy: predominantly sensory axonopathy; may be demyelinating, mixed
- Myelopathy
- Myoclonus
- Intracerebral calcification, especially occipital
- Encephalopathy: ?cerebral vasculitis
- Dementia
- Disseminated enteropathic T-cell lymphomatosis, presenting with cranial nerve palsies, radiculopathies

Although vitamin deficiencies (e.g., vitamin B_{12}) have sometimes been implicated in the neuropathic features, as a consequence of malabsorption, repletion seldom leads to clinical improvement.

The diagnosis of coeliac disease is based on the clinical picture of malabsorption, with anti-endomysial (IgA EMA) and anti-tissue transglutaminase antibodies (IgA tTG), and the finding of subtotal villous atrophy on a duodenal biopsy. Anti-gliadin antibodies (AGA) have a lower sensitivity and specificity for diagnosis than other antibodies and tissue biopsy. Response to a gluten-free diet is typical in coeliac disease.

Some patients with cerebellar ataxia have only anti-gliadin antibodies without intestinal changes, so-called gluten ataxia. It has also been suggested that some cases labeled as "idiopathic late-onset cerebellar ataxia" in fact have gluten ataxia, with or without underlying enteropathy, that is, this may be understood as an isolated, immune-mediated disease of brain rather than a subclinical affection of the gut. Hence, the suggestion is that gluten sensitivity may not necessarily require gastroenterological disease, but be brain-specific.

References

Bushara KO. Neurologic presentation of celiac disease. Gastroenterology. 2005;128(4 Suppl 1):S92–S97
Doran M, du Plessis DG, Larner AJ. Disseminated enteropathy-type T-cell lymphoma: cauda equina syndrome complicating coeliac disease. Clin Neurol Neurosurg. 2005;107:517–520
Grossman G. Neurological complications of coeliac disease: what is the evidence? Pract Neurol. 2008;8:77–89
Luostarinen L, Pirttila T, Collin P. Coeliac disease presenting with neurological disorders. *Eur Neurol.* 1999;42:132–135.
Vaknin A, Eliakim R, Ackerman Z, Steiner I. Neurological abnormalities associated with celiac disease. *J Neurol.* 2004;251: 1393–1397.

Coenurosis

Coenurosis results from infection with the larval form of the dog tapeworm *Taenia multiceps* or *Taenia serialis*, a cestode helminth, which may produce space-occupying cysts within the CNS, causing headache, raised intracranial pressure, and focal signs. The grape-like cysts may be visualized by brain imaging, most often in the posterior fossa, and removed surgically. The differential diagnosis includes *echinococcosis*.

Reference

Ing MB, Schantz PM, Turner JA. Human coenurosis in North America: case reports and review. Clin Infect Dis. 1998;27:519–523

Cogan syndrome (1)

Non-syphilitic interstitial keratitis

This is an autoimmune disorder characterized by non-syphilitic interstitial keratitis and vestibuloauditory symptoms such as episodic vertigo, tinnitus, and hearing loss. The most common presentation is with sudden hearing loss. Headache is a common systemic symptom, along with arthralgia and fever. Complete hearing loss may develop in half of patients whilst visual loss is rare. Cochlear implants are beneficial. Topical corticosteroids may be of benefit for the keratitis, but steroids are rarely effective for other features of the illness.

References

Cogan DG. Syndrome of non-syphilitic interstitial keratitis and vestibuloauditory symptoms. Arch Ophthalmol. 1945;33:144–149

Gluth MB, Baratz KH, Matteson EL, Driscoll CL. Cogan syndrome: a retrospective review of 60 patients throughout a half century. Mayo Clin Proc. 2006;81:483–488

Cogan syndrome (2)

Congenital oculomotor apraxia, Oculomotor apraxia of Cogan

This is a congenital condition in which there is an isolated apraxia of ocular movements, primarily in the horizontal direction, hence, a congenital lack of lateral gaze. To overcome this, patients use a thrusting movement of the head in the desired direction of gaze, often overshooting so that the eyes can fixate by slowly drifting back. A similar apraxia of eye movement is also seen in *ataxia telangiectasia*.

Reflex eye movements (e.g., optokinetic nystagmus) can be elicited normally.

Collagen vascular disorders and the nervous system: overview

There is no universally agreed classification for conditions which may be labeled as collagen vascular disorders, connective tissue disorders, and vasculitides, but conditions recognized to fall within these groupings include:

- Connective tissue disease:
  - Rheumatoid arthritis
  - Systemic lupus erythematosus (SLE)
  - Systemic sclerosis (scleroderma)
  - Dermatomyositis
  - Polymyositis
  - Ankylosing spondylitis
  - Sjögren's syndrome
  - Mixed connective tissue disease (MCTD)
- Vasculitides:
  - Polyarteritis nodosa (PAN)
  - Churg–Strauss syndrome
  - Wegener's granulomatosis
  - Temporal arteritis
  - Takayasu's arteritis
  - Isolated angiitis of the nervous system

The potential effects of these conditions upon the nervous system, both central and peripheral, are protean, including encephalopathy, stroke-like episodes, relapsing–remitting syndromes, radiculopathy, neuropathy, and myopathy.

Reference

Scolding N. Neurological complications of rheumatological and connective tissue disorders. In: Scolding N, ed. Immunological and Inflammatory Disorders of the Central Nervous System. Oxford: Butterworth Heinemann; 1999:147–180

Colloid cyst

Neuroepithelial cyst

Colloid cysts are thought to arise from ependymal cells in the vestigial paraphysis in the anterior portion of the third ventricle. In this location colloid cysts may block the third ventricle and cause obstructive hydrocephalus. Presentation from late childhood onwards is with either an intermittent obstructive syndrome ("ball valve" arrangement) causing severe bifrontal–bioccipital headache, unsteady gait, incontinence, visual impairment, and *drop attacks* without loss of consciousness, or with *normal pressure hydrocephalus*. Behavioral changes may also be noted. Some instances are now found incidentally when undergoing brain imaging for other reasons. The differential diagnosis encompasses glioma, choroid plexus papilloma, craniopharyngioma, pineal and pituitary tumors. Surgical resection may be undertaken, although symptoms may be more easily controlled with shunting or stereotactic decompression of the cyst. Damage to the fornix, either from the cyst or as a consequence of surgery may result in persistent amnesic syndrome.

References

Hodges JR, Carpenter K. Anterograde amnesia with fornix damage following removal of a third ventricle colloid cyst. J Neurol Neurosurg Psychiatry. 1991;54:633–638
Jeffree RL, Besser M. Colloid cyst of the third ventricle: a clinical review of 39 cases. J Clin Neurosci. 2001;8:328–331

Coma: overview

Coma is a state of unresponsiveness, with eyes closed, from which a patient cannot be roused by verbal or mechanical stimuli. It represents a greater degree of impairment of consciousness than stupor or obtundation, all three forming part of a continuum, rather than discrete stages, between being fully alert and being comatose. The causes of coma are multiple, including:

- Drugs and toxins
- Metabolic causes: hypoglycemia, hepatic failure
- Infections
- *Epilepsy*: nonconvulsive status epilepticus
- Cerebrovascular insults: hemorrhage, infarction
- *Traumatic brain injury*

Clinical features

- Although coma may be graded by means of a lumped "score," such as the Glasgow Coma Scale, description of the individual aspects of neurological function in unconscious patients, such as eye movements, limb movements, vocalization, and response to stimuli, may be preferable since this conveys more information.
- Signs should be documented serially to assess any progression of coma. Changes in eye movements and response to central noxious stimuli indicate change in depth of coma: roving eye movements are lost before oculocephalic responses followed by caloric responses; pupillary reflexes are the last to go. The switch from flexor to extensor posturing (decorticate vs. decerebrate rigidity) also indicates increasing depth of coma.

Investigation

Bloods: electrolytes, glucose, arterial blood gases; drug screen.
Imaging: CT, MRI for intracranial lesion (infarct, hemorrhage).
CSF: if meningitis or encephalitis possible.
Neurophysiology: EEG: if nonconvulsive status epilepticus a possibility.

Differential diagnosis

- Abulia
- Akinetic mutism
- Catatonia
- *Locked-in syndrome*
- *Vegetative state*

Treatment and prognosis

General supportive treatment of respiration, circulation. Specific treatments dependent on cause. Some drug-induced comas may be promptly reversible, for example, benzodiazepines with flumazenil, opiates with naloxone.

References

American Congress of Rehabilitation Medicine. Recommendations for use of uniform nomenclature pertinent to patients with severe alterations of consciousness. Arch Phys Med Rehabil. 1995;76: 205–209
Posner JB, Saper CB, Schiff ND, Plum F. Plum and Posner's Diagnosis of Stupor and Coma. 4th ed. Oxford: Oxford University Press; 2007
Wijdicks EFM. Coma. Pract Neurol. 2010;10:51–60
Young GB, Ropper AH, Bolton CF, eds. Coma and Impaired Consciousness: a Clinical Perspective. New York: McGraw-Hill; 1998

Common variable immunodeficiency (CVID)

Common variable immunodeficiency (CVID) is one of the most common syndromes of primary antibody deficiency, characterized by profound hypogammaglobulinemia. Various neurological complications have been described in association with CVID, including pneumococcal *meningitis*, acute and chronic meningoencephalitis due to enteroviral infection, and *subacute combined degeneration of the spinal cord* due to *vitamin B$_{12}$ deficiency* secondary to chronic gastritis or pernicious anemia.

Reference

Hermaszewski RA, Webster ADB. Primary hypogammaglobulinaemia: a survey of clinical manifestations and complications. Q J Med. 1983;86:31–42

Compartment syndromes

Swelling of muscles, for example following ischemia or trauma, within a semi-rigid fibro-osseous compartment may compromise capillary blood flow, leading to a vicious circle of further ischemic damage and swelling. Such compartment syndromes are particularly described for the anterior tibial muscles and the volar muscles of the forearm. Sensory and motor features following compression of peripheral nerves within the compartment may occur. Excessive muscle damage results in *rhabdomyolysis*, myoglobinuria, and possibly renal failure. Eventual fibrosis of damaged muscle may lead to contracture (Volkman's ischemic contracture). Acute treatment is subcutaneous fasciotomy to relieve pressure. Compartment syndrome has sometimes been described after ischemic forearm exercise testing in individuals with metabolic myopathies such as *McArdle's disease* and *glycogen storage disease*.

Reference

Niepel GG, Lowe J, Wills AJ. Compartment syndrome during an ischaemic forearm exercise test. Pract Neurol. 2004;4:242–245

Complex regional pain syndromes

Algodystrophy, Causalgia, Causalgia-dystonia syndrome, Reflex sympathetic dystrophy (RSD)

Complex regional pain syndrome is the term now used to describe ill-understood chronic pain disorders, first described by S. Weir Mitchell in 1864 as a consequence of traumatic peripheral nerve injury (causalgia, complex regional pain syndrome type 2), although there may be no definable nerve injury (complex regional pain syndrome type 1). Potential mechanisms for pain include maintained sympathetic nerve activity in the early (but not the late) stages of the disease, trauma-related cytokine release, exaggerated neurogenic inflammation, and cortical reorganization in response to chronic pain.

Clinical features

- Pain: greater than expected for the degree of tissue damage; chronic burning pain, often initially dermatomal but gradually spreading to be regional; hyperalgesia, allodynia, hyperpathia, leading to sleep disturbance, and secondary depression
- Autonomic dysfunction: sudomotor, vasomotor change
- Edema: limb swelling (?neurogenic inflammation)
- +/– Dystrophy/Atrophy: nails, hair, skin (livedo reticularis, mottling), bone (cystic and subchondral erosion, diffuse osteoporosis [Sudeck's atrophy, Sudeck–Leriche syndrome])
- Movement disorder: inability to initiate movement, weakness, tremor, muscle spasms, *dystonia*

Investigation

Clinical diagnosis; no specific tests. EMG/NCS may be used to define underlying nerve injury.

Differential diagnosis

If movement disorder is prominent, other causes of dystonia may need to be excluded.

Treatment and prognosis

The natural history varies from stability to progression. The evidence base for treatments is weak. Of the many approaches tried, benefit has been reported with steroids, epidural clonidine, intrathecal baclofen, spinal cord stimulation, dimethyl sulfoxide, and intravenous immunoglobulin.

Diagnostic criteria

Van de Beek WJT, Schwartzman RJ, van Nes SI, et al. Diagnostic criteria used in studies of reflex sympathetic dystrophy. Neurology. 2002;58:522–526

References

Birklein F. Complex regional pain syndrome. J Neurol. 2005;252:131–138
Bush D. Complex regional pain syndrome. In: Bennett MI, ed. Neuropathic Pain. Oxford: Oxford University Press; 2006:57–66
Goebel A, Baranowski A, Maurer K, et al. Intravenous immunoglobulin treatment of the complex regional pain syndrome: a randomized trial. Ann Intern Med. 2010;152:152–158
Shenker N, Shaikh MF, Lee M. Central mechanisms in complex regional pain syndrome (CRPS). Adv Clin Neurosci Rehabil. 2009;9(1):37–39
Tran de QH, Duong S, Bertini P, Finlayson RJ. Treatment of complex regional pain syndrome: a review of the evidence. Can J Anaesth. 2010;57:149–166

Congenital cranial dysinnervation disorders (CCDDs): overview

Congenital cranial dysinnervation disorders (CCDDs) are developmental abnormalities of one or more cranial nerves or nuclei with primary or secondary dysinnervation, leading to abnormal eye, eyelid, or facial movement. The rubric includes:

- Predominantly vertical disorders of ocular motility:
  - Congenital fibrosis of extraocular muscles (CFEOM): oculomotor +/– trochlear nerves
  - Congenital ptosis: oculomotor nerve
- Predominantly horizontal disorders of ocular motility:
  - *Duane syndrome*: abducens nerve
  - Horizontal gaze palsy with progressive scoliosis: abducens nerve
- Disorders with abnormalities of facial motility:
  - Facial nerve palsy
  - *Möbius syndrome*: abducens and facial nerves

A number of genetic loci and genes responsible for these disorders have been defined.

Reference

Gutowski N, Ellard S. The congenital cranial dysinnervation disorders (CCDDs). Adv Clin Neurosci Rehabil. 2005;5(3):8–10

Congenital insensitivity to pain

Congenital indifference to pain

Individuals with an inborn indifference or insensitivity to pain, or pain asymbolia, have been described throughout the centuries. It is likely that many of these individuals in fact have a *hereditary sensory and autonomic neuropathy (HSAN)*. Congential insensitivity to pain and anhidrosis (CIPA) is classified as HSAN types IV and V, associated with mutations in a gene encoding a receptor for Nerve Growth Factor (NGF). Clinical features include acroparesthesia and Charcot joints. Although it might be supposed that, since mutilation is painless, it is the loss of pain sensation that results in mutilation, it has been noted that when other sensory modalities persist such deformity does not occur.

Reference

Critchley M. The Divine Banquet of the Brain and Other Essays. New York: Raven; 1979:194–202
Larner AJ, Moss J, Rossi ML, Anderson M. Congenital insensitivity to pain: a 20 year follow up. J Neurol Neurosurg Psychiatry. 1994;57:973–974
Sternbach RA. Congenital insensitivity to pain: a critique. Psychol Bull. 1963;60: 252–264

Congenital muscle and neuromuscular disorders: overview

Many muscle and neuromuscular disorders are inherited and hence might be labeled "congenital," *viz.:*

- Muscular dystrophies
- Spinal muscular atrophies
- Hereditary neuropathies
- Myotonic disorders
- Various myopathies

However, the label "congenital" has been used specifically for

- *Congenital muscular dystrophies*
- *Congenital myasthenic syndromes*
- Congenital myopathies:
  - Central core disease
  - Nemaline myopathy
  - Myotubular/centronuclear myopathy
  - Multi-minicore disease
  - Desmin-related myopathy
  - Ullrich's congenital muscular dystrophy

References

Rakowicz W. Congenital myopathies and muscular dystrophies. Adv Clin Neurosci Rehabil. 2003;2(6):11–13
Taratuto AL. Congenital myopathies and related disorders. Curr Opin Neurol. 2002;15:553–561

Congenital muscular dystrophies: overview

This heterogeneous group of autosomal recessive disorders presents with hypotonia and weakness at birth or in the first few months of life, with or without mental retardation. Some are static, some progress, with or without respiratory muscle involvement. A number of phenotypes are defined within this group, including:

- "Pure" congenital muscular dystrophy.
- Fukuyama-type congenital muscular dystrophy: found almost exclusively in Japan; child is born with profound hypotonia, muscle wasting, and weakness. Additional features include severe mental retardation, seizures, skull asymmetry, and the development of joint contractures. Creatine kinase may be elevated. The condition is linked to chromosome 9q, with deficiency of the protein fukutin.
- Muscle-eye-brain (MEB) disease (of Santavuori): characterized by eye abnormalities in addition to neuronal migration defects. Clinical features are mental retardation, severe myopia, retinal dysplasia, cataracts, and optic atrophy, but children are usually able to stand and walk. Survival to the second decade is common, occasionally to adulthood. Linked to chromosome 1p32–34 and a defect in the protein glycosyltransferase.
- *Rigid spine syndrome.*
- Walker–Warburg syndrome (WWS), also known as cerebro-ocular dysplasia, Chemke syndrome, Pagon syndrome: "HARD + E syndrome" = *H*ydrocephalus (usually aqueduct stenosis), *A*gyria (type II lissencephaly: neuronal migration defect), *R*etinal *d*ysplasia, microphthalmia (thought to be less severe and consistent than in muscle-eye-brain disease), *E*ncephalocoele, +/– cerebellar malformations, severe developmental retardation.

Neurogenetic studies have defined a number of loci and proteins aberrant in these disorders:

	Gene locus	Protein defect
	6q	Laminin α2 (merosin)
	12q	Laminin receptor (α7 integrin)
Fukuyama dystrophy	9q	Fukutin
Rigid spine syndrome	1p	Selenoprotein
Muscle-eye-brain disease	1p	Glycosyltransferase

No specific treatment available. Few walk; contractures may be prominent. Feeding and respiratory problems are the usual cause of death.

References

Dubowitz V. Congenital muscular dystrophies. In: Emery AEH, ed. Diagnostic Criteria for Neuromuscular Disorders. 2nd ed. London: Royal Society of Medicine Press; 1997:23–26
Williams RS, Swisher CN, Jennings M, Ambler M, Caviness VS Jr. Cerebro-ocular dysgenesis (Walker-Warburg syndrome): neuropathologic and etiologic analysis. Neurology. 1984;34:1531–1541

Congenital myasthenic syndromes: overview

The congenital myasthenic syndromes may be classified according to the pattern of inheritance and the site of the defect:

- Type I: Autosomal recessive:
  - CMS type 1a: familial infantile myasthenia syndrome
  - CMS type 1b: limb girdle myasthenic syndrome
  - CMS type 1c: acetylcholinesterase deficiency syndrome
  - CMS type 1d: acetylcholine receptor deficiency syndrome
- Type II: Autosomal dominant:
  - CMS type 2a: slow channel syndrome
- Type III: No family history:
  - CMS type 3: all other patients younger than 12 years with AChR antibody negative fatiguable weakness and neurophysiological evidence of neuromuscular transmission defect and lacking features of any of the other categories

Transient neonatal myasthenia and arthrogryposis multiplex congenita in the offspring of mothers with myasthenia gravis, although presenting at birth, are not included under the rubric of congenital myasthenic syndromes because of the association with anti-AChR antibodies of maternal origin which cross the placenta.

Mutations in 11 different genes have been identified to date in congenital myasthenic syndromes, including ligand-gated nicotinic acetylcholine receptor channels (subunits α_1, β_1, δ, and ϵ), hence *channelopathies*, and DOK7.

Investigation

Bloods: antibodies to AChR are not present and indeed are counted as exclusion criteria for these diagnoses. Neurophysiology (EMG/NCS) is the key investigation, showing decremental response with repetitive stimulation and jitter/block on single fiber studies, indicative of neuromuscular transmission defect. Muscle biopsy may show tubular aggregates in type 1b; morphological evidence of AChE deficiency in type 1c; reduced AChR in type 1d.

Differential diagnosis

Other forms of neonatal/infantile weakness, other defects of neuromuscular transmission.

Treatment and prognosis

No specific treatment available; unlike autoimmune *myasthenia gravis*, CMS do not respond to plasma exchange and immunosuppressive therapy.

Diagnostic criteria

Middleton LT. Congenital myasthenic syndromes. In: Emery AEH, ed. Diagnostic Criteria for Neuromuscular Disorders. 2nd ed. London: Royal Society of Medicine Press; 1997:91–97

References

Engel AG, Ohno K, Sine SM. Congenital myasthenic syndromes: recent advances. Arch Neurol. 1999;56:163–167
Palace J, Beeson D. The congenital myasthenic syndromes. J Neuroimmunol. 2008; 201-202:2–5

Copper deficiency-associated myeloneuropathy

Human Swayback disease

A myeloneuropathy clinically resembling *subacute combined degeneration of the spinal cord* due to *vitamin B$_{12}$ deficiency* has been reported in individuals with acquired copper deficiency due to intestinal resection, sometimes with concurrent hematological abnormalities (microcytic anemia, neutropenia). The diagnosis should be considered in individuals with risk factors for copper deficiency such as malabsorption, prolonged parenteral nutrition, malnutrition, or excessive zinc therapy. Serum copper and ceruloplasmin are low. MR imaging of the spinal cord may show dorsal column increased signal. Oral copper supplementation may halt neurological deterioration. This condition may be the human equivalent of a neurodegenerative disorder of ruminants (enzootic ataxia, Swayback disease) caused by copper deficiency.

References

Kumar N. Copper deficiency myelopathy (human swayback). Mayo Clin Proc. 2006;81:1371–1384

Jaiser SR, Duddy M. Copper deficiency masquerading as subacute combined degeneration of the cord and myelodysplastic syndrome. Adv Clin Neurosci Rehabil. 2007;7(5):20–21

Schleper B, Stuerenburg HJ. Copper deficiency-associated myelopathy in a 46-year old woman. J Neurol. 2001;248:705–706

Corticobasal degeneration (CBD)

Cortical-basal ganglionic degeneration

Corticobasal degeneration (CBD) is a rare late-onset neurodegenerative disorder of unknown etiology that is characterized by a movement disorder, an asymmetric akinetic-rigid syndrome with marked dyspraxia, involuntary movements, and alien limb/hand behavior, in combination with a cognitive disorder (cortical dementia). Early descriptions emphasized the movement disorder, but subsequently the prominence of the cognitive disorder has been increasingly recognized. Neuropathologically the condition is distinct, characterized by nerve cell loss and gliosis in the cortex, underlying white matter, thalamus, lentiform nucleus, subthalamic nucleus, red nucleus, midbrain tegmentum, substantia nigra, and locus ceruleus. Many residual nerve cells are swollen and chromatolyzed with eccentric nuclei (achromasia). Neuronal inclusions resembling the globose neurofibrillary tangles of *progressive supranuclear palsy* may be present in the substantia nigra. This disorder is a *tauopathy*. Phenocopies are not uncommon. There is currently no effective pharmacotherapy.

Clinical features

- Movement disorder:
  - "Classical" clinical picture is of a chronic progressive asymmetric rigidity with apraxia (PARA syndrome):
  - +/– Apraxic limb sometimes displaying an alien limb syndrome
  - +/– Dystonia
  - +/– Myoclonus: action-induced, stimulus-sensitive

- – +/– Less common features include supranuclear gaze palsy, dysarthria, ataxia, chorea, blepharospasm, corticospinal tract signs
  - – +/– Cortical sensory dysfunction
- Cognitive disorder:
  - – Deficits of sustained attention and verbal fluency (as in *Alzheimer's disease*) + deficits of praxis, finger tapping, and motor programming.
  - – Cases presenting with features of *frontotemporal lobar degeneration* without motor disorder have been reported, as have patients with parieto-occipital (Balint-like) cortical dysfunction, and a combination of dementia, parkinsonism, and motor neurone disease.

Neuropsychiatric/behavioral disorders may also occur.

Investigation

Neuroimaging: structural imaging (CT/MRI) may show asymmetric frontoparietal atrophy; functional imaging (SPECT, PET) may show reduced tracer uptake in striatum and medial frontal cortex. CSF may show nonspecific elevation of protein. Neurophysiology: no diagnostic features in EEG, EMG/NCS, SSEP, although nonspecific abnormalities may occur. Neuropsychology may show cortical deficits, especially of frontal type, with deficits of praxis.

Differential diagnosis

- Neurodegenerative conditions with parkinsonian features: idiopathic *Parkinson's disease* (usually begins asymmetrically but then spreads contralaterally); progressive supranuclear palsy; *multiple system atrophy*; *Creutzfeldt–Jakob disease (CJD)*.
- A number of cortical dementias may also enter the differential: Alzheimer's disease (AD), other causes of frontotemporal lobar degeneration.
- Phenocopies with non-CBD pathology are well described, including AD, FTLD of Pick type, and occasional cases of motor neurone disease dementia, CJD, or nonspecific histology. Hence, it is suggested that all clinically diagnosed cases be labeled "corticobasal degeneration syndrome" until histology is available to permit definitive classification.

Treatment and prognosis

The syndrome is essentially unresponsive to levodopa, although a therapeutic trial is often given. Clonazepam may be useful for action tremor/myoclonus.

Severe rigidity with immobility is common within 3–5 years of disease onset. Death usually occurs within 7–10 years of onset.

Diagnostic criteria

Boeve BF, Lang AE, Litvan I. Corticobasal degeneration and its relationship to progressive supranuclear palsy and frontotemporal dementia. Ann Neurol. 2003; 54(Suppl 5): S15–S19
Dickson DW, Bergeron C, Chin SS, et al. Office of Rare Diseases neuropathologic criteria for corticobasal degeneration. J Neuropathol Exp Neurol. 2002;61:935–946

References

Doran M, du Plessis DG, Enevoldson TP, Fletcher NA, Ghadiali E, Larner AJ. Pathological heterogeneity of clinically diagnosed corticobasal degeneration. J Neurol Sci. 2003;216:127–134
Mahapatra RK, Edwards MJ, Schott JM, Bhatia KP. Corticobasal degeneration. Lancet Neurol. 2004;3:736–743

Cough headache

Hindbrain headache

Cough headache may occur as a primary *headache* syndrome, in which a sudden severe headache, usually occipital or suboccipital in location, develops on coughing or other activities, such as sneezing, laughing, or lifting heavy objects, which involve a Valsalva maneuver. Headache lasts seconds to minutes, occasionally hours, and is described as bursting or explosive. It is not associated with persistently raised intracranial pressure and treatment is rarely required; analgesic preparations such as indomethacin or anti-migraine therapies may be tried. This is usually an isolated and benign condition. However, symptomatic, structural causes must be sought for cough headache, particularly lesions of the foramen magnum (e.g., *Chiari malformations*) or posterior fossa (e.g., tumor, AVM).

References

Chen PK, Fuh JL, Wang SJ. Cough headache: a study of 83 consecutive patients. Cephalalgia. 2009;29:1079–1085
Pascual J, Iglesias F, Oterino A, et al. Cough, exertional, and sexual headaches: an analysis of 72 benign and symptomatic cases. Neurology. 1996;46:1520–1524

Cramp fasciculation syndrome

Benign fasciculation with cramps syndrome, Denny-Brown, Foley syndrome

This is the suggested name for the syndrome of benign fasciculations with cramps, with no associated muscle wasting or weakness, which distinguish it from progressive anterior horn cell disease such as *motor neurone disease* (*MND*). However, very occasional cases "evolving" to MND have been reported. Electrophysiologically, there is continuous motor unit activity which differs only quantitatively, rather than qualitatively, from that seen in neuromyotonia (*peripheral nerve hyperexcitability*). If troublesome, cramps may be treated with phenytoin, quinine, or chlorpromazine. The condition may lead to muscle hypertrophy.

Cranial polyneuropathy

Multiple cranial nerve palsies may accompany intrinsic brainstem disease, in which case long tract signs are also usually evident. The differential diagnosis of multiple cranial nerve palsies without evidence of intrinsic brainstem disease is broad, including:

- Infective:
  - Chronic meningitides:
    - Spirochetal (syphilis)
    - Fungal (cryptococcus, aspergillosis)
    - Mycobacterial (tuberculosis)
    - Mycoplasma
    - Viral (EBV, VZV)
- Granulomatous/vasculitis:
  - Neurosarcoidosis
  - Wegener's granulomatosis
  - Giant cell arteritis (rare)
- Metabolic:
  - Diabetes mellitus (usually mononeuropathy)
- Structural:
  - Neoplasia:
    - Primary: chordoma, meningioma of sphenoid ridge, glomus jugulare tumor
    - Secondary: metastasis, carcinomatous/lymphomatous meningitis
  - Aneurysm/dissection (rare)
- Oligosymptomatic Guillain–Barré syndrome
- Idiopathic cranial polyneuropathy: a syndrome characterized by subacute, constant, facial pain, often retro-orbital, followed by multiple cranial nerve palsies, often developing suddenly, including (in order of frequency)

III, IV, VI; V; VII; IX–XII. I and VIII are spared. All investigations for a cause of cranial polyneuropathy are negative. Characteristically, the ESR is raised, whereas the CRP is normal. The syndrome responds to steroids, and may be related to orbital pseudotumor (*"Tolosa–Hunt syndrome"*).

Other diagnoses to consider include Garcin syndrome and jugular foramen syndrome.

Investigation

Bloods: ESR; serology for possible infective agents. Neuroimaging (CT/MRI) may demonstrate structural lesions; enhancement of the meninges may suggest inflammatory or malignant infiltration. CSF: in addition to cell count, protein, and glucose, other studies may be needed, including Indian ink staining, cryptococcal antigen, cytology; may need to repeat CSF if initial study is inconclusive. Meningeal biopsy for tissue diagnosis may be contemplated if other investigations provide no specific answer, particularly if an infiltrative/inflammatory process seems possible.

References

Beal MF. Multiple cranial nerve palsies – a diagnostic challenge. N Engl J Med. 1990;322:461–463
Juncos JL, Beal MF. Idiopathic cranial polyneuropathy: a fifteen year experience. Brain. 1987;110:197–211

Craniopharyngioma

Craniopharyngiomas are tumors of the pituitary region which are thought to arise from the remnant of the embryological pouch of Rathke. Most occur in childhood; they are less common than tumors of the pituitary gland.

Clinical features

Craniopharyngiomas present with local compressive features, *viz.*:

- Visual symptoms: bitemporal hemianopia: often progressing from inferior to superior (cf. pituitary tumors, superior to inferior)
- Hypothalamic dysfunction: growth failure, diabetes insipidus, Froehlich's syndrome (obesity, gonadal underdevelopment)
- Raised intracranial pressure, headache
- Cognitive problems: amnesia due to mammillary body compression is reported

Investigation

Bloods for hypothalamic dysfunction, especially evidence of diabetes insipidus. Neuroimaging (MRI) often shows a tumor with increased signal on T_1-weighted scans due to cholesterol content.

Differential diagnosis

Other *pituitary disease* causing mass lesions.

Treatment and prognosis

The most urgent priority is correction of any endocrine disorders, followed by surgery if vision is threatened. There is a debate as to whether surgery should attempt total resection or partial resection followed by radiotherapy. If the capsule is densely adherent to surrounding structures partial removal is preferred. There is a tendency to recurrence; some authorities advocate periodic postoperative MRI.

Reference

Gottfried ON, Couldwell WT. Craniopharyngiomas. In: Bernstein M, Berger MS, eds. Neuro-oncology. The Essentials. 2nd ed. New York: Thieme; 2008:343–352

Creutzfeldt–Jakob disease (CJD)

Creutzfeldt–Jakob disease (CJD) is the prototypical human *prion disease*, occurring in sporadic, familial, and iatrogenic forms. The inherited (familial) form results from mutations within the prion protein (PrP) gene (*PRNP*). All forms of CJD are associated with accumulation of abnormal isoforms of the cellular prion protein, PrP[Sc] or PrP[Res], within the brain. *Variant Creutzfeldt–Jakob disease* (vCJD) probably results from infection with the agent which caused the epidemic of bovine spongiform encephalopathy (BSE) in British cattle in the 1980s, hence, sometimes known as "human BSE."

Clinical features

Sporadic CJD cases may present subacutely; inherited and iatrogenic variants may have a more insidious onset. Clinical features are heterogeneous and include:

- *Dementia*: subcortical and cortical features
- Cortical blindness (Heidenhain or visual variant)

- Cerebellar syndrome: Brownell–Oppenheimer (ataxic) variant
- Myoclonus
- Encephalopathy (Nevin–Jones syndrome); "epileptic" presentation (mimicking complex partial status epilepticus)
- Extrapyramidal syndrome; akinetic mutism
- Pyramidal signs
- Psychiatric disturbance (more common in vCJD, although may occur in CJD)
- Sensory symptoms and signs (especially vCJD: hyperpathia)
- Amyotrophy (muscle wasting)

If the diagnosis is suspected, a family history of similarly affected relatives should be sought, along with enquiries about exposure to recognized iatrogenic factors: corneal transplantation, dura mater grafts, intracranial electrodes, human pituitary-derived hormones (growth hormone, gonadotrophins).

Investigation

Bloods are normal. Neuroimaging: on CT/MRI brain atrophy may be evident; MR high signal change may be seen in the putamen and caudate head in sporadic CJD, and in posterior thalamus in vCJD (pulvinar sign). Functional imaging (SPECT, PET) may show multiple patchy perfusion abnormalities. CSF may show moderately elevated protein in sporadic CJD; protein markers of neuronal injury (Neuron Specific Enolase, 14-3-3) and glial activation (S100β) may be elevated but this finding is non-specific. EEG may show periodic complexes at a frequency of 1–2/s in a markedly abnormal background; these are the classical changes in CJD, although they may not develop until late in the disease (hence, repeated EEGs may be needed); atypical changes (focal changes, periodic lateralized epileptiform discharges) sometimes reminiscent of complex partial status epilepticus may also be seen. EEG is typically normal in vCJD. Neuropsychology: common features include epsiodic unresponsiveness, interference effects, verbal and motor perseverations, reflecting subcortical disease; +/− cortical features such as cortical blindness, auditory agnosia, language deficits.

Brain biopsy: spongiform vacuolation affecting any part of the cerebral grey matter (cases without spongiform change have also been described); astrocytic proliferation, gliosis; neuronal loss, synaptic degeneration; PrP-immunopositive amyloid plaques. Tonsil biopsy: may be helpful in diagnosis of vCJD if PrP-immunopositive staining is present. (In all biopsy cases, special care is needed to deal with the instruments used for the procedure.) Neurogenetic testing for PrP gene mutations (missense deletions, insertions) in inherited cases; in sporadic CJD gene analysis is normal.

Differential diagnosis

- Paraneoplastic encephalitis
- Complex partial status epilepticus
- Cerebrovascular disease with multi-infarct dementia
- Lithium intoxication
- Dementia with Lewy bodies
- Hashimoto's encephalopathy

Treatment and prognosis

No specific treatment currently known. Disease is uniformly fatal, often within weeks to months in sporadic CJD, although some inherited forms may survive for many years. Survival in vCJD may be more than a year.

Diagnostic criteria

Zerr I, Kallenberg K, Summers DM, et al. Updated clinical diagnostic criteria for sporadic Creutzfeldt-Jakob disease. Brain. 2009;132:2659–2668

References

Mallucci G, Collinge J. Update on Creutzfeldt-Jakob disease. Curr Opin Neurol. 2004; 17:641–647
Meissner B, Kallenberg K, Sanchez-Juan P, et al. MRI lesion profiles in sporadic Creutzfeldt-Jakob disease. Neurology. 2009;72:1994–2001

Critical illness myopathy, critical illness polyneuropathy

Three principal patterns of muscle involvement are recognized in patients requiring intensive care:

- Non-necrotizing "cachectic" myopathy
- Myopathy with selective loss of myosin filaments ("thick filament myopathy")
- Acute necrotizing myopathy of intensive care

The latter two entities may be triggered by use of steroids and neuromuscular blocking agents, but otherwise pathogenesis is obscure, presumed related to mediators of inflammation and multiple organ failure.

   Patients who have protracted stays on intensive care units may develop an acute or subacute symmetrical axonal polyneuropathy, especially if their course is complicated by sepsis and multiple organ failure. The motor nerves seem particularly affected, whereas cranial nerves and autonomic functions are spared. Unlike the situation in *Guillain–Barré syndrome*, which enters the differential diagnosis, CSF is normal. Slow recovery over a period of months may occur. Pathogenesis is not understood, but contributing factors may include drug toxicity, nutritional deficiency, and hyperpyrexia.

Reference

Zink W, Kollmar R, Schwab S. Critical illness polyneuropathy and myopathy in the intensive care unit. Nat Rev Neurol. 2009;5:372–379

Cryoglobulinemia, cryoglobulinemic neuropathy

Cryoglobulins are proteins that precipitate in the cold and dissolve when heated. They can occur in isolation or in association with either lymphoproliferative disorders such as *lymphoma* or chronic viral hepatitis (both hepatitis B and C). Cryoglobulinemia may be asymptomatic, as in mixed essential cryoglobulinemia, or symptomatic. The clinical features of cryoglobulinemia include purpura, polyarthralgia, *Raynaud's phenomenon*, skin vasculitis, and glomerulonephritis. The most common neurological feature is a vasculitic peripheral neuropathy. Central nervous system complications are rare, although a relapsing encephalopathy with abdominal pain, presumed ischemic, has been reported. Management involves avoidance of cold conditions, and treatment of the underlying condition, which in the majority of cases is a lymphoproliferative disorder.

Reference

Ince PG, Duffey P, Cochrane HR, Lowe J, Shaw PJ. Relapsing ischemic encephaloenteropathy and cryoglobulinemia. Neurology. 2000;55:1579–1581

Cryptococcosis

Torulosis

Cryptococcus neoformans is a saprophytic fungus. CNS infections with this organism were formerly rare, but became common in the context of *HIV/AIDS*, where it was the third most common CNS infection (and most common fungal infection) after HIV encephalopathy and *toxoplasma* encephalitis. It occurs most commonly in those with CD4 cell count <200/μL. Organ transplant recipients are also susceptible to cryptococcal infection.

Clinical features

- Cryptococcal meningitis: fever, headache, stiff neck, photophobia, although symptoms may be minimal or absent
- Cryptococcoma (toruloma): mass lesion of brain parenchyma; may cause raised intracranial pressure, cranial nerve palsy, hemiparesis, seizures
- Spinal lesions: rare
- Painful multiple radiculopathies

Investigation

Bloods: main diagnostic test is cryptococcal antigen testing which has high sensitivity and specificity; HIV status; CD4 count. Neuroimaging: CT shows low-density cyst-like lesions in basal ganglia, mesencephalon; MRI shows T_1 low signal intensity, T_2 high signal intensity, lesions +/– meningeal enhancement; enhancement of mass lesions uncommon. CSF may show elevated opening pressure; protein, cell count, and glucose may be normal or only marginally abnormal; Indian ink stain for hyphal threads is necessary, fungal culture; detection of cryptococcal antigen.

Differential diagnosis

- Toxoplasma encephalitis
- CNS *lymphoma*

Treatment and prognosis

Antifungal agents such as amphotericin or fluconazole may be used intravenously for 2–3 weeks or until symptoms resolve. Relapses occur and hence maintenance oral fluconazole may be given.

References

Chuck SL, Sande MA. Infections with Cryptococcus neoformans in the acquired immunodeficiency syndrome. N Engl J Med. 1989;321:580–584
Day JN. Cryptococcal meningitis. Pract Neurol. 2004;4:274–285

Cubital tunnel syndrome

This refers to a form of *ulnar neuropathy*, an *entrapment neuropathy* of the ulnar nerve within the fibro-osseous canal formed by the medial ligament of the elbow joint and the aponeurosis of flexor carpi ulnaris. Compression at this point may occur with ("tardy ulnar palsy") or without a prior history of elbow trauma.

Clinical features

- Sensory:
  - parasthesia, pain in ulnar division of fingers, hand and wrist
- Motor:
  - weakness of interossei, abductor digiti minimi, adductor pollicis, flexor pollicis brevis; atrophy, claw hand; flexor carpi ulnaris remains strong; median/radial innervated muscles unaffected (but beware "all ulnar hand")

Investigation

Neurophysiology (EMG/NCS) shows reduced ulnar SNAP and CMAP, +/– conduction block in motor fibers at the level of the elbow; fibrillation potentials in ulnar-innervated hand muscles.

Treatment and prognosis

Surgical decompression may be considered; splinting.

Reference

Palmer BA, Hughes TB. Cubital tunnel syndrome. J Hand Surg. 2010;35:153–163

Cyanide poisoning

Cyanide poisoning may occur acutely as a deliberate act, or chronically through exposure at work. Acute cases may be rapidly fatal since cyanide disrupts cellular mechanisms for carrying and utilizing oxygen with resultant tissue hypoxia. Survivors may manifest *parkinsonism*, *dementia*, and *dystonia*. In more chronic cases patients may develop epileptic seizures, *delirium*, and visual failure.

Cysts: overview

The term cyst is used to describe a number of fluid-filled lesions which may affect the nervous system.

- Developmental malformations representing trapped embryonic remnants. Lesions with an epithelial lining (mucus secreting columnar epithelium that may vary from low cuboidal to pseudostratified) may be called:
  - Neuroenteric cyst: in the spinal cord, posterior fossa; presumably of enteric origin
  - Neuroepithelial cyst: in the hemispheres; of ependymal origin
  - *Colloid cyst*: in the third ventricle
  - Rathke cleft cyst: in the sella; stomodeal origin
  - Dermoid, epidermoid cysts: misplaced ectoderm (may also be acquired)
  - *Tarlov cyst*: sacral nerve root
- Cystic space bounded by arachnoid membranes: *arachnoid cyst*, most commonly in region of sylvian fissure, anterior temporal lobe
- Cysts associated with parasitic infection: Cysticercosis, coenurosis, echinococcosis, paragonimiasis, trichinosis.
- Cystic swellings associated with tumors, for example, glioma, hemangioblastoma.

Many cysts are discovered incidentally when neuroimaging is performed for other indications. Occasionally arachnoid cysts, which are usually asymptomatic, may be associated with epileptic seizures, cognitive impairment, or raised intracranial pressure due to fluid accumulation.

Investigations

Neuroimaging: CT usually shows cysts as low attenuation lesions; contrast enhancement may be absent or confined to the rim. There may be compression of adjacent structures. Neuropathology: developmental cysts immunostain positive for cytokeratin or epithelial membrane antigen (EMA) but not for glial fibrillary acidic protein (GFAP).

Differential diagnosis

Cysts may present as space-occupying lesions, requiring differentiation from tumor, hematoma, and abscess.

Treatment and prognosis

Surgical decompression or removal may be required if there are compressive symptoms. Parasitic cysts require appropriate chemotherapy; there may be difficulties with surgical approach (e.g., echinococcosis).

Reference

Sartor K, Haehnel S, Kress B. Brain Imaging. Stuttgart: Thieme; 2008:181–198

Cytomegalovirus (CMV) infection: overview

Infection with cytomegalovirus (CMV), a member of the herpesvirus family, may be associated with various neurological syndromes:

- Intrauterine infection:
  - Stillbirth, prematurity; granulomatous encephalitis
  - Epileptic seizures, focal signs, mental retardation in survivors
  - Periventricular calcification seen on skull radiographs, brain CT
  - Meningitis, myelitis, deafness and vertigo
- Adult infection (rare):
  - Infectious mononucleosis-like illness
  - *Encephalitis*
  - *Meningitis*
  - *Guillain–Barré syndrome*

CMV has also been implicated in some cases of Reye's syndrome, and *Rasmussen's syndrome.*

Opportunistic cytomegalovirus infection in HIV/AIDS may cause retinitis, encephalitis, mononeuritis multiplex, cauda equina syndrome. Complement fixation tests, neutralization tests, and polymerase chain reaction tests are available for diagnosis, as well as culture from urine, saliva, or liver biopsy specimens. Ganciclovir may be beneficial for some CMV infections.

D

Dandy–Walker syndrome

The Dandy–Walker syndrome is a developmental abnormality characterized by a failure of development of the midline portion of the cerebellum, which results in a cyst-like enlargement of the fourth ventricle, with bulging of the occipital bone posteriorly and upward displacement of the tentorium and torcula. There may be associated agenesis of the corpus callosum, dilatation of the central aqueduct and third and lateral ventricles, and aplasia of the cerebellar vermis. There is sometimes a tendency for radiologists to overdiagnose a large cisterna magna in adult patients as "Dandy–Walker syndrome."

Danon disease [OMIM#300257]

LAMP-2 deficiency

Danon disease is an X-linked disorder due to mutations in the gene encoding the lysosomal associated membrane protein LAMP-2 and is characterized by marked clinical heterogeneity, including cardiomyopathy, vacuolar myopathy, variable learning disability and asymptomatic hyperCKemia. The myopathy is proximal and often mild in comparison with the cardiomyopathy. Creatine kinase may be elevated (ca. 1000 U/L). Muscle biopsy shows a vacuolar myopathy and there may be deposition of membrane attack complex on vacuolated fibers. Muscle biopsies and cultured skin fibroblasts show a lack of LAMP2 immunostaining. Clinically, the condition may appear similar to Pompe disease, but the α-glucosidase levels are normal. Affected males often die in the second to third decade; carrier females may manifest a cardiomyopathy and die in the third to fifth decade.

References

Di Mauro S, Tanji K, Hirano M. LAMP-2 deficiency (Danon disease). Acta Myologica. 2007;26:79–82
Nishino I, Fu J, Tanji K, et al. Primary LAMP-2 deficiency causes X-linked vacuolar cardiomyopathy and myopathy (Danon disease). Nature. 2000;406:906–910

Dawidenkow syndrome

Kaeser syndrome, Scapuloperoneal syndrome

Dawidenkow's syndrome is a rare neurogenic *scapuloperoneal syndrome*, with amyotrophy and associated distal sensory loss, nerve hypertrophy, and pes cavus. It resembles myogenic scapuloperoneal syndromes, for example, in *facioscapulohumeral dystrophy*, *Emery–Dreifuss syndrome*, and phosphofructokinase deficiency but is thought to be related to the hereditary motor and sensory neuropathies.

References

Schwartz MS, Swash M. Scapuloperoneal atrophy with sensory involvement: Dawidenkow's syndrome. J Neurol Neurosurg Psychiatry. 1975;38:1063–1067
Serratrice G, Pélissier JF, Pouget J. Trois cas d'amyotrophie scapulopéronière neurogène (syndrome de Dawidenkow): situation nosologique par rapport à la maladie de Charcot-Marie-Tooth. Revue Neurol. 1984;140:738–740

Deafferentation pain syndrome

Deafferentation, for example, after brachial root avulsion in a motorcycle accident, may result in a syndrome of spontaneous painful dysaesthesia without allodynia or hyperalgesia, known as deafferentation syndrome. Management of the painful useless limb is difficult; amputation does not result in pain relief. If pharmacotherapy for neuropathic pain fails, surgical options include dorsal root entry zone section.

Degos Disease

Kohlmeier–Degos disease, Malignant atrophic papulosis

Degos disease is a very rare cause of cerebral and spinal cord (and gut) ischemic events due to endothelial proliferation in small arteries, along with characteristic skin lesions consisting of crops of painless, occasionally itchy, pinkish papules on the trunk and limbs, which heal as circular porcelain-white scars (atrophic papulosis).

Reference

Subbiah P, Wijdicks E, Muenter M, et al. Skin lesion with a fatal neurologic outcome (Degos' disease). Neurology. 1996;46:636–640

Déjerine–Mouzon syndrome

Pseudothalamic syndrome

The Déjerine–Mouzon syndrome, first described in 1914–1915, is one of the sensory syndromes with parietal lobe lesions (cf. *Verger–Déjerine syndrome*). Déjerine–Mouzon syndrome is characterized by hypoaesthesia for all primary sensory modalities (touch, pain, temperature, vibration, and joint position sense) contralateral to the lesion, sometimes associated with hyperpathia. Circumscribed lesions producing sensory deficits with an apparently radicular or truncal distribution are recognized, these being examples of false-localizing signs. Déjerine–Mouzon syndrome is usually due to a vascular event involving the parietal branch of the middle cerebral artery, and often improves with time. It is easily confused with the sensory loss seen with a thalamic lesion affecting the sensory relay nuclei (the *Déjerine–Roussy syndrome*) and hence is sometimes known as the pseudothalamic syndrome.

Reference

Capasso M, Manzoli C, Ciccocioppo F, Caulo M, Uncini A. A misleading sensory level. J Neurol. 2009;256:1769–1770

Déjerine–Roussy syndrome

The Déjerine–Roussy syndrome, first described in 1906, is characterized by contralateral sensory loss due to a lesion, typically vascular but occasionally neoplastic, in the ventroposterolateral (VPL) and posteromedial (VPM) nuclei of the thalamus. The sensory loss is most frequently for joint position sense, pain, and temperature. There may be associated transient hemiparesis with or without homonymous hemianopia, with on occasion taste distortion, athetosis of the hand, and depression. With partial recovery the patient may be left with spontaneous pain or discomfort in the region of the sensory loss, so-called thalamic pain, which has an unpleasant, diffuse, and lingering quality, often resistant to standard analgesia. Delayed onset of involuntary movements following stroke in the posterolateral thalamus was also reported by Déjerine and Roussy. This may take the form of dystonia, athetosis, and chorea, associated with position sensory loss (hence, appropriately designated "pseudochoreoathetosis"); or tremor and myoclonus, associated with cerebellar ataxia. Central post-stroke pain syndromes may occur with lesions outside the thalamus, and only about a quarter of patients with classic VPL thalamic strokes develop central post-stroke pain.

References

Déjerine J, Roussy J. Le syndrome thalamique. Revue Neurol (Paris). 1906;14: 521–532

Kim JS. Delayed onset mixed involuntary movements after thalamic stroke. Clinical, radiological and pathophysiological findings. Brain. 2001:124:299–309

Déjerine–Sottas syndrome (DSS) [OMIM#145900]

Hereditary motor and sensory neuropathy type III (HMSN III)

Déjerine–Sottas syndrome describes a severe peripheral demyelinating (or more correctly "hypomyelinating") neuropathy that falls within the rubric of *hereditary motor and sensory neuropathy*. Clinical features include early age at onset, reduced motor nerve conduction velocities (<12 m/s), absent sensory nerve action potentials (usually), and pronounced demyelination in nerve biopsy specimens. The phenotype is genetically heterogeneous, with autosomal dominant and recessive forms, and associated mutations identified in the genes encoding PMP22, MPZ (P_0), EGR2, and PRX, known to be associated with types of *Charcot–Marie–Tooth disease*, particularly CMT1 and CMT4. Although most patients have a severe disorder and become wheelchair-dependent, others remain ambulant into later life.

Reference

Gabreëls-Festen, A. Dejerine-Sottas syndrome grown to maturity: overview of genetic and morphological heterogeneity and follow-up of 25 patients. J Anat. 2002;200:341–356

Delirium: overview

Acute brain syndrome, Acute confusional state, Toxic-metabolic encephalopathy

Delirium (from the Latin meaning "out of furrow") is an organic neurobehaviorial disorder characterized by the acute onset of a fluctuating level of attention; there is disorganized thinking accompanied by global cognitive or behavioral abnormalities, with or without an altered level of consciousness (ranging from drowsiness to hypervigilance). It is a common occurrence in hospital in-patients, especially in the elderly and in the ITU setting. It is more likely to occur in individuals with preexisting cerebral pathology or cognitive impairment, and therefore overlaps with dementia. No consistent pathological abnormalities are seen at postmortem examination.

The pathogenesis of delirium is usually multifactorial, although no cause is identified in 5–20% of cases:

- Metabolic and endocrine abnormalities: hypoglycemia, diabetes mellitus, renal failure, hyponatremia, liver failure, anemia, hypercalcemia, thyroid disease, disseminated intravascular coagulopathy, thrombotic thrombocytopenic purpura (TTP), hyperviscosity states
- Infection:
  - Systemic: urinary tract infection, septicemia, pneumonia (especially the atypical pneumonias), particularly in the elderly; malaria
  - CNS: meningitis, encephalitis; occasionally AIDS
- Vascular: cerebrovascular accidents in the elderly, especially right middle cerebral artery and left posterior cerebral artery territory events; hypertensive encephalopathy
- Epileptic: either post-ictally or in some cases of non-convulsive status epilepticus
- Drug-induced:
  - Drug/solvent abuse in the younger patient
  - Sedatives, hypnotics, antidepressants, anticholinergics, anti-parkinsonian, and steroid therapy, especially in the elderly
- Drug withdrawal: for example, alcohol (Wernicke's encephalopathy) with delirium tremens; barbiturates, benzodiazepines, amphetamine, and cocaine
- Significant head injury
- Brain tumors
- Others: fractured bones +/− fat emboli; paraneoplastic (limbic) encephalitis; systemic lupus erythematosus; porphyria; vitamin B_{12} deficiency; heavy metal poisoning

Recognized risk factors for the development of delirium include:

- Older age groups (biological age more significant than chronological age)
- Preexisting cerebral pathology or cognitive impairment
- Previous history of delirium
- History of substance abuse or dependency
- Use of psychotropic and analgesic medication
- Medical procedures
- Active infective processes
- AIDS
- Serious burns
- Numerous co-morbid conditions

Overall, delirium occurs in 10–35% of all patients in a general hospital.

Clinical features

- Acute onset with fluctuating course, developing over hours or days; often with periods of normality, but typically worse at night.
- Attentional deficits: the patient is distractable, shows disorganized thinking, may have rambling incoherent speech with a degree of perseveration. This is associated with disorientation (in time > place > person) and memory disturbances.
- There are often perceptual disturbances with misidentifications (= illusions), more common than hallucinations (usually visual).
- Altered level of consciousness may occur, varying from hypoactivity and mutism to hyperactivity and general motor overactivity (e.g., in cases of alcohol withdrawal), sometimes with aggressive behavior. In addition, there is often disruption of the normal sleep–wake cycle.
- Mood disturbances are common, often with marked lability.
- Collateral history from the family, friends (e.g., cognitive state prior to admission); drug history.

Investigation

Bloods: first-line investigations in all patients: FBC, ESR, blood film, U+Es, glucose, liver function tests, calcium and phosphate, blood cultures, arterial blood gases. Additional investigations if no cause identified with first-line investigations: clotting, fibrin degradation products (FDPs), blood viscosity, ammonia, thyroid function tests, and serology (infection; syphilis; HIV disease; autoantibodies including anti-neuronal antibodies).
Urinalysis: infection, porphyria screen, drug screen, fat.
Imaging: CXR; CT/MRI head, +/– search for fractured bones/neoplasia.
Neurophysiology: EEG may typically show slowing, the degree of which correlates well with the clinical status of the patient. Occasionally, faster activity (e.g., in delirium tremens), or ictal activity is seen.
CSF: cell count, protein, glucose, oligoclonal bands, Gram stain, culture (infection, inflammation); fat.

Differential diagnosis

- Dementia: chronic confusional state; but may underlie episodes of delirium. Delirium may be the presenting feature of an underlying dementia syndrome.
- Psychiatric disorders: for example, schizophrenia, depression, mania, attention deficit disorder, autism, dissociative disorders, Ganser's syndrome.
- Aphasic syndromes (especially Wernicke-type aphasia).

Treatment and prognosis

Find reversible causes and correct them; particularly, give thiamine and/or glucose if there is any possibility of alcoholism or hypoglycemia. Reduce conflicting and changing sensory stimuli: patient should ideally be nursed in a simple, uncluttered, unchanging immediate environment, and remain in the same bed while on the ward, with adequate lighting and limited noise. Contact should be restricted to a few nurses and doctors; all instructions should be clear and simple; ensure glasses, hearing aids, dentures are all in place. Relatives and friends may visit regularly and encourage patient with questions on orientation and objects from home. Do not interrupt sleep.

Drug therapy: avoid if possible because there is no evidence base. If needed (especially in the hyperactive patient at risk to him/herself or to others), agents that may be used include haloperiodol (~1.5–20 mg/day orally) or lorazepam (initially 0.5–1 mg od).

The outlook is generally good but dependent on the precipitating and predisposing conditions in each patient. Overall, the diagnosis of delirium carries with it an increased mortality rate, especially if it is not recognized and treated. Prevention, by identifying at-risk patients at the time of admission to hospital, is possible.

References

Inouye SK. Current concepts: delirium in older persons. N Engl J Med. 2006;354:1157–1165

Larner AJ. Delirium: diagnosis, aetiopathogenesis and treatment. Adv Clin Neurosci Rehabil. 2004;4(2):28–29

Lindesay J, Rockwood K, Macdonald A, eds. Delirium in Old Age. Oxford: Oxford University Press; 2002

Royal College of Physicians. The Prevention, Diagnosis and Management of Delirium in Older People. London: Royal College of Physicians; 2006

Royal College of Psychiatrists. Who Cares Wins: Improving the Outcome for Older People Admitted to the General Hospital. Report of a working group for the Faculty of Old Age Psychiatry. London: Royal College of Psychiatrists; 2005

Siddiqi N, House AO, Holmes JD. Occurrence and outcome of delirium in medical in-patients: a systematic literature review. Age Ageing. 2006;35:350–364

Dementia: overview

Chronic brain syndrome

Dementia has been variously defined as a progressive loss of cognitive function, usually, but not invariably, with memory impairment, without a deficit of arousal or attention (cf. *delirium*), which is sufficient to interfere with social or occupational function. Hence, by this definition, dementia may be absent in some disorders with a diagnostic label of "dementia" (e.g., early in the course of dementia with Lewy bodies, frontotemporal dementia).

Dementia occurs in many conditions, most often (over 90% of cases) due to neurodegeneration, as in *Alzheimer's disease (AD)* and *frontotemporal lobar degeneration (FTLD)* syndromes, or due to cerebrovascular disease, for example, due to multiple infarcts. Overlap of pathologies (e.g., AD plus cerebrovascular disease) is also common. The prevalence of dementia increases exponentially with age: 1% of people aged 60 years are affected, and up to 50% by the age of 85 years. Although rare, treatable causes of dementing illness must be sought.

Dementia may be classified according to the pattern of neuropsychological deficits, which correlate with areas of involvement within the CNS, and by histopathology (although this is seldom available antemortem). A distinction is sometimes made on neuropsychological grounds between cortical and subcortical dementia syndromes. Cortical dementias are characterized by amnesia, aphasia, apraxia, agnosia, in isolation or combination: examples include AD and FTLD. Subcortical dementias are associated with slowing of cognitive speed with a frontal pattern of cognitive deficits (ranging from apathy to disinhibition, with or without extrapyramidal signs such as akinesia); examples include *progressive supranuclear palsy (PSP)* and *Huntington's disease (HD)*. However, the division between cortical and subcortical dementias is not absolute and this terminology is not universally used.

The clinical picture does not always reliably predict the neuropathological substrate. Neuroimaging techniques and neurophysiological studies may sometimes assist in the diagnosis of dementing disorders.

Dementia may be classified according to etiology:

- Neurodegeneration:
  - Relatively pure dementia syndrome:
    - Alzheimer's disease, or dementia of the Alzheimer type (DAT): accounts for ~70% of all dementia cases
    - Frontotemporal lobar degeneration (encompasses *Pick's disease*): accounts for ~ 1–5% of all cases of dementia
  - "Dementia plus" syndromes:
    - + Motor neurone involvement:
      - Frontotemporal lobar degeneration with motor neurone disease (FTLD/MND)
    - + Basal ganglia involvement:
      - Parkinson's disease dementia (PDD)
      - Dementia with Lewy bodies (DLB)
      - Huntington's disease (HD)
      - Progressive supranuclear palsy (PSP)
      - Corticobasal degeneration (CBD)
    - + Cerebellar involvement:
      - Some autosomal dominant cerebellar ataxias (ADCA type I)

- Cerebrovascular diseases:
  - Multiple infarcts
  - Strategic infarcts, for example, bilateral paramedian thalamic infarction
  - *Binswanger's disease*/encephalopathy
  - Recurrent hemorrhages (e.g., *cerebral amyloid angiopathy*)
  - *CADASIL*
- Metabolic disorders:
  - *Wilson's disease*
  - *Leukodystrophies*
  - *Mitochondrial disease*
  - Lipid-storage disorders
  - *Obstructive sleep apnea-hypopnea syndrome (OSAHS)*
  - Aminoacidopathies
- Endocrine and nutritional disorders:
  - Thiamine deficiency
  - Hypothyroidism
  - Cushing's disease
  - *Vitamin B$_{12}$ deficiency*
- Cell-mediated inflammatory CNS disease:
  - *Multiple sclerosis*
  - *Neurosarcoidosis*
  - *Behçet's disease*
  - Cerebral vasculitis or vasculopathy (e.g., Sjögren's syndrome)
- Antibody-mediated encephalopathies:
  - *Hashimoto's encephalopathy*
  - *Limbic encephalitis* with anti-Voltage Gated Potassium channel (VGKC) antibody
  - *NMDA receptor encephalitis*
  - Neuropsychiatric *systemic lupus erythematosus*
- Neoplasia:
  - Brain tumors
  - Paraneoplastic syndromes (limbic encephalitis)
- Structural disorders:
  - *Dural arteriovenous fistula*
  - *Normal pressure hydrocephalus (NPH)*
  - *Subdural hematoma*
  - Strategically placed tumors (e.g., fornix)
- Infection:
  - *Neurosyphilis*
  - *HIV/AIDS*, and complications thereof: cryptococcus, *progressive multifocal leukoencephalopathy (PML)*
  - *Whipple's disease*
  - *Prion disease*

- Drug-induced:
  - Alcoholism, +/– thiamine deficiency
  - Drug-induced cognitive impairment (especially anticholinergic agents)

Clinical features

- History of memory difficulties, behavioral change, impaired functional capacities (instrumental and basic activities of daily living), psychiatric symptoms (hallucinations, delusions).
- Collateral history from spouse, relative, carer, or someone who knows the patient well is an essential part of the assessment, as the patient may not be aware of problems if amnesic (cognitive anosognosia).
- Drug history, dietary history.
- Family history of cognitive disorder.

Investigation

Neuropsychology or psychometry: simple bedside screening tests (e.g., Mini-Mental State Examination [MMSE], Addenbrooke's Cognitive Examination-Revised [ACE]) may be sufficient; sometimes more detailed and time-consuming assessments, including IQ (e.g., WAIS-R), memory, language, perception, frontal lobe, or executive function tests may be required.

Bloods: first-line investigations in all patients: FBC, ESR, U+Es, glucose, liver function tests, calcium and phosphate, thyroid function tests: usually negative. Additional investigations in certain circumstances: blood film; vitamin B_{12}, autoantibodies, red blood cell transketolase, syphilis serology (VDRL-TPHA), full vasculitic screen, copper and caeruloplasmin, white cell enzymes, urinary amino acids and organic acids, HIV test, *Borrelia* serology, anti-thyroid peroxidase or anti-thyroglobulin antibodies; anti-VGKC antibodies.

Neuroimaging: Structural: CT/MRI to exclude structural causes (NPH, subdural hematoma, tumor, lymphoma), which may potentially be reversible; for global or focal atrophy (AD, FTLD); vascular disease (may be incidental). Functional: SPECT/PET scan may reveal perfusion deficits of possible diagnostic value, for example, temporoparietal in Alzheimer's disease, frontal in frontotemporal dementia

CSF: to exclude infective or inflammatory causes.

Neurogenetics: familial AD (APP, presenilin-1, presenilin-2), FTLD (tau, progranulin), prion disease (PrP), subcortical dementias (HD), and some autosomal dominant cerebellar ataxias.

Neurophysiology: not often helpful, except in cases of suspected prion disease (periodic EEG changes in sporadic CJD) or seizure disorders; EEG generally remains normal in FTLD whereas slowing is usually seen in AD.

Brain biopsy: reserved for cases in which there is a high suspicion of potentially reversible causes, such as inflammatory conditions.

Other tests, according to suspected cause: carotid artery ultrasonography, echocardiography (multi-infarct disease), duodenal biopsy (Whipple's disease).

Differential diagnosis

- Delirium
- Psychiatric illness, especially depression and anxiety states
- Drug-induced cognitive impairment
- Poorly controlled epilepsy, non-convulsive status
- Purely subjective memory impairment, "worried well."

Treatment and prognosis

Reversible causes of dementia are rare. Specific treatments for dementia are few (e.g., cholinesterase inhibitors, memantine for AD). Treatment is most often supportive (information, advice, Day Center, respite care) and palliative. Prognosis in terms of survival depends on the underlying cause.

References

Burns A, O'Brien J, Ames D, eds. Dementia. 3rd ed. London: Hodder Arnold; 2005

Doran M. Diagnosis of presenile dementia. Br J Hosp Med. 1997;58:105–110

Knopman DS, DeKosky ST, Cummings JL, et al. Practice parameter: diagnosis of dementia (an evidence-based review). Report of the Quality Standards Subcommittee of the American Academy of Neurology. Neurology. 2001;56:1143–1153

Kurlan R, ed. Handbook of Secondary Dementias. New York: Taylor & Francis; 2006

Larner AJ. Neuropsychological Neurology. The Neurocognitive Impairments of Neurological Disorders. Cambridge: Cambridge University Press; 2008

Mendez MF, Cummings JL. Dementia: A Clinical Approach. 3rd ed. Boston, MA: Butterworth Heinemann; 2003

Waldemar G, Dubois B, Emre M et al. Recommendations for the diagnosis and management of Alzheimer's disease and other disorders associated with dementia: EFNS guideline. Eur J Neurol. 2007;14:e1–e26

Dementia with Lewy bodies (DLB)

Cortical Lewy body disease, Diffuse Lewy body disease, Lewy body dementia, Senile dementia of the Lewy body type

Dementia with Lewy bodies (DLB) is a neurodegenerative disorder causing a syndrome of dementia and parkinsonism, claimed by some to be second in frequency only to *Alzheimer's disease (AD)* as a cause of dementia.

Clinical features

- Cognitive disorder: usually the presenting feature; cortical dementia similar to AD but with more severe and early impairment of visuospatial function and visual memory. Also, cognitive performance tends to fluctuate from day to day, thought to represent an "unstable platform of attention."
- Visual hallucinations: very common; usually nonthreatening; often children or animals, often the patient retains insight that these are not really there ("pseudohallucinations"); a report of figures emerging from the television into the room may be given.
- Marked neuroleptic sensitivity: these drugs may cause clinical deterioration of both cognition and the extrapyramidal syndrome, and may hasten death (this sensitivity is not exclusive to DLB, but much more common in it than in other dementia syndromes).
- Parkinsonism: usually mild, and follows cognitive disorder; rarely asymmetrical, tremor not prominent (cf. idiopathic Parkinson's disease).
- Falls, syncopal episodes: autonomic failure, due to Lewy body pathology in autonomic ganglia, is the presumed cause, and autonomic failure may on occasion precede the emergence of DLB.
- *REM sleep behavior disorder (REMBD)*: may precede the onset of cognitive impairment by many years.
- Myoclonus may be observed.
- Depression may occur.

A very similar neuropsychological and neuropsychiatric picture may emerge in individuals with established idiopathic *Parkinson's disease*, and it seems likely that the pathological substrate of Parkinson's disease dementia (PDD) is identical to that in DLB, but with differing regional predominance at clinical onset.

Very rare cases with a DLB phenotype have been associated with genetic mutations in the genes encoding presenilin-1 gene (Δ440), α-synuclein (especially those with duplication and triplication of the gene), and in some LRRK2 positive cases of PD, but generally this is a sporadic condition.

Investigation

Bloods are unremarkable. Neuroimaging (CT/MRI) may show medial temporal lobe atrophy as in AD, or more generalized atrophic change. Functional imaging (SPECT/PET) may show the temporoparietal deficits said to be typical of AD but with additional occipital changes, perhaps reflecting the visuospatial dysfunction in DLB. Neurophysiology: EEG may show nonspecific abnormalities such as diffuse slowing; very occasionally, a periodic EEG similar to that seen in sporadic *Creutzfeldt–Jakob disease*, may be seen, which may lead to diagnostic confusion. CSF is usually normal. Neuropsychology: visuospatial deficits may be prominent, as may attentional deficits (leading to fluctuating performance), more so than memory deficits. Other investigations: sleep studies may be indicated if there is a clinical history suggesting REM sleep behavior disorder.

Pathology: Lewy bodies, positive for ubiquitin and α-synuclein, are evident throughout the cerebral cortex as well as in the brain stem; neuritic changes (Lewy neurites) are also seen, primarily in the hippocampus. Concurrent Alzheimer and cerebrovascular pathology may also be seen.

Differential diagnosis

Other cognitive disorders: AD, vascular dementia (fluctuations), prion disease (myoclonus; periodic EEG). Other parkinsonian syndromes: *progressive supranuclear palsy (PSP)* has a different clinical and cognitive profile.

Treatment and prognosis

Anti-parkinsonian medication may help parkinsonian features but exacerbate hallucinations. Cholinesterase inhibition with rivastigmine has been shown in a randomized double-blind placebo-controlled trial to improve attentional deficits and reduce hallucinations. Memantine may be of benefit. Symptomatic treatment may be given for concurrent sleep disorder (e.g., clonazepam for REM sleep behavior disorder). Avoid neuroleptics in any patient in whom the diagnosis of DLB is suspected. Untreated, the pace of the illness is said to be quicker than AD, with survival of 5–8 years.

References

McKeith I, Mintzer J, Aarsland D, et al. Dementia with Lewy bodies. Lancet Neurol. 2004;3:19–28
O'Brien J, McKeith I, Ames D, Chiu E, eds. Dementia with Lewy Bodies and Parkinson's Disease Dementia. London: Taylor & Francis; 2006

Dementia pugilistica

Boxer's dementia, Pugilistic encephalopathy, "Punch drunk syndrome"

Originally described in boxers (hence "punch drunk syndrome"), this is a syndrome of cognitive impairment following repeated head trauma; it may also occur in steeplechase jockeys after repeated falls. In addition to cognitive impairment, there may be dysarthria and a *parkinsonian syndrome* dominated by akinesia and variably responsive to levodopa. Brain imaging may show ventricular dilatation and a cavum septum pellucidum. Pathologically the condition is reminiscent of *Alzheimer's disease*, with neurofibrillary tangles, deposition of amyloid β-peptide, and diffuse neuronal loss.

Reference

Schmidt ML, Zhukareva V, Newell KL, Lee VM, Trojanowski JQ. Tau isoform profile and phosphorylation state in dementia pugilistica recapitulate Alzheimer's disease. Acta Neuropathol. 2001;101:518–524

Demyelinating diseases of the nervous system: overview

Demyelinating disorders may affect the CNS, PNS, or both:

- CNS demyelinating disorders:
  - Acquired:
    - *Multiple sclerosis* and its variants
    - *Acute disseminated encephalomyelitis (ADEM)* and its variants
    - *Neuromyelitis optica* (Devic's disease)
    - Toxic demyelination: *Marchiafava–Bignami syndrome* secondary to alcohol or heroin/cocaine)
    - *Bickerstaff's brain stem encephalitis (BBE)*
    - *Progressive multifocal leukoencephalopathy (PML)*
  - Inherited:
    - *Leukodystrophies*
    - *Harding's syndrome*
- PNS demyelinating disorders:
  - Acquired:
    - *Chronic inflammatory demyelinating poly(radiculo)neuropathy (CIDP)*
    - *Guillain–Barré syndrome (GBS)* and its variants
  - Inherited:
    - Leukodystrophies
    - Inherited demyelinating peripheral neuropathies such as *hereditary motor and sensory neuropathy (HMSN)*
- Combined central and peripheral demyelinating disease may occur:
  - Chronic demyelinating neuropathy with multifocal CNS demyelination, with features of both MS and CIDP; the latter tends to dominate the clinical picture
  - Leukodystrophies
  - EBV-associated ADEM

Myelin damage may be the principal neuropathological finding in other disorders such as *central pontine myelinolysis* and *subacute combined degeneration of the spinal cord*, secondary to vitamin B_{12} deficiency.

Reference

Thomas PK, Walker RWH, Rudge P, et al. Chronic demyelinating peripheral neuropathy associated with multifocal central nervous system demyelination. Brain. 1987;110:53–76

Dengue

Dengue is the most common arthropod-borne viral disease of humans, and is caused by a flavivirus of the togaviridae family, which is transmitted by the mosquito *Aedes aegypti*. It occurs predominantly in the tropics and subtropics, especially Asia, but it is also seen in Africa, Australia, and the Americas. There is a 3–7-day incubation period before the development of fever, with a relative bradycardia, arthralgia, myalgia, and a macular rash that blanches on pressure. This may progress to a more severe form of the disease, dengue hemorrhagic fever, especially in children, in which the patient develops vomiting, collapse, and spontaneous hemorrhages. This is thought to be a vascular leak syndrome.

Neurological complications are uncommon (1% of dengue admissions in one series), and include:

- Encephalopathy/encephalitis: seizures, coma, stiff neck, and paresis
- Cranial and peripheral neuropathies: VII, IX-X, ulnar, sciatic
- Guillain–Barré-like syndrome
- Reye's syndrome

There may be a mild CSF leukocytosis. Diagnosis is by serology or PCR.

Treatment is supportive and symptomatic. The prognosis for pure dengue fever is very good, but the more fulminant forms of the disease have 50% mortality in the untreated state.

Reference

Solomon T, Dung NM, Vaughn DW, et al. Neurological manifestations of dengue infection. Lancet. 2000;355:1053–1059

Dentatorubral-pallidoluysian atrophy (DRPLA) [OMIM#125370]

Dentatorubropallidoluysian atrophy, "Haw River" syndrome

Dentatorubral-pallidoluysian atrophy (DRPLA) is an autosomal dominant condition characterized by a variable phenotype encompassing cerebellar ataxia, an extrapyramidal disorder (dystonia, parkinsonism, or choreoathetosis), myoclonus, seizures, and dementia. This is a *trinucleotide repeat disease*, with an exonic CAG expansion in the atrophin-1 gene on chromosome 12p13.31 (normal = 3–36 repeats, expansion = 49–88 in DRPLA), encoding a polyglutamine tract. Occasional sporadic forms have been described. It is most commonly reported in Japanese families, but not exclusively.

Clinical features

Can present at any age (mean age of onset ~32 years old) with:

- Cerebellar ataxia.
- Extrapyramidal disorder: dystonia, parkinsonism, or choreoathetosis.
- Myoclonus which may be associated with epileptic seizures.
- Psychiatric manifestations.
- Dementia.
- Positive family history.
- It may present as a phenocopy of *Huntington's disease*.

There is a correlation between longer triplet repeat expansion, usually inherited from an affected father, and both early onset disease and the *progressive myoclonus epilepsy* phenotype.

Investigation

Bloods are normal, apart from neurogenetic testing for the expanded triplet repeat, which is diagnostic. Neuroimaging (MRI) shows atrophy of basal ganglia, midbrain, and cerebellum. CSF is usually normal. EEG may show spike and wave abnormalities especially in those patients with epilepsy. Pathology: neuronal loss with atrophy and gliosis of the dentate nucleus in the cerebellum and the red nucleus in midbrain (dentatorubral system); pallidum (especially GP_e) and subthalamic nucleus (pallidoluysian system).

Differential diagnosis

Huntington's disease, especially in older patients. Other autosomal dominant cerebellar ataxias. In the absence of a family history, other conditions to consider include conditions causing progressive myoclonus epilepsy (*neuronal ceroid lipofuscinosis* and *Lafora body disease* in younger patients; *mitochondrial disease*). Also *prion disease, Whipple's disease*.

Treatment and prognosis

Symptomatic treatment only, for example, for seizures, myoclonus.

References

Ikeuchi T, Koide R, Tanaka H, et al. Dentatorubral-pallidoluysian atrophy: clinical features are closely related to unstable expansions of trinucleotide (CAG) repeat. Ann Neurol. 1995;37:769–775
Ross CA, Ellerby LM, Wood JD, Nucifora FC Jr. Dentatorubral-pallidoluysian atrophy (DRPLA): model for Huntington's disease and other polyglutamine diseases. In: Beal MF, Lang AE, Ludolph A, eds. Neurodegenerative Diseases: Neurobiology, Pathogenesis and Therapeutics. Cambridge: Cambridge University Press; 2005:861–870
Tsuji S. Dentatorubral-pallidoluysian atrophy (DRPLA). J Neural Transm Suppl. 2000;58:167–180

Dermatomyositis

Dermatomyositis is an inflammatory disorder of skeletal muscle and dermis, the former being of B-cell origin. The condition involves complement-mediated microvascular injury by antibodies within blood vessels of the dermis and muscle. Classically, patients present with proximal muscle weakness; in addition, a purple discoloration of the skin around the eyes, and extensor surfaces of the arms and fingers may be evident. Dermatomyositis typically requires aggressive immuno-therapy. In older patients, there may be an associated underlying malignancy.

Dermatomyositides may be classified as:

- Childhood dermatomyositis with vasculitis
- Adult dermatomyositis
- Adult dermatomyositis associated with connective tissue disorders, especially systemic sclerosis (scleroderma), rheumatoid arthritis, Sjögren's syndrome, and mixed connective tissue disease: overlap syndrome, for example, sclerodermatomyositis.
- Adult dermatomyositis with underlying malignancy, typically breast, lung, ovary, stomach (i.e., a *paraneoplastic syndrome*).

Clinical features

Children > Adults, F > M.
Muscle involvement may begin with myalgia before progressing to frank weakness:

- Typically symmetrical, proximal muscle involvement of subacute onset (6–12 weeks), progressing with time to proximal muscle weakness, firstly of the lower limbs (e.g., difficulty getting up from chairs, climbing stairs).
- Respiratory, neck, bulbar, and facial muscles may be involved in severe cases.
- Muscle wasting gradually develops; muscles may be swollen and tender with acute disease (inflammation), or firm and indurated with chronic disease (fibrosis and fatty infiltration) with calcification in some instances.

- Occasionally, the disease can present in a florid fashion with development of acute renal failure secondary to myoglobinuria, in which case the muscles are often swollen and tender.
- Extraocular muscles, sphincter function, and sensation are typically spared, and the reflexes are present unless muscles are severely atrophied.

Skin involvement often precedes or accompanies muscle weakness, and may take the form of

- Purple discoloration over the upper eyelids with edema (heliotrope rash).
- Flat red rash on face and upper trunk.
- Erythema on knuckles with a raised violaceous scaly eruption (Gottron's sign), which can spread to involve elbows, knees, malleoli, neck (V-sign), back, and shoulders (shawl sign).
- Rash can be made worse by sunlight.
- In the nailbed, there are looped and dilated capillaries in association with either small hemorrhages or thrombosed vessels.
- In time, the skin may become fragile and shiny with pigmentary changes. In children, there can be marked soft tissue calcification.

Systemic involvement may occur: fever, malaise, fatigue, weight loss, arthralgia, Raynaud's phenomenon (especially with underlying connective tissue disorder).

Investigation

Bloods may reveal leukocytosis, markedly raised ESR, positive ANA; none are diagnostic. Creatine kinase is elevated in over 95% of cases; if this is markedly raised, there may be secondary renal failure. Serology for autoantibodies may reveal an underlying connective tissue disorder. A similar myopathy may occur with *HIV/AIDS* and with HTLV1 in appropriate geographical areas; hence, it is sensible to check for these. Neurophysiology (EMG) shows myopathic changes, but these may be patchy, requiring sampling of more than one site; fibrillation potentials, excessive insertional activity, and spontaneous discharges may also be seen. Indolent disease with fibrotic muscle may not show characteristic EMG changes. Muscle biopsy is the definitive test, showing perifascicular atrophy with other fibers undergoing degeneration and necrosis so that they lose the staining characteristics with many enzyme reactions (so-called ghost fibers). There is also an intense inflammatory infiltrate centered on the blood vessels with endothelial hyperplasia, fibrin thrombi, intracapillary tubular inclusions, and obliteration of capillaries. Neuroimaging is not usually necessary, although MRI of muscle does show some abnormalities. CSF analysis is not necessary. Other investigations may include a search for an underlying malignancy, especially in patients (especially men) presenting after the age of 50 years; this may include CXR, pelvic ultrasound, CT chest and abdomen, barium swallow, GI endoscopy, as appropriate. Check ECG to exclude cardiomyopathy; respiratory function (spirometry) to exclude respiratory muscle involvement.

Differential diagnosis

- *Polymyositis* (+/– overlap syndrome)
- Sporadic *inclusion body myositis*
- Drug induced myopathies (e.g., amiodarone, statins)
- Muscular dystrophies (especially *limb girdle muscular dystrophies*)
- *Polymyalgia rheumatica*

Treatment and prognosis

High-dose prednisolone in the first instance: 100 mg/day, or 2 mg/kg/day in children, reducing to 60 mg/day (or 1 mg/kg/day in children) over the next 2 months. Thereafter, the dose should be reduced by about 5–10 mg a month according to disease activity; this may be measured according to clinical symptoms, quantitative myometry, and creatine kinase level. Anticipate maintenance of steroid therapy for 8–18 months. If symptoms recur or are not controlled, then options include the introduction of

- Azathioprine 1.5–2 mg/kg/day (monitor FBC, LFT weekly in first instance).
- Methotrexate (15–25 mg/week orally).
- Intravenous immunoglobulin (0.4 g/kg/day for 5 days; repeated every 6–8 weeks).
- Ciclosporin, cyclophosphamide and plasma exchange have all been tried, with only marginal benefit.

Supportive treatment may also be necessary (e.g., respiratory support, nasogastric feeding). Physiotherapy is essential to avoid disuse atrophy and development of contractures. Persistent subcutaneous calcifications are difficult to treat.

References

Dalakas MC, Hohlfeld R. Polymyositis and dermatomyositis. Lancet. 2003;362: 971–982
Dalakas MC, Karpati G. Inflammatory myopathies. In: Karpati G, Hilton-Jones D, Bushby K, Griggs RC, eds. Disorders of Voluntary Muscle. 8th ed. Cambridge: Cambridge University Press; 2010:427–452
Mammen AL. Dermatomyositis and polymyositis: clinical presentation, autoantibodies, and pathogenesis. Ann N Y Acad Sci. 2010;1184:134–153

Dermoid

Dermoids are benign cystic tumors, similar to *epidermoid* tumors, the exception being that they contain skin appendages and hair follicles as well as the keratin found in epidermoids. They tend to be more common in children, presenting as midline lesions anywhere from the cerebellum to the lower spinal cord; presenting symptoms depend on location. Like epidermoids, they may rupture into the CSF causing chemical (aseptic) *meningitis*.

Reference

Cohen-Gadol AA, Al-Mefty O. Skull base tumors. In: Bernstein M, Berger MS, eds. Neuro-Oncology. The Essentials. 2nd ed. New York: Thieme; 2008:320–333

Desmin-related myopathy [OMIM#601419]

Myofibrillar myopathy

Desmin is a structural protein of muscle. Although diffuse and focal nonspecific increases in desmin may be seen in biopsies from a variety of muscle diseases, the term desmin-related myopathy or desminopathy is largely reserved for an autosomal dominant *distal myopathy* of middle adulthood associated with frequent cardiac involvement caused by mutations in the desmin gene. Leg weakness leading to gait disturbance is followed over 5–10 years by weakness of all extremities, bulbar, facial, and respiratory muscle weakness, and cardiac problems (arrhythmia, conduction block, congestive failure). EMG shows prominent spontaneous activity, short duration motor unit potentials, and polyphasia. Muscle biopsy shows central nuclei, and intrasarcoplasmic aggregates of desmin in both type I and type II fibers. Electron microscopy shows aggregates of granular and filamentous material arising from the Z-bands. There is no specific treatment. Supportive treatment may include anti-arrhythmic drugs or cardiac pacing for heart block.

Rigid spine syndrome, caused by mutation in the SEPN1 gene, is also a desmin-related myopathy.

References

Goebel HH. Desmin-related neuromuscular disorders. Muscle Nerve. 1995;18:1306–1320
Udd B. Distal myopathies. In: Karpati G, Hilton-Jones D, Bushby K, Griggs RC, eds. Disorders of Voluntary Muscle. 8th ed. Cambridge: Cambridge University Press; 2010:323–340

Diabetes insipidus (DI)

Diabetes insipidus (DI) is a syndrome of polyuria and polydipsia, resulting from failure of antidiuretic hormone (ADH, vasopressin) production or secretion from the hypothalamo-posterior pituitary axis (central DI) or of renal response to secreted ADH (nephrogenic DI). There is an inability to concentrate the urine (failure to increase urine osmolality to >750 mosmol/L after a water deprivation test), which in the case of central DI may be corrected by exogenous DDAVP; plasma osmolality is high with hypernatremia.

Most instances of central DI are idiopathic, but various disease processes affecting the hypothalamus and/or posterior pituitary gland may cause DI, including:

- Trauma, local surgery
- Local tumors, for example, *craniopharyngioma, pineal tumors*
- Inflammatory or granulomatous disease, for example, *neurosarcoidosis*, histiocytosis X
- Vascular lesions
- Other causes: *Froehlich syndrome, Wolfram syndrome, Friedreich's ataxia*, anorexia nervosa, *Langerhans cell histiocytosis* (LCH)

Reference

Baylis PH. Investigation of suspected hypothalamic diabetes insipidus. Clin Endocrinol. 1995;43:507–510

Diabetes mellitus and the nervous system: overview

Diabetes mellitus results from a failure either of adequate insulin production from the endocrine pancreas or of end-organ responsiveness to insulin (insulin resistance), with resultant hyperglycemia, polyuria, and polydipsia. Diabetes mellitus may affect both the PNS and CNS. In the PNS, hyperglycemia causes capillary damage with nerve ischemia, glycosylation of structural nerve proteins, depletion of myoinositol, and accumulation of sorbitol and fructose, leading to reduced axonal transport and axonal loss. In the CNS, the main consequences of diabetes mellitus occur as a result of the etiological role of hyperglycemia in atherosclerosis.

Clinical features

PNS complications:
    Seven to 80% of patients with diabetes mellitus develop neuropathies but only about a fifth are symptomatic. Neuropathies include:

- Symmetrical polyneuropathies:
    - Distal sensory or sensorimotor polyneuropathy is the most common type of diabetic neuropathy. It is predominantly sensory, producing a glove and stocking sensory loss with some distal weakness and wasting. Two major types of this form of neuropathy exist: one in which large

fibers are predominantly involved produces a nonpainful loss of joint position sense and vibration perception. The other type affects the small fibers and is often painful, with allodynia, loss of pinprick, and temperature sensation and a degree of autonomic involvement. These neuropathies can progress to ulceration and destruction of soft tissue and joints (neuropathic or Charcot joints); the picture may resemble tabes dorsalis (pseudotabes). An acute painful neuropathy is occasionally seen after treatment initiation with insulin, so-called insulin-induced neuropathy. This may persist for a number of weeks or months and is thought to represent active axonal degeneration/regeneration.
  - Diabetic neuropathic cachexia is a condition in which there is an acutely painful diabetic polyneuropathy associated with a sudden and severe weight loss, typically in the context of a depressive illness. It is more common in men, especially when the control of diabetes is poor. Recovery occurs with better control of the blood glucose and weight gain.
- Focal and multifocal neuropathies:
  - Lumbosacral radiculoplexopathy (diabetic amyotrophy; Brun–Garland syndrome) typically presents in the older non-insulin-dependent diabetic, when it may be the first presentation of the condition. The patient presents with a painful asymmetric weakness and wasting of proximal leg muscles, typically the quadriceps femoris and hip flexors, with loss of the knee jerk. The onset is either abrupt or stepwise and is often seen in conjunction with a distal symmetrical polyneuropathy (additional loss of ankle jerks). There may be a prodrome of weight loss and malaise. The sensory deficits are mild and recovery is slow (up to 2 years) and incomplete. It is thought to be due to vasculitic infarction of the proximal nerve roots as they emerge from the spinal canal or in the plexus itself.
  - Limb mononeuropathy is usually due to nerve entrapment or infarction. Typically when a nerve infarcts the patient presents with pain and a focal nerve deficit, whereas in *entrapment neuropathy* the sensorimotor loss occurs more insidiously and without pain. On occasion patients may present with a mononeuritis multiplex.
  - Truncal neuropathy/radiculopathy is typically seen in older NIDDM patients and often occurs with the lumbosacral radiculoplexopathy. It presents with a sudden onset of root pain and dysaesthesia in the T4–T12 dermatomes, which spontaneously resolves over several months, but may leave a degree of abdominal wall weakness.
  - Cranial neuropathy may occur, involving especially the third, sixth, and fourth cranial nerves. Occasionally other cranial nerves can be involved, for example, the seventh.
- Autonomic neuropathy:
  - This usually correlates with the severity of the somatic neuropathy and results in orthostatic hypotension, fixed heart rate, delayed gastric emptying and constipation with fecal incontinence, and urinary retention with impotence. The symptoms develop insidiously and this may result

in blunted responses to hypoglycemia. Occasionally, sudomotor abnormalities produce distal anhidrosis, which may be associated with a compensatory hyperhidrosis including "gustatory sweating," profuse facial sweating following food intake.

CNS complications:

- Strokes secondary to accelerated atherosclerosis; hypertension secondary to diabetic renal disease may also contribute, as well as embolic phenomena if there has been a history of myocardial infarction.
- Encephalopathy secondary to hyperosmolar states (hyperosmolar non-ketotic syndrome, HONKS) which may be complicated by hemichorea, sagittal sinus thrombosis.
- Hypoglycemic focal deficits (hemiparesis especially), epileptic seizures and coma, secondary to excessive treatment.
- Retinopathy.
- There is an association between IDDM and *stiff person syndrome*; it may also be a feature of *Friedreich's ataxia, mitochondrial disease, myotonic dystrophy type 1, Wolfram syndrome*.
- Fungal infection (*mucormycosis*) may occur in the context of diabetic acidosis or poorly controlled DM along with malignant otitis media.
- A focal amnesic syndrome, sometimes with hippocampal changes on MR brain scanning, may occur with intensive glycemic control, leading to profound hypoglycemia.

Investigation

Bloods to confirm diabetes: fasting glucose >8 mmol/L, random (non-fasting) glucose >11 mmol/L. If results are equivocal, an oral glucose tolerance test may be performed. Glycemic control may be assessed by measurement of glycated hemoglobin (HbA$_{1c}$). Neurophysiology (EMG/NCS) typically reveals a mixed axonal-demyelinating polyneuropathy, with more sensory than motor involvement and with a predilection for the lower limbs. EMG shows denervation, which is particularly useful in the diagnosis of the lumbosacral radiculoplexopathy. Nerve biopsy (if required) confirms axonal-demyelinating polyneuropathy, with some inflammatory infiltrate of uncertain significance. Neuroimaging (CT/MRI), if required, may reveal multiple cerebral infarcts.

Treatment and prognosis

- Optimal control of hyperglycemia.
- Symptomatic treatment of painful neuropathies with either tricyclic antidepressants (amitriptyline) or carbamazepine, gabapentin, pregabalin, duloxetine.

- Symptomatic treatment of autonomic neuropathies.
- Many patients improve when the above therapies are followed.
- There is limited evidence that some cases of diabetic amyotrophy have a diabetes-related vasculitic origin and that immunotherapies such as IVIg, may have a therapeutic role.

References

Chaudhuri KR. The neurology of diabetes. Br J Hosp Med. 1997;58:343–347
Selvarajah D, Tesfaye S. Central nervous system involvement in diabetes mellitus. Curr Diabetes Rep. 2006;6:431–438
Wong MC, Chung JW, Wong TK. Effects of treatments for symptoms of painful diabetic neuropathy: systematic review. BMJ. 2007; 335:87–90
Zochodne DW. Diabetes mellitus and the peripheral nervous system: manifestations and mechanisms. Muscle Nerve. 2007;36:144–166

Dialysis syndromes

A number of neurological conditions have been associated with dialysis for renal failure:

- Dialysis disequilibrium syndrome: this presents acutely either during or immediately after dialysis with features of cerebral irritation (headache, irritability, disorientation, agitation, somnolence and generalized tonic–clonic seizures), and muscle cramps, tremor, nausea, and vomiting; exophthalmos may occur. It is probably due to cerebral edema, as the urea concentration within the brain remains much higher than that in the blood during rapid dialysis. Characteristically, the EEG shows slowing and there is raised CSF opening pressure on lumbar puncture.
- Dialysis dementia syndrome: now very rare, this syndrome used to be seen in chronic dialysis patients and is thought to have been related to aluminium, in the dialysate; the reduction of aluminium in dialysate fluids has greatly reduced the incidence of this condition. Clinically, patients developed hesitant speech and even speech arrest, which progressed to cognitive decline with delusions, hallucinations, fits, myoclonus, asterixis, and gait abnormalities. The EEG showed slowing, with multifocal bursts of more profound slowing and spikes. Patients typically died within 6–12 months.
- Wernicke's encephalopathy: probably related to nutritional deficiencies, especially protein intake.
- *Carpal tunnel syndrome*: due to ischemia/venous congestion and/or amyloidosis.

References

Chui HC, Damasio AR. Progressive dialysis encephalopathy ("dialysis dementia"). J Neurol. 1980;222:145–157

Harrington CR, Wischik CM, McArthur FK, Taylor GA, Edwardson JA, Candy JM. Alzheimer's-disease-like changes in tau protein processing: association with aluminium accumulation in brains of renal dialysis patients. Lancet. 1994;343:993–997

Diaphragmatic flutter

Leeuwenhoek's disease

The Dutchman Anthony van Leeuwenhoek (1632–1723), seventeenth-century pioneer of microscopy, also described a respiratory myoclonus (diaphragmatic flutter) in himself, epigastric pulsation, and fullness associated with rhythmic activity of the inspiratory muscles not in time with the pulse.

Reference

Larner AJ. Antony van Leeuwenhoek and the description of diaphragmatic flutter (respiratory myoclonus). Mov Disord. 2005;20: 917–918

Diastematomyelia

Split notochord syndrome

Diastematomyelia is a congenital malformation of the spinal cord in which there is sagittal division of part of the cord into two hemicords, usually in the lower thoracic or lumbar region. Usually, there is a bony or cartilaginous spur and dura in the cleft between the two parts of the cord to which the hemicords are tethered, and often there are overlying skin abnormalities, and sometimes hemivertebrae. Diastematomyelia may occur in the context of congenital atlanto-axial dislocation. Although often asymptomatic, neurological dysfunction of lower limbs and sphincters may develop in adolescence or adulthood, and may be progressive. MR imaging confirms the diagnosis. Surgical attempts to untether the cord may be undertaken.

Reference

Sami H, Ross E, Walter M, Goli S. Split spinal cord (diastematomyelia). Neurology. 2003;60:491

Diogenes syndrome

Diogenes of Sinope (ca. 412–323 BC), not to be confused with Diogenes of Apollonia (fl. fifth century BC) and Diogenes Laertius (fl. second century AD), was a cofounder of the Cynic school of philosophy in Athens, and was noted for his austere asceticism and self-sufficiency, and his disregard for domestic comforts: he lived in a barrel or tub. Hence, the term Diogenes syndrome was coined to refer to a syndrome characterized by severe self-neglect, domestic squalor, hoarding behavior, and social withdrawal. Most patients are elderly, single or living alone, of average or above average intelligence, and often with a good income (i.e., the condition is not the result of poverty). A distinction is drawn between primary Diogenes syndrome, when it is unrelated to any mental illness (50–70%), and secondary, when it is related to depression, schizophrenia, dementia (particularly of *frontotemporal lobar degeneration* type), or alcoholism. There may be concurrent physical illness; indeed this may prompt admission to hospital. Management is often difficult because of patients' refusal to cooperate, perhaps a reflection of the suspicious, quarrelsome, and even aggressive traits said to be associated with the syndrome. Treatment of underlying mental and physical illness, involvement of social worker/health visitor or nurse, and attendance at a day center to develop a social network may help, but long-term outlook is generally poor ("relapse," death).

References

Clarke ANG, Manikar GO, Gray I. Diogenes syndrome. A clinical study of gross neglect in old age. Lancet. 1975;i:366–368
Cooney C, Hamid W. Review: diogenes syndrome. Age Ageing. 1995;24:451–453

Diphtheria

Diphtheria is an acute infectious disease, now very rare in the developed world because of the introduction of widespread vaccination, but still encountered in the underdeveloped world. It is caused by the organism *Corynebacterium diphtheriae*, the effects of which may be local or, more seriously, remote, the latter due to the production of a pathogenic exotoxin. Toxigenic *Corynebacterium diphtheriae* causes neurological illness by inhibiting protein synthesis through ADP ribosylation and inactivation of ribosomal GTPase by toxin subunit A. This produces a gradual onset of bulbar palsy followed by a demyelinating neuropathy, both of which recover fully over similar time periods.

Clinical features

Initial infection may be asymptomatic, or symptomatic with malaise, irritability, anorexia, headache, arthralgia. Primary infection may be faucial, cutaneous, vaginal, or, in neonates, umbilical.

- Primary (faucial) infection: inflamed throat with patchy white exudate and membrane, +/– cervical lymphadenopathy ("bull neck") after incubation period of 2–6 days.
- Secondary toxic features: Early local: after 3–6 weeks, bulbar problems: palatal paralysis, lower cranial neuropathies but facial weakness rare (cf. *Guillain–Barré syndrome*).
- Autonomic (myelinated parasympathetic) involvement can produce blurred vision (bilateral ciliary paralysis with loss of accommodation), impaired pupillary reactions, and vagal block, 3–4 weeks into the illness. Cardiomyopathy with congestive cardiac failure, arrhythmias, and death may occur without appropriate supportive therapy.
- Secondary toxic features: Late remote: after around 8 weeks, following hematogenous dissemination, a generalized sensorimotor demyelinating peripheral neuropathy develops, with a proximal to distal spread of weakness (cf. Guillain–Barré syndrome). There may be additional oculomotor nerve palsy and phrenic nerve palsy. The severity of the neuropathy varies from sensory symptoms to a severe large fiber sensory neuropathy (so-called diphtheritic pseudotabes), with inability to walk and the need for ventilatory support.
- Rarely, infection is localized to the skin (primary cutaneous diphtheria) in which case there is an anesthetic zone around the skin ulcer +/– muscle weakness in the surrounding muscles. In just under 50% of such cases, the patient goes on to develop more generalized disease.
- CNS involvement in diphtheria has only rarely been described and in these cases, a vascular origin, secondary to the cardiomyopathy, is the most likely explanation.

Investigation

Bloods are typically unhelpful, apart from pointing toward an infective process. Throat swabs can be taken but special media are required to culture the organism. Neurophysiology (EMG/NCS) is normal in the early stages of the illness, but after 4 weeks, a demyelinating peripheral neuropathy with features similar to Guillain–Barré syndrome is found. Imaging is not usually helpful, although CXR may reveal cardiomegaly in cases of cardiac involvement. CSF is usually normal except in severe cases when there is an elevated white cell count and protein level. In the case of the delayed neuropathy the protein is typically raised. Nerve biopsy shows a demyelinating neuropathy.

Differential diagnosis

- Guillain–Barré syndrome/CIDP in the case of the delayed neuropathy
- Botulism
- Brain stem lesion/demyelination
- Basal meningitis (infective/inflammatory/malignant)
- Myasthenia gravis
- Polymyositis

Treatment and prognosis

Prevention is the primary aim, with diphtheria toxoid given in childhood as part of the triple vaccination. Booster shots of the toxoid should be given every 10 years. In the established case, antitoxin should be given as soon as possible within the first 48 h (although this can produce anaphylactic reactions). Antitoxin reduces the incidence and severity of the neuropathic complications. Antibiotics should be given (penicillin or erythromycin) even when the effect of the toxin is apparent. Supportive therapy may be required once neurological features occur, and this may include ventilatory support. Only very occasionally have patients been described having more than one attack of diphtheria.

References

McAuley JH, Fearnley J, Laurence A, Ball JA. Diphtheritic neuropathy. J Neurol Neurosurg Psychiatry. 1999;67:825–826
McDonald WI, Kocen RS. Diphtheritic neuropathy. In: Dyck PJ, Thomas PK, Griffin JW, Low PA, Podulso JF, eds. Peripheral Neuropathy. 3rd ed. Philadelphia, PA: W.B. Saunders; 1995: 1412–1417

Diphyllobothriasis

Infection with the cestode fish tapeworm *Diphyllobothrium latus* from ingestion of undercooked fish can lead to *vitamin B$_{12}$ deficiency*, with the hematological and neurological consequences thereof due to absorption of this vitamin by the parasite.

Discitis

Discitis is an inflammatory, usually infective, process affecting the intervertebral discs, with sparing of the vertebral body (although the discovertebral junction may be affected). The process may also spread to the epidural space and paraspinal soft tissues, producing neurological features. The clinical picture is one of severe localized back pain with fever, with or without neurological signs, which may be radicular, meningeal, or myelopathic. There may be a history of recent instrumentation of the spine (e.g., epidural anesthesia) or evidence for underlying immunosuppression. Bloods may show a raised ESR. Imaging with plain radiographs may suggest the diagnosis but MRI is the investigation of choice. Commonly encountered organisms are staphylococci, salmonella, and *Mycobacterium tuberculosis*. Direct biopsy may be required to establish the microbiological diagnosis and decide on appropriate antibiotic therapy. Clincal outcome is usually good.

Reference

Hopkinson N, Stevenson J, Benjamin S. A case ascertainment study of septic discitis: clinical, microbiological and radiological features. Q J Med. 2001;94:465–470

Disconnection syndromes

Disconnection syndromes may be defined as conditions in which there is an interruption of inter- and/or intra-hemispheral fiber tracts, either within the corpus callosum or commissures (interhemispheric disconnection syndromes), or within a hemisphere (intra-hemispheric disconnection syndromes). The concept dates originally to the 1890s, but was taken up and modernized by Norman Geschwind in the 1960s.

Clinical features

- Interhemispheric disconnection:
  - Complete, for example, tumor or surgical section of the corpus callosum:
    - A blindfolded patient can correctly name objects placed in the right hand, but not those in left, and objects in the left hemifield cannot be named or matched to a similar object in the right hemifield.
  - Posterior callosal section (at splenium; e.g., left posterior cerebral artery occlusion):
    - Patient cannot read or name colors, as information cannot pass to the left hemispheric language areas. Copying of words and writing, both spontaneously and to dictation, is intact as the information passes to the left hemisphere anterior to the site of damage.
- Intra-hemispheric disconnection syndromes:
  - Conduction aphasia:
    - The patient has fluent but paraphasic speech and writing, with greatly impaired repetition despite relatively normal comprehension of the spoken and written word. This is traditionally explained as due to a lesion in the arcuate fasciculus (supramarginal gyrus).

- Ideomotor apraxia in Broca's aphasia:
  ○ An apraxia of left-hand movements to command. It is due to lesions disconnecting the cortical motor areas anterior to the primary motor cortex.
- Pure word deafness:
  ○ Patients are able to hear and identify nonverbal sounds but unable to understand spoken language. This is due to a lesion in the white matter of the left temporal lobe which isolates Wernicke's area from the auditory cortex.

Speculations that unusual delusional syndromes (Capgras', Cotard's) are also disconnection syndromes have been advanced as well. *Alzheimer's disease* may be viewed as a disconnection syndrome as the pathology isolates the hippocampus from association cortices, basal forebrain, thalamus, and hypothalamus.

Investigation

Neuroimaging may disclose the structural cause for disconnection (stroke, tumor).

Treatment and prognosis

Of underlying cause, where identified.

References

Absher JR, Benson DF. Disconnection syndromes: an overview of Geschwind's contributions. Neurology. 1993;43:862–867
Catani M, ffytche DH. The rises and falls of disconnection syndromes. Brain. 2005;128:2224–2239
Delbeuck X, van der Linden M, Collette F. Alzheimer's disease as a disconnection syndrome? Neuropsychol Rev. 2003;13:79–92
Geschwind N. Disconnexion syndromes in animals and man. Brain. 1965;88:237–294;585-644
Sperry RW. Some effects of disconnecting the cerebral hemispheres. Science. 1982;217:1223–1226

Dissection: overview

Dissection of the cervical arteries (carotid, vertebral) within the neck or extending into the skull may occur spontaneously or as a result of predisposing events such as neck trauma. Dissection per se may cause neck and/or occipital head pain or be asymptomatic, but neurological complications may result from thrombosis and artery-to-artery embolism from the dissected vessel wall (*transient ischemic attacks*).

Clinical features

- Carotid:
  - Unilateral facial pain, often periorbital, +/- Horner's syndrome +/- anterior circulation stroke (e.g., hemispheric infarct with "stuttering" onset) +/- compression of lower cranial nerves by expansion of carotid at skull base.
- Vertebral:
  - Neck and/or occipital head pain, leading to posterior circulation TIA/ stroke (especially lateral medullary syndrome) in hours to 2 weeks.
  - Ophthalmic findings common: diplopia (45% of episodes), nystagmus (37%), ocular misalignment (cranial nerve palsy or skew; 33%), Horner's syndrome (27%), visual field defects (10%), internuclear ophthalmoplegia (4%).
  - *Subarachnoid hemorrhage* may sometimes complicate dissection if this spreads to involve the intracerebral portion of the artery.

+/- History of neck trauma, possibly including osteopathic/chiropractic manipulation of the neck.

Other associations of carotid dissection include *fibromuscular dysplasia*, *Ehlers–Danlos syndrome* (type IV), *Marfan's syndrome*, *pseudoxanthoma elasticum*.

Investigation

Imaging: intra-arterial catheter angiography was formerly the investigation of choice, showing narrowing of the artery lumen; but MRI may now be used, showing an eccentric signal void surrounded by semilunar hyperintensity on spin echo images, characteristic of mural hematoma, although the shape may vary, sometimes being oval or circumferential. This approach has now largely superseded intra-arterial angiography.

Differential diagnosis

The constellation of symptoms and signs may be recognized as of vascular origin but ascribed to ischemia without dissection being thought of. Some cases of "*Raeder's paratrigeminal syndrome*" may in fact be cases of dissection, which are missed by imaging.

Treatment and prognosis

Anticoagulation, initially with heparin followed by oral warfarin, is recommended in those deemed at risk of further embolic events; although, there is as yet no randomized controlled trial evidence currently available to support this policy.

References

Baumgartner RW, Bogousslavsky J, Caso V, Paciaroni M, eds. Handbook on Cerebral Artery Dissection. Basel: Karger; 2005

Debette S, Leys D. Cervical-artery dissections: predisposing factors, diagnosis, and outcome. Lancet Neurol. 2009;8:668–678

Schievink WI. Spontaneous dissection of the carotid and vertebral arteries. N Engl J Med. 2001;344:898–906

Distal myopathy: overview

A number of myopathic disorders may manifest with predominantly distal weakness and muscle wasting. These include:

- Distal muscular dystrophies:
    - Late adult onset (>40 years):
        o Type 1: autosomal dominant, Welander's disease
        o Type 2: autosomal dominant, Markesbery–Griggs/Udd disease
    - Early adult onset (<30 years):
        o Type 1: autosomal recessive, Nonaka type
        o Type 2: autosomal recessive, Miyoshi type (dysferlinopathy)
        o Type 3: autosomal dominant, Laing type
- *Myotonic dystrophy type 1 (DM1)*
- *Desmin-related myopathy*
- *Facioscapulohumeral (FSH) muscular dystrophy, scapuloperoneal myopathy*
- *Inclusion body myositis*/myopathy (IBM)
- Metabolic myopathies: *acid maltase deficiency*, debrancher deficiency
- Congenital myopathies: central core disease, nemaline myopathy

Occasionally myasthenic limb weakness may be predominantly distal. Neuropathies and neuronopathies may present with isolated distal weakness, for example, Charcot–Marie–Tooth disease, distal spinal muscular atrophy, and motor neuropathies (e.g., *porphyria*).

Reference

Udd B. Distal myopathies. In: Karpati G, Hilton-Jones D, Bushby K, Griggs RC, eds. Disorders of Voluntary Muscle. 8th ed. Cambridge: Cambridge University Press; 2010:323–340

Dolichoectasia

Dilatative arteriopathy

Dolichoectasia describes the presence of dilated, elongated, or tortuous intracranial arteries (vertebrobasilar, carotid, or both) with or without thrombus or calcification. Dolichoectasia may cause brain infarction by thrombosis, embolism, stenosis, or occlusion of deep-penetrating arteries. There may be a combination of focal brain stem findings (e.g., sixth nerve palsy) due to local compression from a dilated vessel, and embolic cerebral hemisphere events. Hydrocephalus is also reported. The most common cause of dolichoectasia is atherosclerosis, but it has also been noted in *Fabry's disease* and late-onset *Pompe's disease*.

A retrospective study of nearly 400 cases of first cerebral infarction identified dolichoectasia on CT or MRI in 3% of patients, the majority in the vertebrobasilar circulation. These patients were more likely to have a lacunar pattern of infarction, and a better rate of survival but higher rate of recurrence. Natural history is of progression in about half of patients, who have a worse outcome. Anticoagulation with warfarin may have a place in the management of some of these cases, although no controlled trials have been performed.

References

Ince B, Petty GW, Brown RD Jr, Chu C-P, Sicks JD, Whisnant JP. Dolichoectasia of the intracranial arteries in patients with first ischemic stroke: a population-based study. Neurology. 1998; 50:1694–1698

Passero SG, Rossi S. Natural history of vertebrobasilar dolichoectasia. Neurology. 2008;70:66–72

Pico F, Labreuche J, Touboul PJ, Leys D, Amarenco P. Intracranial arterial dolichoectasia and small-vessel disease in stroke patients. Ann Neurol. 2005;57:472–479

Dopamine-β-hydroxylase deficiency [OMIM#223360]

A rare inborn error of metabolism, which presents with autonomic dysfunction. Dopamine-β-hydroxylase (DBH) synthesizes noradrenaline from dopamine; its deficiency, due to mutations in the gene encoding DBH, leads to virtual absence of circulating noradrenaline and adrenaline. Clinically, there is postural hypotension and partial ptosis, but sweating, bladder function, and cognitive function are preserved.

Reference

Mathias CJ, Bannister R. Dopamine-β-hydroxylase deficiency – with a note on other genetically determined causes of autonomic failure. In: Mathias CJ, Bannister R, eds. Autonomic Failure. A Textbook of Clinical Disorders of the Autonomic Nervous System. 4th ed. Oxford: Oxford University Press; 1999:387–401

Dopa-responsive dystonia (DRD) [OMIM#128230]

DYT5, Hereditary dystonia with marked diurnal fluctuations,
Segawa syndrome

This rare hereditary *dystonia* usually presents before the age of 10 years and is more common in females (F:M = 2:1). It shows autosomal dominant inheritance with variable penetrance and is linked to chromosome 14q22.1-q22.2. It has been shown to result from mutations in the gene encoding GTP cyclohydrolase I (GTPCH I), which is responsible for the synthesis of tetrahydrobiopterin, an essential cofactor for a number of enzymes, including tyrosine hydroxylase which is the first enzyme in the synthetic pathway of dopamine. There is, therefore, a functional dopamine denervation but, unlike the situation in *Parkinson's disease* (PD), without anatomical loss of the dopaminergic neurones in the nigrostriatal tract. DRD is exquisitely sensitive to small doses of levodopa and, again unlike the situation in PD, response fluctuations generally do not develop over time. For these reasons, it is advocated that all children with dystonia of unknown cause, or "dystonic cerebral palsy," should be given an adequate trial of levodopa.

Clinical features

- Dystonic posturing; initially of foot, spreads eventually to all limbs.
- May be associated with a tremor, postural retrocollis, and hyperreflexia with a striatal toe.
- Pyramidal signs and spasticity may be present in addition to the extrapyramidal features.
- Patients typically complain of difficulty walking and of falls.
- Cognitive impairment and epileptic seizures do not occur.
- In many (but not all cases) the dystonia shows diurnal variation, at its best in the morning and worsening during the day or with exertion; if present, this historical point is highly suggestive of DRD.
- In some family members disease manifests with adult onset *parkinsonism* or a tremor.

Investigation

Neuroimaging is normal. CSF shows reduced dopamine metabolites and tetrahydrobiopterin; these tests now superseded by neurogenetic testing for mutations in the GTP cyclohydrolase I gene, both deletions and point mutations. Therapeutic response to levodopa confirms the diagnosis.

Differential diagnosis

DRD may be misdiagnosed as cerebral palsy of athetoid or spastic diplegic type, or *hereditary spastic paraplegia (HSP)*.

Treatment and prognosis

There is a dramatic and sustained improvement with low-dose levodopa (100–300 mg/day), without the development of response fluctuations or loss of efficacy over time. DRD progresses until the age of 20 years, then stabilizes or improves and may be inapparent after the fourth decade.

References

Hagenah J, Saunders-Pullman R, Hedrich K, et al. High mutation rate in dopa-responsive dystonia: detection with comprehensive GCH1 screening. Neurology. 2005;64:908–911

Ichinose H, Ohye T, Takahashi E, et al. Hereditary progressive dystonia with marked diurnal fluctuations caused by mutations in the GTP cyclohydrolase I gene. Nat Genet. 1994;8:236–242

Segawa M, Hosaka A, Miyagawa F, Nomura Y, Imai H. Hereditary progressive dystonia with marked diurnal fluctuation. Adv Neurol. 1976;14:215–233

Down syndrome [OMIM#190685]

Trisomy 21

This common chromosomal dysgenesis, due to either a triplication of chromosome 21 or a translocation, is usually easily recognized clinically because of its morphological features: round head, palpebral fissures slanting upward and outward ("mongoloid slant"), medial epicanthi, low set ears, hypoplastic maxilla, macroglossia, Brushfield spots, palmar simian crease, short stature.

Neurologically, there is learning disability, which may range from mild to severe. Congenital heart disease is a feature, which may lead to embolic strokes or brain abscesses. Atlanto-axial anomalies may lead to spinal cord compression. There is an increased incidence of hypothyroidism in children with Down syndrome. With age, all Down syndrome patients develop the typical neuropathological changes of *Alzheimer's disease*, presumably due to overexpression of the amyloid precursor protein (APP) gene on chromosome 21 and hence excess production of amyloid β-peptide, and many will also have progressive cognitive deficits. Epileptic seizures may also be a feature, and it is for the latter that most referrals of Down syndrome patients to adult neurology clinics are made. A number of these patients have an epilepsy syndrome that may be unique to the condition, namely late-onset myoclonic epilepsy in Down syndrome (LOMEDS). Onset of, or increase in, seizures may be a marker for the development of cognitive decline.

References

Larner AJ. Down syndrome in the neurology clinic: Too much? Too little? Too late? Downs Syndr Res Pract. 2007;12:69–71
Prasher VP. Alzheimer's Disease and Dementia in Down Syndrome and Intellectual Disabilities. Oxford: Radcliffe Publishing; 2005

Dracunculiasis

Infection with the nematode Guinea worm *Dracunculus medinensis* through ingestion of infected water (Africa, Arabia, Asia) can lead to burning dysesthesia at the ulcer site where the female worm emerges after migrating through the subcutaneous tissues; compressive mononeuropathy may result. Up to 120 cm in length, these worms can cause periorbital and spinal epidural abscesses, as well as peripheral nerve thickening. A global eradication program is in progress.

Drop attacks: overview

Drop attacks may be defined as sudden falls, with or without a loss of consciousness: the term has also been used to describe sudden falls without warning, secondary to either a transient ischemic attack or intracranial tumor in the third ventricle or posterior fossa. Drop attacks may be due to a loss of muscle tone (atonic attacks) or abnormal muscle contraction (tonic drops), although in clinical practice it is difficult to distinguish these two conditions. Likewise, it can be surprisingly hard to distinguish attacks associated with brief loss of consciousness and those occurring with retained consciousness. A large number of conditions are associated with drop attacks, of which the most common causes are cardiac arrhythmias. However, many patients do not yield a diagnosis after thorough investigation. Such idiopathic drop attacks are more common in the elderly, and have sometimes been labeled as due to "cerebrovascular insufficiency," although there is no particular evidence to support such a pathogenesis.

Recognized causes of drop attacks include:

- Symptomatic drop attacks (20–30%):
  - *Syncope*:
    - Cardiac arrhythmias, including Stokes–Adams attacks.
    - Postural hypotension and vasovagal attacks: always have preceding symptoms. These episodes may include convulsive syncope, where a patient who has fainted exhibits tonic–clonic movements, which are not epileptic. This is especially associated with breath-holding attacks in children, *long QT syndromes*, blood donation, and *trigeminal neuralgia*.
    - Congenital cyanotic heart disease.

- *Epilepsy*:
  - ○ Lennox–Gastaut syndrome, infantile spasms, and, occasionally, *juvenile myoclonic epilepsy*.
  - ○ Complex partial seizures of frontal or temporal lobe origin.
- Myoclonic jerks:
  - ○ Post-hypoxic action myoclonus (*Lance–Adams syndrome*) and *progressive myoclonus epilepsy* syndromes.
- Transient ischemic attacks (TIA):
  - ○ Bilateral anterior cerebral artery ischemia, which is usually secondary to carotid artery disease.
  - ○ Vertebrobasilar ischemia, which may be precipitated by certain head movements in patients with degenerative cervical spine disease. There may be no warning in such attacks, but often the patient complains of other posterior circulation TIA symptoms.
- Peripheral vestibular disorder:
  - ○ Ménière's disease, including Tumarkin's otolithic crisis, where there is sudden falling without vertigo.
- Startle reactions:
  - ○ Exaggerated normal physiological startle reaction
  - ○ Hyperekplexia
  - ○ Stiff man syndrome
- Cataplexy, typically associated with *narcolepsy*
- *Paroxysmal dyskinesias* such as paroxysmal kinesigenic choreoathetosis
- Structural lesions of the CNS:
  - ○ Brain stem and posterior fossa lesions: tumor, arachnoid cyst, *Chiari malformation*, odontoid process fracture
  - ○ Cerebral hemisphere lesions such as frontal lobe tumors
- Hydrocephalus:
  - ○ *Normal pressure hydrocephalus*
  - ○ Obstructive hydrocephalus due to third ventricular *colloid cyst* or *meningioma*, fourth ventricular ependymoma and aqueduct stenosis
- Neurodegenerative disorders:
  - ○ Alzheimer's disease, Parkinson's disease, progressive supranuclear palsy, Huntington's disease, multiple system atrophy, corticobasal degeneration
- Neuromuscular:
  - ○ Muscle disease, myasthenia gravis, neuropathy, myelopathy and intermittent spinal ischemia
- Psychogenic attacks.
- Idiopathic ("cryptogenic") drop attacks (60–70%)
  - Typically these attacks first occur in patients between the ages of 40 and 60 years, and increase in frequency with advancing age. Some, but not all, studies find the condition to be more common in middle-aged females. Patients typically collapse to the ground with no impairment of consciousness and get up immediately with no sequelae. More than 90% of such patients have recurrent attacks (on average 2–12 per year),

but the remission rate is not known accurately, figures vary from 25% to 80%, depending on the study.

Investigation

Bloods: FBC, ESR, U+E, glucose, LFTs, lipids. Additional tests may be requested if a specific symptomatic cause is suspected.
Imaging: CXR, CT/MRI brain. May need to consider MRA, catheter angiography, or myelography depending on suspected cause.
CSF: not usually necessary.
Neurophysiology: EEG; may need ambulatory EEG recordings +/− telemetry if epilepsy suspected.
Other investigations: ECG, 24-h ECG, echocardiography; neuro-otological assessment.

Treatment and prognosis

Prognosis with symptomatic drop attacks is dictated by the coexistent medical condition, and thus is poorest in patients with cardiac disease. Patients with idiopathic drop attacks usually suffer only minor injuries and have a favorable prognosis, with no increased risk of stroke or death compared to an age- and sex-matched population. However, in older patients the drop attacks cause more serious injuries, including fractures of the femur. No symptomatic treatment is available for patients with idiopathic drop attacks.

References

Meissner I, Wiebers DO, Swanson JW, O'Fallon WM. The natural history of drop attacks. Neurology. 1986;36:1029–1034
Stevens DL, Matthews WB. Cryptogenic drop attacks: an affliction of women. BMJ. 1973;i:439–442

Dropped head syndrome

Floppy head syndrome, Suarez–Kelly syndrome

This is a disorder in which there is weakness of neck extension, such that the head may fall forward on to the chest. This may occur in a number of disorders, most commonly in *myasthenia gravis* and *motor neurone disease*, and also in inflammatory myopathies, facioscapulohumeral muscular dystrophy, inflammatory neuropathies (GBS, CIDP), and carnitine deficiency. A rare isolated neck extensor myopathy has been described in middle-aged to elderly people, which may on occasion be responsive to corticosteroids. Dropped head syndrome may appear similar to the "bent spine syndrome" or *camptocormia*, but is distinguished in that the excessive kyphosis disappears with rest in these latter conditions.

References

Katz JS, Wolfe GI, Burns DK, Bryan WW, Fleckenstein JL, Barohn RJ. Isolated neck extensor myopathy. A common cause of dropped head syndrome. Neurology. 1996;46:917–921
Nicholas RS, Lecky BRF. Dropped head syndrome: the differential diagnosis. [abstract 26]. J Neurol Neurosurg Psychiatry. 2002;73:218

Duane's syndrome

Duane's (retraction) syndrome is a congenital eye movement abnormality causing strabismus, in which there is paradoxical anomalous lateral rectus innervation by misdirected oculomotor nerve axons destined for the medial rectus. Effectively, there is loss of the abducens nerve innervation to the lateral rectus. This is a syndrome of anomalous axonal guidance, which has been classified as one of the *congenital cranial dysinnervation disorders (CCDDs)*. Clinically, there is palpebral fissure narrowing and retraction of the affected eyeball on attempted adduction, with a variable degree of horizontal eye movement limitation: in type I, abduction is defective, in type II adduction is defective, and in type III both abduction and adduction are defective. Up to 10% of cases are familial with autosomal dominant inheritance. Linkage to chromosome 2q31 has been reported.

References

Duane A. Congenital deficiency of abduction, associated with impairment of adduction, retraction movements, contraction of the palpebral fissure and oblique movements of the eye. Arch Ophthalmol. 1905;34:133–136
Gutowski NJ. Duane's syndrome. Eur J Neurol. 2000;7:145–149

Duchenne muscular dystrophy (DMD) [OMIM#310200]

Meryon's disease, Pseudohypertrophic muscular dystrophy

Duchenne muscular dystrophy (DMD) is the most common of the *muscular dystrophies*. This X-linked condition was first described in detail by Meryon in the 1850s but his work was neglected. DMD is linked to chromosome Xp21 and results from deficiency of dystrophin, a sarcolemmal protein; it is allelic with *Becker muscular dystrophy*.

Clinical features

- Affected boys are clinically normal at birth, and develop normally until about 5–7 years, when they develop progressive difficulty running and climbing stairs; proximal myopathy is then evident, along with calf enlargement (pseudohypertrophy).
- Gowers maneuver may be observed in rising from the floor: "climbing up the legs."
- Boys usually become wheelchair bound around 12 years.
- Scoliosis.
- +/– Mild mental impairment (IQ <70 in 20% of boys).
- Cardiac involvement: cardiac conduction defects, dilated cardiomyopathy.
- Nocturnal hypoventilation in later disease may lead to excessive daytime somnolence.
- 5–10% of female carriers (heterozygotes) have muscle weakness, enlarged calves, +/– dilated cardiomyopathy.

Investigation

Blood creatine kinase is raised from birth, usually in the thousands. EMG shows a myopathy. ECG shows prominent R waves in right precordial leads, deep Q waves in left precordial and limb leads; echocardiogram may be required if cardiomyopathy is suspected. Muscle biopsy shows variation in fiber size, fiber necrosis (broken down sarcolemma), macrophage invasion, muscle replaced with fat and connective tissue; there is deficient dystrophin on immunohistochemistry.

Neurogenetics shows mutations in dystrophin gene. Lung function may be measured (FVC) if there is excessive daytime somnolence, +/– sleep studies considered.

Differential diagnosis

The clinical picture is so characteristic that it is not likely to be mistaken for other disorders.

Treatment and prognosis

Prognosis is poor: most boys die in their 20s from pneumonia +/– cardiac complications. Cardiac conduction defects may require pacemaker insertion. Respiratory problems: scoliosis surgery may help to preserve lung function (but succinylcholine should be avoided during anesthesia as this may cause myoglobinuria); elective tracheostomy and/or nocturnal intermittent positive pressure ventilation may be required for nocturnal hypoventilation.

References

Bushby K, Finkel R, Birnkrant DJ, et al. Diagnosis and management of Duchenne muscular dystrophy, part 1: diagnosis, and pharmacological and psychosocial management. Lancet Neurol. 2010;9:77–93
Bushby K, Finkel R, Birnkrant DJ, et al. Diagnosis and management of Duchenne muscular dystrophy, part 2: implementation of multidisciplinary care. Lancet Neurol. 2010;9:177–189
Emery AEH, Muntoni F. Duchenne Muscular Dystrophy. 3rd ed. Oxford: Oxford University Press; 2003
Sinnreich M. Dystrophinopathies. In: Karpati G, Hilton-Jones D, Bushby K, Griggs RC eds. Disorders of Voluntary Muscle. 8th ed. Cambridge: Cambridge University Press; 2010:205–229

Dural arteriovenous fistula (DAVF)

Dural arteriovenous fistula (DAVF) is an acquired type of *vascular malformation* characterized by a direct high flow connection between artery and vein (cf. *arteriovenous malformations*). These may occur intracranially or in the spinal cord. *Carotico-cavernous fistula (CCF)* is usually considered separately from other intracranial DAVF. There are various classifications, such as that of Borden, recognizing three types based on drainage into dural venous sinuses and meningeal veins, with or without retrograde flow, or directly into subarachnoid veins. Pathophysiology is related to venous congestion causing venous hypertension.

Clinical features

- Intracranial: presents either with hemorrhage (intracerebral, subdural, subarachnoid) or with venous hypertension, manifested as pulsatile tinnitus, dementia, epileptic seizures, encephalopathy, parkinsonism.
- Spinal: presents with spinal subarachnoid hemorrhage or progressive myelopathy, which may mimic a polyradiculopathy or anterior horn cell disease in its early stages. Most patients are middle-aged men (cf. AVM).

Investigation

MRI and MR angiography are likely to reveal the abnormal fistula, although sometimes catheter angiography is required to define precise angio-architecture. In the spinal cord, cord swelling with centrally located hyperintense signal on T_2 with hypointense flow voids dorsal to the cord (enlarged tortuous veins) may be seen; more sensitive still is peripheral cord enhancement with gadolinium. Spinal angiography is a long and complex procedure. Lumbar puncture is best avoided since it may be associated with sudden deterioration.

Differential diagnosis

DAVF may be unrecognized as the source of *subarachnoid hemorrhage* or *intracerebral hemorrhage*. Other causes of venous hypertension.

Treatment and prognosis

Treatment is individualized, requiring endovascular, surgical, and radiotherapeutic approaches either singly or in combination, dependent on the location and exact form of the DAVF. Tinnitus, cognitive deficits, encephalopathy, parkinsonism, and myelopathy may be rapidly ameliorated or reversed, and the risk of future hemorrhage reduced.

References

Borden JA, Wu JK, Shucart WA. A proposed classification for spinal and cranial dural arteriovenous fistulous malformations and implications for treatment. J Neurosurg. 1995;82:166–179. [Erratum: J Neurosurg 1995;82:705–706]

Jellema K, Tijssen CC, van Gijn J. Spinal dural arteriovenous fistulas: a congestive myelopathy that initially mimics a peripheral nerve disorder. Brain. 2006;129: 3150–3164

Wilson M, Doran M, Enevoldson TP, Larner AJ. Cognitive profiles associated with intracranial dural arteriovenous fistula. Age Ageing. 2010;39:389–392

Wilson M, Menezes B, Enevoldson P. Intracranial dural arterio-venous fistula. Pract Neurol. 2008;8:362–369

Dysembryoplastic neuroepithelial tumor (DNET)

Dysembryoplastic neuroepithelial tumors (DNET) are low-grade tumors, possibly even hamartomas, of mixed neuronal/glial cell lineage, although they are often categorized with neuronal tumors, which are an important cause of *epilepsy*. They occur throughout childhood, most often in the temporal lobe, as a focal circumscribed cortical mass, which may indent the overlying skull. DNETs may cause intractable complex partial and secondary generalized seizures without other neurological signs, and may account for 10–30% of resected temporal lobe tumors. They are multinodular and may be associated with cortical dysplasia. Brain imaging shows a circumscribed mass, which may calcify and may show contrast enhancement. Prognosis after surgical resection is generally good.

Ganglioglioma and other low-grade tumors with a predilection for the temporal lobe, causing an intractable seizure disorder, enter the differential diagnosis.

References

Burneo JG, Tellez-Zenteno J, Steven DA, et al. Adult-onset epilepsy associated with dysembryoplastic neuroepithelial tumors. Seizure. 2008;17:498–504
Daumas-Duport C. Dysembryoplastic neuroepithelial tumors. Brain Pathol. 1993;8: 283–295

Dysferlinopathy

Dysferlinopathy is a generic term for allelic disorders associated with mutations in the gene encoding dysferlin located on chromosome 2p13. The clinical phenotype of these conditions is variable, including at least three allelic disorders:

- *Limb girdle muscular dystrophy* (type 2B)
- *Miyoshi myopathy*
- Distal anterior compartment myopathy

References

Pradhan S. Clinical and magnetic resonance imaging features of "diamond on quadriceps" sign in dysferlinopathy. Neurol India. 2009;57:172–175
Ueyama H, Kumamoto T, Nagano S, et al. A new dysferlin gene mutation in two Japanese families with limb-girdle muscular dystrophy 2B and Miyoshi myopathy. Neuromusc Disord. 2001;11:139–145

Dystonia: overview

Dystonia is defined as a motor syndrome of sustained involuntary muscle contractions causing twisting and repetitive movements and/or abnormal postures. Dystonic movements may be slow and twisting (athetosis), rapid or rhythmic (dystonic tremor), or apparent only with certain actions (action dystonia) or skilled tasks (task-specific dystonia). Hence, examination of the dystonia and the actions that induce it is important. Pathophysiology remains ill-understood; central and peripheral mechanisms may be relevant, involving both motor and sensory systems, perhaps to different degrees in different syndromes and resulting in some form of maladaptive plasticity in sensorimotor cortex.

The dystonias may be defined by their anatomical extent, in terms of which body parts are involved:

- Focal, that is, involving a single body part
- Segmental, that is, two or more adjacent body parts

- Multifocal, that is, two or more noncontiguous body parts
- Generalized

Focal dystonias typically occur in adult life and are idiopathic in origin. A clue to the dystonic origin of these movements, which, particularly in the past, were sometimes labeled as "hysterical," is the observation of transient relief of the movements by the use of sensory tricks (*geste antagoniste*).

- Focal dystonias include:
  - Cranial dystonia:
    - Meige's syndrome
    - Blepharospasm +/– oromandibular dystonia (Brueghel syndrome)
  - Cervical dystonia (spasmodic torticollis)
  - Writer's cramp (graphospasm)
  - Spasmodic dysphonia
  - Axial dystonia:
    - Spasms of the trunk, which interfere with lying, sitting, standing, or walking
  - Leg dystonia:
    - Inversion and plantar flexion of the foot causing the patient to walk on their toes (toe-walking)
  - Anismus:
    - A focal dystonia of the external anal sphincter during attempted defecation, leading to fecal retention and a complaint of constipation
  - Dystonic dysphagia:
    - A rare dystonia of pharyngeal muscles causing dysphagia; dystonic body movements in children may be induced by gastro-esophageal reflux (Sandifer syndrome or dyspeptic dystonia)
  - Other task-specific or occupational dystonias ("craft palsies"):
    - Scrivener's palsy (= writer's cramp)
    - Auctioneer's jaw, "greeter's cramp"
    - Musician's dystonia: playing various musical instruments, for example, fingers with piano, hand with violin, drum; mouth with brass, woodwind (embouchure dystonia)
    - Typists: hand
    - Sport: "the yips," golf, darts, boules
    - Prayer-induced focal dystonia

Status dystonicus is an unusual syndrome of increasingly frequent and relentless episodes of generalized dystonia. It may be precipitated by infection or drugs. Because of bulbar and respiratory complications patients may need ventilation and sedation; *rhabdomyolysis* may occur. Outcome may vary from return to prior clinical situation, worsened clinical features, or death.

The dystonias may also be classified according to their etiology; hence, family history and perinatal history are important:

- Primary or idiopathic dystonias
  - Hereditary:
    - Generalized dystonia (primary torsion dystonia, dystonia musculorum deformans, idiopathic torsion dystonia: usually autosomal dominant). No hypoxic-ischemic birth injury or kernicterus, normal early developmental milestones. Variable phenotype: spectrum ranges from mild focal dystonia to disabling generalized dystonia. Variable age at onset: with childhood onset, the majority will develop generalized dystonia; usually limb onset (leg > arm), with toe walking, bizarre dystonic gait, falls; with adult onset, may present with writer's cramp, cranial dystonia. Cognition, sphincters, vision, hearing, sensory function all normal; no epileptic seizures. Stable once generalized dystonia present; relentless progression suggests secondary dystonia.
    - X-linked dystonia-parkinsonism syndrome (Lubag disease).
    - Alcohol responsive dystonia, myoclonus-dystonia syndrome (autosomal dominant).
    - Dopa-responsive dystonia (Segawa syndrome; autosomal dominant).
    - Paroxysmal kinesigenic or non-kinesigenic dystonia (?autosomal dominant).
    - Dystonia in mitochondrial disease.
  - Nonhereditary:
    - Sporadic generalized dystonia
    - Sporadic paroxysmal non-kinesigenic dystonia
    - Focal dystonias (see listing above)
- Symptomatic or secondary dystonia:
  - Inherited metabolic causes:
    - Wilson's disease, Menkes disease
    - Gangliosidoses: GM1, GM2
    - Metachromatic leukodystrophy
    - Lesch–Nyhan disease
    - Organic acidurias, for example, glutaric aciduria type I
    - Homocystinuria
    - Hexosaminidase A and B deficiency
    - Hartnup's disease
    - Rett syndrome
    - Triose phosphate isomerase deficiency
  - Noninherited metabolic causes:
    - Kernicterus
  - Inherited possible metabolic causes:
    - Neurodegeneration with brain iron accumulation (formerly known as Hallervorden–Spatz disease)
    - Basal ganglia calcification

- ○ Leigh's syndrome
- ○ Bilateral necrosis of basal ganglia (+/– Leber's hereditary optic neuropathy)
- ○ Niemann–Pick disease
- Inherited non-metabolic causes:
  - ○ Ataxia telangiectasia
  - ○ Neuroacanthocytosis
  - ○ Neuronal ceroid lipofuscinosis
  - ○ Huntington's disease
  - ○ Spinocerebellar ataxias (especially Machado–Joseph disease)
- Noninherited, non-metabolic causes:
  - ○ Degenerative disorders:
    - Parkinson's disease and its treatment
    - Progressive supranuclear palsy
    - Multiple system atrophy
    - Pallidopyramidal degeneration
  - ○ Trauma:
    - Head trauma, cervical cord, and peripheral nerve injury, often with a delay before the onset of the dystonia. In peripheral nerve damage, focal dystonia may develop in conjunction with complex regional pain syndrome (reflex sympathetic dystrophy, Sudeck's atrophy)
  - ○ Anoxia/ischemia:
    - Perinatal anoxia causing immediate and delayed (i.e., up to 20 years) dystonia
    - Cerebrovascular disease
  - ○ Arteriovenous malformations
  - ○ Tumors: of the basal ganglia can present with hemidystonia
  - ○ Toxins: manganese, carbon monoxide, carbon disulphide, methanol, mercury
  - ○ Infections, postinfectious disorders:
    - Encephalitis
    - Reye's syndrome
    - Subacute sclerosing panencephalitis (SSPE)
  - ○ Postoperative: especially after thalamotomy
  - ○ Multiple sclerosis (often paroxysmal)
  - ○ Drug-induced:
    - Neuroleptics
    - Dopamine agonists
    - Antiepileptic drugs
    - Selective serotonin reuptake inhibitors
    - Tetrabenazine
    - Flecainide
    - Propranolol
    - Cimetidine
  - ○ Psychogenic

The dystonias may also be classified according to their age of onset:

- Childhood onset (<13 years of age):

65% generalize; leg involvement common; cause found in ca. 40%

- Adolescent onset (13–20 years of age):

35% generalize, leg involvement often, cause found in ca. 30%

- Adult onset (>20 years of age):

3% generalize, leg involvement very rare, cause found in ca. 13%.

Increasingly dystonias may now be classified according to their genetic basis; a number of genetic mutations and chromosomal linkages have been defined:

Gene	Locus	Inheritance	Clinical classification	Protein
DYT1	9q34	AD	Primary torsion dystonia (PTD)	Torsin A
DYT2	Unknown	AR	Autosomal recessive PTD	Unknown
DYT3	Xq13.1	X-linked	X-linked dystonia-parkinsonism, lubag	Unknown
DYT4	Unknown	AD	Whispering dysphonia + dystonia	Unknown
DYT5	14q22.1-q22.2	AD	Dopa-responsive dystonia (DRD)	GTP cyclohydrolase 1
DYT6	8p21-q22	AD	Cranial cervical dystonia	THAP1
DYT7	18p	AD	Focal dystonia, predominantly cervical	Unknown
DYT8	2q	AD	Paroxysmal nonkinesigenic dyskinesia with dystonia and choreoathetosis	Unknown

(continued)

Gene	Locus	Inheritance	Clinical classification	Protein
DYT9	1p	AD	Paroxysmal choreoathetosis with episodic ataxia, spasticity	Unknown
DYT10	16p11.2	AD	Paroxysmal kinesigenic dyskinesia with generalized dystonia, chorea, athetosis	Unknown
DYT11	7q21	AD	Myoclonus-dystonia	ε-Sarcoglycan
DYT12	19q13	AD	Rapid onset dystonia-parkinsonism	Unknown
DYT13	1p36	AD	Generalized dystonia with variable presentation	Unknown
DYT14	14q13	AD	Dopamine responsive dystonia	Unknown
DYT15	18p11	AD	Myoclonic dystonia	Unknown
DYT16	2q31	AR	Generalized dystonia-parkinsonism	PRKRA
DYT17	20p11.22-q13.12	AR	Focal torsion dystonia	Unknown

Investigation

A large number of investigations may be appropriate in a patient with a dystonia, particularly if the dystonia is generalized.

- Bloods: FBC, 3 (fresh) blood films for acanthocytes
  - ESR
  - Biochemical screen (U&E; glucose; liver and thyroid function tests)
  - Copper/Caeruloplasmin (to exclude *Wilson's disease*, potentially treatable)
  - Lactate/Pyruvate ratio
  - Syphilis serology

- – Creatine kinase
- – Antinuclear antibodies, rheumatoid factor, and immunoglobulins
- – Uric acid
- – α-Fetoprotein
- – White cell enzymes
- – Plasma amino acids
- – Toxicology screen
- Urine: Organic acids
  - – Amino acids
  - – Twenty-four hours protein excretion; creatinine clearance; copper excretion
  - – Mucopolysaccharides/oligosaccharides
- Neuroimaging: MRI brain +/– cervical cord
- CSF: including lactate, oligoclonal bands, +/– lactate/pyruvate ratio
- Neurophysiology: EMG/NCS; EEG; ERG; evoked potentials
- Ophthalmology: Kayser–Fleischer rings, retinal vasculitis
- Neurogenetic testing: a number of specific tests are now fairly readily available, for example, DYT1, DYT5, DYT11. Testing for Huntington's disease, spinocerebellar ataxias may also be appropriate in some circumstances.
- Other: Bone marrow aspirate; Skin/muscle biopsy.

Differential diagnosis

Generalized dystonia in childhood may be misdiagnosed as *cerebral palsy;* hence, the diagnostic importance of ascertaining normal birth and early developmental milestones. Some cases labeled as cerebral palsy may in fact have a dystonic syndrome, for example, dopa-responsive dystonia, glutaric aciduria type I. Odd gait and falls in childhood may be labeled "psychiatric." Adult (>20 years): very rare to develop generalized dystonia; usually onset in axial or cranial muscles.

Treatment and prognosis

Focal dystonias respond poorly to drug therapy and the mainstay of treatment is therefore with local injections of botulinum toxin.

Treatment and prognosis

Treat cause if possible, that is, secondary dystonia, for example, Wilson's disease.

Because of the exquisite and long-lasting sensitivity of dopa-responsive dystonia to levodopa preparations, it is recommended that all patients with young-onset generalized dystonia should receive a trial of levodopa (e.g., two tablets of Sinemet plus or Madopar 125 tds).

In other generalized dystonias, treatment is often disappointing and involves polypharmacy. Other agents that can be used in generalized dystonias include:

- Anticholinergic agents:
  - Benzhexol (trihexyphenidyl) 1 mg bd increasing by 1 mg/day every 1–2 weeks to a maximum dose of 180 mg. Treatment is usually limited by side effects, although most benefit is seen with very high doses of these agents.
- Benzodiazepines:
  - Diazepam, often in high dose.
- Others:
  - Baclofen.
  - Carbamazepine (may be useful for paroxysmal kinesigenic or non-kinesigenic dystonia).
  - Haloperidol, phenothiazines.
  - Tetrabenazine.
  - Pimozide.

In difficult cases, patients may require high-dose anticholinergic drugs with diazepam, tetrabenazine +/– pimozide.

Focal dystonia best treated with botulinum toxin injections.

Other treatments such as physiotherapy and supportive psychotherapy are useful but mechanical braces and other surgical appliances are useless.

Prognosis is linked to age at onset; 5% of all idiopathic dystonias have spontaneous improvement or even resolution of movement disorder, typically within the first 5 years of the illness. However, subsequent relapses are common. Childhood dystonias tend to stabilize in adulthood. Most adult dystonias are focal in nature and remain so; they respond poorly to drug therapy and are best treated with local injections of botulinum toxin.

Stereotactic surgery for dystonia is the subject of resurgent interest; pallidotomy seems to be more effective than thalamotomy in alleviating dystonia (likewise dyskinesia). Deep brain stimulation to the GPi may be effective, especially in those with DYT1 dystonia.

References

Albanese A, Barnes MP, Bhatia KP, et al. A systematic review on the diagnosis and treatment of primary (idiopathic) dystonia and dystonia plus syndromes: report of an EFNS/MDS-ES Task Force. Eur J Neurol. 2006;13:433–444

Altenmüller E. Focal dystonia: advances in brain imaging and understanding of fine motor control in musicians. Hand Clin. 2003;19:523–538

Breakefield XO, Blood AJ, Li Y, Hallett M, Hanson PI, Standaert DG. The pathophysiological basis of dystonia. Nat Rev Neurosci. 2008;9:222–234

Fahn S, Marsden CD, Calne DB. Classification and investigation of dystonia. In: Marsden CD, Fahn S, eds. Movement Disorders 2. London: Butterworth; 1987:332–358
Manji H, Howard RS, Miller DH, et al. Status dystonicus: the syndrome and its management. Brain. 1998;121:243–252
Warner TT, Bressman SB, eds. Clincal Diagnosis and Management of Dystonia. Abingdon: Informa Healthcare; 2007

Dystrophinopathy

The term dystrophinopathy has been used to describe conditions in which the primary genetic disorder is in the gene encoding the sarcolemmal protein dystrophin, for instance, *Duchenne muscular dystrophy* and *Becker muscular dystrophy*, in which there is immunohistochemical evidence of absence or deficiency, respectively, of dystrophin in muscle biopsies.

References

Muntoni F, Torelli S, Ferlini A. Dystrophin and mutations: one gene, several proteins, multiple phenotypes. Lancet Neurol. 2003;2:731–740
Sinnreich M. Dystrophinopathies. In: Karpati G, Hilton-Jones D, Bushby K, Griggs RC, eds. Disorders of Voluntary Muscle. 8th ed. Cambridge: Cambridge University Press; 2010:205–229

E

Eating disorders

Anorexia nervosa and bulimia have been considered as psychiatric diseases, but in light of the known roles of the hypothalamus in controlling feeding behavior, some consider them hypothalamic diseases. Both occur predominantly in young women. Anorexia nervosa is characterized by extreme emaciation as a result of voluntary starvation, related to a distorted body image with fear of gaining weight. Occasional cases have been described in association with hypothalamic tumors, akin to the diencephalic syndrome of infants with hypothalamic mass lesions. Mild diabetes insipidus may occur. There are no characteristic neurological signs, although "hung-up" tendon reflexes have been described. Bulimia (literally "ox-eating") is characterized by binge eating followed by induced vomiting and excessive use of laxatives. Antidepressant medications may help in both anorexia nervosa and bulimia. Hyperphagia akin to that seen in bulimia may occur as one feature of the *Kleine–Levin syndrome*. Disorders of eating may also occur in *frontotemporal lobar degeneration* syndromes of behavioral/disinhibited type. The neuroanatomical substrates of eating disorders are debated: hypothalamic and brainstem lesions may be associated with changes in appetite and eating behavior, but more complex syndromes are associated with right frontal (e.g., *Gourmand syndrome*) and temporal lobe damage.

References

Fairburn CG, Harrison PJ. Eating disorders. Lancet. 2003;361:407–416
Uher R, Treasure J. Brain lesions and eating disorders. J Neurol Neurosurg Psychiatry. 2005;76:852–857

Echinococcosis

Hydatid disease

Infection with the cestode larval tapeworms of the genus *Echinococcus* (*E. granulosus, E. multilocularis*, or *E. vogeli*) may cause cystic lesions (hydatid cysts). The disease occurs in areas where dogs (definitive host) and sheep or cattle (intermediate hosts) are common, hence it occurs mostly in Wales, Australia, Eastern Europe, Argentina and Chile, Africa, and the Middle East. The ova are found in canine feces and, on human ingestion, escape from their eggs, enter the portal circulation, and spread to various organs, including, on occasion, brain and muscle. In these sites, as in other organs, cysts cause symptoms by local compression, for example, seizures, compressive myelopathies (spinal epidural abscess; hydatid Pott's disease). Imaging reveals single or multiple cysts, often with scolices evident within them; different cysts may be at different stages of maturity. There may be a peripheral eosinophilia. Serology (ELISA, indirect hemagglutination) may assist with diagnosis but is not reliable. Differential diagnosis includes *neurocysticercosis*. Treatment of choice is surgical resection of the cyst(s), taking care to avoid rupture as this can be associated with anaphylaxis or recurrent disease. Treatment with albendazole or mebendazole may shrink cysts, and nonresectable cysts may be treated with albendazole (400 mg bd).

Eclampsia

Eclampsia is the most feared neurological complication of pregnancy, defined as the development of seizures with or without coma on the background of preeclampsia, the latter defined as raised blood pressure (>140/90 mmHg), proteinuria, and edema after 20 weeks of gestation. Hence, eclampsia requires the onset of symptoms, specifically seizures. Eclampsia may be subdivided as

* Antepartum (three-quarters of all eclampsia: before 28 weeks = "early")
* Intrapartum (no pre-eclampsia prior to labor)
* Postpartum (within 7 days of delivery)

Eclampsia may complicate as many as 1:2,000 deliveries and is a significant cause of maternal deaths during pregnanacy (~10%). The pathophysiology is uncertain; presumably, hypertension in some way triggers hemorrhages and microinfarcts within cerebral white matter. Seizures are best treated with high doses of parenteral magnesium. Eclampsia may occasionally be seen with hydatiform moles.

Clinical features

- Preeclampsia: hypertension (>140/90 mmHg), proteinuria, and edema after 20 weeks of gestation.
- Headache.
- Epileptic seizures; usually tonic–clonic.
- Obtundation, stupor, and coma.
- Focal neurological signs may develop, including visual scintillations, visual loss, and hemiparesis.
- HELLP syndrome: hemolysis, elevated liver function tests, low platelet count.

Investigation

Bloods may show pregnancy-induced anemia; clotting studies may show the development of disseminated intravascular coagulopathy, an alarming finding. Renal function may be abnormal. Urine shows proteinuria. Neuroimaging (CT/MRI) may be normal, but may show white matter (especially occipital) hypodensity/T_2-weighted hyperintensity; occasionally, multiple small hemorrhages may be seen. EEG is abnormal in 80% of cases, with slowing +/– spikes. CSF examination is not usually necessary.

Differential diagnosis

Other causes of seizures during pregnancy: preexisting epilepsy, cerebral venous thrombosis, cerebrovascular events, space-occupying lesion, infection, metabolic disorder (e.g., hypoglycemia). Other intracranial pathologies: subarachnoid hemorrhage, pituitary apoplexy, and *posterior reversible leukoencephalopathy syndrome (PRES)*.

Treatment and prognosis

Maternal-fetal monitoring for preeclampsia, since prevention is the best treatment. Adequate oxygenation, control of blood pressure (hydralazine, labetalol, nifedipine if rapid control required) and of seizures: magnesium sulfate is now the treatment of choice (preferable to phenytoin, benzodiazepines), for example, as 4 g i.v. over 5–20 min, then an infusion of 1 g/h for 24 h, or 5 g each buttock + single 5 g injection every 4 h, and if seizures recur, then 2–4 g magnesium over 5 min i.v. Need continuous monitoring of ECG, blood pressure, and clinical signs; look for evidence of hypermagnesemia (loss of knee jerks, weakness, nausea, sensation of warmth, flushing, drowsiness, diplopia, and dysarthria), if present treat with calcium gluconate. Management/prevention of organ failure. Safe delivery of the fetus. Eclampsia is a significant cause of maternal perinatal mortality. Prevention cannot therefore be too heavily emphasized.

References

Sibai B, Dekker G, Kupferminc M. Pre-eclampsia. Lancet. 2005;365:785–799
The Eclampsia Trial Collaborative Group. Which anticonvulsant for women with eclampsia? Evidence from the Collaborative Eclampsia Trial. Lancet. 1995;345: 455–1463
Thomas SV. Neurological aspects of eclampsia. J Neurol Sci. 1998;155:37–43

Ehlers–Danlos syndrome

This inherited disorder of connective tissue, of which several subtypes are recognized, may be complicated by various neurological features, in addition to the well-known dermatological manifestations (hyperelasticity of skin, hyperextensibility of joints, and easy bruising). Type IV associated with mutations in the COL3A1 gene on chromosome 2, which codes for the α-1 chain of type III collagen [OMIM#130050], is particularly associated with neurovascular complications:

- Dissection/rupture of intra- and extracranial arteries (usually spontaneous)
- Intra- and extracranial aneurysm formation; subarachnoid hemorrhage (SAH)
- Carotid–cavernous fistula (CCF).
- Mitral valve prolapse

Myotonia and peripheral neuropathy have also been described. Other serious complications include uterine rupture during pregnancy, and arterial or visceral rupture.

References

North KN, Whiteman DAH, Pepin MG, et al. Cerebrovascular complications in Ehlers-Danlos syndrome Type IV. Ann Neurol. 1995; 38:960–964
Pepin M, Schwarze U, Superti-Furga A, Byers PH. Clinical and genetic features of Ehlers-Danlos syndrome type IV, the vascular type. N Engl J Med. 2000;342:673–680

Ehrlichiosis

Infection with tick-borne *Ehrlichia*, an intraleukocytic bacterium which resembles the *Rickettsiae*, may cause meningitis, epileptic seizures, and encephalopathy. Early treatment with doxycycline may reduce complications and reduce duration of hospital stay.

Reference

Fishbein DB, Dawson JE, Robinson LE. Human Ehrlichiosis in the United States, 1985–1990. Ann Intern Med. 1994;120:736–743

Hamburg BJ, Storch GA, Micek ST, Kollef MH. The importance of early treatment with doxycycline in human ehrlichosis. Medicine (Baltimore). 2008;87:53–60

Eighteen q deletion syndrome [OMIM#601808]

De Grouchy syndrome, 18q- syndrome

Deletion of the long arm of chromosome 18 produces a multiple-anomaly mental retardation syndrome of variable phenotype encompassing learning disability, sometimes with nondevelopment of language, short stature, and variable dysmorphism, such as microcephaly, midfacial hypoplasia, prominent antihelix, and long tapering fingers. Hearing loss, sensorineural or conductive, is common, the latter due to congenital aural atresia. Neurological symptoms and signs, such as hypotonia, nystagmus, and incoordination, are also common. Movement disorders such as tremor and dystonia have been reported, as have seizure disorders of variable semiology, including complex partial seizures with prominent autonomic features, apneic seizures, and benign focal seizures, most usually with childhood onset but sometimes presenting in adults. Neuroimaging (MRI) typically shows confluent or multifocal white matter abnormalities with poor differentiation of the grey/white matter interface on T_2-weighted images due to increased white matter signal, reflecting abnormal myelination of the white matter. Neuropathological studies confirm the abnormal myelination seen on brain imaging.

Reference

Larner AJ. Deletion of 18q. In: Lang F, ed. Encyclopedia of Molecular Mechanisms of Disease. 3 vols. Berlin, Germany: Springer; 2009:503–504

Electrical injuries and the nervous system

Electrical injury to the nervous system can occur through lightning strikes or accidental contact with mains electricity. In many cases, it is fatal due to heat damage to the brain or ventricular fibrillation.

The injury sustained with electrical insults is dependent on the course of the current through the body; flow from the head to limbs will damage brain and spinal cord, while current between one arm and the other or to the leg will only affect the spinal cord.

Minor electrical injuries produce pain and paresthesiae that quickly resolve. More serious injuries may induce a number of neurological deficits, some of which are expressed at the time of the injury, others of which are delayed by 1–6 weeks. These include:

- Brain: loss of consciousness; headache, tinnitus, and seizures in the immediate postinjury period with recovery in a few days. Occasionally patients have a delayed vascular event that presents acutely and is thought to be thrombotic in origin. Occasionally patients have been described who develop parkinsonism. Recurrent seizures are rare, but an encephalopathy may develop in some patients with electrical injuries traversing the head, often in association with spinal cord and limb signs.
- Spinal cord: clinical manifestation of cord injury is often delayed: a syndrome of segmental wasting (spinal atrophic paralysis) may occur, progression of which may mimic *motor neurone disease* or a transverse myelopathy.
- Peripheral nervous system: damage may be so severe that repair does not occur, resulting in the development of a chronic pain syndrome.

Indirect neurological consequences of electrical injury may include traumatic brain and cord injury in falls after electrical injury.

A syndrome of diffuse electrical injury has also been reported with some symptoms remote from the current pathway, such as fatigue, exhaustion, low mood, personality change, in other words overlapping with the symptoms seen in disorders such as fibromyalgia, chronic fatigue syndrome, whiplash, and chronic pain syndromes.

References

Berg JS, Morse MS. Diffuse electrical injury. Pract Neurol. 2004;4:222–227
Duff K, McCaffrey RJ. Electrical injury and lightning injury: a review of their mechanisms and neuropsychological, psychiatric, and neurological sequelae. Neuropsychol Rev. 2001;11:101–116
Sirdofsky MD, Hawley RJ, Manz H. Progressive motor neuron disease associated with electrical injury. Muscle Nerve. 1991;14:977–980

Elsberg syndrome

Infectious polyradiculitis, Sacral myeloradiculitis

Elsberg syndrome is characterized by urinary retention with sensorimotor dysfunction (pain, hypoalgesia) affecting lumbosacral dermomyotomes due to polyradiculitis. This is a self-limiting condition, of viral etiology, more common in young women. There may be CSF pleocytosis, with skin eruption due to genital herpes, as HSV-2 is probably the most commonly identified infection. The syndrome may resemble idiopathic lumbosacral plexopathy. It may on occasion be associated with other disorders, such as *primary angiitis of the CNS*.

References

Eberhardt O, Küker W, Dichgans J, Weller M. HSV-2 sacral radiculitis (Elsberg syndrome). Neurology. 2004;63:758–759
Elsberg CA. Experiences in spinal surgery. Observations upon 60 laminectomies for spinal disease. Surgery, Gynecol Obstet. 1931;16:117–135

Emery–Dreifuss muscular dystrophy (EDMD)

This *muscular dystrophy* characterized by the early onset of contractures may be X-linked recessive [OMIM#310300], autosomal dominant [OMIM#181350], or autosomal recessive (rare), resulting from mutations in emerin and lamin A/C (hence allelic with *limb girdle muscular dystrophy* type 1B), respectively. Cardiac complications are common and may account for early death, sometimes in young adults without other evidence of muscular disorder; hence screening is important.

Clinical features

- Early development of joint contractures, sometimes even before clinical signs of weakness are apparent, affecting elbows, Achilles tendons, neck extensors.
- Slowly progressive wasting and weakness, initially in a humeroperoneal distribution, then extending to scapula and pelvic girdle.
- Cardiac disease in adulthood: cardiomyopathy, conduction defects (e.g., prolonged PR interval, complete heart block) by age 30 years. Cardiac manifestations may occur in the absence of muscle disease, and in female carriers of the disease, presenting with sudden death.

Investigation

Blood creatine kinase may be moderately elevated. EMG is myopathic. ECG should be performed to look for cardiac conduction abnormalities: sinus bradycardia, prolonged PR interval, complete heart block. Muscle biopsy shows dystrophic change, with scattered necrotic and regenerating fibers; variation in fiber diameter, increased number of hypertrophic fibers, splitting fibers, internal nuclei; disorganized intermyofibrillary networks producing a "moth-eaten" appearance. Neurogenetic testing may be undertaken, dependent on pattern of inheritance (from the family history), with analysis for mutations in the emerin or lamin A/C genes.

Differential diagnosis

Unlikely to be confused with other muscular dystrophies because of the prominence of contractures: these also occur in *Ullrich's congenital muscular dystrophy* and *Bethlem myopathy*, but the latter lacks cardiac involvement.

* *Rigid spine syndrome*
* *Scapuloperoneal syndrome*

Treatment and prognosis

EDMD is a progressive, incurable condition. Cardiac involvement is the most common cause of death through arrhythmia and cardiac failure. Pacemaker insertion may prolong life.

References

Bonne G, Lampe AK. Muscle diseases with prominent muscle contractures. In: Karpati G, Hilton-Jones D, Bushby K, Griggs RC, eds. Disorders of Voluntary Muscle. 8th ed. Cambridge: Cambridge University Press; 2010:299–313

Emery AEH, Dreifuss FE. Unusual type of benign X-linked muscular dystrophy. J Neurol Neurosurg Psychiatry. 1966;29:338–342

Emery AEH. Emery-Dreifuss muscular dystrophy – a 40 year retrospective. Neuromuscul Disord. 2000;10:228–232

Empty sella syndrome

The empty sella syndrome, or non-tumorous enlargement of the sella, is a radiological diagnosis in which there appears to be no pituitary gland in an expanded pituitary fossa. The presumed pathogenesis is a defect in the dural diaphragm which allows arachnoid to bulge downward, gradually enlarging the sella, possibly as a consequence of pressure pulsations in the CSF. This radiological appearance is sometimes seen in *idiopathic intracranial hypertension* and is not associated with clinical or biochemical evidence of pituitary insufficiency, as the gland remains functional as a thin ribbon of tissue along the wall of the expanded sella. Downward herniation of the optic chiasm may also occur, producing visual disturbances similar to those seen with a pituitary adenoma. In other cases, the radiological finding is incidental.

Encephalitis: overview

Encephalitis is inflammation of the brain parenchyma. This inflammation is usually due to direct invasion of brain tissue by infectious agents, most usually viral but sometimes protozoan, rickettsial, or fungal; there may be concurrent meningitic features (meningoencephalitis). Postinfectious encephalitis, due to allergic or immune reactions, may be clinically indistinguishable. Clinical clues as to the causative agent may be found, but often no specific microbe is identified. Encephalitis is also described with underlying malignancy (paraneoplastic *limbic encephalitis*). Infective encephalitides usually present acutely or subacutely, although chronic presentations and sequelae are not infrequent. Encephalitides may be classified in a number of ways:

- Location:
  - Diffuse: panencephalitis
  - Focal, for example, *herpes simplex encephalitis*, *Rasmussen's encephalitis*, paraneoplastic (limbic) encephalitis, transmissible spongiform encephalitis, brainstem encephalitis, *encephalitis lethargica*.
- Disease incidence:
  - Epidemic encephalitis:
    - Arboviral: including dengue, Russian spring-summer, *Japanese encephalitis*, St. Louis encephalitis, Eastern equine and Western equine encephalitis
    - (Von Economo's) encephalitis lethargica
  - Sporadic encephalitis:
    - Herpes simplex type 1
    - Mumps virus
    - *Epstein–Barr virus*
    - Adenovirus (especially type 7 in children)
    - Other viruses (including hepatitis, rotavirus, CMV)
  - Zoonotic encephalitis:
    - *Rabies*
    - Others including lymphocytic choriomeningitis
  - Chronic encephalitides:
    - *Subacute sclerosing panencephalitis (SSPE)*
    - Progressive measles encephalitis
    - Progressive rubella encephalitis
    - AIDS encephalopathy
    - *Progressive multifocal leukoencephalopathy (PML)*
    - Rasmussen's encephalitis

Specific encephalitides include:

- Viral:
  - Herpes simplex (HSV)
  - Varicella zoster (VZV)
  - Cytomegalovirus (CMV)
  - Epstein–Barr virus (EBV)
  - Measles
  - Mumps
  - Arboviruses: Japanese, California, St. Louis, Murray Valley, Eastern equine, Western equine, Russian spring-summer
  - Human immunodeficiency virus (HIV)
- Protozoal:
  - *Malaria*
  - Rabies
- Bacterial:
  - *Brucellosis*
  - *Legionnaire's disease*
  - *Mycoplasma pneumonia*
  - *Listeria monocytogenes*
  - *Neuroborreliosis* (Lyme disease)
  - Mycobacteria
- Fungal:
  - *Nocardia*
- *Rickettsial*:
  - *Coxiella burnetii*
  - Ehrlichiosis
- Paraneoplastic: limbic, brain stem
- Transmissible spongiform encephalitis (*prion disease*)
- Inflammatory disorders: sarcoid, SLE, *antiphospholipid syndrome*
- Autoimmune: with anti-VGKC channel antibodies, *NMDA-receptor encephalitis*

Clinical features

The presentation can be very dramatic with the patient becoming profoundly unwell and unconscious in a few hours. More typically, the patient presents with:

- Prodrome (days): myalgia, fever, malaise, anorexia; rash (may be characteristic for varicella or measles); parotitis suggests mumps
- Headache, mental change, drowsiness (i.e., encephalopathy), with or without meningitic features
- Coma
- Epileptic seizures

- +/– Focal signs, for example, hemiparesis, aphasia, cerebellar deficits, neuropsychological deficits (memory)
- +/– Raised intracranial pressure

Inquiries should be made about travel to areas where certain encephalitides are endemic.

Investigation

Bloods: evidence of systemic infection (raised ESR, CRP; leukocytosis; blood cultures, immunoglobulins, electrophoretic strip); other organ involvement (U+E, LFTs); viral serology; film for malaria if recent travel to endemic areas. Neuroimaging (CT/MRI) to exclude mass lesions, edema, infarction; may well be normal in the first 2–3 days. Bilateral temporal lobe hyperintensity may be seen in herpes simplex encephalitis (HSE), the commonest encephalitic illness in nontropical countries. EEG may show nonspecific diffuse slow-wave activity +/– epileptic activity; focal temporal lobe spike-and-wave activity is suggestive of HSE. CSF: standard investigations may be normal. Blood may be seen in some cases of severe encephalitis where there is hemorrhagic infarction of the brain. CSF may be under increased pressure; white count may be raised (tens to several thousands/μL), usually lymphocytes, sometimes polymorphs. Protein raised, glucose normal, organisms not seen on Gram stain. Indian ink stain if fungal infection suspected. CSF PCR for common viral causes of encephalitis (HSV, VZV, CMV, EBV). Brain biopsy is favored in some centers, but not others; may be a case for it in immunocompromised patients where diagnosis is not forthcoming by other means, or if there is a focal lesion on neuroimaging. Other tests are usually not necessary unless the presentation is atypical. Autoantibodies (including anti-neuronal, antithyroid, and anti-ENA antibodies) may be sent. Investigations appropriate to rare causes of an encephalitic illness may need to be considered, for example, prion disease, *Whipple's disease*, coeliac disease.

Differential diagnosis

Other encephalopathies, for example

- Infection:
  - Meningitis, especially bacterial
  - Septicemia
  - *Endocarditis*
  - Intracranial *abscess*
- Recreational drug use
- CNS *vasculitis*
- Epilepsy
- Organ failure, for example, liver failure

Treatment and prognosis

Assess patient and decide on level of dependency: may require supportive therapy on ITU.

Aciclovir (antiviral chemotherapy): start as soon as diagnosis is contemplated, especially HSE.

Antiepileptic medications for seizures.

Treat any secondary infections with antibiotic therapy, or if meningitis cannot be excluded.

Consider steroids if a vasculitis cannot be excluded.

Cerebral edema: hyperventilation; glycerol; mannitol; dexamethasone.

Symptomatic treatment: oxygenation (ventilation if necessary), hydration, nutrition.

Condition may be fatal; this was commonly the case before the advent of aciclovir. Recovery may be complete or there may be neurological and/or neuropsychological sequelae, especially an amnesic syndrome after HSE.

References

Anderson M. Encephalitis and other brain infections. In: Donaghy M, ed. Brain's Diseases of the Nervous System. 11th ed. Oxford: Oxford University Press; 2001: 1117–1180

Solomon T, Hart IJ, Beeching NJ. Viral encephalitis: a clinician's guide. Pract Neurol. 2007;7:288–305

Steiner I, Budka H, Chaudhuri A, et al. Viral encephalitis: a review of diagnostic methods and guidelines for management. Eur J Neurol. 2005;12:331–343

Encephalitis lethargica

Postencephalitic parkinsonism, Von Economo disease

Encephalitis lethargica is a parkinsonian syndrome of unknown cause, presumed viral, which occurred in epidemic form in the years after World War I, but is now rare. Clinical features are initially of fever, somnolence, personality changes, and cranial nerve involvement, especially ophthalmoplegia. There may be a CSF leukocytosis and anti-basal ganglia antibodies may be positive. Basal ganglia hypermetabolism may be demonstrated with ^{18}F-FDG PET. A prolonged convalescent period is characterized by parkinsonism and oculogyric crises; myoclonus, dystonia, bulimia, obesity, and sleep disturbances are also reported. Imaging findings are nonspecific: bilateral substantia nigra changes may be seen. Response to levodopa has been demonstrated, and in refractory cases intravenous methylprednisolone has been reported of benefit. Myoclonus may be treated with clonazepam.

Although presumed to be related to the influenza pandemic following World War I, archival brain tissue examined for influenza RNA has been negative. This virus may not have been neurotropic and hence not directly responsible.

References

Dickman MS. Von Economo encephalitis. Arch Neurol. 2001;58:1696–1698
Lopez-Alberola R, Georgiou M, Sfakianakis GN, Singer C, Papapetropoulous S. Contemporary encephalitis lethargica: phenotype, laboratory findings and treatment outcomes. J Neurol. 2009;256:396–404

Encephalopathies: overview

Encephalopathy describes a state of diffuse or global cerebral dysfunction in which patients are typically confused, delirious, or comatose, with abnormal eye movements and asterixis (flapping tremor). Epileptic seizures may occur. Encephalopathies most commonly result from acute (or acute on chronic, or decompensated) metabolic disturbances or toxic insults (including drugs) to the CNS, although the term has also been used in the context of vascular (e.g., Binswanger), epileptic, or neurodegenerative (e.g., Alzheimer's, Creutzfeldt–Jakob) disease.

The differential diagnosis of encephalopathy is broad, but essentially the causes fall into three large groups: metabolic, infective (septic), and drug/toxin induced.

- Metabolic encephalopathies:
  - Hepatic encephalopathy: liver failure.
  - Wernicke's encephalopathy: thiamine deficiency.
  - Uremic encephalopathy.
  - Anoxic-ischemic encephalopathies: may be acute (at the time of the original or ongoing insult), or delayed, emerging after a number of days to weeks (postanoxic encephalopthy, e.g., *carbon monoxide poisoning*).
  - *Lactic acidosis*: for example, *mitochondrial disease*; typically these patients (usually children) become encephalopathic with an intercurrent illness such as a viral infection.
  - Electrolyte disturbances: for example, Na^+, Ca^{++}, Mg^{++}; disorders of glucose homeostasis, for example, hyperosmolar state.
  - Hypertensive encephalopathy: for example, with uncontrolled hypertension.
  - Endocrine encephalopathies: for example, Cushing's disease, hyper- and hypothyroidism, *Hashimoto's encephalopathy* (irrespective of thyroid status).
  - Mitochondrial disorders, urea cycle enzyme defects.
- Septic encephalopathies:
  - Marked brain dysfunction in the context of systemic sepsis with or without multiorgan failure, for example, infective *endocarditis*.

- Drug-/toxin-induced encephalopathies: not uncommon; may be precipitated by a number of agents including:
  - Alcohol.
  - Sedatives, for example, benzodiazepines, opiates.
  - Antidepressants.
  - Metals: lead in children; bismuth.
  - Radiation.

Clinical features

History of prior illness (hepatic, renal, respiratory); drug/toxin exposure.

- Global signs:
  - Disturbance of consciousness: drowsy to comatose.
  - Epileptic seizures.
  - Delirium.
- Focal signs:
  - Hemiplegia, hemisensory signs, ataxia, myoclonus.
  - Aphasia, apraxia.
  - Brainstem signs: orofacial automatisms, posturing, asterixis, tremor.

Investigation

Bloods: consider FBC + film, ESR, clotting including FDPs, urea and electrolytes, glucose, calcium, magnesium, other electrolytes, thyroid function tests, blood cultures, serology, ammonia, lactate, and arterial blood gases. Imaging: includes CXR, CT/MRI (+ MRV) brain +/- echocardiography, abdominal ultrasound. CSF analysis may be required, including lactate. Neurophysiology (EEG) may show nonspecific slowing.

Differential diagnosis

- *Encephalitis/meningitis*
- Nonconvulsive status epilepticus
- Cerebral *vasculitis*
- Cerebral *venous sinus thrombosis*
- Hypothalamic damage

Treatment and prognosis

Of cause where identified. If in doubt, there is little to be lost and possibly much to be gained by administration of thiamine. Therapeutic trials of naloxone (opiate antagonist) and flumazenil (benzodiazepine antagonist) may also be considered if the clinical picture is compatible. Otherwise, supportive care; symptomatic treatment of seizures.

Reference

Angel MJ, Chen R, Bryan Young G. Metabolic encephalopathies. Handb Clin Neurol. 2008;90:115–166

Endocarditis: overview

Infective endocarditis is a microbial infection of the endocardial surface of the heart, most commonly on valves (especially if prosthetic or deformed) but also on chordae tendinae or mural endocardium. The characteristic lesions are vegetations formed of platelets, fibrin, microorganisms, and inflammatory cells. Distinction is sometimes made between acute and sub-acute-chronic endocarditis, dependent on the pace of the disease. Various microorganisms may be involved, including:

- Bacteria: *Streptococci*; if *bovis*, investigate for bowel neoplasm
- Staphylococci
- Pseudomonas, other Gram-negative bacilli
- Brucella
- Enterobacteria
- Fungi: for example, *Candida*
- Rickettsia: for example, *Coxiella* (Q fever)

Intravenous drug abuse and prolonged intravenous access (e.g., for parenteral nutrition) may predispose to endocarditis by providing a route for infection to enter the circulation.

Neurological consequences of endocarditis occur in about a third of cases and typically are embolic in nature, with vegetations embolizing to the cerebral circulation causing infarcts or the development of mycotic *aneurysms* that can rupture. Multiple septic emboli may cause a meningoencephalitis or *encephalopathy*. Treatment is with antibiotics.

Noninfective endocarditis may be seen in *systemic lupus erythematosus*.

Clinical features

- Cardiac:
  - Fever, variable heart murmurs, cardiac failure.
  - Embolic stigmata: nail bed infarcts (cf. nail trauma), Roth spots, Janeway lesions, Olser's nodes.
- Neurological:
  - 10–30% of patients with infective endocarditis present with neurological symptoms.
  - Focal deficits: secondary to embolic infarcts, due to vessel occlusion by septic embolus. May undergo hemorrhagic transformation. Most occur early in course of disease. Patients with *Q fever* are thought particularly prone to embolism.

- *Intracerebral hemorrhage*: secondary to rupture of a cerebral mycotic aneurysm; infected emboli lodge at the distal bifurcation points in the cerebral circulation, and typically are multiple. On occasions, the vessel may rupture with hemorrhage in the absence of aneurysm formation, due to a septic arteritis.
- Meningoencephalitis or diffuse encephalopathy: due to multiple septic emboli, presenting with confusion, meningism, and headache.
- Epileptic seizures.
- *Abscess*: brain, paraspinal.

Of those patients with infective endocarditis and neurological complications, infection with *S. aureus* and history of IV drug abuse are overrepresented compared to those with endocarditis and no neurological features.

Investigation

Bloods: FBC (anemia), ESR (elevated), CRP (elevated), and repeated blood cultures (x 3–6); INR if anticoagulated.

- Imaging:
  - CXR.
  - Echocardiogram: transthoracic, transesophageal.
  - CT/MRI +/– MR/catheter angiography when intracranial hemorrhage has occurred.

CSF: often normal, although a slight polymorph leukocytosis with some red cells and normal glucose is not uncommon. Large numbers of red cells may be seen in cases of intracerebral hemorrhage.

Cardiological and microbiological advice is often required.

Differential diagnosis

There is usually little doubt about the diagnosis, but in patients with a high ESR and cerebral events consider:

- Atrial myxoma
- Marantic or nonbacterial endocarditis (e.g., lupus, Libman–Sacks)
- Vasculitis (including *giant cell arteritis*)
- *Intravascular lymphoma* (angioendotheliomatosis)
- Hyperviscosity syndromes (e.g., Waldenström's macroglobulinemia)
- Cholesterol embolization syndrome
- Paraneoplastic encephalitis

Treatment and prognosis

Untreated the condition is fatal. Aggressive intravenous antimicrobial therapy appropriate for the infective agent is the mainstay of treatment, which may be required for several weeks, and with which most symptoms improve or resolve, including the neurological abnormalities. Embolic phenomena do not mandate anticoagulant treatment in patients with native valve endocarditis. In patients already receiving anticoagulation (e.g., for prosthetic valves), this should not be stopped unless there is intracerebral hemorrhage, when cessation of treatment for a short period (?2 days) is thought advisable. Mycotic aneurysms usually resolve with antibiotic therapy and do not require surgical intervention. Involvement of cardiologists and cardiothoracic surgeons is necessary, as the patient may require treatment for heart failure +/– valve replacement. Despite treatment, overall mortality remains 20–25%; mortality is twice as high in group with neurological complications.

References

Baig W, Sandoe J. Infective endocarditis. Clin Med. 2010;10:188–191

Derex L, Bonnefoy E, Delahaye F. Impact of stroke on therapeutic decision making in infective endocarditis. J Neurol. 2010;257:315–321

Kanter MC, Hart RG. Neurologic complications of infective endocarditis. Neurology. 1991;41:1015–1020

Lerner PI. Neurological manifestations of infective endocarditis. In: Aminoff MJ, ed. Neurology and General Medicine. The Neurological Aspects of Medical Disorders. 2nd ed. New York: Churchill Livingstone; 1995:97–117

Mylonakis E, Calderwood SB. Infective endocarditis in adults. N Engl J Med. 2001;345:1318–1330

Endocrine disorders and neurology: overview

Disorders of the endocrine system can affect the nervous system in a number of different ways. This may be developmental (e.g., in hypothyroidism), or acquired, global (e.g., *encephalopathy*), or focal (e.g., *carpal tunnel syndrome*).

- *Thyroid disease*:
  - Hypothyroidism:
    - In children:
      - Cretinism: manifest as prolonged neonatal jaundice, followed a few weeks later by the development of coarse facial features, thick tongue, protruding abdomen, irritability, and a coarse cry. If untreated it causes permanent mental retardation, with spasticity and cerebellar ataxia. Screening programs in the UK, the USA, and most developed countries have greatly reduced the incidence.
    - In adults:
      - Myopathy, sluggish reflexes, hypothermia, mental slowing, dementia.
      - Rare (and sometimes debatable) accounts of cerebellar syndrome, peripheral neuropathy, and pyramidal syndrome responding to thyroxine therapy.

- Hyperthyroidism:
  - Myopathy.
  - Tremor.
  - Ocular involvement: chemosis, proptosis, and ophthalmoplegia in Graves' disease.
  - Cognitive and mental changes, delirium.
  - Epileptic seizures.
  - Headache: migraine or tension type.
  - Polyneuropathy (distal sensorimotor).
  - Chorea.
- *Hashimoto's encephalopathy* may occur with hypo-, hyper-, or euthyroidism.
- Thyroid disease may be associated with other neurological disorders, for example, *myasthenia gravis*, *periodic paralysis*.
- Embolic phenomena may occur secondary to paroxysmal atrial fibrillation.
- Adrenal gland:
  - Deficiencies in adrenocortical hormones: Addison's disease may present with fatigue, generalized weakness, weight loss, headache, skin hyperpigmentation, and *syncope*. Adrenal failure is a feature of X-linked *adrenoleukodystrophy*.
  - Excessive adrenocortical secretion: Cushing's disease may present with *hypertension*, proximal myopathy, a psychiatric syndrome, or with an encephalopathy.
- *Pituitary disease*:
  - Anterior:
    - Growth Hormone:
      - Deficiency: in children causes a reduction in growth that responds to replacement therapy. Recombinant GH is now used; use of GH from cadaveric pituitaries was discontinued after some children developed iatrogenic *Creutzfeldt–Jakob disease*.
      - Excess: in children this causes gigantism, in adults *acromegaly*. In both cases, there may be secondary *diabetes mellitus*, proximal myopathy, and carpal tunnel syndrome.
      - In the diencephalic syndrome, GH secretion can be increased or decreased.
    - Gonadotrophins:
      - Deficiency: causes delayed puberty and amenorrhea in women; delayed puberty, reduced libido, and body hair in men.
      - Excess: precocious puberty in children, as seen in a number of conditions affecting the hypothalamic–pituitary axis (e.g., hamartomas, germinomas).
  - Posterior:
    - Antidiuretic Hormone:
      - Deficiency: causes *diabetes insipidus*, with polyuria and polydipsia; seen in children and adults when there is damage to the hypothalamus and/or posterior pituitary.
      - Excess: *syndrome of inappropriate ADH secretion*.

- *Parathyroid* glands:
  - Hypoparathyroidism (parathormone deficiency) leads to hypocalcemia, which causes tetany, paresthesia, muscle cramps, laryngeal spasm, and even epileptic seizures. In adults, it may be associated with intracranial calcification involving the basal ganglia and cerebellum, usually incidental but in some cases the patient may manifest a movement disorder (e.g., *parkinsonism*).
  - Hyperparathyroidism, usually due to a parathyroid adenoma, may on occasion be complicated by proximal and bulbar myopathy, ataxia, ophthalmoplegia, and pyramidal signs.

Reference

Schipper HM, Abrams GM. Other endocrinopathies and the nervous system. In: Aminoff MJ, ed. Neurology and General Medicine. The Neurological Aspects of Medical Disorders. 2nd ed. New York: Churchill Livingstone; 1995:383–400

Entrapment neuropathies: overview

Entrapment or compression is the most common cause of mononeuropathy. Various entrapment neuropathies are described, some due to compression within anatomical structures (e.g., carpal tunnel syndrome), many more involving extraneous pressure. Concomitant alcohol use greatly increases the risk of nerve entrapment due to external compression, as does any diffuse clinical or subclinical neuropathy. Pressure on nerves during anesthesia for surgical procedures is a potentially avoidable cause of entrapment. More than one episode of entrapment neuropathy, or a strong family history, should raise suspicion of an underlying *hereditary neuropathy with liability to pressure palsies.*

Commonly occurring peripheral nerve entrapment syndromes include the following:

- Upper limb:

Median nerve	Forearm	*Anterior interosseous syndrome*
		Pronator teres syndrome
	Wrist	*Carpal tunnel syndrome*
Ulnar nerve	Elbow	Medial epicondyle (ulnar groove)
		Cubital tunnel syndrome
	Hand	Canal of Guyon (Ramsay Hunt syndrome)
Radial nerve	Arm	Spiral groove of the humerus ("Saturday night palsy")
	Forearm	*Posterior interosseous syndrome*
		Superficial sensory branch
Suprascapular nerve		Suprascapular notch
Dorsal scapular nerve		Scalene muscle
Lower brachial plexus		(Neurogenic) *thoracic outlet syndrome*

- Lower limb:

Ilioinguinal	Abdominal wall
Lateral cutaneous nerve of the thigh	*Meralgia paresthetica* (Bernhardt–Roth syndrome)
Femoral nerve	Psoas sheath hematoma, abscess
	Inguinal ligament
Obturator nerve	Obturator canal
Sciatic nerve	Sciatic notch
	Piriformis syndrome
	Popliteal fossa
Tibial nerve	Medial malleolus (posterior tibial)
	Tarsal tunnel
Common peroneal nerve	Fibular head; prolonged squatting (e.g., strawberry pickers)
	Anterior compartment
Plantar interdigital nerves	Morton's metatarsalgia

- Other possible nerve entrapment syndromes:

  Cheiralgia paresthetica: radial side of thumb; distal dorsal digital nerve.
  Notalgia paresthetica: medial margin of scapula; dorsal branches of roots T2 to T6.
  Gonyalgia paresthetica: patella; infrapatellar branch of saphenous nerve.

Investigation

Diagnosis is often possible on clinical grounds alone, but if in doubt NCS showing focal slowing or even conduction block and EMG showing denervation of muscles innervated by the nerve in question may be helpful.

Differential diagnosis

Mononeuropathies are unlikely to be confused with peripheral polyneuropathies or radiculopathies but may overlap with inflammatory neuropathy (mononeuritis, mononeuritis multiplex).

Treatment and prognosis

Many entrapment neuropathies due to external pressure ("neurapraxia") recover spontaneously. For anatomical entrapment, surgical decompression may be possible, for example, carpal tunnel syndrome. Often symptomatic treatment with local splinting and/or analgesic medications may suffice. Drugs with particular efficacy for neuropathic pain include pregabalin, gabapentin, carbamazepine, duloxetine, and amitriptyline.

References

Dawson DM, Hallett M, Wilbourn AJ, eds. Entrapment Neuropathies. 3rd ed. Philadelphia, PA: Lippincott, Williams & Wilkins; 1999

Nakano KK. The entrapment neuropathies. Muscle Nerve. 1978;1:264–279

Pećina MM, Krmpotić-Nemanić J, Markiewitz AD. Tunnel Syndromes: Peripheral Nerve Compression Syndromes. 3rd ed..Boca Raton, FL: CRC Press; 2001

Staal A, van Gijn J, Spaans F. Mononeuropathies: Examination, Diagnosis and Treatment. London: W.B. Saunders; 1999

Winfree CJ, Kline DG. Intraoperative positioning nerve injuries. Surg Neurol. 2005;63:5–18

Eosinophilic syndromes: overview

Prominent eosinophilic infiltration of muscle or fascia may occur in a number of conditions:

- Eosinophilic polymyositis: predominantly proximal weakness, evolving over weeks, as part of a systemic illness typical of the *hypereosinophilic syndrome*, hence with other manifestations such as involvement of lung, heart, skin, and blood (eosinophilia, anemia, hypergammaglobulinemia). Creatine kinase is moderately elevated, along with raised ESR, +/– positive rheumatoid factor and antinuclear antibody. EMG usually reveals a myopathic pattern with fibrillation potentials. Pathology is similar to that in *polymyositis* aside from the conspicuous presence of eosinophilic polymorphonuclear leukocytes in the inflammatory infiltrates. An eosinophilic (mono)myositis with painful swelling, often of the calf muscle(s), is also described. Steroids may be used, usually with benefit to the muscle symptoms and signs, but overall prognosis depends on involvement of other organs (hypereosinophilic syndrome).
- Eosinophilic fasciitis (Shulman's syndrome): a rare entity of unknown etiology, predominantly seen in men between 30 and 60 years of age, in which fever and myalgia, often after exercise, wounds or surgery, precedes diffuse cutaneous thickening, likened to scleroderma, and limitation of joint movement which may develop into contractures. Proximal muscle weakness may occur. Blood tests reveal raised ESR, eosinophilia (in most cases), and raised gammaglobulins. Subcutaneous tissues (fascia) are infiltrated with plasma cells, lymphocytes and eosinophils; eosinophilic infiltration of muscle may be seen in those with proximal weakness (hence the condition may overlap with eosinophilic myositis). Clinical improvement may occur spontaneously, or may follow use of steroids or IVIg. Sometimes the condition is hyperacute ("flesh eating disease") and requires aggressive intervention with antibiotics and surgery, including amputation if necessary.

- Eosinophilia-myalgia syndrome: following prolonged consumption of L-tryptophan as a hypnotic agent.
- Eosinophilia and muscle symptoms +/− signs may also coexist in drug-induced muscle disorders (phenobarbitone, tranilast, as well as L-tryptophan), parasitic diseases, Lyme disease, vasculitis, and mixed connective tissue disease.

References

Hertzmann PA, Blevins WL, Mayer J, Greenfield B, Ting M, Gleich GJ. Association of the eosinophilia-myalgia syndrome with the ingestion of tryptophan. N Engl J Med. 1990;322:869–873
Layzer RB, Shearn MA, Satya-Murti S. Eosinophilic polymyositis. Ann Neurol. 1977;1:65–71
Shulman LE. Diffuse fasciitis with hypergammaglobulinemia and eosinophilia: a new syndrome? J Rheumatol. 1984;11:569–570

Ependymoma

Ependymomas are tumors derived from the ependymal cells which line the surface of the ventricular system of the brain and the central canal of the spinal cord; hence they may be classified as a subtype of glioma. They account for about 5% of all brain tumors. They are typically found in the posterior fossa in childhood, but may occur at any age and involve the spinal cord as commonly as the brain in adults. They present insidiously and generally respond to surgical debulking and radiotherapy. Contact with CSF pathways permits seeding of ventricular surfaces and subarachnoid pathways.

Pathologically ependymomas are often grey-pink exophitic growths, often well demarcated. Microscopically tumor cells form rosettes and pseudorosettes (circular arrangements around blood vessels). Distinction may be drawn between benign, well-differentiated tumors which form papillae, and more malignant, anaplastic lesions with high mitotic activity, which may be termed ependymoblastomas; some classify these with primitive neuroectodermal tumors (PNET). Subependymona has features of both ependymoma and astrocytoma.

Clinical features

- Supraspinal tumors: most arise in the fourth ventricle, hence patients present with posterior fossa signs and raised intracranial pressure from obstructive hydrocephalus: headache, nausea, vomiting, ataxia and nystagmus. Cerebral lesions present as space-occupying lesions with seizures.

- Spinal ependymomas: most occur in the lumbosacral region, conus or filum terminale. Unlike supraspinal ependymomas these tumors are only found in adults, and in men more commonly than women (M:F = 2:1). They typically present with a slowly progressive spinal cord syndrome and back pain, with the spinothalamic tract in particular being affected.

Investigation

Neuroimaging (CT/MRI) typically shows tumor which enhances homogeneously with gadolinium contrast.

Differential diagnosis

Other tumors: medulloblastoma in fourth ventricle, *glioma* in cerebral cortex, astrocytoma in spinal cord.

Treatment and prognosis

Treatment is surgical debulking with radiotherapy, except in the case of the benign myxopapillary tumor of the filum terminale where surgery alone can be curative. Chemotherapy with platinum-containing regimens has been shown to induce remission at tumor recurrence. Prognosis depends on the location of the tumor, the degree of seeding (which occurs in about 5–10% of tumors), the age of the patient (better prognosis in adult patients) and the grade of the tumor.

References

Lyons MK, Kelly PJ. Posterior fossa ependymomas: report of 30 cases and review of the literature. Neurosurgery. 1991;28:659–665
Taylor MD, Rutka JT. Pediatric posterior fossa tumors. In: Bernstein M, Berger MS, eds. Neuro-oncology. The Essentials. 2nd ed. New York: Thieme; 2008:287–298

Epidermoid

Cholesteatoma, Pearly tumor

Epidermoids are benign cystic tumors which develop from misplaced ectodermal tissue. They may be congenital, one of the most common embryonal intracranial tumors, or acquired. The congenital forms are often found in association with dysraphism, whereas acquired forms occur secondary to invasive procedures (e.g., lumbar puncture) or infection (e.g., *cholesteatoma*: these may also be congenital).

Epidermoids may be found in a variety of CNS sites: they are one of the recognized causes of a *cerebellopontine angle syndrome*, but also occur in the suprasellar region, skull base, brainstem or intraventricular cavity, presenting with symptoms and signs of local pressure effects. They are usually encapsulated and contain keratin-producing squamous epithelium with or without partly calcified collagenous walls. Rupture of the cyst into the CSF may produce a syndrome akin to *Mollaret's meningitis* (recurrent aseptic meningitis).

On CT, epidermoids are hypodense relative to brain parenchyma. On MR imaging, lesions are hypointense on T_1-weighted and hyperintense on T_2-weighted scans with minimal or no enhancement

Surgical excision is possible, sometimes complete, although the tendency to envelop neurovascular structures may make this difficult. Recurrences may occur.

Reference

Cohen-Gadol AA, Al-Mefty O. Skull base tumors. In: Bernstein M, Berger MS, eds. Neuro-oncology. The Essentials. 2nd ed. New York: Thieme; 2008:320–333

Epilepsy: overview

Epileptic seizures are currently classified, using the International League Against Epilepsy (ILAE) classification, according to seizure phenomenology and EEG findings:

- Partial (focal, localization-related) seizures:
  - Simple partial seizures, with motor, or somatosensory, or autonomic, or psychic symptoms.
  - Complex partial seizures: simple partial seizure followed by impaired consciousness, or with impairment of consciousness at onset, with or without automatisms.
  - Partial seizures evolving to secondarily generalized seizures (tonic-clonic, tonic, or clonic).
  - Nonconvulsive status epilepticus.
- Generalized seizures (convulsive and nonconvulsive):
  - Absence seizures: these may be characterized as:
    ○ Typical: a brief interruption of consciousness with unresponsiveness, with abrupt onset/offset. The attacks may be barely noticeable, without postictal confusion or awareness that an attack has occurred. Such typical absence seizures characterize idiopathic generalized epilepsies such as childhood absence epilepsy (CAE; pyknolepsy; "petit mal") and juvenile absence epilepsy (JAE). Typical absence seizures may also be seen in: Idiopathic generalized epilepsy with absences of early childhood; perioral myoclonia with absences; *Jeavons syndrome*.

- o Atypical: There is a more obvious distancing, "clouding," or "glazing over," possibly with associated automatisms such as lip smacking, as in a complex focal seizure of temporal lobe origin. Activities may continue (cf. typical absence), albeit slowly, sometimes with clumsiness or mistakes. Atypical absences may be seen in Lennox-Gastaut syndrome, Dravet syndrome.
  - Myoclonic seizures (e.g., *juvenile myoclonic epilepsy, progressive myoclonus epilepsy*)
  - Clonic seizures.
  - Tonic seizures.
  - Tonic-clonic seizures.
  - Atonic seizures.
  - Combinations.
  - *Status epilepticus.*
- Unclassified epileptic seizures

Essentially, all epileptic seizures are thought to reflect abnormal, hypersynchronous, electrical discharges within neuronal circuits. Seizure threshold may be lowered by sleep loss, irregular meals, alcohol, hormonal changes (e.g., associated with menstrual periods, pregnancy). Some forms may be precipitated by specific factors (*reflex epilepsies*).

Clinical features

A clear history of seizure morphology is the most important factor in reaching a correct diagnosis, but may be difficult or impossible to obtain if there is impairment or loss of consciousness. Collateral (witness) history may (or may not) add useful information. If possible, a video of a seizure should be obtained by family, friends. Additional neurological signs may suggest an underlying symptomatic cause for epilepsy, e.g., *tuberous sclerosis.*

Investigation

Diagnosis is essentially clinical, based on a description of the seizure. Other investigations seek to identify seizure type and etiology.

Neurophysiology: routine interictal EEG is often normal, it cannot "exclude" or "confirm" epilepsy, unless by chance it coincides with a clinical seizure. Occasional typical changes may be seen, for example in typical absence epilepsy EEG typically shows 3 Hz spike and slow wave abnormalities, which may be elicited by hyperventilation. Sleep-deprived EEG may offer more information. Prolonged recording with telemetry may increase the chance of recording a seizure; if performed in an in-patient setting, this may be combined with video recording. Depth electrodes may be helpful in identifying a focus of seizure onset, not evident from surface recording.

Imaging: MRI is increasingly of value, especially in focal seizures, to identify underlying structural lesions, e.g., indolent temporal lobe tumors (e.g., *ganglio-glioma*), neuronal migration disorders (*heterotopia*). Wada test: if surgery is contemplated, intracarotid phenobarbital may be used to anesthetize one temporal lobe during which neuropsychological functioning may be assessed to determine lateralization of language and memory. This test is less commonly used as functional brain imaging improves and becomes more commonplace.

Despite extensive investigation, many seizures remain cryptogenic.

Differential diagnosis

- *Syncope.*
- *Drop attacks.*
- Cataplexy.
- *Non-epileptic attack disorder* (*NEAD*), "pseudoseizures."
- Concussive convulsions/Immediate convulsions (in mild *traumatic brain injury*).
- Panic attacks.
- Microsleeps.
- Movement disorders, e.g., *paroxysmal dyskinesias*.

Treatment and prognosis

Prognosis for many seizures is good, with spontaneous remission (*benign epilepsy syndromes*) and no requirement for long-term medication or follow-up. Anti-epileptic medications are the mainstay of management. Monotherapy is preferred, since no anti-epileptic drug is without side effects and the potential for interactions is high. First line medications are carbamazepeine and sodium valproate; although the evidence from randomized controlled trials is inconclusive, carbamazepine is probably the most effective drug for seizures of partial onset, sodium valproate for seizures of generalized onset. Second line medications include older drugs such as phenytoin and phenobarbitone, and newer add-on therapies such as lamotrigine, gabapentin, topiramate, levetiracetam, oxcarbazepine, zonisamide, lacosamide. Some of these newer drugs have now obtained licenses for monotherapy, but whether they are better than the established medications remains to be determined. Certain seizure types are best treated with particular anti-epileptic drugs, e.g., juvenile myoclonic epilepsy responds best to sodium valproate; ethosuximide and/or sodium valproate are the treatments of choice for idiopathic generalized absence epilepsies. With focal seizures caused by a focal lesion (tumor, neuronal migration defect), surgery is sometimes possible which may reduce or abolish seizures. Mortality in epilepsy is higher than for a matched seizure-free population: some of these deaths are attributable to seizures, in others the cause is uncertain (*Sudden unexplained death in epilepsy* (*SUDEP*)).

References

Crawford P. Best practice guidelines for the management of women with epilepsy. Epilepsia. 2005;46(Suppl 9):117–124

Crunelli V, Leresche N. Childhood absence epilepsy: genes, channels, neurons and networks. Nat Rev Neurosci. 2002;3:371–382

Manford MR. A Practical Guide to Epilepsy. London: Butterworth Heinemann; 2003

Panayiotopoulos CP. A Clinical Guide to Epileptic Syndromes and Their Treatment: Based on the ILAE Classifications and Practice Parmeter Guidelines. 2nd ed. London: Springer; 2007

Shorvon S. Handbook of Epilepsy Treatment. 2nd ed. Oxford: Blackwell Science; 2005

Smith D, Chadwick D. The management of epilepsy. J Neurol Neurosurg Psychiatry. 2001;70(Suppl II):ii15–ii21

Stokes T, Shaw EJ, Juarez-Garcia A, Camosso-Stefinovic J, Baker R. Clinical Guidelines and Evidence Review for the Epilepsies: Diagnosis and Management in Adults and Children in Primary and Secondary Care. London: Royal College of General Practitioners; 2004

Episodic ataxias

The episodic ataxias are syndromes in which incoordination occurs intermittently, either spontaneously or in association with factors such as stress, fatigue, or certain foods. Two types of autosomal dominant paroxysmal cerebellar ataxia, episodic ataxia types 1 and 2, have been recognized on clinical grounds, and subsequently characterized at the molecular level as channelopathies.

Clinical features

- Episodic ataxia type 1 (EA1), Episodic ataxia/myokymia syndrome:
  - Autosomal dominant disorder characterized by brief (minutes) attacks of cerebellar ataxia, usually without abnormal eye signs (cf. EA2). Attacks may be provoked by stress, emotion, sudden movement. Myokymia or neuromyotonia may be evident as continuous spontaneous repetitive discharges on EMG, but this is not always evident clinically. Some families have seizures. Linkage to chromosome 12p13 and associated with mutations in the potassium channel KCNA1 gene.
- Episodic ataxia type 2 (EA2):
  - Autosomal dominant paroxysmal cerebellar disorder; attacks of longer duration (hours to days) than in EA1, provoked by stress, exercise, fatigue but not startle. In addition there may be migraine-like symptoms (allelic with one form of familial hemiplegic *migraine*), interictal nystagmus, cerebellar atrophy (allelic with spinocerebellar ataxia type 6). Linkage to chromosome 19p13 and associated with mutations in the calcium channel CACNA1A gene. Attacks responsive to acetazolamide. There may be progressive cerebellar dysfunction.

Investigation

Neurogenetic testing is diagnostic. Neuroimaging (MRI) may show cerebellar atrophy in EA2, but not EA1. Neurophysiology (EMG) may show neuromyotonia in EA1.

Differential diagnosis

Other conditions in which intermittent episodes of ataxia have been described include:

- Basilar-type migraine.
- *Neurocysticercosis.*
- Inborn errors of metabolism, especially "small molecule disorders" such as urea cycle enzyme defects (e.g., ornithine transcarbamoylase deficiency), organic acidopathies, variants of maple syrup urine disease, pyruvate dehydrogenase deficiency.

Treatment and prognosis

EA1: some families respond to carbamazepine, acetazolamide; phenytoin. Some families are drug-resistant. EA2: some families respond to acetazolamide.

Reference

Jen JC, Graves TD, Hess EJ, et al. Primary episodic ataxias: diagnosis, pathogenesis and treatment. Brain. 2007;130:2484–2493

Epstein–Barr virus (EBV) infection and the nervous system: overview

Epstein–Barr virus (EBV) is a DNA virus which causes infectious mononucleosis (IM), the syndrome of glandular fever, with fever, pharyngitis and lymphadenopathy. Diagnosis is based on blood tests which reveal a lymphocytosis with atypical lymphocytes and a positive monospot test. Serology for EBV can also be performed.

EBV has been associated with the development of a number of neurological conditions, which can occur in the absence of overt IM:

- *Encephalitis* with predominant cerebellar involvement (imaging and CSF analysis is typically normal in such patients).
- Myelitis.
- *Aseptic meningitis.*

- *Guillain-Barré syndrome.*
- Lumbosacral plexopathy.
- Facial palsy.
- Neuropathy: sensory, autonomic: rarely described.
- Postviral fatigue syndrome.

There is no specific treatment, other than supportive care. Although recovery is the norm, there may be neurological sequelae after encephalitis.

In immunocompromised individuals, Epstein–Barr virus infection is implicated in the development of primary CNS lymphoma, as well as Burkitt's lymphoma.

References

Cohen JI. Epstein-Barr virus infection. N Engl J Med. 2000;343:481–492
Majid A, Galetta SL, Sweeney CJ, et al. Epstein-Barr virus myeloradiculitis and encephalomyeloradiculitis. Brain. 2002;125:159–165

Erb's palsy, Erb-Duchenne palsy

Superior plexus paralysis

Erb's palsy or Erb-Duchenne palsy describes a form of *brachial plexopathy* affecting the upper part of the plexus involving fibers from the C5/C6 roots, as a consequence of which the affected arm hangs at the side, internally rotated and extended at the elbow ("waiter's tip" posture). There is sensory loss down the lateral arm to the hand; biceps and supinator jerks may be lost or depressed (cf. *Klumpke's paralysis*, lower plexus palsy).

Erb-Duchenne palsy typically occurs in traumatic injuries when there is a sudden and severe increase in the angle between the neck and shoulder, for example during a traumatic delivery or, more commonly, with motorcycle accidents. A similar picture may occur after carrying a heavy rucksack for prolonged periods ("*rucksack paralysis*"). If severe trauma has occurred then little recovery may be expected but often there is only neurapraxia or a short distance for axon regrowth. Occasionally exploratory surgery and microsurgical nerve repair may be necessary. Good recovery may occur, aided by physiotherapy.

Erdheim-Chester disease

Erdheim-Chester disease is a rare sporadic non-*Langerhans cell histiocytosis* which may affect multiple organs, including the CNS, manifesting most commonly as a cerebellar syndrome or a pyramidal syndrome. Epileptic seizures, headaches, cranial nerve palsies, cognitive impairment and asymptomatic lesions are also reported. Concurrent extraneural disease is common, especially of bones and diabetes insipidus. Orbital, extra-axial (*meningioma*-like) or intra-axial masses may occur.

Reference

Lachenal F, Cotton F, Desmurs-Clavel H, et al. Neurological manifestations and neuroradiological presentation of Erdheim-Chester disease: report of 6 cases and systematic review of the literature. J Neurol. 2006;253:1267–1277

Essential tremor (ET)

Essential tremor (ET) is one of the most common movement disorders. Some argue that there must be a family history (autosomal dominant condition with variable penetrance), with at least three generations affected, for the diagnosis of ET to apply, others are prepared to accept sporadic cases. ET may present at any age, and tends to worsen with age. Although not life threatening, it may nevertheless be very disabling, both physically and psychologically; hence the previous name of "benign essential tremor" has fallen into disuse. Hands, head, and voice are commonly involved, and the tremor often improves following modest alcohol consumption. The pathophysiology is not well understood: PET studies suggest tremor may originate in the cerebellum. The current treatment of choice is with β-blockers.

Clinical features

- Upper limb involvement: distal, may be asymmetric. Tremor may be present at rest but worsens with action and posture (e.g., writing, holding cups) but is not an intention tremor. As the patient gets older the frequency of the tremor often decreases but the amplitude increases. Classically the tremor improves with alcohol.
- Head titubation occurs in about 50% of cases, and voice may also be involved. This may precede the upper limb tremor, but more typically follows it.
- Tongue, trunk and lower limbs are rarely involved.
- There are no other abnormal findings aside from tremor in patients with ET. The presence of mild extrapyramidal features has been described, but this is very unusual and may suggest that the tremor is symptomatic of another disorder. Eye movements are normal.

Investigation

Bloods are usually normal; may need to exclude *Wilson's disease* and other metabolic causes of an extrapyramidal syndrome in young patients. Thyroid function tests, serum electrophoresis, immunoglobulins may be done to exclude symptomatic causes of tremor.

Liver function tests may also require checking if there is a history of heavy alcohol consumption.

Neuroimaging is normal; may need to exclude other causes of a tremor (e.g., *multiple sclerosis*). CSF is not usually required. Neurophysiology is not required unless the tremor is thought to be secondary to a demyelinating peripheral neuropathy (e.g., *paraproteinaemic demyelinating neuropathy*). In some centers where tremor analysis is undertaken, EMG may reveal a tremor frequency of 5–8 Hz (in PD: 4–5 Hz; physiological tremor 8–12 Hz).

Differential diagnosis

- Parkinson's disease: many patients come to clinic fearing this diagnosis, sometimes in part because other family members are affected, itself a clue to the diagnosis of ET.
- Other extrapyramidal disorders, such as Wilson's disease.
- Demyelinating peripheral neuropathies (neuropathic tremor).
- Exaggerated physiological tremor (endocrine abnormalities, especially thyroid overactivity; drug-induced).
- Cerebellar or midbrain tremor (typically seen in multiple sclerosis).
- Certain toxins may induce a coarse action tremor (e.g., methyl bromide, bismuth).
- Drug induced tremors (e.g., lithium, sodium valproate, SSRIs).

Treatment and prognosis

Most therapies probably act centrally, including alcohol. Options include: propanolol (80–240 mg/day, contraindicated in patients with asthma or peripheral vascular disease); topiramate (50–100 mg/day); clonazepam may help, especially in cases of severe kinetic tremor (i.e., worse with action) or orthostatic tremor; primidone starting at very low dose 25 mg/day, increasing slowly to a maximum of 750 mg/day if tolerated (soporific side effects are problematic); nicardipine 30 mg/day. Occasionally stereotactic surgery is indicated (refractory cases with severe disability): ventrolateral thalamotomy or the use of thalamic stimulators is the surgical treatment of choice. Therapy is often unsatisfactory.

Diagnostic criteria

Louis ED, Ford B, Lee H, Andrews H, Cameron B. Diagnostic criteria for essential tremor: a population perspective. Arch Neurol. 1998;55:823–828

References

Deuschl G, Bain P, Brin M and an Ad Hoc Scientific Committee. Consensus statement of the Movement Disorder Society on tremor. Mov Disord. 1998;13(Suppl 3):2–23
Louis ED. Essential tremor. Lancet Neurol. 2005;4:100–110
Plumb M, Bain P. Essential Tremor: The Facts. Oxford: Oxford University Press; 2007

Exploding head syndrome

The "exploding head syndrome" is characterized by a terrifying sensation of a painless explosion in the head, experienced as a crack, snap or bang, occurring often at sleep onset, but sometimes during sleep. It is classified amongst the parasomnias in the 2005 International Classification of Sleep Disorders (ICSD2). It may be regarded as a physiological phenomenon in the transition from wakefulness to sleep, akin to nocturnal myoclonus, probably representing a disturbance in sensory control in relation to sleep, but it is not clear whether it is related to the migraine mechanism. Although frightening, the syndrome is benign, and reassurance may be the only treatment required. Reports of benefit with clomipramine and nifedipine have appeared. The clinical description differs from hypnic headache although both occur at night. Concurrence with other paroxysmal neurological disorders, such as other primary headache disorders and epilepsy, may be significant.

References

Larner AJ. Exploding heads in the neurology clinic [Abstract 2836]. Eur J Neurol. 2009;16(Suppl 3):623
Pearce JM. Clinical features of the exploding head syndrome. J Neurol Neurosurg Psychiatry. 1989;52:907–910

F

Fabry's disease [OMIM#301500]

Anderson–Fabry disease, Angiokeratoma corporis diffusum, Hereditary dystopic lipidosis

Fabry's disease is a rare X-linked disorder, linked to chromosome Xq22.1, due to α-galactosidase A deficiency, which results in the accumulation of glycosphingolipids, specifically ceramidetrihexoside (also known as globotriaosylceramide or Gb$_3$), in most visceral tissues and body fluids, especially the lysosomes of the vascular endothelium, hence this is a *lysosomal storage disorder*. It is a multisystem disorder affecting skin, eyes, heart and circulation, kidneys, gastrointestinal tract, respiratory tract, and bone, as well as the peripheral, central, and autonomic nervous systems. Patients typically present in childhood and adolescence with characteristic skin lesions, angiokeratomas, and intermittent lancinating pains or dysesthesias in the limb. Heterozygote females may be asymptomatic or exhibit some symptoms and signs of the disease if they have partial deficiency of α-galactosidase. Diagnosis is by assay of enzyme activity in white cells.

Clinical features

Typically affects males in childhood or adolescence, although it does display variable expression in men. Female carriers may be asymptomatic or have limited forms of the disease. Diagnosis may require questioning and examination of female family members who may be carriers with mild symptoms, as well as a dermatological examination for angiokeratomas (cf. *fucosidosis*).

- Neurological features:
  - Peripheral nervous system: a small fiber polyneuropathy is often an early feature of the disease, presenting with distal limb pain and dysesthesia (acroparesthesia) often with autonomic involvement; the lancinating pains are often made worse by exertion, hot weather, or a fever. In children, these symptoms may be erroneously labeled as "growing pains."

- Central nervous system: cerebrovascular events, typically infarcts, affecting the posterior more than the anterior circulation around the fourth decade. Cognitive decline as a result of vascular events may occur. Dolichoectasia may be present, and occasional patients have been described with focal cranial nerve problems related to the abnormal dolichoectatic intracranial arteries, including optic atrophy, oculomotor paralysis, *trigeminal neuralgia*, eighth nerve dysfunction, and hypoglossal nerve palsy.
- Autonomic nervous system: this is often involved early, usually manifest as diminished sweating, impaired tear and saliva formation and gut hypomotility.
- Non-neurological features:
  - Skin: angiokeratoma corpus diffusum universale, dark red telangiectasia, is a skin lesion that is primarily found on the scrotum, buttocks, thighs, and back +/− mucosal involvement.
  - Kidney: progressive renal failure leads to hypertension, which can accelerate the cardiac and cerebrovascular complications of disease.
  - Eye: whorl-like corneal opacifications (cornea verticillata) are characteristic; slit-lamp examination may be required. Anterior cataracts and tortuous retinal vessels (tortuositas vasorum) may also be seen.
  - Heart: cardiac arrhythmias due to involvement of pacemaker tissue. Later, myocardial ischemia and infarction, cardiac failure, and mitral regurgitation may occur. There is also a relatively high incidence of mitral leaflet prolapse, which may play a role in the cerebral ischemia seen in younger patients.
  - Other: a facial appearance akin to acromegaly, lymphedema of the arms and legs, respiratory compromise from obstructive airways disease (late), and arthritis have all been described. A characteristic deformity of the distal interphalangeal joint of the fingers limiting joint extension is described.

Investigation

Bloods: the definitive test is assay of the white cell enzymes for α-galactosidase activity. Renal function tests (urea, creatinine, creatinine clearance) may indicate the degree of renal damage. Imaging: CXR may reveal cardiomegaly, heart failure. Skeletal radiography may show degenerative changes in distal interphalangeal joints. Neuroimaging (CT/MRI) may reveal multiple infarcts (hemorrhages are rare), dolichoectasia. Angiography may reveal irregular abnormal vessels with both stenoses and dilatation, for example, renal artery. Urine microscopy may reveal Maltese cross-shaped crystals. CSF examination is not usually necessary. Neurophysiology (EMG/NCS) may be required if neuropathy is present. ECG may reveal ischemia/infarcts and hypertensive changes. Skin biopsy may show lipid inclusions in vascular epithelial cells.

Differential diagnosis

Other causes of painful peripheral neuropathy, or of young stroke. Similar angiokeratoma may occur in fucosidosis, sialidosis.

Treatment and prognosis

Enzyme replacement therapy with genetically engineered α-galactosidase A (agalsidase alfa, beta), given as an intravenous infusion, is now available, and may improve cardiac and renal function and ameliorate neuropathic pain in some patients. Symptomatic treatment of painful dysesthesias may be required with pregabalin, gabapentin, carbamazepine, phenytoin, or amitriptyline. Heart rhythm abnormalities may require antiarrhythmics and/or a pacemaker. Hypertension must be controlled. Renal failure may require dialysis. Renal transplantation is feasible, the transplanted organ is not affected, but its production of normal enzyme is insufficient to treat other features of the condition, although the neuropathy may improve. Cardiac involvement may now be the most common cause of death, superseding renal failure. Genetic counseling is essential; prenatal screening through chorionic villous biopsies is possible.

References

Beck M, Ries M. Fabry Disease: Clinical Manifestations, Diagnosis and Therapy. Oxford: TKT Europe, 2001
Ginsberg L, Valentine A, Mehta A. Fabry disease. Pract Neurol. 2005;5:110–113
Mehta AB. Anderson-Fabry disease: developments in diagnosis and treatment. Int J Clin Pharmacol Ther. 2009;47(Suppl 1):S66–S74

Facial pain: overview

Facial pain has a broad differential diagnosis:

- *Trigeminal neuralgia (TN)*
- *Migraine*
- *Cluster headache (CH)*, other *trigeminal autonomic cephalalgias*
- *Giant cell arteritis*
- Postherpetic neuralgia
- *Dissection* of the carotid artery, *Raeder paratrigeminal syndrome*
- *Cavernous sinus disease*
- Glossopharyngeal neuralgia
- Geniculate neuralgia
- Otalgia

- *Neck–tongue syndrome*
- *Occipital neuralgia*
- *Gasserian ganglion syndrome*
- Atypical facial pain

Clinical features

History taking is generally the most important factor in reaching a specific diagnosis.

Certain headache syndromes may produce pain which is distributed over the face, in addition to or rather than the head: migraine, cluster headache, tension-type headache, meningitis, meningeal irritation (e.g., after a subarachnoid hemorrhage), raised intracranial pressure and giant cell arteritis.

Local disease of the teeth, sinuses, nasopharynx, temporomandibular joint (Costen's syndrome), ear (otalgia), and bones may also cause facial pain. Vascular pathology must also be considered (dissection of carotid artery), including disease within the cavernous sinus.

Investigation

Bloods: ESR if giant cell arteritis suspected; standard hematological and biochemical screening tests. Imaging: CT if bony lesion suspected; MRI if meningeal disease, cavernous sinus, or brainstem pathology suspected; MRA/ angiography if carotid artery dissection suspected. CSF is only necessary if meningeal disease suspected. May also require ENT, maxillofacial, oral surgical, psychiatric opinion. May cases elude specific diagnosis, the diagnosis of exclusion being atypical facial pain.

Facioscapulohumeral (FSH) muscular dystrophy [OMIM#158900]

Landouzy–Déjerine dystrophy

Facioscapulohumeral muscular dystrophy (FSH) is an autosomal dominant *muscular dystrophy*, with weakness in the areas described by the name, which may be asymmetric and of variable expression within families. It typically presents with facial weakness and winging of the scapulae, and then spreads to involve other proximal muscles of the upper limb. It has been linked to a deletion of an integral number of 3.3 kb KpnI repeats (D4Z4) in the subtelomeric region of chromosome 4 (4q35) in many, but not all, families; the actual genetic defect awaits clarification. Bigger deletions may be associated with younger onset and more severe forms of the disease.

Clinical features

- Weakness, often asymmetric, affects:
  - Facial muscles: often the first feature of disease, although facial expression is relatively well preserved. The mouth may have a pouting quality: *bouche de tapir*. A facial-sparing variant of FSH is described.
  - Shoulder muscles: particularly the scapular fixators, so that winging of the scapulae is an early feature. However, the deltoid muscle is normally well preserved, while biceps and triceps are weak and wasted, giving rise to an appearance of so-called "Popeye arms" or "chicken wings" in the upper limbs.
  - Quadriceps and hip flexor muscle involvement is not uncommon; ankle dorsiflexion, wrist extensors may be involved as the disease progresses.
- A severe form of FSH exists in infancy in which there is typically no facial movement and severe limb weakness, confining the child to a wheelchair by the age of about 10 years. In addition, there may be a severe high tone hearing loss and vascular degeneration of the retina (Coats' disease).
- Scapulohumeral and scapuloperoneal muscular dystrophies may, in some instances, represent variants of FSH.
- Extraocular and pharyngeal muscles are not involved; there is no cardiac involvement; mentation is normal.
- Family history may be positive for the disorder, although intrafamilial heterogeneity is recognized.
- The condition has very variable expression within families but has 95% penetrance by the age of 20 years.

Investigation

Blood creatine kinase is raised to several times above the normal range. Neurophysiology (EMG) shows myopathic change. Muscle biopsy shows general dystrophic features +/– scattered tiny fibers, with an inflammatory infiltrate which may on occasion lead to confusion with *polymyositis*. Changes are sometimes minimal. Neurogenetic testing for the typical deletion of chromosome 4q35 is very helpful in diagnosis, although it is not found in all cases with the clinical phenotype of FSHD, and may obviate the need for EMG and muscle biopsy. ECG is normal.

Differential diagnosis

- *Myotonic dystrophy*
- Polymyositis
- *Nemaline myopathy*

- *Mitochondrial disease*
- Congenital muscular dystrophies
- The severe childhood form may be mistaken for *Möbius syndrome*

Treatment and prognosis

There is no specific treatment. Supportive treatment with physiotherapy and surgical procedures may be helpful, such as stabilization of the scapulae; ankle-foot orthosis; transposition of the posterior tibial tendon to the dorsum of the foot. Immunosuppressive therapy is usually of no value. In its most severe form, the patient may become wheelchair bound in the first decade of life. However, the disease often follows a more benign course and overall only 20% of patients with FSH are wheelchair bound by the age of 40 years.

References

Upadhyaya M, Cooper D, eds. Facioscapulohumeral Muscular Dystrophy (FSHD). Clinical Medicine and Molecular Cell Biology. London: Routledge; 2004
Venance SL, Tawil R. Facioscapulohumeral dystrophy. In: Karpati G, Hilton-Jones D, Bushby K, Griggs RC, eds. Disorders of Voluntary Muscle. 8th ed. Cambridge: Cambridge University Press; 2010:314–322

Fahr's disease

Striatopallidal calcification

Fahr's disease is a rare neurodegenerative disorder characterized by the deposition of calcium symmetrically in the basal ganglia, +/– cerebellar hemispheres and periventricular white matter, with the clinical correlate of *parkinsonism*, cognitive impairment or dementia, seizures, cerebellar signs, or dysarthria. Cases may be sporadic or autosomal dominant. Other causes of *basal ganglia calcification* need to be excluded. Treatment is symptomatic, the parkinsonism is poorly responsive to levodopa preparations.

References

Kobari M, Nogawa S, Sugimoto Y, Fukuuchi Yl. Familial idiopathic brain calcification with autosomal dominant inheritance. Neurology. 1997;48:645–649
Manyam BV. What is and what is not "Fahr's disease." Parkinsonism Relat Disord. 2005;11:73–80

Familial amyloid polyneuropathies (FAP)

Andrade disease

Familial amyloid polyneuropathy (FAP) is a form of hereditary generalized amyloidosis, characterized clinically by a small fiber polyneuropathy and autonomic dysfunction, resulting from formation of amyloid fibrils by variant forms of various proteins (transthyretin, apolipoprotein A-I, gelsolin). Distinction may be drawn between:

- FAP type I (Andrade, Portuguese type): deposition of abnormal transthyretin [OMIM#105210].
- FAP type II (Indiana/Swiss/Maryland/German type): deposition of abnormal transthyretin [OMIM#105210].
- FAP type III (Iowa/Van Allen type): deposition of mutant apolipoprotein A-I [OMIM#105200]
- FAP type IV (Finnish): deposition of gelsolin [OMIM#105120].

Clinical features

The clinical picture is similar (but not identical) in all types:

- Autonomic dysfunction: impotence, postural hypotension, pupillary abnormalities; gastrointestinal abnormalities (constipation, diarrhea)
- Paresthesia, neuropathic pain; *carpal tunnel syndrome*
- Muscle weakness: distal to proximal spread; areflexia
- Bulbar involvement: dysphagia, dysarthria
- No nerve thickening (cf. *primary systemic amyloidosis*)
- Variations:
  - FAP type II: carpal tunnel syndrome; no renal, sphincter involvement.
  - FAP type IV: corneal lattice dystrophy; facial and auditory nerve involvement.

Amyloid deposition may also occur in other organs:

- Heart: cardiomyopathy
- Vitreous body: opacities
- Kidney: nephrotic syndrome
- Leptomeninges: subarachnoid hemorrhage

Investigation

Neurophysiology (EMG/NCS) shows axonal neuropathy (nonspecific). CSF protein is often raised. Tissue diagnosis by biopsy of nerve, rectal mucosa, skin, abdominal fat pad, may show amyloid deposits; in nerve, unmyelinated and small myelinated fibers may be lost, and amyloid preferentially accumulates around endoneurial vessels. Neurogenetic testing for mutations in genes encoding transthyretin (chromosome 18q11.2-q12.1) and gelsolin (chromosome 9q34). In addition, ECG and echocardiography may be undertaken to detect arrhythmia and cardiomyopathy (enlarged interventricular septum); slit-lamp examination for vitreous opacities.

Differential diagnosis

Other axonal and autonomic *neuropathies*.

Treatment and prognosis

Liver transplantation is curative, if performed early in the course of disease, that is, no improvement in neuropathy but no further axonal loss.

References

Adams D. Hereditary and acquired amyloid neuropathies. J Neurol. 2001;248: 647–657
Shimojima Y, Morita H, Kobayahsi S, Takei Y, Ikeda S. Ten-year follow-up of peripheral nerve function in patients with familial amyloid polyneuropathy after liver transplantation. J Neurol. 2008;255:1220–1225

Familial British dementia (FBD) [OMIM#176500]

Familial cerebral amyloid angiopathy, Worster–Drought syndrome

Familial British dementia is an autosomal dominant progressive *dementia* syndrome with associated cerebellar ataxia and spastic paraparesis, due to deposition of a novel cerebrovascular amyloid. The condition is linked to a mutation in the stop codon of the ABri gene on chromosome 13. The C-terminus of this enlarged protein forms the amyloidogenic peptide.

Clinical features

- Family history of presenile dementia.
- Progressive dementia (presenting sign, onset age 40–57 years).
- Cerebellar ataxia (early).
- Spastic paraparesis (late).

Investigations

Neuroimaging (CT/MRI) shows mild ventricular dilatation, with low attenuation/high signal intensity in frontoparietal white matter. Pathology shows severe cerebrovascular amyloid involving vessels of brain grey and white matter, spinal cord and leptomeninges; non-neuritic plaques, perivascular plaques, some neurofibrillary tangles, and white matter changes with myelin loss and small cystic infarcts are also seen. Neurogenetic testing for mutations in ABri gene is diagnostic.

Differential diagnosis

Other familial (autosomal dominant) dementias, especially familial *Alzheimer's disease*, although the other signs largely rule this out (spastic paraparesis may be a feature in early-onset AD with certain mutations in the presenilin-1 gene, especially but not exclusively exon 9 deletions). Inflammatory dementias such as vasculitides, Sjögren's syndrome, may have spastic paraparesis but lack a family history, as does *von Winiwarter–Buerger's disease*.

Treatment and prognosis

Uniformly fatal prognosis, death occurring at age 50–66 years. Currently no specific treatment.

References

Vidal R, Frangione B, Rostagno A, et al. A stop-codon mutation in the BRI gene associated with familial British dementia. Nature. 1999;399:776–781
Worster-Drought C, Hill TR, McMenemey WH. Familial presenile dementia with spastic paralysis. J Neurol Psychopathol. 1933;14:27–34

Familial Danish dementia (FDD) [OMIM#117300]

Heredopathia ophthalmo-oto-encephalica

This novel form of cerebral amyloidosis is associated with mutations in a gene (BRI2) on chromosome 13, which leads to the production of an extended precursor protein and of an amyloidogenic fragment (A-Dan), similar to the involvement of A-Bri in the pathogenesis of *familial British dementia* (Worster–Drought syndrome).

Clinical features are:

- Cataracts and ocular hemorrhages (30s)
- Impaired hearing and hearing loss (40s–50s)
- Cerebellar ataxia (40s)
- Paranoid psychosis and *dementia* (50s)

Pathologically there is *cerebral amyloid angiopathy*, parenchymal amyloid protein deposits, and neurofibrillary change.

Reference

Holton JL, Lashley T, Ghiso J, et al. Familial Danish dementia: a novel form of cerebral amyloidosis associated with deposition of both amyloid-Dan and amyloid-b. J Neuropathol Exp Neurol. 2002;61:254-267

Familial encephalopathy with neuroserpin inclusion bodies (FENIB) [OMIM#604218]

An autosomal dominant disorder characterized clinically by progressive *dementia* with frontal and frontal-subcortical deficits and relative sparing of recall memory, and neuropathologically by cytoplasmic neuroserpin inclusions (Collins bodies) within the deep cortical layers, substantia nigra and subcortical nuclei. It is linked to a point mutation in the gene on chromosome 3 encoding neuroserpin, a serine proteinase inhibitor, the mutant protein undergoing polymerization. Mutations causing greater conformational change (G392E) cause early-onset *progressive myoclonus epilepsy*, whereas lesser degrees of conformational change (S49P) cause dementia in the fifth decade.

References

Davis RL, Shrimpton AE, Carrell RW, et al. Association between conformational mutations in neuroserpin and onset and severity of dementia. Lancet. 2002;359:2242–2247
Davis RL, Shrimpton AE, Holohan PD, et al. Familial dementia caused by polymerization of mutant neuroserpin. Nature. 1999;401:376–379

Familial Mediterranean fever (FMF) [OMIM#249100]

Familial Mediterranean fever (FMF) is an inherited inflammatory disorder associated with mutations in the pyrin gene, characterized clinically by recurrent febrile polyserositis and secondary amyloidosis. Aseptic meningitis may be a feature. There is also some evidence for an increased prevalence of definite *multiple sclerosis* or other demyelinating CNS disease.

Reference

Akman-Demir G, Gul A, Gurol E, et al. Inflammatory/demyelinating central nervous system involvement in familial Mediterranean fever (FMF): coincidence or association? J Neurol. 2006;253:928–934

Familial periventricular heterotopia [OMIM#300049]

Periventricular nodular heterotopia (PVNH)

This is an X-linked dominant disorder with contiguous symmetrical nodular *heterotopia* lining the lateral ventricles, and manifesting in affected females with *epilepsy*. Cognitive levels may range from mild retardation to normal. The condition is prenatally lethal in hemizygous males. It is associated with mutations (missense or distal truncations, the former causing milder consequences) in the *filamin 1 (FLN1)* gene.

Reference

Moro F, Carrozzo R, Veggiotti P, et al. Familial periventricular heterotopia: missense and distal truncating mutations of the FLN1 gene. Neurology. 2002;58:916–921

Fat embolism syndrome (FES)

The fat embolism syndrome is a post-traumatic neurological syndrome occurring in 3–4% of patients with long bone fractures, typically 12 h to 3 days after trauma (although cases after up to 11 days have been reported). Diagnosis is based on clinical criteria, the features being respiratory distress, encephalopathy, retinal hemorrhages, and cutaneous petechiae; in addition, anemia, coagulopathy, fever, or urinary fat globules may be found. Some patients may have neurological focal deficits in addition to encephalopathy. MR imaging may show transient patchy lesions of low intensity on T_1-weighted imaging and high intensity on T_2-weighted imaging in the white matter and subcortical grey matter; these may represent transient perivascular edema. FES is a self-resolving illness and most patients make a full recovery if provided with supportive therapy at the time of respiratory distress.

Reference

Dominguez-Morán JA, Martinez-San Millán J, Plaza JF, Fernández-Ruiz LC, Masjuan J. Fat embolism syndrome: new MRI findings. J Neurol. 2001;248:529–532

Fatal familial insomnia (FFI) [OMIM#600072]

This is a rare, inherited autosomal dominant *prion disease* that presents with progressive insomnia and autonomic dysfunction, with motor and cognitive abnormalities developing later in the course of the illness. The sleep disorder is characterized by loss of slow-wave sleep and abnormal rapid eye movement sleep behavior. Endocrine and vegetative circadian rhythms are lost. The dysautonomia may cause hyperhidrosis, hypertension, hyperthermia, tachycardia, and sphincter disturbances. Similar features have been observed in *Morvan's syndrome*, mediated by autoantibodies directed to voltage-gated potassium channels. Motor features of FFI include ataxia, myoclonus, pyramidal features, and tremor. The condition occurs in middle age and is progressive, causing coma and death in 1–2 years. There is no specific treatment. Pathologically, thalamic nuclei seem to be predominantly affected (anterior ventral, dorsomedial). Mutations in codons 178 and 200 of the prion protein (PrP) gene have been reported in FFI. Occasional cases of sporadic fatal insomnia have also been reported. The condition has also been transmitted to primates by experimental inoculation.

References

Lugaresi E, Medori R, Montagna P, et al. Fatal familial insomnia and dysautonomia with selective degeneration of thalamic nuclei. N Engl J Med. 1986;315: 997–1003
Max DT. The Family That Couldn't Sleep. Unraveling a Venetian Medical Mystery. London: Portobello Books; 2007

Fatty acid oxidation disorders (FAOD): overview

A number of inborn errors of fatty acid oxidation are recognized, affecting transport and β-oxidation of long-, medium-, and short-chain fatty acids which takes place in the mitochondrial matrix:

- Medium-chain acyl-CoA dehydrogenase (MCAD) deficiency: the most common of these disorders, presenting in older infants with recurrent episodes of acute encephalopathy with hepatocellular dysfunction, or a Reye-like syndrome; rarely a cause of severe illness in the newborn
- Systemic carnitine deficiency: Reye-like syndrome with evidence of skeletal myopathy and cardiomyopathy (cf. MCAD)
- Long-chain acyl-CoA dehydrogenase (LCAD) deficiency: Reye-like syndrome with evidence of skeletal myopathy and cardiomyopathy (cf. MCAD)

- Short-chain acyl-CoA dehydrogenase (SCAD) deficiency: very rare, presenting in the newborn period with nonspecific encephalopathy, poor feeding, failure to thrive, hypotonia, seizures, myopathy, and cardiomyopathy, with metabolic acidosis
- Long-chain hydroxyacyl-CoA dehydrogenase (LCHAD) deficiency: as for LCAD but with very prominent cardiomyopathy (cf. MCAD)
- Carnitine palmitoyltransferase I (CPT I) deficiency
- Carnitine palmitoyltransferase II (CPT II) deficiency
- Carnitine-acylcarnitine translocase deficiency (CACT)

Clinical features

- Symptoms are provoked by fasting, exercise, or infection, commonly hypoketotic hypoglycemia. Metabolic myopathy may be evident, sometimes complicated by exercise-induced *rhabdomyolysis*.
- MCAD, LCAD, and SCAD have infantile presentation; CPT I and LCHAD have childhood presentation; CPT II may present in infancy or adulthood (classical exercise-induced myoglobinuria).
- FAOD have been associated with sudden infant death syndrome (SIDS), severe liver injury, and complications of pregnancy (e.g., HELLP syndrome). Search for evidence of FAOD is recommended in these situations, and screening of siblings.

Investigation

Enzyme analysis in cultured skin fibroblasts is the diagnostic test. Bloods show hypoglycemia, hyperammonemia, hepatocellular dysfunction; plasma acylcarnitines; α-fetoprotein is normal (cf. tyrosinemia).
Urine: organic acid abnormalities, but these may be evanescent, for example:

- MCAD: large amounts of dicarboxylic acids: adipic, suberic, sebacic; very low levels of 3-hydroxybutyrate
- SCAD: large amounts of ethylmalonic acid, glutarate, butyrylglycine, and hexanoylglycine (similar to glutaric aciduria type II)
- LCAD, LCHAD: long-chain dicarboxylic and monocarboxylic acids

Differential diagnosis

- *Aminoacidopathies*, for example, hepatocellular dysfunction and cardiomyopathy resembles hepatorenal tyrosinemia (but hypoalbuminemia and coagulopathy are not prominent in FAOD)
- Neonatal hepatitis, hemochromatosis

- *Hereditary fructose intolerance*
- Reye's syndrome

Treatment and prognosis

No specific treatment, but reduction of fatty acid oxidation by ensuring avoidance of fasting. A high-calorie high-carbohydrate diet, and elimination of fat from the diet, is recommended. Riboflavin, polyunsaturated fatty acid supplementation may be recommended.

References

Angelini C, Federico A, Reichmann H, Lombes A, Chinnery P, Turnbull D. Task force guidelines handbook: EFNS guidelines on diagnosis and management of fatty acid mitochondrial disorders. Eur J Neurol. 2006;13:923–929

Kerner J, Hoppel C. Genetic disorders of carnitine metabolism and their nutritional management. Annu Rev Nutr. 1998;18:179–206

Febrile seizures

Febrile convulsions

Febrile seizures may be defined as epileptic seizures occurring between the ages of 3 months and 5 years, in association with a temperature of $\geq 38°C$, in the absence of CNS infection or metabolic disturbance. These are the most common form of childhood seizures, affecting up to 5% of infants.

Clinical features

Febrile convulsions may be classified clinically as:

- Simple: primary generalized, usually tonic-clonic seizure, lasting no more than 15 min and not recurring within 24 h.
- Complex: prolonged, focal, and/or recurrent within 24 h.

A number of genetic susceptibility loci for febrile seizures have been defined, and mutations have been identified in genes encoding voltage- or ligand-gated ion channels (hence *channelopathies*) in some families with *generalized epilepsy with febrile seizures plus* (*GEFS+*), an autosomal dominant syndrome of variable phenotype characterized by multiple febrile seizures and various afebrile generalized seizures (tonic-clonic, absence, myoclonic, atonic).

Investigation

CSF examination is recommended in infants below 18 months of age to exclude meningitis. Bloods, EEG, neuroimaging not mandatory in a child with a first simple febrile seizure, although these may be indicated in the context of complex febrile seizure(s).

Differential diagnosis

Meningitis, especially in those under 18 months.

Treatment and prognosis

During fever antipyretics may be given; prophylactic antiepileptic drugs such as diazepam may reduce the risk of febrile seizure. A febrile seizure lasting more than 2–3 min may be treated with diazepam. Regular phenobarbitone may reduce the risk of further seizures, but this benefit needs to be balanced against the risk of cognitive and behavioral adverse effects. Febrile seizures are a risk factor for the development of *epilepsy* later in life, occurring in about 2–7% of children, predictors being complex febrile seizures, neurodevelopmental abnormalities, family history of epilepsy, recurrent febrile seizures.

References

Mikati MA, Rahi AC. Febrile seizures in children. Pract Neurol. 2003;3:78–85
Nakayama J, Arinami T. Molecular genetics of febrile seizures. Epilepsy Res. 2006;70(Suppl 1):S190–S198

Femoral neuropathy

Palsy of the femoral nerve, which arises from L2-4 roots, most often follows surgical trauma, stretch or traction injuries, or direct compression.

Clinical features

- Motor: weak quadriceps, absent or diminished patellar reflex; adductor muscles should not be affected (innervated by obturator nerve; this is useful in differentiating a femoral neuropathy from L2-L4 radiculopathy)
- Sensory: loss over anterior thigh and, if the saphenous branch is involved, medial aspect of leg and foot

Investigation

Neurophysiology (EMG/NCS) is diagnostic. EMG involvement of paraspinal muscles or adductor muscles refutes the diagnosis of femoral neuropathy.

Differential diagnosis

L2-4 radiculopathy; "diabetic amyotrophy"; lumbosacral plexopathy.

Reference

Staal A, Van Gijn J, Spaans F. Mononeuropathies: Examination, Diagnosis and Treatment. London: W.B. Saunders; 1999:103–108

Fibromuscular dysplasia (FMD)

Fibromuscular dysplasia is a rare, non-atheromatous and noninflammatory, segmental disease of small- and medium-sized arteries, first described in renal arteries but which can affect craniocervical arteries, especially the internal carotid artery. Intracranial involvement is rare. It is usually bilateral, much more common in women aged 15–50 years. It may be associated with transient ischemic attacks, strokes, arterial dissection, and intracranial aneurysm formation.

Clinical features

- May be asymptomatic; probably most cases. There may be an asymptomatic carotid bruit, or pulsatile tinnitus.
- May cause cerebral ischemia, possibly embolic (e.g., following a dissection) or occlusive.
- Concurrent saccular intracranial aneurysms (in ca. 25%) may cause *subarachnoid hemorrhage*.
- May be concurrent hypertension from renal artery involvement.

Investigation

Imaging: carotid arteriography shows multifocal stenoses (characteristic "string of beads" appearance), tubular narrowing, usually bilateral; +/– intracranial aneurysms. Histology shows degeneration of elastic tissue, proliferation of fibroblasts, smooth muscle hyperplasia, +/– atherosclerosis.

Differential diagnosis

Other causes of cerebral ischemia; atheromatous carotid artery disease.

Treatment and prognosis

Antiplatelet therapy is recommended for asymptomatic individuals. In symptomatic individuals, endovascular dilatation (percutaneous balloon angioplasty) may be indicated. Aneurysms may require coiling or surgery.

Reference

Olin JW, Pierce M. Contemporary management of fibromuscular dysplasia. Curr Opin Cardiol. 2008;23:527–536

Fibromyalgia syndrome (FMS)

Myofascial pain syndrome

Although the fibromyalgia syndrome is not a neurological disorder, patients with this condition are not infrequently referred to neurology clinics. It is characterized by diffuse muscle aches and pains ("myalgia"), with an emphasis on the shoulder girdle musculature, with focal tender spots in the muscle. There is no associated clinical or investigative abnormality to indicate a disease of joints, bones, connective tissue, muscle, or nervous system. Symptoms of fatigue, sleep disturbance, and headache are common; there may be an underlying depressive illness. Symptomatic treatment may be helpful; the condition may be self-limiting, lasting for a period of weeks to months. The possibility of concurrent *somatoform disorder* should be considered.

Diagnostic criteria

Wolfe F, Smythe HA, Yunus MB, et al. The American College of Rheumatology 1990 Criteria for the classification of fibromyalgia. Report of the Multicenter Criteria Committee. Arthritis Rheum. 1990;33:160–172

References

Hauser W, Thieme K, Turk DC. Guidelines on the management of fibromyalgia syndrome – A systematic review. Eur J Pain. 2010;14:5–10
Lyseng-Williamson KA, Siddiqui MA. Pregabalin: a review of its use in fibromyalgia. Drugs. 2008;68:2205–2223

Fibrous dysplasia

Small areas of bone destruction or massive sclerotic overgrowth involving the skull vault and/or base may occur in isolation, causing headache and cranial nerve involvement (e.g., visual loss, hearing loss), or as part of the McCune–Albright syndrome (with café-au-lait spots, endocrinopathy such as precocious puberty, thyrotoxicosis, primary hyperparathyroidism, hyperprolactinemia). Malignant transformation to fibrosarcoma may occur. Surgical resection or radiation therapy may be used to relieve symptoms.

Filariasis

Lymphatic or Bancroftian filariasis results from infection with nematodes (e.g., *Wuchereria bancrofti*) spread by mosquito bite in equatorial Africa and Southeast Asia, causing fever and lymphadenitis. Lymphedema may follow resulting in swelling of limbs (elephantiasis) or genitalia. Nerve compression palsies may occur as a consequence of enlarged or calcified lymph nodes or dilated lymphatic channels, and Guillain-Barré syndrome has been reported in the context of acute filariasis. Diagnosis may be based on clinical features, or use of antibody detection tests, or visualization of adult worms or microfilariae in tissue sections.

Focal retrograde amnesia

Rare cases of focal retrograde amnesia with relative sparing of anterograde memory have been described, sometimes following head injury or an encephalitic illness. Retrograde amnesia following recovery from non-paraneoplastic *limbic encephalitis* with voltage-gated potassium channel antibodies has been reported. More usually, brain insults result in anterograde amnesia with a temporal gradient.

References

Kapur N. Focal retrograde amnesia in neurological disease. A critical review. Cortex. 1993;29:219–234
Larner AJ, Ghadiali EJ, Doran M. Focal retrograde amnesia: clinical, neuropsychological and neuroimaging study [abstract P1-116]. Neurobiol Aging. 2004;25(S2):S128

Foix–Alajouanine syndrome

Subacute necrotizing myelopathy

First described in 1926, this is a slowly or subacutely progressive paraparesis, often asymmetrical, with distal pain and sensory disturbance and with sphincter and sexual dysfunction. It results from a vascular malformation leading to impaired venous outflow from the cord causing a necrotic myelopathy. A rereading of the original paper has suggested that the original reports may in fact have been due to spinal *dural arteriovenous fistula.*

References

Ferrell AS, Tubbs RS, Acakpo-Satchivi L, Deveikis JP, Harrigan MR. Legacy and current understanding of the often-misunderstood Foix-Alajouanine syndrome. Historical vignette. J Neurosurg. 2009;111:902–906

Mirch DR, Kucharuczyk W, Weller MA, et al. Subacute necrotizing myelopathy: MR imaging in four pathologically proved cases. Am J Neuroradiol. 1991;12:1077–1083

Foix–Chavany–Marie syndrome

Anterior opercular syndrome

This is an acquired syndrome in which there is bilateral anterior perisylvian damage involving the primary motor cortex and parietal opercula. There is loss of voluntary control of the facial, pharyngeal, lingual, masticatory +/– ocular muscles, while retaining normal reflexive and automatic functions of these muscles. Patients can therefore yawn, blink, and laugh spontaneously but cannot close their eyes or open their mouths to command. Cerebrovascular disease is the commonest cause. This may be a paretic rather than an apraxic disorder.

A similar syndrome may be seen in children following bilateral opercular damage: the perisylvian syndrome is sometimes designated "developmental Foix–Chavany–Marie syndrome," as well as the Worster–Drought syndrome.

References

Mao C-C, Coull BM, Golper LAC, Rau MT. Anterior operculum syndrome. Neurology. 1989;39:1169–1172

Weller M. Anterior opercular cortex lesions cause dissociated lower cranial nerve palsies and anarthria but no aphasia: Foix-Chavany-Marie syndrome and "automatic voluntary dissociation" revisited. J Neurol. 1993;240:199–208

Worster-Drought C. Suprabulbar paresis. Dev Med Child Neurol. 1974;16(Suppl 30):1–30

Foot drop: overview

Foot drop is not an uncommon neurological presentation. The differential diagnosis is potentially broad, reflecting the extensive neuroanatomical pathway subserving foot movement, but division of cases into upper motor neurone ("stiff foot drop") and lower motor neurone ("floppy foot drop") facilitates diagnosis and focuses investigation.

The neural pathway controlling ankle dorsiflexion is:

- Motor cortex (parasagittal region)
- Descending motor pathways (corticospinal pathway: internal capsule, cerebral peduncles, corticospinal tracts)
- Anterior horn cells of spinal cord (neuronopathy)
- L4-S1 roots containing motor axons (radiculopathy)
- Lumbosacral plexus (plexopathy)
- Sciatic nerve, common peroneal nerve (mononeuropathy)
- Neuromuscular junction
- Muscles (myopathy):
  - Tibialis anterior
  - Extensor digitorum and hallucis longus
  - Extensor digitorum brevis

Pathology anywhere along this pathway may potentially cause foot drop.

Clinical features

- Upper motor nerve lesion: "stiff foot drop"
  - Appearance: wasting may be minimal unless lesion is chronic
  - Tone: spasticity of leg, foot; may be sustained ankle clonus
  - Reflexes: hyperreflexia, extensor plantar response
  - Gait: circumduction of leg on walking
  - Sensory findings: may be absent

Potential causes:
- Cerebral (e.g., parasagittal) lesion: usually unilateral, for example, meningioma; stroke
- Spinal cord lesion: usually bilateral, for example, demyelination
- Dystonia
- Lower motor nerve lesion: "floppy foot drop"
  - Appearance: wasting of leg, intrinsic foot muscles may be evident
  - Tone: hypotonia, flaccidity of foot, leg
  - Power: sparing of ankle inversion in foot plantar flexion differentiates common peroneal nerve palsy from L5 radiculopathy
  - Reflexes: depressed or absent ankle jerk; plantar response flexor or mute.
  - Gait: dragging of foot on walking
  - Sensory findings: may be root, plexus, or peripheral nerve pattern of sensory impairment/loss

Potential causes	Unilateral	Radiculopathy (L5/S1 root)
		Plexopathy
		Mononeuropathy: sciatic, common peroneal
	Bilateral	Polyneuropathy
		Muscular dystrophy: scapuloperoneal type

- A combination of upper and lower motor signs may be seen, suggesting anterior horn cell disease or *spinal muscular atrophy* (e.g., fasciculations, weakness, but brisk reflexes, upgoing plantar); absent ankle jerks with extensor plantar responses may be seen in *Friedreich's ataxia* and *subacute combined degeneration of the cord* due to vitamin B_{12} deficiency.

Investigation

Bloods required only if malignancy or peripheral neuropathy is suspected. Imaging requirements vary: for upper motor neurone type foot drop, imaging of whole neuraxis may be required, unless other features point to a more specific localization; in lower motor neurone type, MRI of lumbar spine and/ or lumbosacral plexus may be appropriate. CSF is required if infiltrative meningitic process is suspected. Neurophysiology (EMG/NCS) is often diagnostic in floppy foot drop.
Muscle/nerve biopsy may be required as appropriate.

Differential diagnosis

Dorsal column lesions (e.g., tabes dorsalis) or large fiber sensory neuronopathies (ganglionopathies) causing sensory ataxia may be mistaken for foot drop as the patient slams foot to ground because of the proprioceptive loss.

Treatment and prognosis

Dependent on cause.

Foramen magnum syndrome

The foramen magnum syndrome is characterized by neck stiffness and suboccipital pain which may be associated with sensorimotor abnormalities from the neck downward and neuro-ophthalmological abnormalities. It may result from extrinsic or intrinsic lesions. Recognition of the syndrome is important as many of the tumors responsible for it are benign and readily excised, without long-term sequelae. However, the signs are often subtle even with large lesions. The advent of MR imaging has made diagnosis easier.
Causes of the foramen magnum syndrome include:

- Extrinsic compressive lesions:
  - Meningioma
  - Neurofibroma
  - Metastasis

- – Skull base tumor (e.g., teratoma, chordoma)
- – Tonsillar ectopia in *Chiari malformation*
- – Cervical spondylosis
- – Atlantoaxial dislocation (e.g., rheumatoid arthritis)
- – Other craniovertebral junction bony abnormalities
- Intrinsic lesions:
  - – Glioma
  - – Demyelination (e.g., multiple sclerosis)
  - – Syrinx (typically with Chiari malformation)

Clinical features

- The history is often indolent and nonspecific with progression over years.
- Neck-occipital stiffness and pain with radiation to the shoulder or arm, with Lhermitte's phenomenon. Pain is typically made worse by head movement; the patient may hold the head at an angle, or even develop torticollis.
- Weakness of the limbs, which may be upper and/or lower motor neurone in type. The UMN presentation typically begins in the ipsilateral arm and then spreads sequentially to involve the ipsilateral leg before the contralateral leg and then contralateral arm ("around-the-clock" presentation), eventually producing hemiparesis, triparesis, or quadriparesis. The LMN presentation is with wasting, weakness, and areflexia in the upper limb which may be false-localizing, suggesting involvement of cord segments well below the level of the lesion, posssibly as a result of compromise of the anterior spinal artery blood supply to the cervical cord.
- Numbness and clumsiness of the hands and arms, with a sensory loss to all modalities. There may be a dissociated and suspended sensory loss akin to that seen in *syringomyelia*, and there may be pseudoathetosis if posterior columns are affected. Occasionally there may be patches of sensory loss or dysesthesia on the trunk.
- Lower cranial nerve palsies (e.g., IX–XII) are rare, although facial sensory loss may be present.
- Down beating nystagmus is highly suggestive of a lesion at the cervicomedullary junction (although this can be an isolated finding in elderly patients without foramen magnum lesion).
- Papilledema may be seen if there is obstruction to CSF circulation.
- Occasionally patients with foramen magnum tumors have a relapsing-remitting course.

Investigation

Bloods are not usually helpful; serology for rheumatoid arthritis may be appropriate. Neuroimaging with MRI is the most appropriate modality. CSF is only necessary if demyelination is suspected.

Neurophysiology (EMG/NCS) is not usually necessary, unless there are marked lower motor neurone findings in the arms, although these may be false-localizing.

Treatment and prognosis

This is dependent on cause. Mass lesions require a complicated neurosurgical approach and as such may have a relatively high morbidity. However, benign tumors may be associated with few neurological sequelae.

Reference

Symonds CP, Meadows SP. Compression of the spinal cord in the neighbourhood of the foramen magnum. Brain. 1937;60:52–84

Fotopoulos syndrome

A syndrome of uncertain nosology, characterized by the association of chorea and lower motor neurone disease causing neurogenic atrophy. *Neuroacanthocytosis*, *mitochondrial disease*, and *trinculeotide repeat disorders* may account for many, but not all, cases.

Reference

Pageot N, Vial C, Remy C, Chazot G, Broussolle E. Progressive chorea and amyotrophy without acanthocytes: a new case of Fotopoulos syndrome? J Neurol. 2000;247:392–394

Fowler's syndrome

Fowler's syndrome is characterized by otherwise unexplained urinary retention in women who show EMG evidence of external urethral sphincter abnormalities. Such EMG findings are a positive predictive factor for the efficacy of neuromodulation with sacral nerve stimulation to restore voiding, unlike the situation in idiopathic urinary retention.

References

De Ridder D, Ost D, Bruyninckx F. The presence of Fowler's syndrome predicts successful long-term outcome of sacral nerve stimulation in women with urinary retention. Eur Urol. 2007;51:229–233
Swinn MJ, Fowler CJ. Isolated urinary retention in young women, or Fowler's syndrome. Clin Auton Res. 2001;11:309–311

Fragile X syndromes (FRAX, FRAXE) [OMIM#300624; #309548]

Martin–Bell syndrome, Renpenning's syndrome

Fragile X syndromes are believed to be the most common cause of mental retardation in males. The name originates from the identification of an unusual, folate-sensitive, fragile site on the X chromosome, evident during karyotype preparation in folate free culture medium. Fragile X syndromes are *trinucleotide repeat diseases*: FRAX is usually caused by an expansion of a trinucleotide repeat (CGG) in the 5' untranslated region of the *FMR1* gene at Xq27.3-Xq28; deletions and point mutations have also been identified. The gene product is an RNA binding protein important in fetal development where it is found in dendrites: immature dendritic spine morphology is seen pathologically in patients with FRAX. FRAXE is also a trinucleotide repeat disorder with expansion of the trinculeotide CCG in the gene *FMR2*; children are less severely affected.

FRAX is characterized clinically by:

- Mental retardation (IQ 40–55)
- Somatic abnormalities: long narrow face, strabismus, prominent long ears, thick nasal bridge, dental malocclusion, prognathism, +/− excessive joint laxity, pectus excavatum, kyphoscoliosis, single palmar crease, pes planus, macrocephaly; after puberty macroorchidism
- Behavioral phenotype: pronounced gaze aversion, language delay, echolalia, perseveration, stereotypies, need for sameness, hypersensitivity to sensory stimuli, preoccupations with restricted interests, social anxiety; a small percentage meet full autism criteria

Female carriers may sometimes be affected but only to a slight degree.

Neuroimaging may show structural abnormalities in the caudate nucleus and cerebellum, and functional deficits in the caudate, frontal-striatal circuits, and limbic system.

References

Bensaid M, Melko M, Bechara EG, et al. FRAXE-associated mental retardation protein (FMR2) is an RNA-binding protein with high affinity for G-quartet RNA forming structure. Nucleic Acids Res. 2009;37:1269–1279

Irwin SA, Galvez R, Greenhough WT. Dendritic spine structural anomalies in fragile-X mental retardation. Cereb Cortex. 2000;10:1038–1044

Jacquemont S, Hagerman RJ, Hagerman PJ, Leehey MA. Fragile-X syndrome and fragile X-associated tremor/ataxia syndrome: two faces of FMR1. Lancet Neurol. 2007;6:45–55

Fragile X tremor ataxia syndrome (FXTAS) [OMIM#300623]

Fragile X tremor ataxia syndrome (FXTAS) results from small numbers of repeats (50–200), termed premutations, in the FMR1 gene, larger expansions of which are responsible for the most common of the *fragile X syndromes*. A wide neurological phenotype may be seen in males, usually over the age of 50 years, with the FMR1 premutation, including:

* Progressive cerebellar ataxia, especially of gait
* Tremor (action > postural, rest)
* Parkinsonism
* Peripheral neuropathy
* Autonomic dysfunction
* Cognitive impairment and dementia
* Psychiatric features: anxiety, depression, disinhibition

FXTAS has also been described in women.

Neuroimaging (MRI) typically shows high signal lesions on T_2-weighted scans in the cerebellar peduncles and in the white matter inferior and lateral to deep cerebellar nuclei.

References

Hall DA, Berry KE, Jacquemont S, et al. Initial diagnoses given to persons with the fragile X associated tremor/ataxia syndrome (FXTAS). Neurology. 2005;65:299–301

Jacquemont S, Hagerman RJ, Hagerman PJ, Leehey MA. Fragile-X syndrome and fragile X-associated tremor/ataxia syndrome: two faces of FMR1. Lancet Neurol. 2007;6:45–55

Willemsen R, Mientjes E, Oostra BA. FXTAS: a progressive neurologic syndrome associated with Fragile X premutations. Curr Neurol Neurosci Rep. 2005;5:405–410

Friedreich's ataxia (FA) [OMIM#229300]

Friedreich's ataxia (FA), described first by Friedreich in 1861, is the most common of the autosomal recessive ataxias with an incidence of 1–2 per 100,000 population. The disease typically presents before the age of 20 years with a combination of ataxia, axonal polyneuropathy, optic atrophy, dysarthria, pyramidal weakness of the legs, scoliosis, and cardiac abnormalities. The discovery that FA is a *trinucleotide repeat disease* due to an intronic trinucleotide repeat (GAA) in the frataxin gene on chromosome 9q13 (FRDA1; normal = 8–22 repeats, affected = 90–1,700 repeats) has led to an expansion of the clinical phenotype. Some FA patients are compound heterozygotes, with GAA expansion on one allele and point mutation on the other. Genetic changes cause reduced expression of frataxin protein, localized in the mitochondrial matrix (hence FA may be regarded as a mitochondrial disorder), resulting in production of reactive oxygen species, inactivation of iron-sulfur proteins in various complexes (I, II, III) of the oxidative phosphorylation pathway, and iron accumulation. Another locus for the disorder has been mapped to chromosome 9p (FRDA2). FA is currently incurable and 95% of patients are wheelchair bound by 45 years of age.

Clinical features

- FA typically presents between the ages of 8 and 15 years, but since the discovery of the frataxin gene the age range has expanded, with case onset even into the seventh decade being recorded.
- Progressive limb and gait ataxia with dysarthria (slow, jerky speech) and abnormal eye movements (nystagmus in less than 50%, but fixation instability with square-wave jerks almost always present); symptoms may begin abruptly after a febrile illness.
- Axonal sensory polyneuropathy with absent tendon reflexes (but preserved abdominal reflexes early in the disease), loss of proprioception and vibration perception, with distal wasting and pes cavus +/– equinovarus deformity of the feet.
- Pyramidal weakness of the legs with extensor plantar responses (90% in later stages of the disease).
- Optic atrophy (25%).
- Sensorineural deafness (10%).
- Head titubation is relatively common and there may be irregular ataxic respiration.
- Sphincter abnormalities are not a major feature of disease.
- Kyphoscoliosis (50%) can precede neurological deficits.
- Heart disease is seen in 65% of cases, including heart failure with arrhythmias late in the disease; in the early stages, the main abnormality is on ECG with widespread T-wave inversion and left ventricular hypertrophy.
- *Diabetes mellitus* (10%), with an additional 10–20% having an impaired glucose tolerance test.
- Diabetes insipidus is also reported.
- Mentation is preserved, although emotional lability is not uncommon.
- Atypical presentations are also reported, with late-onset spastic ataxia, pure sensory ataxia, ophthalmoplegia, myoclonus, or chorea.

Investigation

Bloods are usually noncontibutory; diabetes mellitus and vitamin E deficiency should be excluded. Neuroimaging (CT and/or MRI) of the brain and spinal cord usually reveals a degree of cerebellar and spinal cord atrophy. CSF is usually normal; investigation is not obligatory. EMG/NCS shows an axonal polyneuropathy; severe reduction or loss of sensory action potentials without involvement of motor conduction velocities. This pattern is very useful in distinguishing FA from *hereditary motor and sensory neuropathy (HMSN)* type I, in which motor nerve conduction velocity is slowed, and autosomal dominant ataxias such as SCA3 in which sensory neuropathy may not be clinically apparent. Visual evoked potentials are abnormal in most cases, as are limb SEPs. ECG may show widespread T-wave inversion, left ventricular hypertrophy. Neurogenetic testing to search for trinucleotide expansion and mutation in the frataxin gene is now the definitive test. Other consults may be required, including echocardiography, cardiac opinion, respiratory studies, and orthopedic opinion. Pathology shows degeneration with gliosis of the dorsal columns, especially in cervical cord, dorsal root ganglia, pyramidal tracts, especially in lower spinal cord, and spinocerebellar tracts with secondary mild atrophy of cerebellum and neuronal loss in the dentate nucleus and inferior olivary nucleus. Optic and peripheral nerves show loss of large myelinated fibers. Nuclei of cranial nerves VIII, X, and XII all show reduced cell counts.

Differential diagnosis

- Hereditary motor and sensory neuropathy (HMSN), especially type I
- *Ataxia with vitamin E deficiency (AVED)*
- Other inherited cerebellar syndromes, autosomal recessive or dominant, especially adult onset *ataxia with oculomotor apraxia* type II
- *Mitochondrial disease*
- *Abetalipoproteinemia*
- Complicated *hereditary spastic paraplegia (HSP)*
- *Wolfram syndrome*

Treatment and prognosis

The rate of progression is very variable: death may occur in the 30 s but patients can live into sixth and seventh decades. Mean time to become wheelchair bound is ~15 years, 95% are wheelchair bound by age of 45 years. Mean survival time from onset is ~36 years. Symptomatic treatment includes management of diabetes mellitus and cardiac abnormalities. Surgery may be needed for foot deformities. There is currently no treatment for the underlying condition but improved understanding of pathogenesis suggests that antioxidants may be helpful. A trial of idebenone did not suggest significant benefit in terms of neurological progression.

References

Dürr A, Cossee M, Agid Y, et al. Clinical and genetic abnormalities in patients with Friedreich's ataxia. N Engl J Med. 1996;335:1169–1175
Pandolfo M. Friedreich ataxia. Arch Neurol. 2008;65:1296–1303

Froin's syndrome

Froin's syndrome is the name given to exceptionally high CSF protein concentration, which may be sufficient to cause the CSF to clot, sometimes associated with low CSF opening pressure, as may be seen with spinal block, malignancy, *Guillain-Barré syndrome*, and *vestibular schwannoma*.

Frontotemporal lobar degeneration (FTLD)

Neurodegenerative disorders with circumscribed atrophy of the frontal and/ or temporal regions were first described by Pick (1892, 1906). These account for perhaps 20% of cases of primary cerebral atrophy occurring in the presenium, and in younger age groups (<60 years) may be as common as *Alzheimer's disease (AD)*. A number of subsyndromes are recognized on clinical grounds, dependent upon the precise anatomical distribution of pathology, although there is a tendency for clinical merging as disease progresses:

- Behavioral variant of frontotemporal dementia (bvFTD), frontal variant of frontotemporal dementia (fvFTD), frontotemporal dementia, dementia of frontal type, frontal lobe degeneration
- *Progressive non-fluent aphasia (PNFA)*, primary progressive aphasia (PPA), temporal variant of frontotemporal dementia (tvFTD)
- *Semantic dementia*
- Frontotemporal lobar degeneration with motor neurone disease (FTLD/ MND), motor neurone disease dementia, MND-dementia

Classifications in terms of pathological appearances and/or predominant abnormal proteins also exist:

- Tau positive pathology, although not all cases have the typical pathology of "Pick's disease," as originally described by Alzheimer.
- Ubiquitinated inclusions, which may or may not be TDP-43 positive; this may be typical of the pathological inclusions seen in *motor neurone disease*.
- "Dementia lacking distinctive pathology."

Familial occurrence of FTLD is more common than in AD. A genetic classification is possible for some families:

- Mutations in the tau gene and the progranulin gene, both on chromosome 17 (*frontotemporal dementia with parkinsonism linked to chromosome 17 (FTDP-17)*) [OMIM#600274, #607485]
- Chromosome 3-linked frontotemporal dementia (CHMP2B) [OMIM#600795]
- *Inclusion body myositis* with early-onset *Paget's disease* and frontotemporal dementia (IBMMPFD) (valosin-containing protein, VCP) [OMIM#167320]

Clinical features

* Behavioral variant of frontotemporal dementia (bvFTD): a neurobehavioral syndrome with change in personality, impaired judgment (dysexecutive syndrome); patient may be apathetic and lack motivation, or be disinhibited, overactive, and fatuous. Reduced ability to show emotion or empathize with the emotions of others. Stereotyped and perseverative behaviors; rituals, clockwatching. Gluttony, food fads, especially a predilection for sweet or sticky foods to the exclusion of other food. Speech economic, concrete. No amnesia or disorientation. Late akinesia, rigidity.
* Progressive non-fluent aphasia: progressive decline in language production with relative absence of other neuropsychological deficits; comprehension relatively preserved, as are activities of daily living.
* Semantic dementia: loss of word meaning leading to fluent but empty speech.
* Fasciculation of shoulder girdle muscles may suggest an underlying pathological diagnosis of FTLD/MND.

Investigation

Neuropsychology: deficits appropriate to anatomical distribution of pathology: attentional difficulties in bvFTD, language problems in progressive non-fluent aphasia, semantic difficulties in semantic dementia. Neuroimaging (CT/MRI) may show focal frontotemporal atrophy, often asymmetric; SPECT may show focal (frontal) deficits of perfusion. EEG is typically normal (cf. Alzheimer's disease). CSF is unremarkable. EMG/NCS may be undertaken to look for subclinical evidence of anterior horn cell disease.

Differential diagnosis

Cases of bvFTD have probably been labeled as mania or manic-depressive psychosis in the past; many patients with bvFTD are initially referred to psychiatric services because of neuropsychiatric features, but psychosis is rare (with the possible exception of FTLD/MND). Language disorders need to be distinguished from focal presentations of AD or cerebrovascular disease. Semantic dementia is sometimes confused with AD.

Treatment and prognosis

No specific treatment is currently available. Behavioral agitation may be treated empirically with anticonvulsant medication (carbamazepine, valproate) or "atypical" antipsychotics such as risperidone, olanzapine, or quetiapine. Survival is variable, best in PNFA and worst in FTLD/MND.

Diagnostic criteria

Cairns NJ, Bigio EH, Mackenzie IRA, et al. Neuropathologic diagnostic and nosologic criteria for frontotemporal lobar degeneration: consensus of the Consortium for Frontotemporal Lobar Degeneration. Acta Neuropathol. 2007;114:5–22

McKhann GM, Albert MS, Grossman M, Miller B, Dickson D, Trojanowski JQ. Clinical and pathological diagnosis of frontotemporal dementia. Report of the Work Group on Frontotemporal Dementia and Pick's disease. Arch Neurol. 2001;58: 1803–1809

References

Alzheimer Disease and Frontotemporal Dementia Mutation Database, www.molgen. ua.ac.be/Admutations

Hodges JR ed. Frontotemporal Dementia Syndromes. Cambridge: Cambridge University Press; 2007

Mackenzie IRA, Neumann M, Bigio EH, et al. Nomenclature for neuropathologic subtypes of frontotemporal lobar degeneration: consensus recommendations. Acta Neuropathol. 2009;117:15–18

Mackenzie IR, Neumann M, Bigio EH, et al. Nomenclature and nosology for neuropathologic subtypes of frontotemporal lobar degeneration: an update. Acta Neuropathol. 2010;119:1–4

Mendez MF, Lauterbach EC, Sampson SM, ANPA Committee on Research. An evidence-based review of the psychopathology of frontotemporal dementia: a report of the ANPA Committee on Research. J Neuropsychiatry Clin Neurosci. 2008;20:130–149

Mendez MF, Shapira JS, Woods RJ, Licht EA, Saul RE. Psychotic symptoms in frontotemporal dementia: prevalence and review. Dement Geriatr Cogn Disord. 2008;25:206–211

Frontotemporal dementia with parkinsonism linked to chromosome 17 (FTDP-17) [OMIM#600274, #607485]

The term "frontotemporal dementia with parkinsonism linked to chromosome 17" (FTDP-17) was coined to describe autosomal dominant kindreds linked to chromosome 17q21-22 with a highly penetrant disorder characterized clinically by a phenotype of frontotemporal dementia and parkinsonism. The FTDP-17 nomenclature superseded various clinical and clinicopathological labels previously applied to some of these kindreds, which included:

- Disinhibition-dementia-parkinsonism-amyotrophy complex
- Hereditary dysphasic disinhibition dementia
- Pallido-ponto-nigral degeneration
- Progressive subcortical gliosis
- Multiple system tauopathy with presenile dementia

Pathogenic mutations within the gene encoding the microtubule associated protein tau (MAPT) have been described in some of these families; over 40 are recognized to date, with significant clinical heterogeneity, some presenting with a phenotype of *Alzheimer's disease, progressive supranuclear palsy, corticobasal degeneration*, or *Parkinson's disease* as well as frontotemporal dementia. Subsequently, mutations were also identified in the progranulin gene, also located on chromosome 17q21-22, again with considerable clinical heterogeneity, but with non-tau pathology unlike the situation with tau gene mutations. Progranulin mutations seem to occur at a similar frequency to tau mutations in large cohorts of patients fulfilling clinical diagnostic criteria for frontotemporal lobar degeneration, but family history of dementia is not always present in progranulin cases, unlike tau, disease onset is later, and certain phenotypic features (progressive nonfluent aphasia, limb apraxia) are more common.

References

Alzheimer Disease and Frontotemporal Dementia Mutation Database, www.molgen. ua.ac.be/Admutations

Foster NL, Wilhelmsen K, Sima AAF, et al. Frontotemporal dementia and parkinsonism linked to chromosome 17: a consensus conference. Ann Neurol. 1997;41:706–715

Larner AJ, Doran M. Clinical heterogeneity associated with tau gene mutations. Eur Neurol Rev. 2009;3(2):31–32

Pickering-Brown SM, Rollinson S, Du Plessis D, et al. Frequency and clinical characteristics of progranulin mutation carriers in the Manchester frontotemporal lobar degeneration cohort: comparison with patients with MAPT and no known mutations. Brain. 2008;131:721–731

Van Swieten JC, Heutink P. Mutations in progranulin (GRN) within the spectrum of clinical and pathological phenotypes of frontotemporal dementia. Lancet Neurol. 2008;7:965–974

Fucosidosis [OMIM#230000]

Fucosidosis is a rare autosomal recessive inherited *lysosomal storage disorder* due to a deficiency of α-fucosidase. Although most cases are diagnosed in infancy and childhood, occasional cases only come to light in adolescence or adulthood. Cases may be classified as:

- Type I (infantile): with onset between 3 and 18 months; in which epileptic seizures may occur and progression is rapid.
- Type II (juvenile): with onset from 1 to 2 years in which ataxia and behavioral problems may feature, progression somewhat slower.
- Type III: signs noted in the first few years of life, but adolescence or adulthood reached before severe mental and motor deterioration.

However, some authors do not support this classification, finding a wide and continuous clinical spectrum.

"Storage facies" (enlarged salivary glands, coarse facial features, gargoylism, excessive sweating) may be a feature, likewise angiokeratoma (cf. *Fabry's disease*) and recurrent infections. Blood smears may show vacuolated mononuclear cells; assay of white cell enzymes for fucosidase activity is the diagnostic test. Skin biopsy electron microscopy may reveal intralysosomal laminated structures and axonal spheroids. There is no specific treatment; the condition is usually fatal within 4–6 years of onset.

Reference

Willems PJ, Gatti R, Darby JK, et al. Fucosidosis revisited: a review of 77 patients. Am J Med Genet. 1991;38:111–131

G

Gait disorders: overview

Disorders of gait are relatively common in neurological practice and may have a number of different causes, acting either individually or collectively: gait disorder may be multifactorial. A thorough neurological examination is indicated in any patient with a gait disorder. Various forms of gait disorder are recognized:

- Myopathic gait:
  - Waddling; difficulty climbing stairs, rising from chairs; proximal weakness.
- Neuropathic gait:
  - May be unsteady, cautious; high stepping gait (steppage); distal weakness and sensory loss, foot drop, areflexia. Focal neuropathies may cause gait difficulties, for example, lateral popliteal or femoral neuropathies.
- Spastic gait:
  - Most commonly unilateral, with circumduction of extended leg, +/− ipsilateral arm held in abduction, internally rotated at the shoulder and flexed at the elbow (hemiplegic); +/− other upper motor neurone signs, aphasia. May be bilateral, with scissoring gait, spastic paraparesis +/− impaired bladder function, sensory level.
- Ataxic gait:
  - Cerebellar ataxia: broad-based, staggering +/− nystagmus, dysarthria, limb ataxia; midline cerebellar lesions cause a gait/truncal ataxia with little in the way of limb or eye signs.
  - Sensory ataxia: broad based, staggering, Romberg sign positive, often high stepping with slapping down of foot; distal sensory loss +/− weakness.
- Extrapyramidal gait:
  - *Parkinson's disease*: stooped posture, slow initiation, shuffling/festinant ambulation, reduced or absent arm swing, freezing +/− hypomimia, tremor, quiet voice.
  - Progressive supranuclear palsy: as for PD but axial rigidity with neck extension (retrocollis); early history of falls, especially on turning; +/− supranuclear gaze palsy.

- Dystonia: abnormal leg posture, often with walking: typically inversion and plantar flexion of the foot but may involve hip; toe-walking; minimal neurological signs examining on the couch, except possibly dystonia; differential diagnosis includes dopa-responsive dystonia (DRD), and paroxysmal kinesigenic choreoathetosis (PKC).
  - Choreiform: often only hand and head chorea seen, but typically also involves the legs and causes a lurching or stumbling gait which is irregular and unpredictable; +/- cognitive abnormalities (Huntington's disease).
  - Postanoxic action myoclonus: bouncing gait, collapsing; bizarre give-way type walking may be labeled "psychiatric."
  - *Primary orthostatic tremor (POT)*: "shaky legs syndrome," unsteady on standing still, often better with walking or sitting; minimal signs; leg tremor is not uncommonly seen in essential tremor (ET) but rarely causes a gait disorder.
- Rigid gait:
  - Stiff man syndrome: stiff but not scissoring, often described as walking through treacle; lumbar hyperlordosis, abdominal rigidity, no abnormal limb signs.
- *Marche à petit pas*:
  - Short, small steps, upright posture; +/- subcortical dementia, pseudobulbar palsy, history of strokes.
- Gait apraxia:
  - Unable to start walking = gait ignition failure, associated with frontal lobe involvement; normal examination on bed, can pretend to cycle on bed. This may also be seen in *normal pressure hydrocephalus*.
- Painful, antalgic gait:
  - Staggering, limping; no neurological deficits, may be Trendelenburg sign positive.
- Psychogenic gait disorders:
  - Often bizarre, staggering but always able to compensate, never falling; inconsistent neurological deficits; consider chorea and action myoclonus as possible causes before applying this diagnosis.
- Cautious gait:
  - Holding on to objects (e.g., furniture), small steps, fear of falling; no abnormal signs.
- Impaired vision/diplopia, vestibular disorders:
  - May produce cautious gait, ataxic gait.

Gait disorders may be multifactorial, particularly in the elderly (any combination of painful hips, poor vision, mild neuropathy, vestibular dysfunction, etc.).

A number of different gait disorders have been described with frontal lobe pathology, including:

- Subcortical disequilibrium
- Frontal disequilibrium

- Isolated gait ignition failure
- Frontal gait disorder

Neurological gait disorders are risk factors for falls, especially in elderly patients.

References

Axer H, Axer M, Sauer H, Witte OW, Hagemann G. Falls and gait disorders in geriatric neurology. Clin Neurol Neurosurg. 2010;112:265–274

Baezner H, Hennerici M. From trepidant abasia to motor network failure – gait disorders as a consequence of subcortical vascular encephalopathy (SVE): review of historical and contemporary concepts. J Neurol Sci. 2005;229–230:81–88

Bronstein AM, Brandt T, Woollacott MH, Nutt JG, eds. Clinical Disorders of Balance, Posture and Gait. 2nd ed. London: Hodder Arnold; 2004

Nutt JG, Marsden CD, Thompson PD. Human walking and higher-level gait disorders, particularly in the elderly. Neurology. 1993;43:268–279

Verghese J, Ambrose AF, Lipton RB, Wang C. Neurological gait abnormalities and risk of falls in older patients. J Neurol. 2010;257:392–398

Galloping tongue syndrome

Galloping tongue syndrome is an episodic, rhythmic, involuntary movement of the tongue following head and neck trauma. The episodes begin as posterior midline focal tongue contractions at a frequency of 3 Hz and last for around 10 s. The movements differ from branchial myoclonus, are innocuous and self-limiting, resolving in 2–4 months. They do not spread and are not associated with any EEG abnormality.

Reference

Keane JR. Galloping tongue: post-traumatic, episodic, rhythmic movements. Neurology. 1984;34:251–252

Ganglioglioma

Gangliogliomas are benign tumors, occurring typically in childhood and early adulthood, often occurring in the temporal lobe and causing partial *epilepsy*. They are occasionally found in other lobes of the cerebral hemisphere, cerebellum, and spinal cord. They are composed of both neuronal and glial elements and are well delineated from surrounding tissues; calcification is common. MR imaging is nonspecific, lesions may be cystic, solid, or mixed. Local surgical excision is often possible.

References

Lang FF, Epstein FJ, Ransohoff J. Central nervous system ganglioglioma, II: clinical outcome. J Neurosurg. 1993;79:867–873

Zentner J, Wolf HK, Ostertun B, et al. Gangliogliomas: clinical, radiological and histopathological findings in 51 patients. J Neurol Neurosurg Psychiatry. 1994;57:1497–1502

Gangliosidoses: overview

Gangliosides are made up of ceramide and sialic acid, and are important components of CNS and PNS lipid. Accumulation of various gangliosides, in the CNS as well as systemically, occurs in the inherited gangliosidoses, of which two main types are recognized:

- GM1 gangliosidosis: due to deficiency of lysosomal β-galactosidase
- GM2 gangliosidosis: due to deficiency of hexosaminidase activity, though more complex, since three genes may be involved (for the α-locus, the β-locus, and for a heat-stable protein cofactor), and two enzymes, hexosaminidase A (α- and β-subunits) and B (only β-subunit)

Although most often disorders of infants, occasional adult cases occur.

Clinical features

- GM1 gangliosidosis (familial neurovisceral lipidosis); no ethnic tendencies
  Type 1/Infantile: (birth to <6 months old) [OMIM#230500]:
  - Coarsened facies at birth, enlarged tongue, hepatosplenomegaly, umbilical hernia; pseudo-Hurler's phenotype
  - Neurology: Micro- or macrocephaly
    ○ No psychomotor development after 3–6 months
    ○ Blind with macular cherry-red spots (50%) and nystagmus; corneal clouding unusual
    ○ Deafness
    ○ Hypotonia then spasticity
    ○ Epileptic seizures (late)
    ○ +/− Cardiomyopathy
  Type 2/Late infantile, Juvenile: (7 months to 3 years old) [OMIM#230600]:
  - No systemic features (i.e., no visceral storage or bone involvement)
  - Neurology: Weakness (progressive)
  - Incoordination
  - Spasticity
  - Mental retardation
  - Epileptic seizures
  - Vision preserved

Type 3/Adult: (mid-childhood to adolescence) [OMIM# 230650]:
 - No systemic features
 - Neurology: Marked variability
   o Gait disorder with spasticity
   o Dystonia and other extrapyramidal features
   o Dysarthria and ataxia
   o Mental retardation; may progress to dementia
   o No visceral or skeletal changes
- GM2 gangliosidosis: predilection for Ashkenazi Jews
 - Type 1: Tay–Sachs disease; Infantile (α-locus: total hexosaminadase A deficiency) [OMIM#272800]
 - Type 2: Sandhoff disease (β-locus: hexosaminidase A and B deficiency) [OMIM#268800]
 - AB variant: inability to form a functional GM2 activator complex, normal hexosamindiase A and B [OMIM#272750]

Investigation

- GM1 gangliosidosis:
 - Blood: vacuolated lymphocytes; deficiency of β-galactosidase in leukocytes, fibroblasts
 - Urine: oligosaccharides abnormal
 - Imaging: plain radiographs: dysostosis multiplex
 - CT/MRI: putaminal lesions in adult form
 - Neurophysiology: VER delayed or absent, ERG abnormal with retinal involvement

Differential diagnosis

GM1 gangliosidosis, type III: other forms of *dystonia*

Treatment and prognosis

Neither condition has specific treatment. In GM1 gangliosidosis, prognosis in type 1 and type 2 disease is poor, with death in childhood. In type 3, survival is typically prolonged.

References

Navon R. Molecular and clinical heterogeneity of adult GM2 gangliosidosis. Dev Neurosci. 1991;13:295–298
Roze E, Paschke E, Lopez N, et al. Dystonia and parkinsonism in GM1 type 3 gangliosidosis. Mov Disord. 2005;20:1366–1369
Suzuki K. Neuropathology of late onset gangliosidosis. A review. Dev Neurosci. 1991;13:205–210

Garcin syndrome

Hemibasal syndrome

Garcin syndrome refers to unilateral palsy of all cranial nerves, often occurring successively. It is most commonly seen with skull base tumors (chordoma, chondrosarcoma of the clivus), rhinopharyngeal tumors (nasopharyngeal carcinoma) or metastases, and basal meningitides. It may mimic the foreign accent syndrome.

References

Hanse MCJ, Nijssen PCG. Unilateral palsy of all cranial nerves (Garcin syndrome) in a patient with rhinocerebral mucormycosis. J Neurol. 2003;250:506–507
Hoffmann M. Foreign accent syndrome mimicked by Garcin syndrome with spontaneous resolution. Behav Neurol. 2008;19:195–197

Gardner's syndrome

A dominantly inherited familial polyposis coli syndrome, associated with multiple osteomas, sometimes of the skull, skin, and soft tissue tumors. Brain tumors may sometimes occur.

Reference

Foulkes WG. A tale of four syndromes: familial adenomatous polyposis, Gardner syndrome, attenuated APC and Turcot syndrome. Q J Med. 1995;88:853–863

Gasperini's syndrome

Gasperini's syndrome is a brainstem syndrome comprising at minimum ipsilateral palsy of the facial (VII) and abducens (VI) nerves with additional involvement of the trigeminal (V) and vestibuloauditory (VIII) nerves and with contralateral sensory disturbance, with additional nystagmus, due to a lesion, usually vascular of the posterior tegmentum of the pons.

Reference

Krasnianski M, Muller T, Zierz S, Winterholler M. Gasperini syndrome as clinical manifestation of pontine demyelination. Eur J Med Res. 2009;14:413–414

Gastrointestinal disease and the nervous system: overview

Neurological and gastroenterological problems may be interrelated in a number of ways. Neurological disorders may cause abnormalities of gut motility; gastroenterological disorders may cause malabsorption with secondary neurological effects.

Clinical features

- Disorders of gut motility:
  - Achalasia: primary, secondary (Chagas' disease)
  - Dysphagia:
    - Neurogenic: stroke (hemisphere, brain stem); extrapyramidal disorders (Parkinson's disease, progressive supranuclear palsy, Huntington's disease, Wilson's disease), multiple sclerosis, Guillain-Barré syndrome, motor neurone disease, myasthenia gravis
    - Myogenic: inflammatory muscle disease (polymyositis, inclusion body myositis), myotonic dystrophy, oculopharyngeal muscular dystrophy
  - Constipation/diarrhea (?autonomic neuropathy): diabetes mellitus
- Malabsorption:
  - Vitamin B1 deficiency: beriberi, Wernicke-Korsakoff syndrome; pellagra
  - Vitamin B12 deficiency: peripheral neuropathy, myelopathy (subacute combined degeneration of the cord), optic neuropathy, disorder of affect or cognition (rarely dementia)
  - Vitamin D deficiency: myopathy
  - Vitamin E deficiency: spinocerebellar syndrome
  - Coeliac disease (gluten-sensitive enteropathy): epilepsy (usually partial, occipital), cerebellar syndrome, peripheral neuropathy, myelopathy, myoclonus, dementia
- Inflammatory bowel disease: thromboembolic complications including venous sinus thrombosis; peripheral neuropathy (possibly related to nutritional deficiency). *Behçet's disease* can present with involvement of the gut and an inflammatory bowel disease-like pathology.
- Whipple's disease: dementia, ophthalmoplegia (supranuclear), myoclonus, hypothalamic features (hypersomnia, polydipsia, hyperphagia).

Treatment and prognosis

Treatment of the underlying cause where possible. Speech therapy advice on appropriate feeding methods and diet; in extreme cases percutaneous endoscopic gastrostomy (PEG) or jejunostomy (PEJ) may be required to ensure adequate nutrition.

Reference

Perkin GD, Murray-Lyon I. Neurology and the gastrointestinal system. J Neurol Neurosurg Psychiatry. 1998;65:291–300

Gaucher's disease

Glucosylceramide lipidosis

This is a rare autosomal recessive *lysosomal storage disorder*, in which there is a deficiency of lysosomal β-glucosidase (or glucocerebrosidase) which leads to the accumulation of glucocerebrosides in cells of the reticuloendothelial system. Three forms of the disease are recognized, of which the most common form, type I, is non-neuronopathic. Type II is a severe form of neuronopathic disease with onset in the first months of life and death usually by 2 years of age. Type III is the late onset adult form of the condition that has a subacute onset with supranuclear gaze palsies, intellectual decline, and spasticity with hepatosplenomegaly. Gaucher's disease is linked to genetic mutations in the glucocerebrosidase gene on chromosome 1q21. An increased frequency of glucocerebrosidase mutations has been identified in *Parkinson's disease*. Rare cases of Gaucher disease are associated with deficiency of saposin C, a heat-stable cofactor required for the normal catalytic activity of glucocerebrosidase, due to mutations in the prosaposin gene on chromosome 10q21 [OMIM#610539], allelic to some forms of *metachromatic leukodystrophy*.

Clinical features

- Type I: non-neuronopathic [OMIM#230800]:
  - Visceromegaly
  - Bone changes
  - Thrombocytopenia: marked bruising, anemia
- Type II: acute infantile neuronopathic [OMIM#230900]:
  - Typically presents in first months of life
  - Neurological features:
    - Developmental arrest
    - Hypertonia (spasticity)
    - Neck retraction, opisthotonos
    - Strabismus, visual impairment; normal fundi; supranuclear gaze palsy
    - Feeding difficulties, unable to swallow: laryngeal stridor, trismus, and dysphagia
    - Microcephaly
    - Epileptic seizures are rare

- – Systemic features:
  - ○ Hepatosplenomegaly: huge
  - ○ Skin and scleral pigmentation
  - ○ +/− lymphadenopathy
  - ○ No bone changes (cf. type I)
- • Type III: subacute neuronopathic [OMIM#231000]:
  - – Typically presents in early to middle childhood, either with neurological features, or with aggressive visceral disease reminiscent of type I which may cause death from hepatic failure before significant neurological problems develop
  - – Neurological features:
    - ○ Epileptic seizures, myoclonus
    - ○ Slowly progressive ataxia
    - ○ Dysarthria
    - ○ Cognitive decline
    - ○ Oculomotor disorder (supranuclear gaze palsy)
  - – Systemic features:
    - ○ Hepatosplenomegaly: almost always

Investigation

Bloods: raised acid phosphatase; pancytopenia if bone marrow significantly involved; deficiency of β-glucosidase (glucocerebrosidase) may be demonstrated in leukocytes or fibroblasts and is diagnostic. Imaging: widened ends of long bones on plain radiography due to infiltration and expansion by glucocerebroside-containing storage cells ("Erlenmeyer flask" in femur). CSF: not usually required, although Gaucher cells (swollen by intracytoplasmic accumulation of cerebrosides giving a foamy appearance) may be found in the CSF. Others: characteristic Gaucher cells may be seen in bone marrow aspirates and liver biopsies.

Differential diagnosis

- • Type I may be clinically indistinguishable from Niemann-Pick disease type B.
- • Type III may be clinically similar to metachromatic leukodystrophy but the presence of hepatosplenomegaly assists in differentiating them. It also enters the differential diagnosis of progressive myoclonus epilepsy.

Treatment and prognosis

Intravenous enzyme replacement therapy may be effective for treating the systemic features in types I and III, for example, to reduce hepatosplenomegaly; however, it delays but does not prevent the neurological complications of type II; outcome uncertain in type III. Treatment of hypersplenism by splenectomy may be required. Prognosis in type II is typically death by the age of 2 years; in type III death by the second to fourth decade.

References

Cox TM. Gaucher's disease – an exemplary monogenic disorder. Q J Med. 2001;94: 399–402
Sidransky E, Nalls MA, Aasly JO, et al. Multicenter analysis of glucocerebrosidase mutations in Parkinson's disease. N Engl J Med. 2009;361:1651–1661

Gelastic epilepsy

In gelastic epilepsy, there are partial epileptic seizures characterized by involuntary laughter. They may be symptomatic, particularly of hypothalamic hamartoma (along with precocious puberty and mental retardation), and of *tuberous sclerosis*, but may also be cryptogenic in some cases, in which case the prognosis for seizure control with antiepileptic medications is better.

Reference

Striano S, Striano P, Sarappa C, Boccella P. The clinical spectrum and natural history of gelastic epilepsy-hypothalamic hamartoma syndrome. Seizure. 2005;14:232–239

Gelsolin amyloidosis [OMIM#105120]

Familial amyloidosis Finnish type (FAF), Meretoja syndrome

This *amyloid disease* is a hereditary systemic amyloidosis, first described in Finland, which results from mutations in the gene encoding gelsolin, an actin binding protein, on chromosome 9, G654A or G654T ("Danish type"), resulting in the Asp187Asn substitution.
The clinical features are characteristic, namely:

- Corneal lattice dystrophy
- Cranial neuropathy, especially facial weakness, +/– atrophic bulbar palsy
- Polyneuropathy: mild, sensory, principally proximal nerve involvement, with preferential large fiber loss
- +/– Gait ataxia
- +/– Cognitive impairment
- +/– skin changes: baggy and atrophic

Pathologically there is meningeal amyloid angiopathy. Familial amyloid polyneuropathy (FAP) enters the differential diagnosis of the neuropathy.

Reference

Kiuru S. Gelsolin-related familial amyloidosis, Finnish type (FAF), and its variants found worldwide. Amyloid. 1998;5:55–66

Generalized epilepsy with febrile seizures plus (GEFS+) [OMIM#604233]

Febrile seizures are relatively common in children, a proportion of whom go on to develop *epilepsy* with afebrile seizures and also have evidence for autosomal dominant inheritance. A number of genetic loci and causative genes have been defined:

	Locus	Gene
GEFS+ type 1	19q13	Voltage-gated sodium channel beta-1 subunit gene, SCN1B
GEFS+ type 2	2q24	α subunit, voltage-gated Na⁺ channel, SCN1A
GEFS+ type 3	5q31.1-q33.1	GABA(A) receptor γ2 subunit, GABRG2
GEFS+ type 4	2p24	
GEFS+ type 5		GABRD
GEFS+ type 6	8p23-p21	
GEFS+ type 7	2q24	SCN9A

Hence, a number of these conditions are *channelopathies*.

Reference

Deprez L, Jansen A, De Jonghe P. Genetics of epilepsy syndromes starting in the first year of life. Neurology. 2009;72:273–281

Geniculate neuralgia

Geniculate neuralgia is a rare cause of otalgia, characterized by severe paroxysmal neuralgic pain centered in the ear, but sometimes the pain is dull and persistent with occasional sharp and stabbing features. The cause of the pain is unknown, and there are no associated neurological signs. Carbamazepine and other anti-neuropathic agents may be of benefit, but in intractable pain surgical intervention may be required, typically involving excision of the nervus intermedius and geniculate ganglion.

Reference

Pulec JL. Geniculate neuralgia: long-term results of surgical treatment. Ear Nose Throat J. 2002;81:30–33

Geniospasm

Chin trembling

Geniospasm is a focal movement disorder involving tremor of the chin and lower lip, sometimes precipitated by stress, concentration, or emotion. The condition begins in early childhood, and sometimes occurs in families with an autosomal dominant pattern of inheritance.

References

Aggarwal A, Warren JE, Warren JD, Thompson PD. Facial reflex hyperexcitability in geniospasm suggests a brainstem origin. Mov Disord. 2009;24:783–784
Jarman PR, Wood NW, Davis MT, et al. Hereditary geniospasm: linkage to chromosome 9q13-q21 and evidence for genetic heterogeneity. Am J Hum Genet. 1997;61:928–933

Genitofemoral neuropathy

Lesions of the genitofemoral nerve, which arises from the L1 and L2 spinal roots, cause pain and paresthesiae in the groin and upper medial thigh ("spermatic neuralgia"). Because of the proximity of the ilioinguinal nerve, *ilioinguinal neuropathy* is also often present. The cremasteric reflex may be absent. Surgery is probably the most commonly identified cause of genitofemoral neuropathy.

Reference

O'Brien MD. Genitofemoral neuropathy. BMJ. 1979;1:1052

Gerhardt syndrome

Gerhardt syndrome is bilateral vagus (X) nerve palsies, due to brainstem or skull base pathology, causing bilateral adductor laryngeal paralysis with severe dysphonia and dyspnea. It may also occur in *multiple system atrophy*.

Germ cell tumors

The group of germ cell tumors encompasses the following histological types:

- Germinoma
- Teratoma

- Embryonal carcinoma
- Yolk sac tumor
- Choriocarcinoma

Although germ cell tumors may occur at many intracranial locations, the pineal gland is the most common. The pineal location may result in the clinical findings of Parinaud's syndrome. There may be elevations of serum and CSF α-fetoprotein, human chorionic gonadotrophin (HCG), and placental alkaline phosphatase, which may facilitate diagnosis, since MR imaging findings are usually nonspecific. If bloods and imaging prove unhelpful, biopsy may be undertaken to establish tumor type. However, clinical and histological diagnoses were often consistent in one series, and treatment with neoadjuvant chemotherapy and radiotherapy without histological verification generally has a good outcome.

References

Glenn OA, Barkovich AJ. Intracranial germ cell tumors: a comprehensive review of proposed embryologic derivation. Pediatr Neurosurg. 1996;24:242–251
Kanamori M, Kumabe T, Tominaga T. Is histological diagnosis necessary to start treatment for germ cell tumours in the pineal region? J Clin Neurosci. 2008;15: 978–987

Germinoma

Germinoma is one of the *germ cell tumors*, accounting for less than 1% of primary intracranial tumors, with a predilection for the pineal gland and suprasellar region, rarely the basal ganglia and thalami, and very uncommonly the posterior fossa, with symptoms and signs appropriate to specific location. This is a tumor occurring most commonly in childhood. There may be elevations of serum and CSF α-fetoprotein, human chorionic gonadotrophin, and placental alkaline phosphatase. MR imaging usually shows a solid lesion, sometimes surrounded by calcium, but there may be cystic areas, with homogeneous or heterogeneous enhancement. Biopsy is the key to management, especially for *pineal tumors* since a variety of histopathological types may occur in this location. Good remission rates with no detectable disease have been achieved with chemotherapy and local, limited, radiotherapy.

Reference

Shibamoto Y. Management of central nervous system germinoma: proposal for a modern strategy. Prog Neurol Surg. 2009;23:119–129

Gerstmann syndrome

Angular gyrus syndrome

The Gerstmann syndrome refers to a constellation of clinical signs:

- Right-left disorientation
- Finger agnosia
- Acalculia
- Agraphia (central type)

These occur with lesions, most usually of vascular origin, in the region of the dominant (usually left) posterior parietal cortex (angular and supramarginal gyri), and thus may be associated with a visual field defect. Partial syndromes occur, indicating that all the signs dissociate, but nonetheless the syndrome is useful for clinical localization.

References

Benton AL. Gerstmann's syndrome. Arch Neurol. 1992;49:445–447
Mayer E, Martory M-D, Pegna AJ, et al. A pure case of Gerstmann's syndrome with a subangular lesion. Brain. 1999;122:1107–1120

Gerstmann–Sträussler–Scheinker disease (GSS) [OMIM#137440]

This is a rare inherited form of *prion disease*, first described in 1928, that presents with a slowly evolving cerebellar syndrome followed by dementia, long tract signs, and an extrapyramidal disorder; myoclonus and psychiatric features may occur, visual and sensory signs are rare. Pathologically it is characterized by multicentric amyloid plaques. Few patients survive for more than 5 years after onset of illness. GSS is associated with mutations in the PrP gene which encodes the prion protein.

Reference

Kovacs GG, Trabattoni G, Hainfellner JA, Ironside JW, Knight RSG, Budka H. Mutations of the prion protein gene: phenotypic spectrum. J Neurol. 2002;249:1567–1582

Geschwind syndrome

Gastaut–Geschwind syndrome

This clinical syndrome comprises:

- Hypergraphia
- Hyperreligiosity
- Hyposexuality

It may occur as part of an interictal psychosis in patients with complex partial seizures of temporal lobe origin, particularly with a nondominant focus.

References

Trimble MR. The Gastaut-Geschwind syndrome. In: Trimble MR, Bolwig TG, eds. The Temporal Lobes and the Limbic System. Petersfield: Wrightson Biomedical; 1992:137–147
Waxman SG, Geschwind N. The interictal behavior syndrome of temporal lobe epilepsy. Arch Gen Psychiatry. 1975;32:1580–1586

Giant axonal neuropathy (GAN) [OMIM#256850]

This is a rare, autosomal recessive, condition, traditionally classified with the hereditary peripheral neuropathies, although both PNS and CNS are affected. It manifests in childhood with:

- Psychomotor retardation
- Progressive axonal peripheral neuropathy
- Ataxia
- Dysarthria
- Nystagmus
- Dementia
- Dull blonde curly hair

In sporadic cases, skeletal and cardiac muscle involvement has been reported. Nerve biopsy shows pathognomonic large focal axonal swellings that contain neurofilamentous masses, which reflect a defect of the cellular intermediate filaments. The condition is linked to chromosome 16q24 and mutations in the gene encoding gigaxonin have been identified. Prognosis is poor, most patients become wheelchair bound with death before age 30 years.

References

Bomont P, Cavalier L, Blondeau F, et al. The gene encoding gigaxonin, a new member of the cytoskeletal BTB/kelch repeat family, is mutated in giant axonal neuropathy. Nat Genet. 2000;26:370–374
Tazir M, Nouioua S, Magy L, et al. Phenotypic variability in giant axonal neuropathy. Neuromusc Disord. 2009;19:270–274

Giant cell arteritis (GCA)

Cranial arteritis, Extracranial arteritis, Granulomatous arteritis, Horton's syndrome, Polymyalgia arteritica, Temporal arteritis

Giant cell or temporal arteritis is an inflammatory disorder most commonly affecting the ophthalmic and superficial branches of the external carotid artery, which usually occurs in people over 50 years of age. It most commonly presents with headache and local tenderness of the temporal artery and is often associated with the features of *polymyalgia rheumatica*. Almost invariably there is a markedly raised ESR, but temporal artery biopsy is required for definitive diagnosis. However, treatment should be initiated early, often before the diagnosis is established with certainty, since occlusion of branches of the ophthalmic artery may result in irreversible blindness. Other arteries may be involved. Treatment is with steroids.

Clinical features

- Headache, with local tenderness over the temporal (and less often occipital) arteries, often noted as scalp tenderness on combing the hair. The temporal artery is typically thickened with reduced pulsation and painful to touch.
- Jaw claudication with eating is relatively rare but almost pathognomonic for this condition. Tongue claudication is very rare.
- Painful proximal muscles and joints with stiffness may be a feature, especially first thing in the morning (polymyalgia rheumatica).
- Lassitude, fatigue, preceding weight loss may occur.
- Amaurosis fugax is an ominous sign as it often heralds impending visual failure.
- Sudden non-painful visual loss is rarely the presenting symptom of this disease, representing an arteritic acute ischemic optic neuropathy.
- Other, rare, associations that occur in less than 10% of patients include:
  - Peripheral neuropathy
  - Extraocular muscle involvement
  - Limb (typically arm) claudication
  - TIA/stroke (more common in posterior vascular territories)
  - Confusional state
  - Acute myelopathy

Incidence is 5–15 per 100,000 in population over the age of 50 years; F:M = 3:1, Caucasians affected more often than Asians, Afro-Caribbeans.

Investigation

Bloods: raised ESR, sometimes in excess of 100 mm/h; very rarely the ESR may be normal in biopsy-proven GCA. Anemia, leukocytosis, and thrombocytosis may occur. Neuroimaging is usually normal; not mandatory. Temporal artery biopsy is the diagnostic test, so should be performed as soon as possible, although inflammation persists for several days after the initiation of steroid therapy. A long segment of artery should be taken, given the patchy nature of the inflammation (skip lesions); a negative biopsy could be due to sampling error. Inflammation of the vessel wall, with lymphocytes, neutrophils, and giant cells, is seen, with intimal proliferation causing vessel stenosis and occlusion.

Differential diagnosis

- Metastatic malignant disease
- Viral illnesses
- Systemic vasculitis
- Other causes of *ischemic optic neuropathy*

Treatment and prognosis

If the diagnosis is suspected, treatment with steroids should be started immediately because of the potential risk to vision; biopsy should be arranged as soon as possible thereafter. Typical doses of prednisolone are 80 mg/day for a week, thereafter 60 mg/day for a month or until ESR falls. The steroids should then be slowly tapered by 5–10 mg/day/month, depending on symptoms and the ESR. If the ESR does not fall within a week, the diagnosis needs reevaluating if the biopsy was noncontributory. In cases with visual loss, some clinicians start with intravenous methylprednisolone (1 g/day for 3 days) before commencing high dose oral steroids. As the population suffering from this disease is elderly, prophylaxis for gastrointestinal ulceration and osteoporosis may be required. Once appropriate therapy is commenced the outlook is good, especially from a visual point of view, assuming the steroids are not reduced too quickly. However, neuropathies and large artery involvement can still occur several months after initiation of the steroid therapy.

Diagnostic criteria

Hunder GG, Bloch DA, Michel BA, et al. The American College of Rheumatology 1990 criteria for the classification of giant cell arteritis. Arthritis Rheum. 1990;33:1122–1128
Hayreh SS, Podhajsky PA, Raman R, Zimmerman B. Giant cell arteritis: validity and reliability of various diagnostic criteria. Am J Ophthalmol. 1997;123:285–296

References

Caselli RJ, Hunder GG, Whisnant JP. Neurologic disease in biopsy-proven giant-cell (temporal) arteritis. Neurology. 1988;38:352–359
Salvarani C, Cantini F, Hunder GG. Polymyalgia rheumatica and giant cell arteritis. Lancet. 2008;372:234–245
Weyand CM, Gorozny JJ. Giant-cell arteritis and polymyalgia rheumatica. Ann Intern Med. 2003;139:505–515

Glioma

Gliomas are tumors consisting of abnormal proliferation of glial cells. Within this rubric may be included both low grade gliomas, consisting of astrocytomas, oligodendrogliomas, and ependymomas; and malignant gliomas including malignant astrocytoma and glioblastoma multiforme (GBM, accounting for perhaps half of all gliomas). Deletions from chromosomes 13, 17, and 22 are found in many gliomas, with tumor suppressor genes being located on chromosomes 13 and 22, and p53 on chromosome 17. *Neurofibromatosis* is associated with the development of gliomas (optic chiasm).

Clinical features

- Epileptic seizures, of focal onset with secondary generalization, are the typical presenting feature of low grade glioma, usually in isolation. High grade tumors are usually accompanied by other features.
- Raised intracranial pressure (ICP): classically with a headache that is worse in the recumbent posture (e.g., at night or first thing in the morning), or related to change in posture; +/− nausea and vomiting, especially with posterior fossa tumors. In these cases, the headache is often occipital in location while supratentorial tumors produce more of a frontal headache. Papilledema is usually present; visual obscurations are an ominous sign, suggesting compromised retinal perfusion pressure. False localizing signs consequent on raised ICP may occur, most commonly sixth nerve palsies, although others may occur, for example, VII nerve palsy; hemiparesis ipsilateral to the side of the lesion when the cerebral peduncle is compressed contralaterally by the herniating cerebral hemisphere (*Kernohan's syndrome*).
- Focal neurological deficits: hemiparesis, aphasia, hemisensory deficits.
- Changes in cognitive function may be the presenting feature.
- Occasionally presentation is acute, as a stroke following a bleed into the tumor.
- In the frontal and temporal lobes gliomas may grow to considerable size without producing any significant neurological deficits ("silent areas").

Investigation

Neuroimaging: MR is imaging modality of choice to define tumor anatomy; enhancement with contrast is usually absent or limited, although ring-enhancement may be seen especially in high grade tumors; cystic elements may be seen (e.g., low grade cerebellar glioma). Imaging of other structures (e.g., lung, kidney) may be undertaken to exclude a primary tumor if metastasis rather than primary brain tumor is suspected, or if neurofibromatosis is suspected. Bloods are usually noncontributory, unless there is a concern about metastatic disease or infective causes. Routine hematological and biochemical screen is sufficient in most cases, but in context of *HIV*, the management is different. CSF: LP is usually contraindicated, especially if evidence of raised intracranial pressure. Brain biopsy +/– excision: may be undertaken if a tissue diagnosis is required, but may not always be necessary with low grade lesions.

Differential diagnosis

Other CNS mass lesions:

- Tumor: *meningioma*, metastatic disease, medulloblastoma
- *Abscess*
- *Cysts*, for example, infection (cysticercosis)
- Granulomatous or vasculitic disease (e.g., *neurosarcoidosis*)
- Infarct with luxury perfusion
- Demyelinating disease occasionally presents as a mass lesion (pseudotumoral)

Treatment and prognosis

Best management of low grade glioma remains uncertain: a policy of waiting and watching (serial clinical and neuroradiological assessment) may be appropriate, but some authorities advocate biopsy +/– radiotherapy (astrocytoma) or chemotherapy (oligodendroglioma).

With high grade tumors, early symptomatic improvement may be obtained using dexamethasone (4 mg tds) to reduce local cerebral edema, which alleviates many of the symptoms of raised intracranial pressure as well as some of the focal deficits. Major resection of tumor is generally favored as the initial neurosurgical option (since extent of resection is a prognostic factor), followed by fractionated radiotherapy. Chemotherapy may be indicated in some circumstances, such as oligodendroglioma with 1p19q chromosome loss, and temozolamide in GBM. Prognostic factors in glioma include age (worse in elderly), histologic grade, extent of resection +/– radiotherapy, Karnofsky Performance Scale score (100–0, higher is better). Recurrence/relapse of high grade glioma is almost inevitable and may require further surgery and/or chemotherapy; most people succumb to the glioma after a relatively short period of time.

References

Jenkinson MD, Du Plessis DG, Walker C, Smith TS. Advanced MRI in the management of adult gliomas. Br J Neurosurg. 2007;21:550–561

Kalkanis SN, Rosenblum ML. Malignant gliomas. In: Bernstein M, Berger MS, eds. Neuro-oncology. The Essentials. 2nd ed. New York: Thieme; 2008:254–265

Karnofsky DA, Abelmann WH, Carter LF, et al. The use of nitrogen mustards in the palliative treatment of cancer. Cancer. 1948;1:634–656

Kongkham PN, Bernstein M. Low-grade gliomas. In: Bernstein M, Berger MS, eds. Neuro-oncology. The Essentials. 2nd ed. New York: Thieme; 2008:245–253
Whittle IR. The dilemma of low grade glioma. J Neurol Neurosurg Psychiatry. 2004;75 (Suppl II):ii31–ii36

Gliomatosis cerebri

Gliomatosis cerebri is a rare neoplastic disorder in which malignant cells, usually astrocytoma but sometimes oligodendroglioma, widely infiltrate the brain without forming mass lesions. The condition may be envisaged as part of the spectrum of diffuse astrocytic *glioma*. Clinically, the condition presents with progressive headache, gait disorder, and epileptic seizures (partial with or without secondary generalization), with signs of raised intracranial pressure (papilledema, ophthalmoparesis), hemiparesis, and neurobehavioral changes. Neuropsychological deficits reflecting the affected brain region(s) may occur. Treatment options include chemotherapy and temozolomide. Prognosis is variable, sometimes as poor as glioblastoma multiforme.

References

Herrlinger U, Felsberg J, Küker W, et al. Gliomatosis cerebri: molecular pathology and clinical course. Ann Neurol. 2002;52:390–399
Kim DG, Yang HJ, Park IA, et al. Gliomatosis cerebri: clinical features, treatment, and prognosis. Acta Neurochirurg. 1998;140:755–762

Glomus jugulare tumor

Chemodactoma, Paraganglioma

Tumors of the glomus jugulare, derived from the glomus body in the jugular bulb lying just below the floor of the middle ear, are rare. Tumors are derived from nonchromaffin paraganglioma cells in the adventitia of the jugular bulb. They grow slowly, over 10–20 years, and may invade locally into the middle ear, cranial nerves, brain stem, and temporal lobe, presenting with slowly evolving lower cranial nerve palsies in association with a vascular polyp in the ear and a mass in the neck. Treatment is with radical surgery and radiotherapy.

Clinical features

- Conductive deafness, otalgia +/– pulsatile tinnitus, with a vascular polyp in the external auditory meatus.
- Local cranial nerve palsies: facial (VII), hypoglossal (XII), glossopharyngeal (IX) and vagus (X) nerves, the latter two causing dysphagia and dysarthria.

- Mass in the neck anterior to the mastoid eminence, with a bruit.
- Occasionally brain stem and temporal lobe involvement, with raised intracranial pressure from partial occlusion of the jugular vein.

Investigation

Imaging (CT/MRI) shows a mass originating from the jugular foramen with erosion of the skull base (CT is often imaging modality of choice initially); angiography to define tumor blood supply may be desirable preoperatively. As these lesions are highly vascular, biopsy is contraindicated. Caution should be exercised when considering biopsy of any mass lesion in the ear.

Differential diagnosis

Metastatic disease, tumors originating from bone, meningioma, inflammatory disease such as cholesteatoma, and Wegener's granulomatosis.

Treatment and prognosis

Surgical resection is the most effective treatment, but may be complicated by lower cranial nerve palsies. Bilateral and/or multiple tumors are more challenging and may be treated with radiotherapy.

References

Al-Mefty O, Teixeira A. Complex tumors of the glomus jugulare: criteria, treatment, and outcome. J Neurosurg. 2002;97:1356–1366
Spector GJ, Druck NS, Gado M. Neurologic manifestations of glomus tumors in the head and neck. Arch Neurol. 1976;33:270–274

Glossopharyngeal neuralgia

Reichert syndrome, vagoglossopharyngeal neuralgia

This condition is characterized by severe, unilateral, paroxysmal pain in the throat, radiating to the neck, nasopharynx, and pinna. Pain is usually triggered by swallowing, talking, and coughing and may cause coughing paroxysms, excessive salivation, and occasionally symptomatic bradycardia with *syncope* (deglutition syncope, swallow syncope). Glossopharyngeal neuralgia most often develops in people over the age of 40 years, for reasons that are not clear. Occasionally it is seen with local malignancies in the skull base and oropharynx, as well as after tonsillar infections. Multiple sclerosis is an exceedingly rare cause of glossopharyngeal neuralgia.

Eagles syndrome has a similar presentation, in which an elongated stylohyoid process and/or calcified stylohyoid ligament compresses the glossopharyngeal nerve, symptoms triggered by chewing, swallowing, and rotating the head. Surgical resection of the ligament may be curative.

Treatment of glossopharyngeal neuralgia is as for *trigeminal neuralgia*, with which glossopharyngeal neuralgia shares many features, using drugs such as carbamazepine, phenytoin, and gabapentin, or surgery (microvascular nerve decompression, or section). A pacemaker may be required to prevent syncopal episodes.

References

Jacobson RR, Ross Russell RW. Glossopharyngeal neuralgia with cardiac arrhythmia: a rare but treatable form of syncope. BMJ. 1979;1:379–380
Rushton JG, Stevens JC, Miller RH. Glossopharyngeal (vagoglossopharyngeal) neuralgia: a study of 217 cases. Arch Neurol. 1981;38:201–205

Glutaric acidurias

Glutaric aciduria may be primary, due to disorders of glutaric acid metabolism (glutaric aciduria types I and II), or, more commonly, secondary, for example, to mitochondrial disease affecting the electron transport chain. Although typically a disorder of the neonate or infant, occasional adult presentations with movement disorders occur.

Clinical features

- Type I: GAI, mitochondrial glutaryl-CoA dehydrogenase (GCDH) deficiency [OMIM#231600].
  - Acute onset in infancy of episodic encephalopathy with vomiting and ketoacidosis, often after an infectious episode, with hypotonia, epileptic seizures, movement disorders (choreoathetosis, dystonia, posturing, arching or opisthotonos, grimacing, tongue thrusting, fisting). Recovery from episodes is incomplete with extrapyramidal features persisting. A Reye-like syndrome may also occur without neurological signs. Adult disease may present with headache, leukoencephalopathy, *dystonia* with prominent orofacial movements, and dysarthria.
- Type II: GAII, multiple acyl-CoA dehydrogenase deficiency [OMIM#231680].
  - Heterogeneous presentation: Neonatal disease is severe, with dysmorphism (face, abdominal wall, hypospadias), hypotonia, hepatomegaly, hypoketotic hypoglycemia, metabolic acidosis, hyperammonemia, +/– cardiomyopathy, odor of sweaty feet. It may also occur without dysmorphism, but with the other metabolic features present. Later-onset disease is mild, with acute metabolic acidosis, failure to thrive, hypoglycemia, hyperammonemia.

Investigation

- Type I:
  - Bloods: metabolic acidosis, ketosis, hypoglycemia, hyperammonemia, hepatocellular dysfunction; plasma carnitine levels reduced, excess glutarylcarnitine.
  - Urine: usually contains large amounts of glutaric acid, + 3-hydroxyglutarate and glutaconic acid; raised glutarylcarnitine.
  - Neuroimaging: early cortical atrophy; attenuation of white matter, basal ganglia (especially caudate, putamen).
  - CSF: mild increase in protein.
  - Neurogenetics: mutations in GCDH gene on chromosome 19p13.2.
- Type II:
  - Bloods: metabolic acidosis, ketosis, hypoglycemia, hyperammonemia, hepatocellular dysfunction; elevations of several amino acids in plasma, especially proline and hydroxyproline.
  - Urine: very large amounts of glutarate, ethylmalonate, dicarboxylic acids; mild GAII is also known as ethylmalonic-adipic aciduria in consequence of the predominant urinary findings.
  - Neuroimaging: MR brain shows disorganized cerebral cortex, reflecting a neuronal migration disorder; ultrasound shows cystic disease of the kidneys in severe disease.

Differential diagnosis

Other causes of neonatal encephalopathy, metabolic acidosis. GAI may be mistaken for meningitis or encephalitis because of acute deterioration in context of infective episode with raised CSF protein (also been observed after immunizations). Some cases labeled as "cerebral palsy" may in fact be GAI. GAII may be difficult to distinguish from severe neonatal carnitine palmitoyltransferase II (CPT II) deficiency.

Treatment and prognosis

GAI: Dietary restriction of tryptophan and lysine recommended in GAI, + L-carnitine, riboflavin, baclofen. Symptomatic treatment of metabolic derangements. Prognosis poor for late diagnosis.

References

Bähr O, Mader I, Zschocke J, Dichgans J, Schulz JB. Adult onset glutaric aciduria type I presenting with a leukoencephalopathy. Neurology. 2002;59:1802–1804
Gitiaux C, Roze E, Kinugawa K, et al. Spectrum of movement disorders associated with glutaric aciduria type 1; a study of 16 patients. Mov Disord. 2008;23:2392–2397

Glycogen storage disorders: overview

Glycogenoses

There are a number of glycogen storage disorders, or glycogenoses, with a confusing nomenclature, which often affect muscle, the most common of which are *Pompe's disease* (acid maltase deficiency) and *McArdle's disease*. Here, a list of the glycogen storage disorders with their specific enzyme defects and clinical features is given. Most are autosomal recessive, with the exception of some X-linked forms and possibly some autosomal dominant forms of type V (McArdle's disease). Most show elevated creatine kinase levels when symptomatic, and have a myopathic EMG. Defective enzyme may be assayed in muscle in most cases, and sometimes also in other tissues such as leukocytes and fibroblasts.

- Type I: von Gierke's disease, GSD I
  - Enzyme defect: four subtypes, 1a-1d, result from glucose-6-phosphatase (G6P) deficiency; deficiency of G6P transporter 1 produces a similar phenotype. Genetic linkage to chromosome 1p21 and 11 [OMIM#232220], respectively.
  - Inheritance: autosomal recessive.
  - Clinical phenotype: hepatomegaly, renal enlargement, infantile hypotonia; raised lipids, low glucose, ketoacidosis. Does not affect skeletal muscle.
- Type II: Pompe's disease, acid maltase deficiency, GSD II [OMIM#232300].
  - Enzyme defect: acid α-glucosidase (acid maltase).
  - Inheritance: autosomal recessive.
  - Clinical phenotype: variable. Infantile: Cardiomegaly and heart failure, +/− hepatosplenomegaly, macroglossia, firm muscles. Late infantile/ Juvenile (Smith's disease): proximal muscle weakness, +/− respiratory difficulty, large calves. Adult (Engel's disease): proximal muscle weakness (slowly progressive), respiratory failure.
- Type III: Cori-Forbes disease, GSD III, debranching enzyme deficiency [OMIM#232400].
  - Enzyme defect: glycogen debrancher enzyme deficiency in liver +/− muscle. Genetic linkage to chromosome 1p21.
  - Inheritance: autosomal recessive.
  - Clinical phenotype: infantile presentation may resemble von Gierke's; progressive skeletal myopathy of childhood and adolescence with hypotonia and contractures; creatine kinase sometimes elevated; liver involvement gradually improves; high protein diet may be helpful.
- Type IV: Andersen disease, GSD IV [OMIM#232500].
  - Enzyme defect: branching enzyme. Genetic linkage to chromosome 3.
  - Inheritance: autosomal recessive.
  - Clinical phenotype: infantile or childhood failure to thrive, growth retardation, hypotonia and wasting with contractures, hepatosplenomegaly. More benign forms in later life. One form of polyglucosan body disease is allelic.

- Type V: McArdle's disease, GSD V [OMIM#232600].
  - Enzyme defect: myophosphorylase deficiency. Genetic linkage to chromosome 11.
  - Inheritance: autosomal recessive; some cases may be autosomal dominant.
  - Clinical phenotype: exercise-induced muscle cramps, sometimes leading to marked creatine kinase elevation, rhabdomyolysis, myoglobinuria, and acute renal failure; no organomegaly.
- Type VI: Hers disease, GSD VI; elsewhere labeled GSD VIII.
  - Enzyme defect: hepatic phosphorylase. Genetic linkage to chromosome 14.
  - Inheritance: autosomal recessive.
  - Clinical phenotype: hepatosplenomegaly, growth retardation, hypoglycemia; no myopathy.
- Type VII: phophofructokinase (PFK) deficiency, Tarui disease, GSD VII [OMIM#232800].
  - Enzyme defect: muscle phophofructokinase. Genetic linkage to chromosome 1.
  - Inheritance: autosomal recessive.
  - Clinical phenotype: as for McArdle's disease
- Type VIII: Hug's disease, Ohtani's disease, GSD VIII; elsewhere labeled GSD IXb [OMIM#300559].
  - Enzyme defect: phosphorylase B kinase.
  - Inheritance: autosomal recessive, some X-linked.
  - Clinical phenotype: as for McArdle's disease but no "second wind phenomenon"; + organomegaly.
- Type IX: Bresolin's disease, GSD IX; elsewhere not so labeled.
  - Enzyme defect: phosphoglycerate kinase. Genetic linkage to chromosome Xq13.
  - Inheritance: X-linked recessive.
  - Clinical phenotype: as for McArdle's disease but no "second wind phenomenon"; + organomegaly.
- Type X: Tonin's disease, GSD X [OMIM#261670].
  - Enzyme defect: phosphoglycerate mutase. Genetic linkage to chromosome 7p12–13.
  - Inheritance: autosomal recessive.
  - Clinical phenotype: as for McArdle's disease but no "second wind phenomenon"; adult onset.
- Type XI: Tsujino's disease, lactate dehydrogenase deficiency, GSD XI [OMIM#612933].
  - Enzyme defect: lactate dehydrogenase. Genetic linkage to chromosome 11.
  - Inheritance: autosomal recessive
  - Clinical phenotype: as for McArdle's disease
- Type XII: Kreuder's disease, GSD XII [OMIM# 611881].
  - Enzyme defect: aldolase. Genetic linkage to chromosome 16p11.2.

- Type XIII: GSD XIII [OMIM#612932].
  - Enzyme defect: Enolase 3 deficiency.
- Type XIV; GSD XIV [OMIM#612934].
  - Enzyme defect: phosphoglucomutase I deficiency.

References

Maertens P, Dyken PR. Storage diseases: neuronal ceroid-lipofuscinoses, lipidoses, glycogenoses, and leukodystrophies. In: Goetz CG, ed. Textbook of Clinical Neurology. 2nd ed. Philadelphia, PA: W.B. Saunders; 2003:601–628

Tarui S. Phosphofructokinase deficiency in skeletal muscle: a new type of glycogenosis. Biochem Biophys Res Commun. 1965;19:517–523

Tsujino S, Servidei S, Tonin P, et al. Identification of three novel mutations in non-Ashkenazi Italian patients with muscle phosphofructokinase deficiency. Am J Hum Genet. 1994;54:812–819

Vissing J, Di Donato S, Taroni F. Metabolic myopathies. Defects of carbohydrate and lipid metabolism. In: Karpati G, Hilton-Jones D, Bushby K, Griggs RC, eds. Disorders of Voluntary Muscle. 8th ed. Cambridge: Cambridge University Press; 2010:390–408

Gnathostomiasis

Gnathostomiasis is a food-borne zoonosis caused by the nematode *Gnathostoma sphingerum*. Risk factors for acquisition include consumption of raw or undercooked freshwater fish and geographical exposure. Previously confined to Southeast Asia and Central and South America, cases are now reported from southern Africa. Infection may cause fever, subcutaneous swellings, eosinophilia, subarachnoid hemorrhage, myelitis, and encephalitis.

Reference

Herman JS, Chiodini PL. Gnathostomiasis, another emerging imported disease. Clin Microbiol Rev. 2009;22:484–492

Godot syndrome

The name Godot syndrome, after Samuel Beckett's play *Waiting for Godot*, has been used to describe anxiety regarding upcoming events, seen for example in Alzheimer's disease: this is one of the symptoms evaluated in the BEHAVE-AD global and carer assessment. Such anxiety may confound repeated assessments of cognitive function, for example, in assessing the efficacy of cholinesterase inhibitor treatment.

Reference

Larner AJ, Doran M. Broader assessment needed for treatment decisions in AD. Prog Neurol Psychiatry. 2002; 6(3):5–6

Godtfredsen's syndrome

Godtfredsen's syndrome refers to combined abducens (VI) nerve and hypoglossal (XII) nerve palsies seen in the context of nasopharyngeal carcinoma; trigeminal numbness may also be counted part of the syndrome. The combination may occur with other clival lesions, particularly tumors, although occasionally lesions within the lower brain stem or meninges may produce this clinical picture.

Reference

Keane JR. Combined VIth and XIIth cranial nerve palsies: a clival syndrome. Neurology. 2000;54:1540–1541

Gonyalgia paresthetica

Gonyalgia paresthetica refers to numbness and paresthesia over the patella due to damage, such as *entrapment neuropathy*, to the infrapatellar branch of the saphenous nerve. It usually develops insidiously after trauma to the knee ("housemaid's knee").

Gourmand syndrome

This term has been used to describe an eating disorder characterized by a preoccupation with food and a preference for fine dining. It has been associated with pathology in the right anterior part of the brain, including tumor, vascular damage, epilepsy, and trauma. There are often associated neuropsychological features such as impaired spatial memory, conceptual thinking, and visual perception (hemispatial neglect). Gourmand syndrome may be a disorder of impulse control.

Reference

Regard M, Landis T. "Gourmand syndrome": eating passion associated with right anterior lesions. Neurology. 1997;48:1185–1190

Gradenigo's syndrome

Gradenigo–Lannois syndrome

Gradenigo's syndrome is characterized by facial pain, particularly in the first division of the trigeminal nerve, and diplopia due to a sixth cranial nerve palsy. It is associated with disease at the apex of the petrous temporal bone where the abducens nerve is closely related to the trigeminal nerve. Some authors also accept facial (VII) palsy and deafness (VIII) as components of the syndrome. Causes include inflammation (petrositis, possibly spreading from a local infection such as otitis or mastoiditis), tumors (cholesteatoma, chordoma, meningioma, nasopharyngeal carcinoma, metastatic disease), and skull base fracture.

Reference

Davé AV, Diaz-Marchan PJ, Lee AG. Clinical and magnetic resonance imaging features of Gradenigo syndrome. Am J Ophthalmol. 1997;124:568–570

Grisel syndrome

As originally described by Grisel, this is the name given to nontraumatic atlantoaxial subluxation, leading to *cervical dystonia* (torticollis), associated with inflammatory processes in the neck. Fever and torticollis may also be seen in children with upper respiratory tract infection, pharyngitis, tonsillitis, cervical lymphadenopathy, but one study found that atlantoaxial subluxation was in fact rare in this syndrome.

References

Grisel P. Enucleation de l'atlas et torticollis nasopharyngien. Presse Med. 1930;38:50–53
Meuze WC, Taha ZM, Bashir EM. Fever and acquired torticollis in hospitalized children. J Laryngol Otol. 2002;116:280–284

Guam amyotrophic lateral sclerosis parkinsonism–dementia complex (ALS/PDC)

Lytico-Bodig

A very high incidence of both amyotrophic lateral sclerosis (*motor neurone disease (MND)*) and of *parkinsonism* associated with a severe progressive *dementia*, sometimes occurring together (ALS/PDC), was noted among the

Chamorro people on the Pacific island of Guam in the 1940s and 1950s. Because of the extensive clinical and neuropathological overlap the two conditions are often considered together. Clinically, the MND is like that found elsewhere in the world. However, there is a frequent familial occurrence, common co-occurrence of parkinsonism-dementia complex (PDC), and an association with an unusual linear retinopathy known as Guam retinal pigment epitheliopathy. Similar foci are found on the Kii peninsula of Japan and among the Auyu and Jakai people of southwestern New Guinea. The cause is unknown. It was hypothesized that it related to the ingestion of a putative neurotoxin, β-methylamino-L-alanine (BMAA), found in seeds of the false sago palm, *Cycas circinalis*, which form part of the staple diet. This idea is now questioned, and the role of genetic factors more favored. The PDC is characterized by parkinsonian rigidity, bradykinesia, with or without resting tremor, and a dementia characterized by memory impairment, disorientation, difficulty with calculation; this may be the presenting feature, or occur in isolation. Neuropathologically there is brain atrophy. The morphological hallmark microscopically is the large number of neurofibrillary tangles seen in hippocampus, entorhinal cortex, amygdala, basal forebrain, and neocortex; the immunohistochemical and ultrastructural features are identical to those seen in *Alzheimer's disease*. Neuronal loss in the substantia nigra and locus coeruleus is prominent in cases with parkinsonism. Eosinophilic rodlike bodies (Hirano bodies) may also be seen but amyloid plaques, congophilic angiopathy, and Lewy bodies are not seen.

References

Morris HR, Al-Sarraj S, Schwab C, et al. A clinical and pathological study of motor neurone disease on Guam. Brain. 2001;124:2215–2222
Perl DP, Hof PR. Western Pacific ALS/parkinsonism-dementia complex. In: Beal MF, Lang AE, Ludolph A, eds. Neurodegenerative Diseases. Neurobiology, Pathogenesis and Therapeutics. Cambridge: Cambridge University Press; 2005:827–843

Guillain-Barré syndrome (GBS)

Acute inflammatory demyelinating polyradiculopathy (AIDP), Landry–Guillain–Barré syndrome

First described in 1859 by Landry (and possibly earlier, by Wardrop), but named after the description by Guillain, Barré, and Strohl in 1916, this is a relatively common acute neuropathy, often following an infective illness (e.g., *Campylobacter jejuni* enteritis, *Mycoplasma pneumoniae*, CMV, EBV). A number of variants is described, but most usually this is a monophasic demyelinating poly(radiculo)neuropathy, the pathogenesis of which is thought to be autoimmune attack directed against antigens in myelin, perhaps as a cross-reaction to antigens in infective agents. Anti-GM1 antibodies are found in ~50% of cases, although these may be epiphenomenal. Disruption of normal nerve impulse conduction ensues. Recovery is slow, but often substantial if the patient can be adequately supported during the acute phase, when respiratory and cardiac problems may occur. Immune modulatory therapy (plasma exchange, intravenous immunoglobulin) speeds recovery.

Acute inflammatory demyelinating polyradiculopathies may be classified as follows:

- Acute postinfectious demyelinating polyradiculoneuropathy (classical GBS)
- Acute post-infectious axonal polyradiculoneuropathy (AMSAN, axonal GBS)
- Pure motor GBS (AMAN; Chinese paralytic syndrome)
- Acute sensory ataxic neuropathy (ASAN)
- *Miller Fisher syndrome*: ophthalmoplegia, ataxia, areflexia
- Relapsing inflammatory demyelinating polyradiculoneuropathy: relapsing over weeks and months with increasing disability at each relapse

In subacute demyelinating polyradiculoneuropathy, the patient continues to deteriorate after 4 weeks but less than 8 weeks, so by definition this is not GBS. In *chronic inflammatory demyelinating polyradiculoneuropathy (CIDP)* symptoms progress for longer than 8 weeks.

Clinical features

- Antecedent infective illness: gastrointestinal, respiratory; may not always be a feature of the history.
- Back pain in 30–50% of cases involving the lower back +/− thighs and buttocks, and so the condition can be misdiagnosed as an acute disc prolapse; abdominal pain may also occur, sometimes of sufficient severity to be confused with an acute abdomen and leading to laparotomy/laparoscopy.
- Ascending numbness and weakness, latter often in so-called pyramidal distribution; areflexia.
- Cranial nerve involvement with bulbar and facial weakness in about 50% of cases.
- Ophthalmoplegia: especially in the Miller Fisher syndrome.
- Weakness may involve the respiratory muscles, leading to insidious onset of respiratory failure; hence monitoring of vital capacity is crucial.
- Sphincter abnormalities occur in 10–20% of cases with involvement of the external urethral sphincter.

- Autonomic instability and autonomic failure may occur: labile blood pressure and cardiac arrhythmias (hence need for monitoring), with gastric paresis.
- Progression of sensorimotor dysfunction reaches a plateau in most patients after 2 weeks, and improvement starts within 4 weeks. Progression beyond 8 weeks falls outside the definition of GBS and into CIDP.

Investigation

Bloods: usually unremarkable; look for evidence of infection (*Campylobacter* serology); anti-ganglioside antibodies, probably of more relevance in variants (Miller Fisher: GQ1b; ASAN: GD1b). Neuroimaging is not usually indicated unless one is worried by the degree of back pain when it should be done to exclude other pathologies such as an epidural abscess. CSF characteristically shows a raised protein, which may take a few days to develop, in the absence of cellular reaction (*dissociation albuminocytologique*). CSF leukocytosis sometimes occurs, but if >50 cells/μL, other diagnoses should be considered. Oligoclonal bands identical to those in serum may be found. Neurophysiology: abnormalities on EMG/NCS depend on when the study is done relative to the disease onset. No abnormalities may be seen in studies performed very early in disease course. The typical picture is of evidence of proximal and distal demyelination with absent F waves. Occasionally a purely axonal picture is seen. Nerve biopsy is rarely needed, unless there is clinical suspicion of *vasculitis*.

Differential diagnosis

Other acute *neuropathies*:

- *Neuroborreliosis* (Lyme disease)
- *Porphyria*
- Vasculitic and nonsystemic vasculitic neuropathy (especially SLE)
- *HIV*
- Paraneoplastic neuronopathy
- *Lead* poisoning

May also need to consider:

- *Poliomyelitis*
- *Botulism* (if there is ophthalmoplegia)
- *Rabies* (paralytic or "dumb" variant)
- Brainstem stroke
- Spinal epidural *abscess* or vascular abnormality
- Somatoform disorder/hysteria

Treatment and prognosis

Supportive treatment: best nursed on ITU or HDU. Monitor vital capacity: if <1 L, elective ventilation may be needed. Monitor cardiac rhythm: if heart block, arrhythmia, pacemaker may be required. Specific therapy: plasma exchange and IVIg (0.4 g/kg/day for 5 days) have been shown equally effective in GBS (oral or intravenous steroids are not helpful). IVIg is simplest to give. About 10% of patients have permanent disability as a result of GBS (e.g., require an aid for walking). About 5% of patients die from GBS. The worse prognostic groups are the elderly, those with severe rapid onset GBS requiring early ventilation, and those with axonal loss on nerve conduction studies.

References

Fish M, Llewellyn G. The Guillain-Barré syndrome. Adv Clin Neurosci Rehabil. 2008;8(4):10–12
Pritchard J. What's new in Guillain-Barré syndrome? Pract Neurol. 2006;6:208–217
van Doorn PA, Ruts L, Jacobs BC. Clinical features, pathogenesis, and treatment of Guillain-Barré syndrome. Lancet Neurol. 2008;7:939–950

H

Hematoma: overview

A hematoma is a focal collection of blood, forming a space-occupying lesion. Blood may be arterial or venous in origin, the former tending to have a more acute presentation. Bleeding may occur at various locations within the nervous system, with varying neurological presentations:

- Cerebral hematoma: *Intracerebral hemorrhage (ICH)*.
- Spinal cord hematoma (hematomyelia): rare compared to cerebral hemorrhage; common causes are trauma, *vascular malformations*, anticoagulation.
- Epidural or extradural hematoma: located between dura and bone, these may be cranial or, less often, spinal
  - Cranial: most commonly follows head trauma in parietal or temporal area, causing tearing of blood vessels, most often the middle meningeal artery; less often, there is a dural venous tear. A history of brief unconsciousness associated with the trauma, followed by a lucid period of hours, a day or, with venous bleeding, several days or a week, followed by increasing drowsiness, aphasia, epileptic seizures, and coma, is typical. Skull X-ray may show a temporoparietal fracture; CT will show the hematoma. If the patient is unconscious, or the level of consciousness is deteriorating, urgent surgical decompression is required.
  - Spinal: may produce spinal cord and/or cauda equina compression; sudden onset of neck or back pain is followed by sensorimotor deficit, progressing to paraplegia or quadriplegia. MRI is imaging modality of choice, followed by surgical decompression.
- *Subdural hematoma.*
  - Cranial > spinal

Hemochromatosis

Primary (hereditary) hemochromatosis is an iron overload disorder causing pathological deposition of iron in liver parenchyma and pancreas, with symptoms of hepatocellular dysfunction, diabetes mellitus, and arthralgia.

At least five types have been distinguished on clinical, biochemical, and genetic grounds. Classic hemochromatosis is most often caused by mutation in the HFE gene on chromosome 6p21.3. Juvenile hemochromatosis or HFE2, also autosomal recessive, is caused by mutation in either the hemojuvelin gene (HFE2A, [OMIM#602390]) or the hepcidin antimicrobial peptide gene (HFE2B [OMIM#613313]). Hemochromatosis type 3 is also autosomal recessive and caused by mutations in the transferrin receptor-2 gene [OMIM#604250]. Hemochromatosis type 4 is autosomal dominant and caused by mutation of the SLC40A1 gene encoding ferroportin [OMIM#606069].

Primary neurological problems are rare in hemochromatosis, but peripheral neuropathy, movement disorder (parkinsonism), and dementia have been reported on occasion. Their exact relationship to the biochemical abnormality, if any, remains unclear. It is possible that *aceruloplasminemia* may be misdiagnosed as hemochromatosis (because of the raised ferritin).

References

Adams PC, Barton JC. Haemochromatosis. Lancet. 2007;370: 1855–1860
Russo N, Edwards M, Andrews T, O'Brien M, Bhatia KP. Hereditary haemochromatosis is unlikely to cause movement disorders. A critical review. J Neurol. 2004;251:849–852

Harding's syndrome

Harding's syndrome is the name given to the coexistence of a *multiple sclerosis*-like illness and *Leber's hereditary optic neuropathy (LHON)* associated with Leber's-related mutations of mitochondrial DNA (e.g., 11778, 14484). Clinically, there is visual loss consistent with LHON before the onset of a demyelinating disorder with features typical for MS.

References

Harding AE, Sweeney MG, Miller DH, et al. Occurrence of a multiple sclerosis-like illness in women who have a Leber's hereditary optic neuropathy mitochondrial DNA mutation. Brain. 1992;115:979–989
Parry-Jones AR, Mitchell JD, Gunarwardena WJ, Shaunak S. Leber's hereditary optic neuropathy associated with multiple sclerosis: Harding's syndrome. Pract Neurol. 2008;8:118–121

HARP syndrome [OMIM#607236]

The rare syndrome of *h*ypoprebetalipoproteinemia, *a*canthocytosis, *r*etinitis pigmentosa, and *p*allidal degeneration is called HARP syndrome. Orofacial dystonia is particularly prominent. The original HARP patient was subsequently shown to have a nonsense mutation in the PANK2 gene, hence this disorder may be allelic with *neurodegeneration with brain iron accumulation* (pantothenate kinase-associated neurodegeneration, Hallervorden–Spatz syndrome).

References

Ching KH, Westaway SK, Gitschier J, Higgins JJ, Hayflick SJ. HARP syndrome is allelic with pantothenate kinase-associated neurodegeneration. Neurology. 2002;58:1673–1674
Orrell RW, Amrolia PJ, Heald A, et al. Acanthocytosis, retinitis pigmentosa and pallidal degeneration: a report of three patients, including the second reported case of hypoprebetalipoproteinemia (HARP syndrome). Neurology. 1995;45:487–492

Hashimoto's encephalopathy

A diffuse encephalopathy may occur in association with Hashimoto's thyroiditis with elevated antithyroglobulin antibody titers: patients may be hyper-hypo-, or euthyroid, but the autoantibodies are probably unrelated to the pathogenesis of the encephalopathy. Clinically, there may be a subacute confusional state, stroke-like episodes, focal deficits, epileptic seizures (myoclonic, partial complex, generalized tonic-clonic), and neuropsychological impairment. CSF may show elevated protein. Although uncommon, identification is important since the condition is steroid-sensitive.

References

Brain L, Jellinek EH, Ball K. Hashimoto's disease and encephalopathy. Lancet. 1966;2:512–514
Chong JY, Rowland LP, Utiger RD. Hashimoto encephalopathy: syndrome or myth? Arch Neurol. 2003;60:164–171
Singh B, Nyatsanza S. Hashimoto's encephalitis and young-onset dementia. Prog Neurol Psychiatry. 2010;14(1):11,13–15

Headache: overview

Headache is the most common reason for patient consultation in the general neurology outpatient clinic, accounting for at least 20% of all consultations. The vast majority of such headaches are benign, although most patients have an underlying concern that their headache reflects a brain tumor. Diagnosis is usually possible on the basis of history and examination alone. The precise causes of headache remain uncertain, but are presumably related to fibers of the trigeminal system innervating the dura.

Headaches may be classified using the *International Classification of Headache Disorders* 2nd edition (ICHD2). This divides headaches into primary and secondary categories, under the following major subheadings:

- Primary headaches:
  - *Migraine*
  - Tension-type headache
  - *Cluster headache* and other *trigeminal autonomic cephalalgias*
  - Other primary headaches
- Secondary headaches:
  - Headache attributed to head and/or neck trauma
  - Headache attributed to cranial or cervical vascular disorder
  - Headache attributed to nonvascular intracranial disorder
  - Headache attributed to a substance or its withdrawal
  - Headache attributed to infection
  - Headache attributed to disorder of homeostasis
  - Headache or facial pain attributed to disorder of cranium, neck, eyes, ears, nose, sinuses, teeth, mouth or other facial or cranial structures
  - Headache attributed to psychiatric disorder
- Cranial neuralgias, central and primary facial pain and other headaches:
  - Cranial neuralgias and central causes of facial pain
  - Other headache, cranial neuralgia, central or primary facial pain

Clinical features

- Features most predictive of migraine when compared to tension-type headache are nausea, photophobia, phonophobia, exacerbation by physical activity.
- Tension-type headache: episodic or chronic headache, generally lasting all day for days or weeks (>50% of the time = chronic daily headache), often worse as the day goes on; no postural features. Although sometimes labeled "featureless," these headaches may be described as generalized aching, especially bifrontal, on the vertex, at the back, with superimposed localized stabbing sensations. A pressure type sensation on top of the head and/or a band like compression or vice around the head is common. Headache may have been intermittently present for months or years; short duration of headache symptoms should increase index of suspicion for symptomatic cause.
- History of medication use: searching for evidence of medication overuse headache.
- Enquire for features of raised intracranial pressure: headache worse with recumbency, morning headache, nausea and vomiting, visual obscurations (particularly alarming).
- Although rare, *giant cell arteritis* should always be thought of since it may cause blindness and is treatable; therefore, enquire for jaw claudication, weight loss, and palpate temporal arteries.

Investigation

Diagnosis is essentially clinical, i.e., based on the history (as in psychiatric diseases). Examination is usually normal. Unexpected findings (e.g., papilledema) mandate further investigation. Check ESR if there is a possibility of giant cell arteritis. Many headache patients (and their general practitioners) expect a brain scan (rather than a clinical diagnosis from a practitioner skilled in the art); opinion is divided as to whether one should accede to or resist these expectations. The patient's desire to "put my mind at ease" by having a scan may backfire if incidental abnormalities are found (the moreso if MR is selected in preference to CT): the obligation to inform the patient of these may serve only to increase anxiety and magnify symptoms.

Treatment and prognosis

Patient (and general practitioner) education is important, by means of an explanation of the headache, its nonserious nature, and its amenability to treatment.

Treatment may be effected with simple analgesia, such as aspirin or paracetamol, or with nonsteroidal anti-inflammatory preparations. Long-term, and opiate, analgesia is best avoided because of the risk of inducing medication overuse headache. Amitriptyline given for some months is an option.

Resistant headache may mandate referral to a pain clinic. The role of underlying psychological and psychiatric issues in headache maintenance is debated (generally neurologists think these important, patients do not), likewise how they are best addressed.

References

International Headache Society Classification Subcommittee. The international classification of headache disorders, second edition. Cephalalgia 2004; 24(Suppl 1):1–160

Sandrini G, Friberg L, Jänig W, et al. Neurophysiological tests and neuroimaging procedures in non-acute headache: guidelines and recommendations. Eur J Neurol. 2004;11:217–224

Silberstein SD, Lipton RB, Dodick DW, eds. Wolff's Headache and Other Head Pain. 8th ed. Oxford: Oxford University Press; 2008

Smetana GW. The diagnositc value of historical features in primary headache syndromes: a comprehensive review. Arch Intern Med. 2000;160:2729–2737

Heatstroke

The cardinal features of exertional heatstroke are:

- Loss of consciousness of variable duration (cf. more common condition of heat exhaustion, where there is no loss of consciousness)
- Hyperthermia despite vigorous sweating

Recognized complications include:

- *Rhabdomyolysis*, myoglobinuria, acute renal failure
- Hepatocellular damage, acute hepatic failure
- Abnormal hemostasis (with or without liver injury)

The syndrome is most often seen in the context of unaccustomed exercise in hot climates (e.g., unconditioned military recruits, novice runners, pilgrims to Mecca). There may be an underlying metabolic myopathy akin to that responsible for *malignant hyperthermia*. Treatment involves reduction of body temperature by cooling: fanning and tepid sponging encourage convective and evaporative heat loss; plunging into ice water is not recommended because the cutaneous vasoconstriction will inhibit, rather than promote, heat loss. Pharmacotherapy with dantrolene, which blocks sarcoplasmic reticulum calcium release channels to uncouple muscle excitation and contraction, may be useful. Human recombinant activated protein C may be beneficial by restoring normal hypothalamic and thermoregulatory functions. If mechanical ventilation is required, paralysis with non-depolarizing neuromuscular blocking agents may help control muscle heat generation. Neurological sequelae in the survivors of heatstroke include cerebellar syndromes and spinal cord lesions with motor neurone loss. Peripheral neuropathy following hyperpyrexia has also been described. The take home message is that "neurones are quickly cooked."

Reference

Pease S, Bouadama L, Kermarrec N, et al. Early organ dysfunction, course, cooling time and outcome in classic heatstroke. Intensive Care Med. 2009;35:1454–1458

Heavy metal poisoning: overview

Various metals may have adverse, toxic effects on nervous system structure and function, whether due to inadvertent exposure or therapeutic use. All are rare. These include (in alphabetical order):

- Aluminium: encephalopathy, "dialysis dementia."
- Arsenic: neuropathy, axonal degeneration in chronic poisoning; *Guillain–Barré syndrome*-like (+/– encephalopathy with pericapillary encephalorrhagia, or brain purpura) with acute poisoning; both accompanied by gastrointestinal symptoms.
- Bismuth: myoclonic encephalopathy.
- Gold: acute or subacute sensorimotor neuropathy; myokymia.
- *Lead*: encephalopathy, peripheral neuropathy.
- *Manganese*: parkinsonism.

- Mercury: Inorganic/elemental: mild sensorimotor peripheral neuropathy; may sometimes resemble motor neurone disease; tremor (often circumoral); personality change: timidity, seclusion, secretiveness (erethism, "Mad Hatter syndrome"). Organic (e.g., Minamata disease): paresthesias, sensory ataxia, visual field constriction.
- Thallium: axonal sensory neuropathy, alopecia.
- Tin: organic tin compounds may cause seizures, muscle weakness, and raised intracranial pressure.

References

Mathew L, Vale A, Adcock J. Arsenical peripheral neuropathy. Pract Neurol. 2010;10:34–38

Ratnaike RN. Acute and chronic arsenic toxicity. Postgrad Med J. 2003;79:391–396

Windebank AJ. Heavy metals and neurological disease. In: Evans RW, Baskin DS, Yatsu FM, eds. Prognosis of Neurological Disorders. New York: Oxford University Press; 1992:571–576

Helminthic diseases: overview

Helminths are multicellular metazoan parasites, with complex life cycles involving human and animal hosts at different stages of development. Helminths causing central nervous system disease may be classified as:

- Cestodes (tapeworms): cysticercosis, echinococcosis, sparganosis; diphyllobothriasis (indirectly through vitamin B_{12} deficiency)
- Nematodes (roundworms): strongyloidiasis, trichinosis, onchocerciasis, angiostrongyliasis, gnathostomiasis, ascariasis, dracunculiasis, toxocariasis
- Trematodes (flukes): schistosomiasis, paragonimiasis

References

Awasthi S, Bundy DAP, Savioli L. Helminthic infections. BMJ. 2003;327:431–433

Nishimura K, Hung T. Current views on geographic distribution and modes of infection of neurohelminthic diseases. J Neurol Sci. 1997;145:5–14

Hemifacial spasm (HFS)

Hemifacial spasm is an involuntary, painless, dyskinetic (not dystonic) movement disorder, characterized by contractions of muscles on one side of the face, sometimes triggered by eating or speaking, and exacerbated by fatigue or emotion. This may be regarded as a peripheral form of myoclonus. The movements may result from compression of the facial (VII) nerve, usually at the root entry zone, often by a tortuous anterior or posterior inferior cerebellar artery (hence a *neurovascular compression syndrome*). Other causes include intrapontine lesions (e.g., demyelination), mass lesions (tumor, arteriovenous malformation) located anywhere from the facial nucleus to the stylomastoid foramen, and following a *Bell's palsy*. Most cases remain idiopathic. Posterior fossa lesions contralateral to the hemifacial spasm (i.e., false-localizing) have occasionally been reported.

Clinical features

- Twitching movements around the eye or the angle of the mouth, sometimes described as a pulling sensation. Movements may continue during sleep. Patients often find the movements embarrassing because it attracts the attention of onlookers ("winking").
- Paradoxical elevation of the eyebrow, as orbicularis oris contracts and the eye closes, may be seen; this synkinesis ("Babinski's other sign") is not reproducible by will.

Investigation

Diagnosis is essentially clinical. If movements are not evident when the patient attends clinic, suggest relatives/friends make a home video. Neuroimaging (MR) may be undertaken to exclude symptomatic lesions.

Differential diagnosis

- Oromandibular dystonia.
- Focal epilepsies may give rise to facial twitching.
- Facial myokymia: "creeping flesh."
- Fasciculation of facial muscles as in spinal and bulbar muscular atrophy (Kennedy's syndrome).

Treatment and prognosis

Symptomatic lesions (e.g., tortuous vessel) may be amenable to surgical resection/correction. For idiopathic hemifacial spasm, or patients declining surgery, botulinum toxin injections are the treatment of choice. These need to be repeated about every 3 months, and are generally very effective.

References

Bentivoglio AR, Fasano A, Ialongo T, et al. Outcome predictors, efficacy and safety of Botox and Dysport in the long-term treatment of hemifacial spasm. Eur J Neurol. 2009;16:392–398

Huh R, Han IB, Moon JY, Chang JW, Chung SS. Microvascular decompression for hemifacial spasm: analyses of operative complications in 1582 consecutive patients. Surg Neurol. 2008;69:153–157

Hepatic encephalopathy

Portal-systemic encephalopathy

Liver disease is one of the most common causes of *encephalopathy* seen in hospital practice. Hepatic encephalopathy may occur in the context of:

- Acute liver failure (fulminant hepatocellular failure), for example, in acute viral hepatitis, *Wilson's disease*, or drug-induced hepatocellular necrosis; due to failure of hepatic detoxifying functions.
- Acute decompensation of chronic liver disease (acute-on-chronic, e.g., cirrhosis); due to the production of ammonia and other related compounds. Decompensation to encephalopathy may be precipitated by drugs, gastrointestinal (especially esophageal variceal) bleeding, increased dietary protein, infection, constipation.

Clinical features

- Encephalopathy: suggestive features may be asterixis (can occur in other forms of encephalopathy), hepatic fetor. Stigmata of chronic liver disease may be evident (jaundice, caput medusae, telangiectasia, ascites).

Investigation

Bloods: FBC (for anemia), clotting screen, electrolytes, glucose (need to exclude hypoglycemia), liver-related blood tests, serum ammonia level; serum copper and ceruloplasmin in young individuals with otherwise unexplained acute hepatic failure, + blood film (for hemolysis), to exclude Wilson's disease. Infection screen including blood cultures.

Examine urine and ascites for infection. EEG may show various abnormalities depending on the degree of encephalopathy, including triphasic complexes. Neuroimaging (MRI) may show pallidal abnormality.

Differential diagnosis

Other causes of encephalopathy.

Treatment and prognosis

In acute decompensation, reverse any precipitants; avoid sedative drugs, restrict dietary protein while administering lactulose, vigorously treat any infection; esophageal variceal bleeding may necessitate sclerotherapy. In acute (fulminant) hepatic failure, full supportive care is required. Some cases gradually improve, but in others liver transplantation may be the only hope of survival. Recurrent bouts of hepatic encephalopathy may give rise to *non-Wilsonian hepatocerebral degeneration* with fixed neurological deficits such as dementia, dysarthria, gait ataxia, and extrapyramidal features +/− myelopathy.

Reference

Bajaj JS. Review article: the modern management of hepatic encephalopathy. Aliment Pharmacol Ther. 2010;31:537–547

Hereditary fructose intolerance (HFI) [OMIM#229600]

Several hereditary disorders of fructose metabolism exist, including hereditary fructose intolerance (HFI), hereditary fructosuria, and fructose-1, 6-diphosphatase deficiency.

- Hereditary fructose intolerance (HFI) is due to a defect in the enzymatic activity of fructose bisphosphate aldolase and may present with severe hypoglycemia and epileptic seizures with vomiting, failure to thrive, hepatorenal disease, and aversion to fructose-containing foods (e.g., fruits). It can be diagnosed by measuring the specific enzyme activities and challenging the patient to a fructose load in hospital. However, the intravenous fructose tolerance test is not without hazard, and has now been largely superseded by genetic diagnosis of mutations in the gene encoding aldolase. The presence of non-glucose reducing substances in the urine is a clue to the diagnosis (also seen in galactosemia); there is also *lactic acidosis*.
- Hereditary fructosuria is asymptomatic and due to a defect in the enzyme fructokinase.
- Fructose-1,6-diphosphatase deficiency presents with fasting hypoglycemia, an encephalopathy with epileptic seizures, and a metabolic acidosis. It may be difficult to distinguish from *glycogen storage disease* type I (von Gierke's disease) since hepatomegaly is common to both, but response to glucagon is found only in fructose-1,6-diphosphatase deficiency.

All of these disorders can be treated by avoidance of dietary fructose. When such a diet is followed, no long-term sequelae occur.

Reference

Ali M, Rellos P, Cox TM. Hereditary fructose intolerance. J Med Genet. 1998;35:353–365

Hereditary hemorrhagic telangiectasia (HHT) [OMIM#187300]

Familial telangiectasia, Osler–Weber–Rendu syndrome, Rendu–Osler–Weber syndrome

Hereditary hemorrhagic telangiectasia is an autosomal dominant condition characterized by telangiectasia in the skin, mucous membranes, gastrointestinal tract, genitourinary system, and occasionally the nervous system. The vascular lesions are of various sizes and have a tendency to bleed, gastrointestinal and genitourinary lesions sometimes leading to iron deficiency anemia. HHT type 1 results from mutations in the gene encoding endoglin located on chromosome 9q34.

Neurological complications of HHT include:

* Brain or spinal cord angiomas; may present acutely with hemorrhage, or with insidious focal features from gradual enlargement to repeated small hemorrhages.
* Cerebral *abscess* as a consequence of pulmonary fistulas (prevalence in HHT ca. 25%).

Embolization of angiomas may be possible.

Diagnostic criteria

Shovlin CL, Guttmacher AE, Buscarini E, et al. Diagnostic criteria for hereditary hemorrhagic telangiectasia (Rendu-Osler-Weber syndrome). Am J Med Genet. 2000;91:66–67

Reference

Kjeldsen AD, Oxhoj H, Andersen PE, Green A, Vase P. Prevalence of pulmonary arteriovenous malformations (PAVMs) and occurrence of neurological symptoms in patients with hereditary haemorrhagic telangiectasia (HHT). J Intern Med. 2000;248:255–262

Hereditary motor and sensory neuropathy (HMSN)

The classification of hereditary neuropathies proposed by Dyck and Lambert in 1968 included the category of hereditary motor and sensory neuropathies (HMSN). These were later subdivided according to those with motor nerve conduction velocities below or above 38 m/s into types I and II respectively, also known as *Charcot Marie Tooth disease* types I and II. The clinical classification of HMSN now encompasses seven groups, namely:

* HMSN I (= CMT I)
* HMSN II (= CMT II)
* HMSN III: *Déjerine–Sottas syndrome*

- HMSN IV: *Refsum's disease*
- HMSN V: HMSN + spastic paraparesis
- HMSN VI: HMSN with optic atrophy
- HMSN VII: HMSN with retinitis pigmentosa

Types I and II are the most common.

The HMSN classification has been superseded to some extent by the increasingly detailed molecular genetic definition of hereditary neuropathies, with a preference for the CMT terminology

Clinical features

- Slowly progressive distal muscle weakness and atrophy: small foot muscles, peroneal muscles, hands, forearms.
- Distal, usually symmetrical, sensory deficits; positive sensory symptoms such as paresthesias make the diagnosis unlikely.
- Foot deformities: pes cavus, claw (or hammer) toes.
- Diminished tendon reflexes.
- Family history.
- In HMSN type I and II males are more likely to be symptomatic, and severely affected, whereas females are more often asymptomatic.

Investigation

Neurophysiology (EMG/NCS): nerve conduction velocities may be severely reduced (HMSN I or CMT I, demyelinating neuropathy), or normal or only slightly reduced (HMSN II or CMT II, predominantly axonal neuropathy). Sensory nerve action potentials are severely reduced or not recordable. EMG of distal muscles often shows chronic denervation. Nerve biopsy is variable according to subtype. Neurogenetic testing is increasingly useful in defining these syndromes.

Differential diagnosis

- Distal *spinal muscular atrophy*
- HMSN I: CIDP; *Friedreich's ataxia* if ataxia also present
- HMSN II: idiopathic axonal polyneuropathy

Treatment and prognosis

No specific treatment with the exception of Refsum's disease. Patients seldom become wheelchair bound.

References

Dyck PJ, Lambert EH. Lower motor and primary sensory neuron diseases with peroneal muscular atrophy. I. Neurologic, genetic and electrophysiologic findings in hereditary polyneuropathies. Arch Neurol. 1968;18:603–618

Harding AE, Thomas PK. The clinical features of hereditary motor and sensory neuropathy types I and II. Brain. 1980;103:259–280

Kuhlenbäumer G, Young P, Hünermund G, Ringelstein B, Stögbauer F. Clinical features and molecular genetics of hereditary peripheral neuropathies. J Neurol. 2002;249:1629–1650

Reilly MM. Sorting out the inherited neuropathies. Pract Neurol. 2007;7:93–105

Hereditary motor neuropathy (HMN)

Distal hereditary motor neuropathy

Distal hereditary motor neuropathies comprise a heterogeneous group of disorders, showing some clinical and genetic overlap with *Charcot Marie Tooth disease.*

	Inheritance	Clinical features	Protein/gene/locus
HMNI	dominant	Juvenile onset	Unknown
HMNII	dominant	Adult onset	HSP27, allelic with CMT2F; HSP22, allelic with CMT2L
HMNIII	recessive	Early onset	11q13
HMN IV	recessive	Juvenile onset, diaphragm involved	11q13
HMN V	dominant	Upper limb onset	GARS, allelic with CMT2D; BSCL2, allelic with SPG17
HMN VI	recessive	Spinal muscular atrophy with respiratory distress	IGHMBP2
HMN VII	dominant	Adult onset, vocal cord paralysis	2q14; DCTN1
HMN/ALS4	dominant	Early onset, pyramidal signs	SETX
HMN-J	recessive	Juvenile onset, pyramidal signs	9p21.1-p12

Reference

Reilly MM. Sorting out the inherited neuropathies. Pract Neurol. 2007;7:93–105

Hereditary neuropathy with liability to pressure palsies (HNLPP) [OMIM#162500]

Tomaculous neuropathy

This autosomal dominant condition manifests, usually between the ages of 20 and 40 years, with painless focal peripheral lesions, often following minimal trauma or compression, including *carpal tunnel syndrome*, common peroneal nerve palsy (*peroneal neuropathy*), and *brachial plexopathy*. Symptoms gradually improve over weeks to months. A slowly progressive neuropathy similar to Charcot Marie Tooth disease type 1 may develop. Neurophysiologically, there is slowing of nerve conduction velocity, prolonged distal motor latencies, and conduction blocks. Pathologically, nerves show characteristic swellings or tomacula ("sausages") with signs of demyelination and remyelination. Neurogenetic studies have revealed deletions of chromosome 17p11.2 encompassing the peripheral myelin protein 22 (PMP22 gene; region duplicated in *Charcot Marie Tooth disease* type 1A), and other cases resulting from point mutations of this gene have also been reported, suggesting genetic homogeneity, although the exact pathogenesis is unknown.

Reference

Chance PF. Inherited focal, episodic neuropathies: hereditary neuropathy with liability to pressure palsies and hereditary neuralgic amyotrophy. NeuroMol Med. 2006;8:159–174

Hereditary sensory and autonomic neuropathy (HSAN)

Hereditary sensory and autonomic neuropathies are, as their name implies, characterized by autonomic and sensory disturbance, with less motor involvement than in *Charcot Marie Tooth disease* (*hereditary motor and sensory neuropathy*). Five variants are described in the classification suggested by Dyck:

- HSAN type I: autosomal dominant, onset second decade; distal pain, painless ulcerations, sensory deficit mainly affecting pain and temperature sensation; nerve biopsy shows axonal loss affecting small fibers more severely. Linked to chromosome 9q22.1–22.3. One form is linked to a point mutation in the gene encoding serine-palmitoyltransferase-1 (SPTLC1) [OMIM#162400]. Clinically, it is very similar to CMT2B secondary to RAB7 mutations [OMIM#600882].
- HSAN type II: autosomal recessive, onset in infancy; acroparesthesia, distal injury and Charcot joint formation, pan-sensory loss. Some cases of "congenital insensitivity to pain" may be examples of HSAN type II. May

be caused by mutation in the HSN2 isoform of the WNK1 gene on chromosome 12p13 [OMIM#201300], HSAN2A, or by mutation in the FAM134B gene on chromosome 5p15.1 [OMIM#613115], HSAN2B.

- HSAN type III: familial dysautonomia, *Riley–Day syndrome*; autosomal recessive; most cases associated with mutations in the inhibitor of kappa light polypeptide gene (IKBKAP) gene [OMIM#223900].
- HSAN type IV: "congenital insensitivity to pain and anhidrosis" (CIPA); autosomal recessive; very early onset with unexplained fever, anhidrosis, self-mutilating behavior and mental retardation; nerve biopsy shows almost complete loss of unmyelinated fibers. Caused by mutations in the neurotrophin receptor tyrosine kinase 1 (NTRK1) gene, previously known as trkA, which encodes a receptor for Nerve Growth Factor (NGF) [OMIM#256800].
- HSAN type V: clinically similar to type IV, but less severe; autosomal recessive; small myelinated fibers lost in nerve biopsies, unmyelinated fibers well preserved. Caused by mutations in the nerve growth factor beta (NGFB) gene [OMIM#608654].

References

Kuhlenbäumer G, Young P, Hünermund G, Ringelstein B, Stögbauer F. Clinical features and molecular genetics of hereditary peripheral neuropathies. J Neurol. 2002;249:1629–1650
Reilly MM. Sorting out the inherited neuropathies. Pract Neurol. 2007;7:93–105

Hereditary spastic paraplegia (HSP)

Hereditary spastic paraplegia (HSP) is the name given to a heterogeneous group of inherited motor system disorders, characterized by lower limb spasticity and weakness (spasticity usually more predominant). This may be:

- Pure or uncomplicated: spasticity, weakness, mild diminution of lower limb vibration sensation +/– proprioception. Most cases are autosomal dominant.
- Complicated: HSP +/– epileptic seizures, dementia, amyotrophy, extrapyramidal signs, peripheral neuropathy. Tend to be autosomal recessive.

Most HSP is inherited as an autosomal dominant condition (ca. 70%), but autosomal recessive and X-linked modes of inheritance have been described. Various genetic loci, labeled SPG (for "spastic gait"), have been defined, and mutations in certain genes identified. Some of these conditions are extremely rare, being confined to a few or single families. SPG4A and SPG31 account for around 40% and 8% of pure autosomal dominant HSP.

	Locus	Inheritance	Clinical classification	Protein/gene
SPG1	Xq28	X-linked	Complicated	L1-CAM [OMIM#303350]
SPG2	Xq22	X-linked	Pure and complicated	PLP [OMIM#312920]
SPG3a	14q12-q21	Dominant	Pure and complicated	Atlastin [OMIM#182600]
SPG4	2p22	Dominant	Pure	Spastin [OMIM#182601]
SPG5a	8q21.3	Recessive	Pure	CYP7B1 [OMIM#270500]
SPG6	15q11.2-q12	Dominant	Pure	NIPA1
SPG7	16q24.3	Recessive	Pure and complicated	Paraplegin [OMIM#607259]
SPG8	8q24	Dominant	Pure	KIAA0196, strumpellin
SPG9	10q23.3-q24.2	Dominant	Pure	??
SPG10	12q13	Dominant	Pure and complicated	KIF5A
SPG11	15q21.1	Recessive	Either	Spatacsin [OMIM#604360]
SPG12	19q13	Dominant	Pure	??
SPG13	2q24-q34	Dominant	Pure	Heat shock protein 60, HPSD1
SPG14	3q27-28	Recessive	Complicated	??
SPG15, Kjellin syndrome	14q24.1	Recessive	Complicated	Spastizin [OMIM#270700]
SPG16	Xq11.2	X-linked	Either	??
SPG17, Silver syndrome	11q12-q14	Dominant	Complicated	BSCL2, seipin
SPG18		Dominant		??
SPG19	9q33-q34	Dominant	Pure	??
SPG20, Troyer syndrome	13q12.3	Recessive	Complicated	Spartin [OMIM#275900]
SPG21, Mast syndrome	15q21-q22	Recessive	Complicated	ACP33, maspardin [OMIM#248900]
SPG22, Allan–Herndon–Dudley syndrome	Xq13.2	X-linked		SCL16A2
SPG23	1q24-q32	Recessive	Complicated	??
SPG24	13q14	Recessive	Pure	??
SPG25	6q23-q24.1	Recessive	Pure	??

(continued)

	Locus	Inheritance	Clinical classification	Protein/gene
SPG26	12p11.1-q14	Recessive	Complicated	??
SPG27	10q22.1-q24.1	Recessive	Pure	??
SPG28	14q21.3-q22.3	Recessive	Pure	??
SPG29	1p31-p21	Dominant		??
SPG30	2q37.3	Recessive	Complicated	??
SPG31	2p11.2	Dominant	Pure	REEP1 [OMIM#610250]
SPG32	14q12-q21	Recessive	Complicated	??
SPG35	16q21-q23	Recessive	Complicated	??
SPG36	12q23-q24	Dominant	Complicated	??
SPG37	8p21.1-q13.3	Dominant	Pure	??
SPG38	4p16-p15	Dominant	Complicated	??
SPG39	19p13	Recessive		PNPLA6
SPG41	11p14.1-p11.2	Dominant		??
SPG42	3q25.31	Dominant	Pure	SLC33A1 [OMIM#612539]
SPG44	1q42.13	Recessive	Complicated	Connexin 47, GJC2
SPG45	10q24.3-q25.1	Recessive	Complicated	??

Other hereditary forms of spastic paraparesis with additional neurological features include:

- *Behr's syndrome*
- *Charlevoix-Saguenay syndrome* (ARSACS) [OMIM#270550]
- Sjögren–Larsson disease [OMIM#270200]

Clinical features

- Variable age at onset, usually in early adulthood with stiffness of legs and difficulty walking, with or without backache and lumbar lordosis. Clinically, spasticity is out of proportion to weakness. Arms, sensation, and sphincter function are generally normal.
- In the "complicated" variants, other features may develop, including epileptic seizures, cognitive decline and dementia, amyotrophy, extrapyramidal signs, peripheral neuropathy.
- Asymptomatic family members may have upper motor neurone signs.
- Although the clinical picture of HSP may be uniform, symptom onset and severity may vary between and within families linked to the same genetic locus.

Investigation

Usually unremarkable. Neuroimaging (MR) of spinal cord is often normal but may show slight atrophy. CSF is acellular, with no oligoclonal bands, but may have slightly elevated protein. Neurophysiological investigation may show prolonged central motor conduction times.

Differential diagnosis

Other causes of myelopathy, for example:

- *Multiple sclerosis*
- Cervical myelopathy
- *Motor neurone disease, Primary lateral sclerosis* (PLS)
- *Myelitis*
- Spinal *dural arteriovenous malformation*
- *Chiari malformation*
- *Adrenoleukodystrophy* (adrenomyeloneuropathy)
- *HTLV-1 myelopathy*

Krabbe's disease has been reported to present in this way.

SPG1 is allelic with *MASA syndrome*; SPG2 is allelic with *Pelizaeus–Merzbacher disease* (PMD); SPG17 is allelic with distal hereditary motor neuropathy V.

Treatment and prognosis

Slow progression is typical, but patients generally remain ambulant for many years. Symptomatic treatment of spasticity: baclofen, tizanidine, dantrolene; intrathecal baclofen; physiotherapy. Genetic counseling to family members may be appropriate.

References

Dion PA, Daoud H, Rouleau GA. Genetics of motor neuron disorders: new insights into pathogenic mechanisms. Nat Rev Genet. 2009;10:769–782
Salinas S, Proukakis C, Crosby A, Warner TT. Hereditary spastic paraplegia: clinical features and pathogenetic mechanisms. Lancet Neurol. 2008;7:1127–1138
Warner T. Hereditary spastic paraplegia. Adv Clin Neurosci Rehabil. 2007;6(6):16–17

HERNS

HERNS is *h*ereditary *e*ndotheliopathy with *r*etinopathy, *n*ephropathy and *s*troke, an autosomal dominant condition linked to chromosome 3p21 in which both cerebral and retinal vessels are affected. Clinically there is early progressive visual loss, focal neurological deficits, dementia and headache, along with renal insufficiency and proteinuria. It resembles others cerebroretinal vasculopathies linked to 3p21 but with the additional renal features.

Reference

Jen J, Cohen AH, Yue Q, et al. Hereditary endotheliopathy with retinopathy, nephropathy and stroke (HERNS). Neurology. 1997;49:1322–1330

Heroin

Heroin use may be associated with various neurological sequelae, including:

- Spinal cord syndrome: acute paraplegia: hypotensive, toxic, anterior spinal artery syndrome; chronic myelopathy
- Cerebral *vasculitis*
- Peripheral neuropathy, mononeuropathy, plexopathy
- Epileptic seizures
- *Rhabdomyolysis*

Reference

De Gans J, Stam J, van Wijngaarden GK. Rhabdomyolysis and concomitant neurological lesions after intravenous heroin abuse. J Neurol Neurosurg Psychiatry. 1985;48:1057–1059

Herpes simplex encephalitis (HSE)

The herpes simplex virus (HSV) is the most common cause of *encephalitis*, most usually (90%) due to HSV type 1; HSV-2 affects neonates and the immunocompromised. The recognition of HSE is crucial since early and appropriate treatment has been shown to reduce mortality and morbidity significantly. However, HSE may present in various ways and investigations in the early stages can be normal, thus a high clinical index of suspicion is needed. In case of doubt, antiviral therapy with aciclovir should be started prior to diagnostic confirmation. Viral invasion of the brain (source uncertain, possibly via spread from olfactory pathways or trigeminal ganglia, possibly de novo infection rather than reactivation of latent viral infection) causes characteristic pathological changes: acute necrotizing encephalitis of orbitofrontal and temporal lobes, +/– insular and cingulate cortices, +/– overlying meningitis; may be asymmetric. Uncal herniation may be seen in fatal cases. Microscopically there is neuronophagia, perivascular inflammatory infiltrates, glial nodules, and intranuclear Cowdry type A inclusion bodies. Immunostaining reveals HSV antigen in brain tissue.

Clinical features

HSE may present in various ways, ranging from a dramatic vascular-type onset to a more chronic indolent disease. Typically, however, patients present with:

- Prodrome: fever, headache, malaise, anorexia +/– behavioral changes
- Confusion, clouding of consciousness, coma
- Epileptic seizures: focal, generalized
- Aphasia, mutism
- +/– Meningism, focal motor weakness, brainstem encephalitic picture

The advent of highly sensitive CSF PCR for the diagnosis of HSE has revealed a variety of unusual presentations of HSV infection, including:

- Mild or subacute encephalitis
- Psychiatric presentations
- Brainstem encephalitis
- Benign recurrent meningitis (of Mollaret type)
- Myelitis (HSV2)

Investigation

Bloods usually normal. Neuroimaging: CT scan is often normal. MR imaging is modality of choice, showing focal edema in the medial temporal lobe, orbital surface of the frontal lobe, insular and cingulate cortex, sometimes asymmetrically, with gadolinium enhancement; occasionally MR imaging may be normal. SPECT may show (nonspecific) focal hypoperfusion. CSF may be normal but in most cases is under raised pressure with a lymphocytic pleocytosis (10–200 cells/mm^3) +/– increased red cell count (or xanthochromia) with a raised protein (0.6–6.0 g/L) but a normal glucose level. CSF PCR for HSV is a highly specific and sensitive test for confirming the diagnosis; false negatives may be encountered in early (<48 h) or late (>10 days) disease. Neurophysiology: EEG is invariably abnormal, showing a nonspecific disorganized and slow background rhythm in the early stages; epileptiform abnormalities such as high-voltage periodic lateralizing epileptiform discharges (PLEDs) may appear later. A normal prolonged EEG should raise doubts as to the diagnosis of HSE. Brain biopsy for confirmation of disease was once popular, particularly in the USA and Europe, but is now seldom required following the advent of CSF PCR for HSV and aciclovir therapy; it is reserved for atypical cases or where a tumor in the temporal lobe is considered part of the differential diagnosis.

Differential diagnosis

- Other viral encephalitides, especially CMV (cf. treatment with ganciclovir)
- *Venous sinus thrombosis*
- *Meningitis*
- *Vasculitis*, small vessel vasculopathy or conventional vascular event in temporal lobe
- *Hashimoto's encephalopathy*
- *Wernicke's encephalopathy*
- *Limbic encephalitis*, paraneoplastic or non-paraneoplastic
- Brain tumor, for example, glioma
- Poorly controlled temporal lobe *epilepsy*
- *Subdural empyema*
- *Acute disseminated encephalomyelitis (ADEM)*

Treatment and prognosis

- Aciclovir (10 mg/kg intravenously every 8 h) should be given as soon as the diagnosis is contemplated (i.e., before confirmation) for 10–14 days; relapse rate is lower with 14 days treatment. In immunocompromised patients, 21 days treatment may be given. Monitoring CSF PCR for HSV may assist with decision making concerning the duration of treatment.
- Symptomatic treatment: anticonvulsants if epileptic seizures complicate the clinical course; supportive ITU care may be required, including ventilation.
- Early treatment greatly improves survival and reduces long-term complications.
- Mortality of untreated cases is 70–80%, falling to 20–30% in cases where treatment is given. The outlook is best in patients treated early, the young, and those with GCS > 6 at onset of treatment.
- The major morbidity results from ongoing epilepsy, cognitive deficits (especially anterograde memory deficits, i.e., amnesia) and behavioral problems.
- Recurrence is reported.

References

Bell DJ, Suckling R, Rothburn MM, et al. Management of suspected herpes simplex encephalitis in adults in a UK teaching hospital. Clin Med. 2009;9:231–235
Cinque P, Cleator GM, Weber T, et al. The role of laboratory investigation in the diagnosis and management of patients with suspected herpes simplex encephalitis: a consensus report. J Neurol Neurosurg Psychiatry. 1996;61:339–345
Kennedy PGE, Chaudhuri A. Herpes simplex encephalitis. J Neurol Neurosurg Psychiatry. 2002;73:237–238

Herpes zoster and postherpetic neuralgia

Shingles

Herpes zoster or shingles develops in patients years (usually decades) after primary varicella zoster virus (VZV) infection as chickenpox. Virus lies dormant in neurones of sensory ganglia, prior to reactivation, sometimes in the context of systemic cancer, immunodeficiency, or trauma, although a precipitating cause is not identified in most cases. Around 10% of herpes zoster cases are complicated by postherpetic neuralgia, a persistent pain in the distribution of the previous zoster rash: this may be burning or paroxysmal and lancinating.

Clinical features

- Herpes zoster:
  - Sharp, burning pain in dermatomal distribution, followed by rash: macular, becoming vesicular, in dermatomal distribution. Some cases lack a rash: zoster sine herpete.
  - Usually unilateral, involving a single dermatome.
  - Distribution: trunk > head (typically first division of the trigeminal nerve) > limbs.
  - Recovery over weeks: residual dermatomal hypo- or hyperalgesia.
- Complications: virus may spread to:
  - Eye: herpes zoster ophthalmicus (HZO).
  - Anterior roots, motor nerves: radiculitis.
  - Spinal cord: myelitis.
  - Brain: encephalomyelitis, a delayed vasculopathy.

Involvement of the geniculate ganglion leads to geniculate herpes or *Ramsay Hunt syndrome*. HZO may be followed by contralateral hemiparesis about 2 months after rash, presumed due to a granulomatous angiitis.

- Postherpetic neuralgia: pain for >1 year in distribution of prior herpes zoster; often disabling pain.

Investigation

Clinical history and examination is usually adequate for diagnosis. Complications may necessitate imaging, neurophysiology, CSF analysis to exclude other causes. Looking for an underlying cause for the reactivation of the virus may be necessary.

Differential diagnosis

Herpes zoster per se is unlikely to be mistaken (unless zoster sine herpete). Complications may require consideration of the differential diagnosis of radiculopathy, myelitis, encephalomyelitis.

Treatment and prognosis

- Herpes zoster: simple analgesics: local measures. Aciclovir in immunocompromised patient. Zoster immune globulin of doubtful efficacy. Steroids controversial.
- Postherpetic neuralgia: agents for neuropathic pain: amitriptyline, gabapentin, pregabalin, carbamazepine, fluphenazine, capsaicin cream, TENS; despite which pain may persist.

References

Gnann JW Jr, Whitley RJ. Herpes zoster. N Engl J Med. 2002;347:340–346
Johnson RW, Dworkin RH. Treatment of herpes zoster and postherpetic neuralgia. BMJ. 2003;326:748–750

Heterotopias

Heterotopias are malformations of the cerebral cortex due to disordered neuronal migration during embryogenesis, which may be a cause of *epilepsy*. Heterotopias may be classified as:

- Subependymal or periventricular:
  - Periventricular nodular heterotopia, for example, X-linked periventricular heterotopia is caused by mutation in the gene encoding filamin-A [OMIM#300049].
  - Periventricular laminar/ribbon heterotopias.
- Subcortical heterotopia:
  - Large subcortical heterotopia with abnormal cortex, hypogenetic corpus callosum.
  - Single subcortical heterotopic nodule.
  - Excessive single neurones in white matter.
- Band heterotopia (double cortex syndrome): demarcated layer of neurones in white matter; mostly sporadic but may be associated with mutations in the doublecortin (DCX) gene on Xq22.3-q23 [OMIM#30067] or, less frequently in lissencephaly 1 caused by mutation in the PAFAH1B1 gene on chromosome 17p13.3 [OMIM#607432].

These conditions may manifest with epileptic seizures, +/– mental and developmental delay. They are best identified with MR imaging.

References

Barkovich AJ, Kuzniecky R, Jackson GG, et al. Classification system for malformations of cortical development. Neurology. 2001;57:2168–2178
D'Agostino MD, Bernasconi A, Das S, et al. Subcortical band heterotopia (SBH) in males: clinical imaging and genetic findings in comparison with females. Brain. 2002;125:2507–2522

Histoplasmosis

A fungal infection causing a chronic nonspecific meningitis, seldom identified from the CSF; culture from extraneural sites may be possible.

Reference

Sprofkin BE, Shapiro JL, Lux JJ. Histoplasmosis of the central nervous system: a case report of Histoplasma meningitis. J Neuropathol Exp Neurol. 1955;14:288–296

HIV/AIDS: overview

The HIV retrovirus is neurotropic, rendering the whole neuraxis vulnerable to damage. Furthermore, the immunosuppression consequent upon development of AIDS may be associated with opportunistic CNS infection and the emergence of neoplastic disease. Multiple pathologies may coexist, an important point in management.

Clinical features

- Seroconversion:
  - Encephalitis
  - Aseptic meningitis
  - Myelitis
  - Cauda equina syndrome
  - Guillain–Barré syndrome
  - Myositis

Up to 10% of patients may present with a neurological disorder at sero-conversion.

- Complications of HIV infection:
  - Opportunistic infection:
    - Toxoplasmosis, causing cerebral abscess, encephalitis
    - Cryptococcosis, causing meningitis
    - Progressive multifocal leukoencephalopathy (PML)
    - Cytomegalovirus, causing retinitis, encephalitis, mononeuritis multiplex, cauda equina syndrome
    - Tuberculosis: tuberculous meningitis, tuberculoma

- Tumors: Primary CNS lymphoma
- HIV-related disorders:
  - Dementia
  - Vacuolar myelopathy
  - Distal sensory polyneuropathy
  - Polymyositis
- Nutritional disorders:
  - Vitamin B$_{12}$ deficiency
  - Wernicke–Korsakoff syndrome (WKS)
- Drug-related toxicity:
  - Mitochondrial myopathy (zidovudine)
  - Peripheral neuropathy
- Stroke:
  - Ischemic: embolic, thrombotic
  - Hemorrhagic: thrombocytopenia, vasculitis
- Clinical neurological disorders associated with HIV infection include:
  - Meningitis:
    - Viral: HIV-related, Herpes simplex, Varicella
    - Bacterial: Mycobacteria, Listeria, Streptococcus pneumoniae, syphilis
    - Fungal: cryptococcosis
    - Aseptic
  - Encephalopathy
  - Myelopathy: vacuolar myelopathy
  - Radiculopathy: especially lumbosacral, cauda equina syndrome
  - Neuropathy: sensory, sensorimotor, autonomic; cranial (Bell's palsy); multiple mononeuropathy
  - Myopathy

Investigation

A high index of clinical suspicion may be required to determine that a particular neurological syndrome is related to HIV seroconversion. In established HIV infection, diagnosis may be simpler. Bloods: HIV test after appropriate counseling, if not already done; CD4 count is helpful, since different neurological syndromes occur at different counts: toxoplasmosis, cryptococcosis < 200/mm^3; CMV < 50/mm^3. Neuroimaging: CNS mass lesions may reflect abscess (toxoplasmosis), lymphoma, tuberculosis. CSF often shows a mild pleocytosis in neurologically normal HIV patients; in context, may require PCR for viruses, TB; Indian ink staining, cryptococcal antigen. Neurophysiology (EMG/NCS) for peripheral neuropathies, myopathy/myositis. Biopsy may be indicated for cerebral mass lesion(s).

Differential diagnosis

Extremely broad, i.e., dependent on context, differential diagnosis of meningitis, encephalopathy, dementia, neuropathy, myopathy.

In a HIV + ve patient with any evidence of focal signs, epileptic seizures, headache, or altered mental status, imaging may reveal focal lesions. In this circumstance, the differential diagnosis encompasses toxoplasmosis, primary CNS lymphoma, tuberculoma, PML, or cryptococcoma.

Treatment and prognosis

If multiple cerebral lesions are identified, then it is probably reasonable to give treatment for toxoplasmosis for a period of 2–6 weeks, with clinical and radiological reevaluation; if there is no improvement, then biopsy may be considered, although the alternative pathologies (lymphoma, PML) are unlikely to be treatable. For a single lesion with negative toxoplasma serology, biopsy is indicated.

For HIV infection per se, HAART (highly active antiretroviral therapy), a combination of nucleoside and non-nucleoside reverse transcriptase inhibitors and protease inhibitors that reduces "virus load" (HIV RNA), has been shown to reduce significantly the incidence of opportunistic infections and prolong survival in AIDS-related PML.

References

Gendelman HE, Grant I, Everall IP, Lipton SA, Swindells S. The Neurology of AIDS. 2nd ed. Oxford: Oxford University Press; 2005
Manji H, Miller R. The neurology of HIV infection. J Neurol Neurosurg Psychiatry. 2004;75(Suppl I):i29–i35
Portegies P, Solod L, Cinque P, et al. Guidelines for the diagnosis and management of neurological complications of HIV infection. Eur J Neurol. 2004;11:297–304
Torok ME. Human immunodeficiency virus associated central nervous system infections. Pract Neurol. 2005;5:334–349

Hoffman's syndrome

Thyroid disease may be associated with various neuromuscular features. Hypothyroidism may be accompanied by a proximal myopathy. Hoffmann's syndrome refers to enlargement of affected muscles, which may demonstrate myoedema, local mounding when percussed.

Reference

Klein I, Parker M, Shebert R, Ayyar DR, Levey GS. Hypothyroidism presenting as muscle stiffness and pseudohypertrophy: Hoffmann's syndrome. Am J Med 1981;70: 891–894

Holmes–Adie syndrome

The Holmes–Adie syndrome refers to the association of a Holmes–Adie (tonic) pupil with other neurological features:

- Holmes–Adie, or tonic, pupil: enlarged pupil, usually unilateral (hence causing anisocoria), unresponsive to a phasic light stimulus in a darkened environment, but slowly responsive to a tonic light stimulus. Accommodation reaction is preserved, hence there is light-near pupillary dissociation. The pupil shows denervation supersensitivity, constricting with application of dilute (0.2%) pilocarpine, indicating a peripheral lesion.
- +/– Loss of lower limb tendon reflexes (especially ankle jerks).
- +/– Impaired corneal sensation.
- +/– Chronic cough.
- +/– Localized or generalized anhidrosis, sometimes with hyperhidrosis (*Ross syndrome*).

The syndrome is more common in women.

Reference

Martinelli P. Holmes-Adie syndrome. Lancet. 2000;356:1760–1761

Homocystinuria [OMIM#236200]

Cystathionine β-synthase deficiency

Accumulation of homocystine, a dimer of homocysteine, is associated with dysmorphism. The most common cause is an autosomal recessive inborn error of metabolism resulting from deficiency of cystathionine β-synthase (CBS). Homocystinuric syndromes with abnormalities of folate or vitamin B_{12} metabolism with or without methylmalonic aciduria are also described.

Clinical features

- Learning disability: moderate.
- Psychiatric problems; psychosis rare.
- Lens dislocation (downward; cf. *Marfan's syndrome*: upward); myopia, retinal detachment, secondary glaucoma.
- Osteoporosis, especially spine; thoracic scoliosis.
- Marfanoid habitus, but no true arachnodactyly, and no cardiac abnormalities.

- Cerebral arterial or venous thrombosis (may also have peripheral arterial, venous and coronary thrombosis).
- +/ Epileptic seizures.

Occasionally associated with dystonia, possibly due to vascular damage in the basal ganglia.

Investigation

Blood plasma amino acids show raised methionine; homocystine and mixed disulfides are also present. Fibroblast enzyme analysis shows reduced activity of cystathionine β-synthase. Urine amino acid analysis shows elevated homocystine. Neurogenetic testing shows mutations in cystathionine β-synthase gene, mapping to chromosome 21q22.3: most are missense, many are private; common mutations are I278T associated with pyridoxine responsiveness, and G307S, associated with pyridoxine unresponsiveness.

Differential diagnosis

Marfan's syndrome; other causes of "young stroke."

Treatment and prognosis

Biochemical abnormalities may be normalized with large doses of pyridoxine (250–500 mg/day) in about half of patients; CBS requires pyridoxine as a prosthetic group for catalytic activity. Pyridoxine 500–1,000 mg/day should be given for several weeks before a patient is deemed pyridoxine unresponsive. Methionine-restricted diet supplemented with betaine is recommended. Folate repletion may be necessary. Symptomatic treatment of vascular syndromes may be appropriate. Without treatment, patients die from thromboembolic complications. Outlook is better in pyridoxine-responsive patients.

References

Carson NA, Cusworth DC, Dent CE, Field CM, Neill DW, Westall RG. Homocystinuria: a new inborn error of metabolism associated with mental deficiency. Arch Dis Child. 1963;38:425–436
Kraus JP, Janosik M, Kozich V, et al. Cystathionine β-synthase mutations in homocystinuria. Hum Mutat. 1999;13:362–375
Testai FD, Gorelick PB. Inherited metabolic disorders and stroke part 2: homocystinuria, organic acidurias, and urea cycle disorders. Arch Neurol. 2010;67:148–153

Hopkins' syndrome

Asthmatic amyotrophy

Cases of a *poliomyelitis*-like syndrome with onset following asthma attacks have been described as Hopkins' syndrome. Most have occurred in children, but adult cases are described. There is a flaccid monoparesis, sometimes with sensory and/or pyramidal involvement, with denervation on EMG studies. The picture suggests widespread involvement of the spinal cord. HyperIgEaemia, with allergen-specific IgE, is reported. Enteroviral infection has been suspected as a cause of both the asthma exacerbation and the neurological syndrome. Recovery after IVIg treatment has been reported.

Reference

Horiuchi I, Yamasaki K, Osoegawa M, et al. Acute myelitis after asthma attacks with onset after puberty. J Neurol Neurosurg Psychiatry. 2000;68:665–668

HTLV-1 myelopathy

HTLV-1-associated myelopathy (HAM), Tropical spastic paraparesis (TSP)

Infection with human T-lymphotropic virus type I (HTLV-1) may cause a chronic progressive myelopathy, seen most often in Japan and equatorial Africa and South America, and more often in women. The virus is transmitted via breast milk, sexual intercourse, and exposure to contaminated blood products (e.g., hypodermic needles).

Clinical features

- Symptoms:
  - Leg weakness, backache, painful legs, paresthesias, bladder symptoms
- Signs:
  - Leg spasticity, walking difficulty/inability, urinary frequency, sensory loss

Investigation

Bloods: serology for HTLV-1: ELISA, PCR; blood film may show atypical lymphocytes with convoluted nuclei (flower cells). Neuroimaging: spinal cord MRI is usually normal; brain MRI may show white matter lesions. CSF may show lymphocytic pleocytosis, elevated protein common; glucose normal; oligoclonal bands common; antibodies to HTLV-1 may be found in CSF. Neurophysiology: lower limb SSEPs may show increased latency, due to central pathology.

Differential diagnosis

Other causes of spastic paraparesis, for example, *multiple sclerosis, hereditary spastic paraplegia*, lathyrism.

Treatment and prognosis

No specific treatment currently available; steroids are not helpful. Symptomatic treatment for spasticity along with bladder care. Prevention, by attention to mode of spread, is possible.

Reference

Engstrom JW. HTLV-I infection and the nervous system. In: Aminoff MJ, ed. Neurology and General Medicine. The Neurological Aspects of Medical Disorders. 2nd ed. New York: Churchill Livingstone; 1995:779–790

Huntington's disease (HD) [OMIM#143100]

Huntington's chorea

This autosomal dominant disorder causing a movement disorder and psychiatric and cognitive dysfunction most often results from a defect in the coding region of the gene encoding huntingtin (IT15) on the short arm of chromosome 4, namely an expansion of a CAG trinucleotide, hence a *trinucelotide repeat disease*. Exactly how this genetic change brings about clinical disease is still uncertain, but anticipation with increasing repeat length is seen. Deletion of the huntingtin gene by telomeric rearrangement on chromosome 4p results in the Wolf–Hirschhorn syndrome or chromosome 4p syndrome, the clinical phenotype of which bears no relation to Huntington's disease, hence a strong argument for the trinucleotide (CAG) repeat that underpins HD producing a toxic gain of function rather than a loss of function.

Clinical features

- Personality change: irritability, apathy, depression, schizophrenia-like features.
- Movement disorder: chorea, initially transient, often progresses to continuous athetotic and dystonic movement; patient unable to feed, dress, use

toilet; gait disorder may also be evident. Juvenile cases may present with parkinsonism (Westphal variant) and may show cortical myoclonus.

- Cognitive disorder: subcortical type dementia leading to a global dementia with time.
- Hypothalamic changes may occur early in the disease course with disturbances in sleep and weight loss.
- Family history of movement disorder, dementia, suicide, may be suggestive of diagnosis.

Investigation

Neuroimaging (CT/MRI) may demonstrate caudate atrophy, with dilatation of frontal horns of lateral ventricles (box-like appearance of ventricles); decreased signal may be seen in globus pallidus and putamen on T_2-weighted MR scans; SPECT/PET may show decreased caudate/striatal perfusion and glucose metabolism. EEG is normal early on; low voltage with poorly developed or absent alpha rhythm may be seen in symptomatic cases. Neurogenetic testing for CAG trinucleotide repeat expansion in the IT15 gene is the diagnostic test, but requires pretest counseling about implications. Neuropathology: brain atrophy, particularly marked in striatum and caudate nucleus. Loss of spiny neurones in the basal ganglia. Brain intranuclear aggregates suggest that abnormal protein handling is a feature of the disease, whether pathogenetic or epiphenomenal.

Differential diagnosis

- Huntington disease-like 1 (HDL1): due to eight extra octapeptide repeats in the PRNP gene [OMIM#603218].
- Huntington disease-like 2 (HDL2): due to CAG/CTG repeat in the junctophilin-3 (JPH3) gene [OMIM#606438].
- Huntington disease-like 3 (HDL3): linked to chromosome 4p15.3.
- Huntington disease-like 4 (HDL4): = *spinocerebellar ataxia* type 17 (SCA17) due to trinucleotide repeat encoding glutamine (CAG or CAA) in the TATA box-binding protein (TBP) [OMIM#607136].
- The choreiform disorder is often characteristic, but other causes of chorea may have to be excluded (e.g., *neuroacanthocytosis, dentatorubral-pallido-luysian atrophy (DRPLA)*); ditto young onset parkinsonism.
- Benign hereditary chorea is also autosomal dominant but the absence of dementia means it is unlikely to be mistaken for HD.
- Familial dementias (e.g., familial *Alzheimer's disease*, FTLD) may be considered, but neuropsychological profile is different and movement disorder absent.

Treatment and prognosis

No specific treatment is currently available. The possibility of gene and cell transplantation is being investigated. Symptomatic treatment for the movement disorders may include olanzapine, sulpiride, or tetrabenazine. Cognitive and behavioral deficits are difficult to manage; the latter may mandate the use of olanzapine or antiepileptic medication. Depression may be treated with SSRIs. Genetic counseling is important in affected families. Support may also be obtained from patient organizations. Prognosis from onset to death is around 15–20 years. In some patients there is a risk of suicide, and this is typically seen early on in the disease course. In advancing cases of HD, consideration needs to be given for PEG feeding and advanced directives.

References

Harper PS ed. Huntington's Disease. 2nd ed. London: W.B. Saunders; 1996
Phillips W, Shannon KM, Barker RA. The current clinical management of Huntington's disease. Mov Disord. 2008;23:1491–1504
Quarrell OWJ, Brewer HM, Squitieri F, Barker RA, Nance MA, Landwehrmeyer GB eds. Juvenile Huntington's Disease and Other Trinucleotide Repeat Disorders. Oxford: Oxford University Press; 2009

Hydrocephalus: overview

Hydrocephalus may be defined as an increase in the production and/or circulation, or impaired absorption, of CSF within the skull. This may be caused by:

- Increased CSF production, for example, choroid plexus papilloma
- Obstruction to CSF flow between secretion from the choroid plexuses and absorption in the arachnoid villi in the sagittal sinus, for example, posterior fossa tumor, aqueduct stenosis, Chiari malformations
- Impaired CSF absorption due to inflammation (e.g., meningitis) or *venous sinus thrombosis*

Hydrocephalus may be classified as:

- Obstructive (internal, noncommunicating, tension): obstruction of CSF circulation
- Communicating (external, nonobstructive): disturbed formation or absorption of CSF

Hereditary or familial forms of hydrocephalus are described, most commonly an X-linked type associated with aqueduct stenosis; this may be associated with mutations in the gene encoding the neural cell adhesion molecule L1-CAM (allelic with *hereditary spastic paraplegia* type 1). Autosomal recessive and, rarely, autosomal dominant, forms of hydrocephalus have also been described.

Clinical features

- Infantile: large head, prominent scalp veins, "setting sun" eye sign; increased intracranial pressure slight or absent due to the deformability of the skull; epileptic seizures, spastic lower limbs; may have impaired cognition.
- Post-infantile: may be asymptomatic. Enlarged head. Alternatively, there may be signs of raised intracranial pressure, conspicuous if obstructive hydrocephalus: headache, nausea, vomiting, papilledema; cranial nerve palsies (VI, VII = false-localizing signs) may occur.

Investigation

Diagnosis may be clinically obvious in infancy. Neuroimaging may be required in adulthood: CT/MRI good for showing obstructive dilated ventricles; MRI better for defining any obstructive lesion.

Differential diagnosis

Radiologically it is important to distinguish ventricular enlargement due to *ex vacuo* brain atrophy from communicating hydrocephalus, for example, in patients with cognitive decline where normal pressure hydrocephalus may be suspected. "Pseudohydrocephalus" in Silver–Russell syndrome.

Treatment and prognosis

Of cause where possible. Shunting to relieve pressure may be necessary. Third ventriculostomy may be an alternative in certain circumstances.

References

Esiri MM, Rosenberg GA. Hydrocephalus and dementia. In: Esiri MM, Lee VMY, Trojanowski JQ, eds. The Neuropathology of Dementia. 2nd ed. Cambridge: Cambridge University Press; 2004:442–456

Gjerris F. Hydrocephalus and other disorders of cerebrospinal fluid circulation. In: Bogousslavsky J, Fisher M, eds. Textbook of Neurology. Boston, MA: Butterworth-Heinemann; 1998:655–674

Pople IK. Hydrocephalus and shunts: what the neurologist should know. J Neurol Neurosurg Psychiatry. 2002;73(Suppl I): i17–i22

Hyperekplexia

Hyperekplexia is an involuntary movement disorder in which there is pathological exaggeration of the startle response, usually to sudden unexpected (often auditory) stimuli.

The hyperekplexias may be classified as:

- Primary:
  - Major form: autosomal dominant or recessive disorder with hyperekplexia and hypertonia, manifested as a hesitant and wide-based gait, and hypnagogic myoclonic jerks. Some families demonstrate a mutation in the α_1 subunit of the inhibitory glycine receptor gene GLRA1 [OMIM#149400]. Mutations in the gene encoding the presynaptic glycine transporter-2, SLC6A5, also cause autosomal recessive hyperekplexia [OMIM#604159], and mutation in the gene encoding the beta-subunit of the glycine receptor GLRB has been identified in autosomal recessive hyperexplexia [OMIM#138492]. Further genetic heterogeneity has been confirmed in rare sporadic cases, with mutations affecting other postsynaptic glycinergic proteins including gephyrin GPHN [OMIM#603930] and RhoGEF collybistin causing hyperekplexia with epilepsy [OMIM#300429].
  - Minor form: excessive startle triggered by acute febrile illness in childhood or stress in adult life.
- Secondary/symptomatic:
  - Perinatal ischemic-hypoxic encephalopathy.
  - Brainstem or thalamic lesions.
  - Drugs (e.g., cocaine, amphetamines).
  - Tourette syndrome.

Clonazepam may be helpful in primary hyperekplexias.

References

Harvey RJ, Topf M, Harvey K, Rees MI. The genetics of hyperekplexia: more than startle! Trends Genet. 2008;24:439–447
Wilkins DE, Hallett M, Wess MM. Audiogenic startle reflex of man and its relationship to startle syndromes. A review. Brain. 1986;109:561–573

Hypereosinophilic syndrome (HES)

The following are the suggested diagnostic criteria for this rare syndrome:

- Persistent eosinophilia ($>1,500/mm^3$)
- No evidence of parasitic infection or other recognized cause of eosinophilia
- Signs and symptoms of organ involvement or dysfunction caused by eosinophil infiltration or another mechanism

The latter may include involvement of the nervous system as well as other organs:

- Nervous system: *polymyositis*-like picture ("eosinophilic polymyositis," see *eosinophilic syndromes*); monomyositis; stroke
- Heart: conduction disturbance, congestive failure
- Vascular system: Raynaud's phenomenon; splinter hemorrhages
- Lung: pulmonary infiltrates
- Blood: anemia, hypergammaglobulinemia

The differential diagnosis encompasses necrotizing vasculitides such as *polyarteritis nodosa* and *Churg–Strauss syndrome*, but tissue biopsies provide no evidence to confirm these diagnoses, whereas inflammatory infiltrates with prominent eosinophilic infiltration are found. Despite the unknown etiology, the syndrome often responds dramatically to steroids, although the long-term outlook is not good, dependent on organ involvement.

Reference

Klion A. Hypereosinophilic syndrome: current approach to diagnosis and treatment. Annu Rev Med. 2009;60:293–306

Hyperostosis cranialis interna

An inherited syndrome, probably autosomal dominant, characterized by intracranial hyperostosis and osteosclerosis of the calvaria and skull base (hence a craniotubular hyperostosis) causing *cranial neuropathy* from nerve entrapment, usually recurrent facial nerve palsy, and, less often, impaired smell, taste, vision, and cochleovestibular symptoms. Serum alkaline phosphatase is normal (cf. *Paget's disease*).

Reference

Waterval JJ, Stokroos RJ, Bauer NJ, De Bondt RB, Manni JJ. Phenotypic manifestations and management of hyperostosis cranialis interna, a hereditary bone dysplasia affecting the calvaria and the skull base. Am J Med Genet Part A. 2010; 152A:547–555

Hypertension and the nervous system: overview

Most hypertension remains "essential," i.e., the ultimate causes are unknown. If resistant to treatment, and particularly in young individuals, possible renal (e.g., renal artery stenosis) or endocrine (e.g., Cushing's syndrome, Conn's syndrome, pheochromocytoma) contributors to hypertension may be sought. If inadequately treated, hypertension may have various adverse effects on the nervous system.

Clinical features

- Hypertension per se may be associated with headache, dizziness.
- Hypertension is a modifiable risk factor for both ischemic and hemorrhagic *stroke*; and both *vascular dementia* and *Alzheimer's disease*. There is a log-linear relationship between usual diastolic blood pressure and stroke throughout the normal range.
- Hypertensive encephalopathy: headache, epileptic seizures, focal neurological deficits, papilledema with retinal hemorrhages and exudates, as well as renal and cardiac impairment; occurs in the context of uncontrolled (may be malignant) hypertension. Search for an underlying cause is mandatory and treatment with antihypertensive agents is needed.
- Chronic encephalopathy (*Binswanger's disease*): may develop in patients with hypertension: picture is of a subcortical dementia, may be in association with other motor deficits.
- Risk factor for microangiopathic sixth (abducens) and third (oculomotor) nerve palsies.

Investigation

Bloods: electrolytes (especially for hypokalemia); renal function; may need to assay cortisol. Urine examination for red cells; presence may suggest ongoing end-organ damage (malignant hypertension); collection for creatinine clearance; may need to assay urinary VMA (pheochromocytoma). Neuroimaging (CT/MRI) may show evidence of subcortical infarcts, lacunar state. Renal imaging may show small kidney, underperfused, renal artery stenosis. CXR for heart enlargement; echocardiography may show left ventricular hypertrophy. ECG may show left ventricular hypertrophy, strain pattern.

Treatment and prognosis

Of cause where possible. Symptomatic treatment includes β-blockers, ACE inhibitors, calcium channel antagonists, and diuretics. Prognosis related to how effective blood pressure control is.

Hypertension can occur in some neurological conditions such as raised intracranial pressure, disorders of the autonomic nervous system (e.g., *Guillain–Barré syndrome*), and *neuroleptic malignant syndrome*.

References

Gelmers HJ. The neurology of hypertension, a neurologist view. Clin Neurol Neurosurg. 1982;84:107–112

Mancia G, Laurent S, Agabiti-Rosei E, et al. Reappraisal of European guidelines on hypertension management: a European Society of Hypertension Task Force document. Blood Press. 2009;18:308–347

Hypnic headache

"Alarm clock" headache, Solomon's syndrome

Hypnic headache is a rare primary *headache* syndrome, mostly seen in the elderly and predominating in women, in which pulsating headache wakes the patient at the same time on most nights, with associated nausea. Unlike *cluster headache*, the pain is generalized and there are no autonomic features. The headache lasts about 30 min (range 5–180) and may occur up to three times per night. There are no associated clinical signs. The clinical description differs from "exploding head syndrome" although both occur at night. The headache may respond to lithium carbonate, indomethacin, or caffeine (as in coffee) taken before retiring.

References

Dodick DW, Mosek AC, Campbell JK. The hypnic ("alarm clock") headache syndrome. Cephalalgia. 1998;18:152–156

Evers S, Goadsby PJ. Hypnic headache. Pract Neurol. 2005;5:144–149

Hypobetalipoproteinemia

Familial hypobetalipoproteinemia is an autosomal dominant condition, which in its homozygous state is clinically indistinguishable from *abetalipoproteinemia*. In the heterozygous state, the disease is often asymptomatic. The defect is an abnormal synthetic rate, and hence lower concentration, of betalipoproteins. As a result, there are secondary reductions in the levels of VLDL and LDL and so plasma cholesterol and triglyceride levels are reduced. Malabsorption is uncommon as chylomicrons are formed.

Reference

Vongsuvanh R, Hooper AJ, Coakley JC, et al. Novel mutations in abetalipoproteinaemia and homozygous familial hypobetalipoproteinaemia. J Inherit Metab Dis. 2007;30:990

Hypothalamic disease: overview

The hypothalamus has key roles in neuroendocrine and autonomic function, and also in controlling circadian and seasonal rhythms and sleep–wake cycles. Clinical clues to the involvement of the hypothalamus in disease processes include disorders of temperature regulation, sleep regulation, water balance, caloric balance, reproductive function, emotional behavior, and affect. Disease of the hypothalamic region may be the consequence of various pathological processes:

- Inflammatory, infiltrative: *neurosarcoidosis*; Langerhans cell histiocytosis; multiple sclerosis (rare)
- Neoplastic: hamartoma
- Infection: *Whipple's disease*

Clinical features

- Temperature regulation: hypothermia (*e.g., spontaneous periodic hypothermia*), hyperthermia
- Sleep regulation: hypersomnia (narcolepsy, *Kleine–Levin syndrome*), insomnia (Whipple's disease)
- Epileptic seizures: "diencephalic," gelastic
- Water balance: *diabetes insipidus, syndrome of inappropriate ADH secretion* (sIADH)
- Caloric balance: obesity, hyperphagia (Prader–Willi syndrome; Laurence–Moon syndrome, Bardet–Biedl syndrome; Kleine–Levin syndrome); emaciation (anorexia nervosa; diencephalic [Russell's] syndrome).
- Endocrine function: precocious puberty (hypothalamic hamartoma); gonadal underdevelopment (Prader–Willi syndrome; Froehlich's syndrome), gynecomastia.
- Emotional affect: rage reactions, fear, disinhibition, apathy.
- Abnormal growth: dwarfism, gigantism.

Investigation

Bloods: dependent on context, may need to assay electrolytes (water balance), hormones (disorders of growth, gonadal development, caloric balance). Neuroimaging with MR is the modality of choice for structural change in hypothalamus.

Treatment and prognosis

Of cause where established.

Reference

Brazis PW, Masdeu JC, Biller J. Localization in Clinical Neurology. 4th ed. Philadelphia, PA: Lippincott Williams & Wilkins; 2001:387–402

I

Idiopathic hyperCKemia

This term was coined for persistently elevated serum levels of creatine kinase (CK) in apparently healthy individuals. A number of such individuals will harbor subclinical neuromuscular disease which may be elucidated by muscle biopsy, but some remain entirely normal, thereby meriting the diagnosis of "idiopathic hyperCKemia." Cases with mutations of the caveolin 3 (CAV3) gene have been described, a condition that is allelic with *rippling muscle disease* (*RMD*), *limb-girdle muscular dystrophy* type 1C, and *long QT syndrome* type 9.

References

Alias L, Gallano P, Moreno D, et al. A novel mutation in the caveolin-3 gene causing familial isolated hyperCKaemia. Neuromuscul Disord. 2004;4:321–324

Prelle A, Tancredi L, Sciacco M, et al. Retrospective study of a large population of patients with asymptomatic or minimally symptomatic raised serum creatine kinase levels. J Neurol. 2002;249:305–311

Idiopathic hypersomnia

Essential hypersomnolence

This name has been given to a syndrome characterized by excessive daytime somnolence with episodes of sleep for which no cause, such as *narcolepsy* or *obstructive sleep apnea-hypopnea syndrome* (*OSAHS*), can be found. Two varieties have been delineated, with or without long sleep time. There is no associated cataplexy or sleep paralysis, and although the condition runs in families there is no obvious HLA association (cf. narcolepsy). Confusional arousal ("sleep drunkenness") may be a feature. Reports of preceding Epstein–Barr virus infection, Guillain–Barré syndrome, and HIV infection have appeared. It may be difficult to distinguish from narcolepsy, usually affecting young adults, but sleep studies show no sleep onset REM. The condition is lifelong, and may be very disabling. Besides other sleep disorders, it is important to exclude a hypothalamic lesion and depression in these patients, since these diagnoses open other possible therapeutic approaches.

Reference

Billiard M. Diagnosis of narcolepsy and idiopathic hypersomnia. An update based on the International classification of sleep disorders, 2nd ed. Sleep Medicine Reviews 2007;11:377–388

Idiopathic intracranial hypertension (IIH)

Benign intracranial hypertension (BIH), Meningitis serosa, Pseudotumor cerebri

Idiopathic intracranial hypertension (IIH) was first described by Quincke in 1897 as "meningitis serosa." It is a relatively common neurological condition in which there is raised CSF pressure, usually with papilledema, but normal brain imaging; there is no CNS mass lesion (hence another appellation, "pseudotumor cerebri") or hydrocephalus. Cerebral venous thrombosis, most often of the sagittal sinus, can produce a similar picture. The aetiopathogenesis of IIH is not understood. Some form of obstruction of CSF outflow, either at the arachnoid villi or in the dural venous sinuses is suspected. Risk factors include female sex (F:M = 4–10:1), reproductive age, menstrual irregularity, obesity, recent weight gain, and hypertension. Various other associations have been described, including vitamin A deficiency and toxicity, and drug use including corticosteroids, oral contraceptives, tetracycline, nitrofurantoin, and nalidixic acid. The papilledema consequent on raised CSF pressure may cause loss of vision if untreated (hence "benign" is an inappropriate epithet). There have been no randomized controlled trials of any of the various medical and surgical treatment modalities. Joint follow-up by neurologist and ophthalmologist may be the optimal management.

Clinical features

Modified Dandy's criteria for the diagnosis of IIH are:

- Signs and symptoms of raised intracranial pressure:
  Headache, +/− nausea, vomiting, and visual obscurations; the latter are characteristically described as momentary loss ("greying out") of vision bilaterally, often on standing up or bending over. They are probably due to reduced perfusion of the optic nerve head and so represent an ominous symptom necessitating urgent investigation.
  Papilledema, which is usually bilateral and can be chronic in appearance; very occasionally patients with IIH have no papilledema.

Visual field mapping shows enlargement of the blind spot, often with constricted peripheral fields. The visual acuity may be normal, impairment developing later (hence not a good test to monitor disease).

- No localizing neurological signs, although false-localizing signs, most commonly sixth nerve palsy (unilateral, bilateral, with diplopia), may occur.
- Normal neuroimaging (small ventricles, empty sella allowed).
- Raised CSF pressure (>250 mmH$_2$O) with normal composition.
- Exclusion of primary structural or systemic cause of raised intracranial pressure, e.g., venous sinus thrombosis, hyperviscosity, right heart failure.

Occasionally patients complain of a number of other minor symptoms including neck stiffness, tinnitus, paraesthesia, and joint pains. Rarely, there are other false-localizing signs in IIH (e.g., facial nerve palsy).

Investigation

Bloods are typically normal, although abnormalities in the thrombophilia screen have been described even in the absence of sagittal sinus thrombosis. Neuroimaging is generally normal, although an empty sella may be observed. CT +/– MRV may be done to exclude other causes for the papilledema. MRI may be indicated to exclude a chronic meningitic process in some cases. CSF opening pressure should be measured.

Differential diagnosis

- Space occupying lesion
- Sagittal or lateral sinus thrombosis
- Meningitic process; either chronic inflammatory or malignant
- Hydrocephalus
- Malignant hypertension
- Bilateral optic neuritis
- Obstructive sleep apnea-hypopnea syndrome

Treatment and prognosis

Medical therapy: in patients with headache only, weight loss and diuretics (e.g., acetazolamide 250 mg tds) +/– analgesia are recommended, as is monitoring of visual fields. Surgical therapy: if there are visual symptoms, or progressive visual field loss, then surgical intervention may be undertaken. Options include ventriculoperitoneal shunting, stenting of the venous sinuses, or optic nerve sheath defenestration. Repeated lumbar punctures are also an option, often unpopular, but may have a place in pregnancy when diuretics are contraindicated. None of these treatments has been submitted to a randomized controlled trial. Natural history of IIH is for 25% of cases to remit spontaneously after the first lumbar puncture.

Diagnostic criteria

Friedman DI, Jacobsen DM. Diagnostic criteria for idiopathic intracranial hypertension. Neurology. 2002;59:1492–1495

References

Dhungana S, Sharrack B, Woodroofe N. Idiopathic intracranial hypertension. Acta Neurol Scand. 2010;121:71–82
Larner AJ. Idiopathic intracranial hypertension: towards an integrated care pathway. J Integr Care Pathways. 2007;11:62–65
Lueck C, McIlwaine G. Interventions for idiopathic intracranial hypertension. Cochrane Database Syst Rev. July 20, 2005;(3):CD003434
Pearce JMS. From pseudotumour cerebri to idiopathic intracranial hypertension. Pract Neurol. 2009;9:353–356

Ilioinguinal neuropathy

Lesions of the ilioinguinal nerve, arising from the L1 and sometimes the L2 spinal roots, cause burning and stabbing pain in the inguinal region, which may radiate to the genitalia and the hip. In the recumbent position, the hip is kept slightly flexed and medially rotated. Because of its proximity, there is often concurrent *genitofemoral neuropathy*. The cremasteric reflex may be absent. Surgery is probably the most common cause of ilioinguinal neuropathy. L1 radiculopathy enters the differential diagnosis, as does primary hip joint pathology.

Reference

Kopell HP, Thompson WA, Postel AH. Entrapment neuropathy of the ilioinguinal nerve. N Engl J Med. 1962;266:16–19

Imerslund–Gräsbeck syndrome

Cubulin deficiency, Selective vitamin B_{12} malabsorption with proteinuria

A rare autosomal recessive disorder characterized by:

• Megaloblastic anemia
• Proteinuria
• Neurological features: spasticity, ataxia, brain atrophy

There is *vitamin B_{12} deficiency* due to low absorption, which is not corrected by administration of intrinsic factor. The syndrome responds to parenteral vitamin B_{12} therapy, and is thought to result from a defective uptake of intrinsic factor-vitamin B_{12} complexes in the terminal ileum due to defects in the receptor for these complexes, due to mutations in one of two genes, cubulin (chromosome 10) and amnionless (chromosome 14).

Reference

Gräsbeck R. Imerslund-Gräsbeck syndrome (selective vitamin B(12) malabsorption with proteinuria). Orphanet J Rare Dis. 2006 May 19;1:17

Inclusion body myositis (IBM)

This is perhaps the most common acquired myopathy of middle-aged and elderly patients, especially men (F:M = 1:5), often presenting with isolated quadriceps weakness. Although classified with the inflammatory myopathies, its pathogenesis is uncertain; it is generally resistant to immunosuppressive therapy. The resemblance of muscle histology to certain of the features seen in *Alzheimer's disease* brain prompts the suggestion that this may be a degenerative condition with an inflammatory component.

Clinical features

* Weakness, often of quadriceps; distal weakness also seen (e.g., finger and wrist flexors, ankle dorsiflexors); involvement is often asymmetric. Individual muscles may seem to be "picked out"
* Dysphagia
* +/– Concurrent autoimmune disorder: e.g., *Sjögren's syndrome*

Investigation

Blood creatine kinase may be moderately elevated. EMG is myopathic, with fibrillation potentials, positive sharp waves. Muscle biopsy is the diagnostic test, showing endomysial inflammatory infiltrates, predominantly of T-cell origin, small groups of atrophic fibers, rimmed vacuoles, eosinophilic cytoplasmic inclusions, ragged red fibers, Aβ amyloid within or next to vacuoles; filaments of phosphorylated tau protein in cytoplasm or nuclei on EM.

Differential diagnosis

Other inflammatory myopathies such as *polymyositis* and *dermatomyositis*. The absence of sensory features makes neuropathic conditions (e.g., brachial, lumbar plexopathy) unlikely.

Treatment and prognosis

A trial of prednisolone and methotrexate or azathiporine is recommended, especially if there is another associated autoimmune disorder, even though only a minority of patients respond. Response to mycophenolate is also recorded. IvIg may be helpful if there is dysphagia. An isometric and aerobic exercise program may be prescribed.

References

Amato AA, Barohn RJ. Inclusion body myositis: old and new concepts. J Neurol Neurosurg Psychiatry. 2009;80:1186–1193

Dalakas MC, Karpati G. Inflammatory myopathies. In: Karpati G, Hilton-Jones D, Bushby K, Griggs RC, eds. Disorders of Voluntary Muscle. 8th ed. Cambridge: Cambridge University Press; 2010:427–452

Needham M, Mastaglia FL. Inclusion body myositis: current pathogenetic concepts and diagnostic and therapeutic approaches. Lancet Neurol. 2007;6:620–631

Incontinentia pigmenti (achromians)

Bloch–Sulzberger syndrome, Hypomelanosis of Ito

Incontinentia pigmenti is a *neurocutaneous syndrome*, third only to *neurofibromatosis* and *tuberous sclerosis* in frequency, yet rare; possibly a disorder of neuroblast migration. It may manifest with neurological (in >50%), dermatological, skeletal, and ocular features:

- Cerebral and cerebellar developmental abnormalities: mental retardation, epileptic seizures
- Arteriovenous malformations
- Tumors: medulloblastoma, *choroid plexus papilloma*
- Macrocephaly, autism
- Hypopigmented/depigmented streaks or whorls in the skin, following the lines of Blaschko and not crossing the midline (best seen using Woods light)
- Dental dysplasia, conical teeth, alopecia

Chromosomal abnormalities are common. Symptomatic treatment for seizures is possible.

Reference

Pascual-Castroviejo I, Roche C, Martinez-Bermejo A, et al. Hypomelanosis of Ito. A study of 76 infantile cases. Brain Dev. 1998;20:36–43

Intervertebral disc prolapse

With increasing age, the intervertebral discs become increasingly dehydrated and liable to herniate into the spinal canal and/or intervertebral foramina, especially in the cervical and lumbar regions, with resultant myelopathy and/or radiculopathy. Concurrent spondylotic change is frequent, although seldom the cause of neurological symptoms and signs per se.

Disc prolapse may be (in order of frequency):

- Posterolateral/paracentral: compressing nerve roots in lateral recess of spinal canal
- Lateral/foraminal: nerve root compressed against vertebral pedicle in intervertebral foramen
- Central: unusual because the posterior longitudinal ligament reinforces this area, hence has to be ruptured for disc to prolapse in this direction; may cause cord compression or *cauda equina syndrome*; former may present with sudden urinary incontinence with paucity of other neurological findings

In terms of frequency, roots affected by disc prolapse are lumbar >> cervical >>> thoracic. As compared to the lumbar and cervical spine, thoracic spinal disc protrusion is extremely rare, principally because the thoracic spine is more rigid. However, the small capacity of the thoracic spinal cord makes compression more critical, and operation more difficult. Concurrence of thoracic disc prolapse with *Scheuermann's disease* may be noted.

Clinical features

Prolapse leading to root compression produces a syndrome of:

- Pain: in radicular distribution (e.g., sciatica); knife-like, aggravated by actions that raise intraspinal pressure (coughing, sneezing, straining at stool)
- Sensory impairment/loss: in dermatomal distribution
- Motor features: weakness in the affected myotome, +/− depression or loss of reflex subserved by affected root

Investigation

Imaging: MRI is modality of choice to visualize herniated disc material and bony anatomy; CT-myelography is an option (e.g., patients too large for MR scanner, claustrophobic individuals). Neurophysiology (EMG/NCS): EMG fibrillation potentials in two or more muscles innervated by the same root, preferably via different peripheral nerves, and no abnormalities in muscles innervated by rostral and caudal neighbors of affected root is diagnostic; especially true for C5, C7, C8. However, fibrillation potentials take 2–3 weeks to develop, so are not useful in the acute situation. Sensory nerve action potentials are preserved in radiculopathies (cf. plexopathy, peripheral neuropathy).

Differential diagnosis

Other causes of limb pain, sensory impairment, and weakness: plexopathy, diabetic polyradiculoneuropathy ("diabetic amyotrophy").

Treatment and prognosis

Conservative treatment: rest, analgesia, gentle exercise; cervical collar for cervical radiculopathy. Surgery: indicated if cord compression or cauda equina syndrome (may be urgent especially if presentation is with loss of sphincter function); severe and/or progressive neurological deficit; severe pain continues after 4–6 weeks of conservative treatment. A randomized controlled trial suggested that mild or moderate spondylotic myelopathy with slow progression and long symptom duration did no better with surgery compared to conservative treatment over a 2-year follow-up.

References

Kadanka Z, Bednarik J, Vohanka S, et al. Conservative treatment versus surgery in spondylotic cervical myelopathy: a prospective randomized study. Eur Spine J. 2000;9:538–544
Nikolaidis I, Fouvas IP, Sandercock PA, Statham PF. Surgery for cervical radiculopathy or myelopathy. Cochrane Database Syst Rev. 2010;(1):CD001466

Intracerebral hemorrhage (ICH)

Intracerebral hemorrhage accounts for around 15% of all strokes (cf. 80% ischemic), and is more common in men than women. Mortality remains high, as does morbidity. Search for a potential cause is important because this may determine treatment.

Recognized causes of intracerebral hemorrhage include:

- Head trauma (may be occult).
- Hypertension: common sites are basal ganglia, thalamus, pons, cerebellum, lobar.
- Hemorrhagic transformation of ischemic stroke.
- *Aneurysm*: usually saccular, but consider also infective (infective *endocarditis*), neoplastic causes.

- *Vascular malformations*: *arteriovenous malformations, cavernous angioma.*
- *Moyamoya.*
- Drugs: amphetamines, cocaine, Ecstasy
- Tumor: primary, metastasis.
- *Cerebral amyloid angiopathy*: typically lobar.
- *Vasculitis*: primary; secondary to drugs, infection (herpes zoster, HIV).
- Cerebral venous (sinus) thrombosis.
- Bleeding diathesis: thrombocytopenia, hemophilia, sickle cell disease; therapeutic anticoagulation: risk factors are intensity of anticoagulation, age, hypertension, insulin dependent diabetes mellitus, leukoaraiosis.

Clinical features

Although there are no completely reliable clinical criteria to distinguish cerebral hemorrhage from cerebral ischemia, the possibility of the former should be considered if there is:

- Sudden onset (simplistically: bleed = event; atherothrombosis = process)
- Intense headache
- Accompanying features: nausea, vomiting, prostration
- Disturbed consciousness

Investigation

Neuroimaging: immediate CT is usually adequate to diagnose intracerebral hemorrhage; it may need to be repeated if there is further clinical deterioration (rebleed, hydrocephalus). Additional investigations are aimed at ascertaining cause and/or managing the consequences:

Bloods: FBC, ESR, electrolytes, glucose, clotting studies; urgent INR if receiving warfarin; arterial blood gases if hypoxia or respiratory failure suspected; blood cultures if infective endocarditis suspected
Neuroimaging: MRI, for age of hemorrhage; MRA, catheter angiography: for possible aneurysms, vasculitis
Urine: levels of recreational drugs
Other: echocardiography if infective endocarditis suspected; brain biopsy if vasculitis suspected

Differential diagnosis

Ischemic stroke.

Treatment and prognosis

Acute: ABC of life support; oxygen for hypoxia; correct hyper- or hypoglycemia, thrombocytopenia if profound; reverse excessive therapeutic anticoagulation.

- Monitor vital signs, neurological signs
- Control arterial hypertension: labetalol, nitroprusside, hydralazine, enalapril
- Treat raised intracranial pressure

The place of hemostatic agents such as recombinant activated factor VII remains uncertain.

Surgical evacuation: indications not certain, other than cerebellar hemorrhage compressing the brainstem or obstructing CSF pathways. Ventricular shunting for secondary hydrocephalus.

Cause-specific treatment: coiling/clipping of aneurysms or AVMs; anticoagulation may be favored for cerebral venous thrombosis even in the presence of cerebral hemorrhage.

References

Al-Shahi Salman R. Haemostatic drug therapies for acute spontaneous intracerebral haemorrhage. Cochrane Database Syst Rev. October 7, 2009;(4):CD005951
Al-Shahi Salman R, Labovitz DL, Stapf C. Spontaneous intracerebral haemorrhage. BMJ. 2009;339:284–289
Carhuapoma JR, Mayer SA, Hanley DF eds. Intracerebral Hemorrhage. Cambridge: Cambridge University Press, 2010
Prasad K, Mendelow AD, Gregson B. Surgery for primary supratentorial intracerebral haemorrhage. Cochrane Database Syst Rev. October 8, 2008;(4):CD000200

Intravascular lymphoma

Intravascular lymphomatosis, Neoplastic angioendotheliomatosis

Intravascular lymphoma or angioendotheliomatosis is an unusual condition in which there is a malignant intravascular proliferation of endothelial cells or lymphocytes. It is more accurately defined as an angiotropic intravascular large-cell *lymphoma* of B-cell type. It may affect vessels in almost all organs but most usually involves the skin and central nervous system. A number of neurological presentations are recognized of which the most common is with multifocal ischemic events, due to vascular occlusion by neoplastic cells within small blood vessels, with subsequent disseminated neurological signs and symptoms (simultaneous events in different vascular territories is typical), or dementia. There are often associated systemic features such as fever, raised ESR, and skin lesions, but the diagnosis can only be made by brain and/or meningeal biopsy.

Clinical features

- Neurological deficits:
  - Progressive multifocal infarcts, may lead to *vascular dementia, vascular cognitive impairment*
  - Paraparesis, pain, and incontinence
  - Subacute encephalopathy
  - Cranial and/or peripheral neuropathy
- Systemic abnormalities include fever.
- Skin lesions resembling thromophlebitis or vasculitis

Investigation

Bloods often show raised ESR. Neuroimaging (MRI/CT) brain may show multifocal infarcts of different ages as well as striking meningeal enhancement. CSF may show raised protein. Brain and/or meningeal biopsy is often required for diagnosis.

Differential diagnosis

- *Primary angiitis of the central nervous system* (*PACNS*)
- Cerebral *vasculitis*
- Behçet's disease
- Bacterial *endocarditis*
- Subacute viral encephalitis
- Gliomatosis cerebri
- CNS lymphoma
- Creutzfeldt–Jakob disease
- Paraneoplastic encephalomyelitis

Treatment and prognosis

The condition is usually fatal, possibly because it is diagnosed late. If detected early, treatment with chemotherapy and radiotherapy may be tried. Steroids may give a temporary benefit. Overall prognosis is poor.

References

Lachance DH, Louis DN. Case records of the Massachusetts General Hospital (Case 31–1995). N Engl J Med. 1995;333:992–999
Lozsadi DA, Wieshmann U, Enevoldson TP. Neurological presentation of intravascular lymphoma: report of two cases and discussion of diagnostic challenges. Eur J Neurol. 2005;12:710–714

Ischemic optic neuropathy (ION)

Ischemic optic neuropathy (ION) may be classified as anterior or posterior.

- Anterior ischemic optic neuropathy:
  - Causes subacute monocular visual loss; it may be non-arteritic (ischemic, atheromatous) or arteritic (*giant cell arteritis (GCA)*) in origin. The main difference between the two forms is age at onset, arteritic ION being a disease of the elderly. There is a high risk of involvement of the contralateral eye within 2 years (ca. 40%). Infarction of the laminar or retrolaminar portion of the optic nerve head, supplied by the short posterior ciliary arteries, is thought to be the cause.
- Posterior ischemic optic neuropathy:
  - Less common, due to retrobulbar optic nerve infarction. May be arteritic (related to GCA), non-arteritic, or related to surgery (severe perioperative hypotension?).

Clinical features

- Painless visual loss, either subacute and/or stepwise, but occasionally sudden (more likely with arteritic cause)
- Systemic symptoms (headache, tender scalp, jaw claudication, aching shoulders and hips, weight loss, fever, night sweats) may suggest arteritic cause
- Visual field defect: central scotoma, altitudinal defect, inferior nasal quadrantic field defect; relative afferent pupillary defect may be present
- Fundoscopy: acute optic disc swelling (edema), may be sectoral rather than general, +/– hemorrhage, followed by atrophy; pseudo-Foster Kennedy syndrome may be seen if there is previous involvement of contralateral eye
- Risk factors: of vascular disease; anatomical predisposition: low hypermetropic eyes with small optic discs with low cup–disc ratio ("the disc at risk")

Investigation

Bloods: ESR, CRP to exclude arteritic cause. Consider biopsy of temporal artery to exclude giant cell arteritis.

Differential diagnosis

- *Optic neuritis*: disc hemorrhages less common than in ION
- Optic nerve compression
- *Leber's hereditary optic neuropathy* (*LHON*)

Treatment and prognosis

Arteritic cases: treatment as for giant cell arteritis, namely, prednisolone 80–120 mg/day, usually resolves symptoms. Non-arteritic cases: reduce intraocular pressure to increase optic nerve head perfusion with oral or topical carbonic anhydrase inhibitors; identify and treat vascular risk factors; steroids are also often given although there is no strong evidence of efficacy. There may be no or incomplete improvement in vision. There is a high risk of involvement of the contralateral eye within 2 years; no prophylactic treatment known, other than control of risk factors.

References

Hayreh SS. Posterior ischaemic optic neuropathy: clinical features, pathogenesis, and management. Eye. 2004;18:1188–1206
Kerr NM, Chew SS, Danesh-Meyer HV. Non-arteritic anterior ischaemic optic neuropathy: a review and update. J Clin Neurosci. 2009;16:994–1000

J

Japanese encephalitis

Japanese encephalitis (formerly known as Japanese type B encephalitis) is a typical example of the zoonotic arboviral encephalitides, all of which produce similar symptoms and signs but differ in their animal reservoir, vector of infection, geographical distribution, and seasonal appearance.

Japanese encephalitis is caused by an RNA flavivirus, which has its reservoir in pigs, birds (heron, egrets), cows and buffalo, and is spread by mosquitoes, most commonly *Culex* (typically *C. tritaenorhyncus* and *C. vishnui*) but also *Anopheles*. Humans are a "dead-end" host. It causes disease epidemics in the monsoon months in Asia. Young children and adolescents are most at risk of infection. After the mosquito bite there is a systemic viremia, the neurotropic virus entering the CNS via vascular endothelium, causing a meningoencephalitic illness characterized pathologically by grey and white matter involvement, neuronolysis, T-cell inflammation, and early intrathecal IgM antibody synthesis. There is a significant mortality (20–30%) and morbidity.

Clinical features

- Few infected individuals develop encephalitis. The incubation period is 1–2 weeks.
- Prodromal phase: headache, malaise, fever, anorexia, vomiting; lasts 2–3 days.
- Acute encephalitic phase: altered consciousness, seizures, meningism (variable) +/− focal neurological deficits; cranial nerve palsies, papilledema, both rare; lasts 2–4 days.
- A poliomyelitis-like illness, with flaccid paralysis, has been reported, which may meet the clinical case definition of Guillain–Barré syndrome.
- Early recovery stage/defervescence: lasts 7–10 days.
- Convalescent stage: 1–2 months, or longer.

Investigation

Blood shows a polymorphonuclear leukocytosis with lymphopenia. Rising antibody titers in serum are the diagnostic tests. Virus may be isolated.

Neuroimaging (CT/MRI) is usually normal, but may show thalamic lesions (low sensitivity, high specificity). CSF shows a leukocytosis, initially neutrophilia, then lymphocytosis, with normal glucose, raised protein; virus may be isolated. EEG may show generalized slowing +/– spikes. Pathology (brain biopsy or autopsy): circumvascular necrolysis, microglial infiltration.

Differential diagnosis

- Other viral encephalitides
- Pyogenic, TB meningitis
- Other bacterial and fungal infections
- Cerebral malaria
- Herpes simplex encephalitis
- Poliomyelitis, Guillain–Barré syndrome

Treatment and prognosis

Supportive therapy only. Fatality rate 5–50%. Neurological sequelae in up to a third of patients, especially the very young and old, usually consisting of seizures, cognitive impairment, ataxia, paralysis (poliomyelitis-like picture), and parkinsonism, personality change. Prevention is the best treatment, but difficult because of the complex ecology of the virus: options include eradication of the mosquito vector, and vaccination of at risk individuals or animal reservoirs. All are difficult to achieve, but vaccination of humans now looks promising.

References

Solomon T. Flavivirus encephalitis. N Engl J Med. 2004;351:370–378
Solomon T. Control of Japanese encephalitis – within our grasp? N Engl J Med. 2006;355:869–871

Jeavons syndrome

Eyelid myoclonia with absences

Jeavons syndrome is a reflex idiopathic generalized epilepsy syndrome characterized by the triad of:

- Eyelid myoclonia with or without absences
- Eye closure-induced seizures, EEG paroxysms, or both
- Photosensitivity

Eyelid myoclonia, marked jerking of the eyelids, is the clinical hallmark, with or without brief absence seizures lasting a few seconds. Generalized tonic-clonic seizures may occur; myoclonic jerks are rare. Investigations are normal with the exception of the EEG, which shows brief high amplitude generalized discharges related to eye closure. Concurrent video may show the eyelid myoclonia with or without absences. Eyelid myoclonia may be confused with facial tics, eye closure in other forms of idiopathic generalized epilepsy, and eyelid jerking in typical absence seizures or juvenile myoclonic epilepsy. Treatment with sodium valproate, with or without clonazepam or ethosuximide, is probably most effective. Although distinctive, Jeavons syndrome does not feature in the current ILAE classification of epileptic seizures.

Reference

Duncan JS, Panayiotopoulos CP eds. Eyelid Myoclonia with Absences. London: John Libbey, 1996

Jugular foramen syndrome

Skull base lesions at or around the jugular foramen may involve various combinations of the lower cranial nerves: glossopharyngeal (IX), vagus (X), and accessory (XI).

Clinical features

- Ipsilateral atrophy +/– weakness of sternocleidomastoid and trapezius due to accessory nerve involvement. Atrophy may be the more evident in sternocleidomastoid, hence the importance of palpating the muscle bellies.
- Dysphagia, dysphonia, palatal droop, impaired gag reflex; ipsilateral reduced taste sensation on the posterior third of the tongue, and anesthesia of the posterior third of the tongue, soft palate, pharynx, larynx, and uvula, due to glossopharyngeal and vagus nerve involvement.

Recognized causes of a jugular foramen syndrome include:

- Skull base trauma/fracture
- Glomus jugulare tumor
- Metastases
- Inflammatory/infective collection at the skull base, e.g., sarcoidosis, varicella zoster
- Ischemia

Investigation

Bloods may show markers of infection/inflammation (leukocytosis, raised ESR). Imaging of skull base identifies mass lesions, collections.

Differential diagnosis

This includes a variety of eponymous syndromes involving the lower cranial nerves (IX to XII), with or without involvement of the sympathetic chain. The eponyms are not of particular value, etiology determining optimal treatment. Nonetheless, these include:

- Vernet's syndrome: unilateral IX, X, XI due to trauma (as in Vernet's original case), tumor, inflammation
- Collet–Sicard syndrome: unilateral IX, X, XI, XII; retroparotid space occupying lesions, either intra- or extracranial, or trauma, vascular disease
- Villaret's syndrome: IX, X, XI, XII + sympathetic chain (i.e., Collet–Sicard syndrome + sympathetic palsy) +/– facial nerve (VII); retropharyngeal or retroparotid space occupying lesions
- Lannois–Jouty syndrome: IX, X, XI, XII; skull base lesion
- Mackenzie syndrome: IX, X, XI, XII + Horner's syndrome: retroparotid space tumor
- Jackson's syndrome: X, XI, XII; usually an extramedullary lesion before the nerve roots leave the skull
- Schmidt's syndrome: X, XI; due to an extramedullary lesion affecting the nerve roots before they leave the skull
- Tapia syndrome: X, XII, +/– XI, sympathetic
- Avellis syndrome: brainstem syndrome with X involvement (one of the *brainstem vascular syndromes*)
- *Garcin syndrome*: all cranial nerves on one side

Fractures of the skull base that extend to the jugular foramen with paralysis of IX, X, and XI may go by the name of Siebenmann's syndrome.

The definition of particular eponymous syndromes is perhaps of little importance for management, which will be based on MR imaging findings.

Treatment and prognosis

Of cause where possible, e.g., tumor resection, drainage of collections.

References

Kawabe K, Sekine T, Murata K, et al. A case of Vernet syndrome with varicella zoster virus infection. J Neurol Sci. 2008;270:209–210

Otto M, Otto V, Gotzinger R, Cordes P, Wessel K. Collet-Sicard's syndrome as a result of jugular vein thrombosis. J Neurol. 2001;248:143–144

Vernet M. Syndrome du trou dechire posterieur. Rev Neurol. 1918;2:117–154

Juvenile myoclonic epilepsy (JME)

Janz syndrome

Juvenile myoclonic epilepsy (JME) is a subtype of idiopathic generalized *epilepsy* with onset usually between 8 and 20 years of age. A genetic linkage to chromosome 6 has been suggested, but is disputed.

Clinical features

- Myoclonic jerks, especially in the morning, of variable intensity ranging from simple twitching ("flying saucer syndrome") to falls; consciousness not impaired.
- Generalized tonic-clonic seizures, especially in the morning, after waking.
- Typical absences may also occur, usually prior to myoclonic jerks.
- Myoclonic and tonic-clonic attacks may be precipitated by alcohol and sleep deprivation.
- Normal intelligence.
- First-degree relatives often have a seizure disorder.

Investigation

EEG shows generalized spikes, 4–6 Hz spike and wave, and multiple spike ("polyspike") discharges.

Treatment and prognosis

Sodium valproate is the drug of choice for both seizures and myoclonus. For those not controlled by valproate, options include lamotrigine and levetiracetam. The syndrome generally has been regarded as unremitting, with treatment required lifelong. However, the longest population study (25-year follow-up) found that one third of patients had seizures vanish, such that antiepileptic drug therapy was no longer required. Concurrent depression, social isolation, and unemployment may impair quality of life.

References

Camfield CS, Camfield PR. Juvenile myoclonic epilepsy 25 years after seizure onset: a population-based study. Neurology. 2009;73:1041–1045

Craig JJ, Hunt SJ. Treating women with juvenile myoclonic epilepsy. Pract Neurol. 2009;9:268–277

Renganathan R, Delanty N. Juvenile myoclonic epilepsy: under-appreciated and under-diagnosed. Postgrad Med J. 2003;79:78-80

Schmitz B, Sander T eds. Juvenile Myoclonic Epilepsy: The Janz Syndrome. Petersfield, UK: Wrightson, 2000

K

Kallmann's syndrome

Olfactogenital dysplasia, X-linked hypogonadotrophic hypogonadism

A syndrome of:

- Congenital anosmia: congenital absence or hypoplasia of primary receptor neurones
- Hypogonadotrophic hypogonadism

Clinically, there may also be mirror movements. Brain imaging may show arhinencephaly. This is a clinically and genetically heterogeneous syndrome. Mutations in five genes have been demonstrated to date, but in less than 30% of patients: KAL1 (X-linked recessive form), FGFR1 and FGF8 (autosomal dominant with incomplete penetrance), and PROKR2 and PROK2 (heterozygous, homozygous, and compound heterozygous states).

References

Dode C, Hardelin JP. Kallmann syndrome. Eur J Hum Genet. 2009;17:139–146
Mayston MJ, Harrison LM, Quinton R, Stephens JA, Krams M, Bouloux P-MG. Mirror movements in X-linked Kallmann's syndrome. I. A neurophysiological study. Brain. 1997;120:1199–1216

Kearns–Sayre syndrome (KSS)

Oculocraniosomatic syndrome

Kearns–Sayre syndrome (KSS) is one of the recognized phenotypes of *mitochondrial disease* usually caused by large rearrangements of the mitochondrial genome. Its clinical features overlap in some ways with the *chronic progressive external ophthalmoplegia (CPEO)* phenotype, but onset is earlier.

Clinical features

Features deemed by some authorities to be invariable are:

- Onset before age 15 or 20 years
- Ophthalmoplegia
- Retinal pigmentary degeneration

Other features include:

- Cerebellar dysfunction
- Cardiac conduction deficits (often heart block)
- Raised CSF protein

These six features have been seen as defining criteria by some authors. Other features may also be present:

- Psychomotor regression
- Sensorineural deafness
- Short stature
- Lactic acidosis
- Epileptic seizures
- Cardiomyopathy (may be delayed for years)
- Diabetes mellitus
- Calcification of the basal ganglia

These features suggest overlap with other mitochondrial disorders. The term "ophthalmoplegia plus" has sometimes been used.

Investigation

Blood shows a raised lactate. On neuroimaging, degenerative change may be seen, e.g., cerebellar atrophy; calcification of the basal ganglia. CSF shows raised lactate, protein. EEG may show various abnormalities. ECG should be performed to look for evidence of cardiac conduction disorder. On muscle biopsy, ragged red fibers may be seen on Gomori trichrome stain; cytochrome c oxidase deficiency may be shown. Neurogenetic testing may show deletions within mtDNA in a wide variety of tissues. Ophthalmology consultation may be indicated for fundus photography, ERG. Audiometry may be indicated.

Differential diagnosis

May be confused with *spinocerebellar ataxia* type 7.

Treatment and prognosis

No specific treatment. Supportive treatment only, e.g., pacemaker for heart block, antiepileptic drugs for seizures.

References

Bindoff L, Brown G, Poulton J. Mitochondrial myopathies. In: Emery AEH, ed. Diagnostic Criteria for Neuromuscular Disorders. 2nd ed. London: Royal Society of Medicine Press; 1997:85–90

Maceluch JA, Niedziela M. The clinical diagnosis and molecular genetics of Kearns-Sayre syndrome: a complex mitochondrial encephalomyopathy. Pediatr Endocrinol Rev. 2006 Dec–2007 Jan:4:117–137

Kernohan's syndrome

Crus syndrome, Kernohan-Woltman syndrome, Notch syndrome

Raised intracranial pressure as a result of an expanding supratentorial lesion (e.g., tumor, subdural hematoma) may cause herniation of brain tissue through the tentorium into the subtentorial space, putting pressure on the midbrain. If the midbrain is shifted against the contralateral margin (free edge) of the tentorium, the cerebral peduncle on that side may be compressed, resulting in a hemiparesis which is ipsilateral to the supratentorial lesion (and hence may be considered a "false-localizing" sign).

There may also be an oculomotor nerve palsy ipsilateral to the lesion, which may be partial (unilateral pupil dilatation); parkinsonism has also been described.

References

Kernohan JW, Woltman HW. Incisura of the crus due to contralateral brain tumor. Arch Neurol Psychiatry. 1929;21:274–287

Mastronardi L, Puzzilli F, Ruggeri A, Guiducci A. Magnetic resonance imaging findings of Kernohan-Woltman notch in acute subdural hematoma. Clin Neurol Neurosurg. 1999;101:122–124

Kjellin's syndrome

Kjellin's syndrome comprises:

- Spastic paraparesis.
- Cerebellar dysarthria + upper limb ataxia.
- Pigmentary macular degeneration, not usually giving rise to visual loss. The fundal appearances may resemble those of Stargardt disease.
- +/– Distal wasting.
- +/– Dementia.

If ophthalmoplegia is also present, the name Barnard-Scholz syndrome may be given, although the cases reported by the latter authors lacked spastic paraparesis. Imaging may show a thin corpus callosum. This condition is one of the complicated *hereditary spastic paraparesis (HSP)* syndromes. Inheritance is autosomal recessive, and it has been associated with the mutations found in SPG11 and SPG15.

Kleine–Levin syndrome

Kleine–Levin–Critchley syndrome, periodic hypersomnia, and megaphagia, "Rip van Winkle disease"

This rare sleep disorder occurs typically in adolescence, more often in males, and is characterized by episodes of hypersomnolence and bulimia lasting days (usually 4–7) to weeks, in which the patient may sleep 16–18 h/day and eat voraciously on awakening. Cycles occur every few months. Other behavioral features include irritability (90%), depression (50%), hypersexuality (40%, more common in males), altered mood, hallucinations, and memory impairment. Cases following head injury have been reported. Structural brain imaging (CT/MRI) is normal, but functional neuroimaging (SPECT) may show hypoperfusion of thalamus, basal ganglia, and frontotemporal regions during attacks. EEG may show nonspecific slow wave background. The multiple sleep latency test shows pathological sleepiness, but unlike narcolepsy, there is no REM sleep at sleep onset. Treatment may be tried with mood stabilizers (lithium, sodium valproate) or stimulants (methylphenidate, modafinil), but there are no controlled trials. The condition seems to remit in adulthood.

References

Arnulf I, Zeitzer JM, File J, et al. Kleine-Levin syndrome: a systematic review of 186 cases in the literature. Brain. 2005;128:2763–2776
Critchley M. The Divine Banquet of the Brain and Other Essays. New York: Raven; 1979:167–171
Lisk DR. Kleine-Levin syndrome. Pract Neurol. 2009;9:42–45

Klippel–Feil anomaly

The Klippel–Feil anomaly consists of abnormality of the cervical vertebrae which may be malformed or fused (congenital synostosis), creating a short neck with limited movement, sometimes with compromise of the cervical spinal cord or roots. Mirror movements may be seen. This may occur in isolation or be associated with other developmental anomalies such as Mullerian duct aplasia (absent vagina and uterus), renal aplasia, other bony defects (cervicothoracic somite dysplasia), deafness, and gastrointestinal defects. One form is linked to chromosome 5q11.2.

Reference

Thomsen MN, Schneider U, Weber M, Johannisson R, Neithard FU. Scoliosis and congenital anomalies associated with Klippel-Feil syndromes types I-III. Spine. 1997;22:396–401

Klippel–Trénaunay–Weber syndrome

In this syndrome, a vascular malformation of the spinal cord is associated with a cutaneous vascular nevus, which may be associated with hypertrophy of connective tissues and bone (hemangiectatic hypertrophy) affecting fingers or a whole limb, and underdevelopment of other parts. Additional features may include ocular abnormalities, visceromegaly, mental retardation, and seizures. *Cobb syndrome* enters the differential diagnosis.

Klumpke's palsy

Déjerine-Klumpke palsy or paralysis, inferior plexus paralysis

Klumpke's palsy or paralyis describes a form of *brachial plexopathy*, a lower brachial plexus lesion involving fibers from the C8/T1 roots as a consequence of which there is weakness of the small hand muscles and flexors of the hand, causing a claw hand. There may additionally be a Horner's syndrome, and trophic changes in the hand and fingers. Causes of Klumpke's paralysis include trauma (road traffic accident, obstetric trauma, post-sternotomy for cardiac surgery, electrical injury), pressure from a cervical rib, and *Pancoast syndrome* (pulmonary sulcus tumor).

Klüver–Bucy syndrome

The Klüver–Bucy syndrome is a neurobehavioral syndrome observed following bilateral temporal lobectomy, initially described in monkeys and subsequently in man. The characteristic features, not all of which may be present, are:

- Visual agnosia (e.g., misrecognition of others); also known as psychic blindness
- Hyperorality

- Hyperphagia, binge eating
- Hypermetamorphosis
- Hypersexuality
- Emotional changes: apathy; loss of fear, rage reactions

Recognized causes of Klüver–Bucy syndrome include:

- Bilateral temporal lobectomy
- Post-ictal: in the context of previous unilateral temporal lobectomy
- Rare complication of herpes simplex encephalitis
- *Frontotemporal lobar degeneration* (Pick's disease)
- *Alzheimer's disease*: especially hyperorality and hyperphagia, but it is rare to have all the features

References

Kile SJ, Ellis WG, Olichney JM, Farias S, DeCarli C. Alzheimer abnormalities of the amygdala with Klüver-Bucy syndrome symptoms: an amygdaloid variant of Alzheimer disease. Arch Neurol 2009;66:125–129

Klüver H, Bucy P. Preliminary analysis of functions of the temporal lobes in monkeys. Arch Neurol Psychiatry. 1939;42:979–1000.

Konzo

Mantakassa

Konzo is a syndrome of symmetrical spastic paraparesis occurring in epidemics in Central Africa. It is believed to be a consequence of poisoning with cyanide (an inhibitor of the mitochondrial enzyme cytochrome oxidase) through the consumption of insufficiently processed roots of cassava (*Manihot esculenta*), a food staple in rural communities. Concurrent low sulfur intake may also be important in pathogenesis, since this may contribute to impaired detoxification of cyanide. Symptoms may develop very acutely, sometimes in less than 1 h, always within 1 week. There is a spastic gait, hyperreflexia, clonus, flexion contractures of the legs, disturbances of vision and eye movements, spastic dysarthria, and bulbar symptoms. No specific or symptomatic therapy has been reported. After some initial improvement, disability remains unchanged over many years. Second episodes have been reported.

References

Rosling H, Tylleskar T. Konzo. In: Shakir RA, Newman PK, Poser CM, eds. Tropical Neurology. London: W.B. Saunders; 1996:353–364

Krabbe's disease [OMIM#245200]

Galactosylceramide lipidosis, globoid cell leukodystrophy

Krabbe's disease is an autosomal recessive *leukodystrophy* in which there is a deficiency of the lysosomal enzyme galactocerebroside β-galactosidase (GALC), resulting from mutations in the GALC gene at chromosome 14q24.3-q32.1. Hence, this may be classed with the *lysosomal storage disorders*. Storage of galactosylceramide within multinucleated macrophages of the CNS white matter forms globoid cells. Destruction of oligodendroglia results from the action of psychosine, a metabolite of galactocerebroside.

Clinical features

Three types distinguished by age at onset:

- Infantile: within first 6 months of life, the most common variant; CNS and PNS demyelination causes implacable irritability, spasticity, opisthotonos, ataxia, seizures; hypotonia, weakness, areflexia; +/– optic atrophy, cortical blindness, hearing loss; no organomegaly.
- Late infantile/juvenile form: onset between ages 2 and 10 years: ataxia prominent in young children, spasticity commoner in older children; bulbar palsy; dementia in children with younger onset.
- Adult form: after age 10 years; may present as a *hereditary spastic paraplegia* without neuroimaging abnormalities.

Investigation

Bloods: white cell or fibroblast enzyme analysis required. Neuroimaging (MR) may show progressive demyelination in periventricular and centrum semiovale regions with sparing of subcortical U fibers, but can be normal in the early stages of disease; MR spectroscopy may show diffuse increases in white matter choline resonances, without change in *N*-acetyl aspartate levels, consistent with myelin breakdown. Neurophysiology (EMG/NCS) may show peripheral nerve demyelination, but may be normal in later onset variants. CSF may show raised protein especially in infantile forms. Neurogenetic testing for mutations in the GALC gene may be undertaken.

Differential diagnosis

Other leukodystrophies

Treatment and prognosis

Progressive psychomotor decline leading to quadriplegia; death within a few years. Bone marrow transplantation may reverse the neurological manifestations.

Reference

Pastores GM. Krabbe disease: an overview. Int J Clin Pharmacol Ther. 2009; 47(Suppl1):S75–S81

Kufor-Rakeb disease [OMIM#606693]

PARK9

Kufor-Rakeb disease is a very rare autosomal recessive condition characterized by a levodopa-responsive *parkinsonian syndrome* with spasticity (as in *pallido-pyramidal syndrome*), plus supranuclear upgaze palsy and *dementia* with onset in teenage and rapid progression. Additional clinical features observed in the original Jordanian family include mini-myoclonus of face, fauces, and fingers, visual hallucinations, oculogyric dystonic spasms, and response fluctuations to levodopa. MR imaging may show atrophy of the globus pallidus and pyramids, progressing to global atrophy. Pathologically, this is a nigrostriatal-pallidal-pyramidal degeneration. The syndrome has been mapped to chromosome 1p36, and mutations identified in the ATP13A2 gene.

References

Al-Din NAS, Wriekat A, Mubaidin A, Dasouki M, Hiari M. Pallido-pyramidal degeneration, supranuclear upgaze paresis and dementia: Kufor-Rakeb syndrome. Acta Neurol Scand. 1994;89:347–352
Williams DR, Hadeed A, al-Din AS, Wreikat AL, Lees AJ. Kufor Rakeb disease: autosomal recessive, levodopa-responsive parkinsonism with pyramidal degeneration, supranuclear gaze palsy, and dementia. Mov Disord. 2005;20:1264–1271

Kufs' disease

Kufs' disease is one of the *neuronal ceroid lipofuscinosis (NCL)* group of *lysosomal storage diseases* characterized by the accumulation of autofluorescent inclusion bodies in neurones and other tissues, with onset usually in adult life rather than infantile and juvenile onset seen with other forms of NCL.

Inheritance of Kufs' disease may be either autosomal recessive (CLN4A), as in other NCLs, or autosomal dominant (CLN4B), although the underlying genetic mutations have not yet been defined.

Clinical features

- Onset 2nd to 3rd decade
- Type A: Seizures: often myoclonic
- Type B: Psychiatric, cognitive features progressing to dementia, progressive spasticity, rigidity, ataxia, choreoathetosis; vision preserved: no retinal changes

Investigation

Bloods: no specific abnormalities. Urine: raised dolichols in urinary sediment (disputed by some authors). Neuroimaging shows brain atrophy. Neurophysiology: EEG may show epileptogenic patterns; ERG normal (cf other NCLs). Biopsy: rectal mucosa, skin biopsy, endothelial cells, blood lymphocytes, and conjunctival cells may show typical inclusion bodies/cytosomes, especially rectilinear bodies, sometimes curvilinear inclusion bodies.

Differential diagnosis

Other causes of *progressive myoclonus epilepsy*, or of neurodegenerative early-onset *dementia*, such as *Alzheimer's disease*

Treatment and prognosis

No specific treatment currently available. Symptomatic control of seizures (valproate), dystonia, myoclonus.

References

Berkovic SF, Carpenter S, Andermann F, et al. Kufs' disease: a critical reappraisal. Brain. 1988;111:27–62
Josephson SA, Schmidt RE, Millsap P, McManus DQ, Morris JC. Autosomal dominant Kufs' disease: a cause of early onset dementia. J Neurol Sci. 2001;188:51–60

Kugelberg–Welander disease

"Arrested Werdnig–Hoffmann disease," spinal muscular atrophy type III, Wohlfart–Kugelberg–Welander disease

Kugelberg–Welander disease is a form of *spinal muscular atrophy (SMA)* of proximal type, akin to type I (*Werdnig–Hoffmann disease*) but with later age at onset (up to 15 years) and generally better prognosis. Presentation is typically with symmetrical proximal weakness, areflexia, and hypotonia, with sometimes additional facial weakness, tongue wasting, weak intercostal muscles, and widespread muscle fasciculation. Lordosis, scoliosis, and contractures may occur, likewise cardiac involvement. Diagnosis is by means of neurophysiology and muscle biopsy. Hexosaminidase deficiency enters the differential diagnosis. Prognosis is very variable, but survival to the 5th or 6th decade may occur. Although there is no specific treatment, the management of skeletal deformity, a major source of morbidity, is important.

Kuru

Kuru is the prototypical *prion disease*, seen in the Fore people of the Eastern highlands of New Guinea, who performed ritual cannibalism of their dead, including consumption of the brain. This was particularly reserved for women and children, in whom this neurodegenerative condition occurred, characterized pathologically by spongiosis and the occurrence of kuru plaques. The condition is now extremely rare, following the cessation of cannibalsim in this tribal group in the 1950s, but occasional new cases occur, suggesting that an extremely long incubation time is possible in this disorder, which may have implications for other prion diseases such as *variant Creutzfeldt–Jakob disease* in which, unlike sporadic *Creutzfeldt–Jakob disease*, kuru-type plaques may be seen.

References

Collinge J, Whitfield J, McKintosh E, et al. Kuru in the 21st century – an acquired human prion disease with very long incubation periods. Lancet. 2006;367:2068–2074
Gajdusek DC. Unconventional viruses and the origin and disappearance of kuru. Science. 1977;197:943–960
Hornabrook R. Early descriptions of kuru: instinct, insects and intellect. Pract Neurol. 2006;6:122–125
Zigas V. Laughing Death: The Untold Story of Kuru. Clifton, NJ: Humana; 1990

L

L-2-Hydroxyglutaric acidemia [OMIM#236792]

This rare autosomal recessive inborn metabolic error may result in mental retardation, pyramidal and extrapyramidal signs, ataxia with cerebellar atrophy, seizures, and cardiomyopathy. Onset is most often in infancy, but adult presentations with migraine and with tremor have been reported. There may be macrocephaly. There is organic acidemia with hyperlysinemia, and increased L-2-hydroxyglutaric acid in urine, plasma, and CSF. MR imaging shows subcortical leukoencephalopathy.

Mutations in the L2HGDH gene on chromosome 14q22.1 can cause this condition.

References

Barth PG, Hoffmann GF, Jaeken J et al. L-2-Hydroxyglutaric acidemia: a novel inherited neurometabolic disease. Ann Neurol. 1992;32:66–71
Karatas H, Sayqi S, Bastan B et al. L-2-Hydroxyglutaric aciduria: report of four Turkish adult patients. Neurologist. 2010;16:44–46

Lactic acidosis: overview

Accumulation of lactate, the end product of anaerobic glucose metabolism, occurs when production exceeds use, as in anaerobic exercise, or pathological states such as ischemia-hypoxia, hepatocellular failure, and uncontrolled diabetes mellitus ("type A lactic acidosis"); there may be an increase in the lactate to pyruvate (L/P) ratio. In inherited metabolic diseases, lactic acidosis may be associated with increased pyruvate production or decreased oxidation of pyruvate (normal or increased L/P ratio). Care is needed in the measurement of venous blood lactate, since false elevations may occur with use of a tourniquet, delay in analyzing the sample, and inadequate mixing of blood with fluoride in the collecting tube. Arterial or CSF samples may overcome some of these difficulties. Fasting samples are required for the measurement of pyruvate.

Examples of conditions associated with lactic acidosis include:

- *Mitochondrial disease*, e.g., MELAS, Leigh's disease
- Disorders of gluconeogenesis:
  - *Glycogen storage disease (GSD)* type I
  - Hereditary fructose intolerance (HFI)
  - PEPCK deficiency
- *Fatty acid oxidation disorders*
- Pyruvate carboxylase (PC) deficiency
- Pyruvate dehydrogenase (PDH) deficiency
- Biotin metabolism defects: Biotinidase deficiency, holocarboxylase deficiency
- Methylmalonic acidemia

Hence confirmation of lactic acidosis without obvious cause should initiate a search for metabolic disorders, which may necessitate analysis of blood glucose, amino acids, and ammonia, urinary organic acids, plus other studies (MRI, muscle biopsy, fibroblast enzymatic studies).

Lacunar syndromes (LACS)

The lacunar syndromes were originally described by Miller Fisher on the basis of pathological findings. Although the term may also be used for clinical-radiological syndromes, associated with small, deep vascular lesions of the corona radiata, internal capsule, thalamus, cerebral peduncle and pons, the term "small, deep infarct" is preferred. Sometimes a clinically defined "lacunar syndrome" may be associated with an infarct in the territory of one of the major cerebral arteries. Typically, there are no cortical (aphasia, visual deficit) or brainstem (diplopia, crossed deficits) features in lacunar syndromes. They are presumed to reflect occlusion of small perforating arteries due to degenerative vascular disease, often in the context of hypertension.

Although a variety of lacunar syndromes have been proposed, the four principal types are:

- Pure motor stroke, pure motor hemiplegia (ca. 50%):
  - Unilateral motor deficit affecting face, upper limb, lower limb; although there may be sensory symptoms, there are no sensory signs. There may be a flurry of preceding *transient ischemic attacks* (the *capsular warning syndrome*). The lesion is usually in the internal capsule or pons, sometimes the corona radiata or cerebral peduncle, rarely in the medullary pyramid.
- Pure sensory stroke (ca. 5%):
  - Symptoms of sensory loss, with or without sensory signs, in the same distribution as for pure motor stroke; the lesion is usually in the thalamus.

- Sensorimotor stroke (ca. 35%):
  - Pure motor stroke plus sensory signs in the affected parts; the lesion is usually in the thalamus or internal capsule but may be in the corona radiata or pons.
- Ataxic hemiparesis: includes "dysarthria-clumsy hand syndrome" and homolateral ataxia with crural paresis (ca. 10%):
  - A combination of corticospinal and ipsilateral cerebellar dysfunction; the lesion is usually in the internal capsule or cerebral peduncle, pons, or corona radiata.

Although debate continues about the utility of such a clinical classification with the advent of neuroimaging, many neurologists continue to find these syndromes clinically useful.

References

Arboix A, Bell Y, Garcia-Eroles L et al. Clinical study of 35 patients with dysarthria-clumsy hand syndrome. J Neurol Neurosurg Psychiatry. 2004;75:231–234
Bamford J. Lacunar syndromes – are they still worth diagnosing? In: Donnan G, Norrving B, Bamford J, Bogousslavsky J eds. Subcortical Stroke. 2nd ed. Oxford, UK: OUP; 2002:161–174
Fisher CM. Ataxic hemiparesis. A pathologic study. Arch Neurol. 1978;35:126–128
Fisher CM. Pure sensory stroke and allied conditions. Stroke. 1982;13:434–447

Lafora body disease [OMIM#254780]

Lafora body disease is an autosomal recessive syndrome of *progressive myoclonus epilepsy*, usually presenting between 6 and 20 years of age, although later onset and protracted course have been described. Besides epileptic seizures (frequently focal occipital attacks), the clinical picture includes personality change and progressive dementia. The characteristic finding is of Lafora bodies, round basophilic PAS-positive intracellular inclusions of 3–30 μm diameter, in CNS neurones and in the excretory ducts of eccrine or apocrine sweat glands; they may also be seen in skin, liver, and muscle biopsies, although all may produce negative findings. Prognosis is generally poor, with death occurring within a few years. Mutations within the laforin (EPM2A) or malin (NHLRC1) genes may cause Lafora body disease. The differential diagnosis includes *Unverricht–Lundborg disease*, *Kuf's disease*, and *mitochondrial diseases*.

Reference

Footitt DR, Quinn N, Kocen RS, Oz B, Scaravilli F. Familial Lafora body disease of late onset: report of four cases in one family and a review of the literature. J Neurol. 1997;244:40–44

Laing myopathy [OMIM#160500]

Early onset distal myopathy (MPD1)

Laing *distal myopathy* is caused by mutations within the slow skeletal muscle fiber myosin heavy chain (MYH7) gene at chromosome 14q12, and is allelic with one form of hypertrophic cardiomyopathy and with myosin storage myopathy. The clinical phenotype is consistent, with initial weakness of big toe and ankle dorsiflexion followed by finger extension and neck flexion, but with variable age at onset, up to the 20s, and slow progression. Mild (up to three times) elevation of creatine kinase may be seen. Muscle biopsy appearances are variable, with type 1 fiber atrophy, and rimmed vacuoles found in only a minority of patients (cf. *Nonaka myopathy*, *Miyoshi myopathy*).

References

Laing NG, Laing BA, Meredith C et al. Autosomal dominant distal myopathy: linkage to chromosome 14. Am J Hum Genet. 1995; 56:422–427
Lamont PJ, Udd B, Mastaglia FL et al. Laing early onset distal myopathy: slow myosin defect with variable abnormalities on muscle biopsy. J Neurol Neurosurg Psychiatry. 2006;77:208–215

Lambert–Eaton myasthenic syndrome (LEMS)

Lambert–Eaton myasthenic syndrome (LEMS) is a rare syndrome of fluctuating muscle weakness with autonomic features, of autoimmune etiology due to antibodies directed against presynaptic P/Q type voltage-gated calcium channels (VGCC), hence a *neuromuscular junction (NMJ) disease*. There is an association with underlying, sometimes occult, malignant disease, particularly small-cell lung carcinoma, hence this is a *paraneoplastic syndrome* in about 60% of cases, the remainder being sporadic.

Clinical features

- Proximal limb weakness, legs > arms (difficulty with stairs, rising from sitting).
- Fatigue, fluctuation of symptoms; improvement with sustained or repeated exercise.
- Autonomic dysfunction: xerophthalmia, xerostomia.
- +/− myalgia, muscle stiffness, distal paresthesia, erectile dysfunction.
- Depressed or absent tendon reflexes may be elicited following sustained muscular contraction.

- Other autoimmune disorders, such as thyroid disease, may develop.
- Unlike myasthenia gravis, LEMS rarely affects the extraocular muscles.

Investigation

Bloods: antibodies to voltage-gated calcium channels (VGCC) in >85% of patients. Neurophysiology (EMG/NCS) shows low amplitude CMAPs, with decrement to slow rates of stimulation, but facilitation after brief exercise. Imaging to search for an underlying neoplasm, especially chest, should be undertaken; if negative whole body PET scan may be undertaken, especially in the more elderly patient presenting with this condition for the first time. Imaging may need to be repeated if initially negative since malignancy may remain occult for many years.

Differential diagnosis

Myasthenia gravis. Weakness and areflexia may be mistaken for *Guillain–Barré syndrome.*

Treatment and prognosis

Specific treatment of underlying neoplasm, if found. Symptomatic therapy: weakness may be improved with 3,4-diaminopyridine (3,4-DAP); immuno-suppression is sometimes used (prednisolone +/− azathioprine, ciclosporin). Plasma exchange or IVIg may be used for severe symptoms, but the effect is transient (weeks). Xerophthalmia may be treated with hypromellose eye drops.

References

O'Neill JH, Murray NM, Newsom-Davis J. The Lambert-Eaton myasthenic syndrome. A review of 50 cases. Brain. 1988;111:577–596

Pourmand R. Lambert-Eaton myasthenic syndrome. Front Neurol Neurosci. 2009;26:120–125

Sathasivam S, Larner AJ. Disorders of the neuromuscular junction. In: Sinclair A, Morley JE, Vellas B eds. Pathy's Principles and Practice of Geriatric Medicine. 5th ed. Chichester, UK: Wiley; 2011: in press

Skeie GO, Apostolski S, Evoli A et al. Guidelines for the treatment of autoimmune neuromuscular transmission disorders. Eur J Neurol. 2006;13:691–699

Weimer MB, Wong J. Lambert-Eaton myasthenic syndrome. Curr Treat Options Neurol. 2009;11:77–84

Lance–Adams syndrome

Post-anoxic (action) myoclonus

Lance–Adams syndrome is the name given to a *posthypoxic syndrome* characterized by myoclonic jerking, observed after brain hypoxia, for example, in the context of resuscitation from respiratory and cardiac arrest. Survivors may be left with action myoclonus, presumably of cortical origin, which may range in severity from mild to disabling. Pharmacotherapy with clonazepam, sodium valproate, piracetam, and baclofen may be tried, sometimes in combination. The movements may initially be confused with epileptic seizures, but consciousness is preserved.

References

Lance JW, Adams RD. The syndrome of intention or action myoclonus as a sequel to hypoxic encephalopathy. Brain. 1963;86:111–136
Larner AJ, Heafield MTE. Post anoxic action myoclonus. J R Soc Med. 1993;86:310

Landau–Kleffner syndrome

Acquired epileptic aphasia

This unusual *epilepsy* syndrome of childhood is characterized by acquired aphasia, with a reduction in spontaneous speech, behavioral (autistic), and psychomotor disturbances. Boys are affected twice as often as girls. Typically, language development is normal for several years until there is loss of comprehension or use of language; the main deficit seems to be a verbal auditory agnosia. The condition may also present with seizures of various types, generalized and focal, although some patients never suffer seizures. A fluctuating course may occur, with remissions and exacerbations. Structural brain imaging is normal although functional imaging may show temporal lobe abnormalities. EEG abnormalities may include multifocal sharp and slow waves, mainly in posterior temporal foci, which may intensify during slow wave sleep.

Seizures and EEG abnormalities often remit in teenage. Treatment with antiepileptic medications may be undertaken in those with frequent seizures, or to reduce EEG abnormalities in the belief that these are responsible for the linguistic (and other) symptoms. Steroids may be used if antiepileptic therapy fails. Ultimate prognosis is variable: some normalize completely, others are left with permanent sequelae which may be severe; seizures may continue, often infrequently.

References

Fifty years of Landau-Kleffner syndrome. Proceedings of an international symposium, November 2–4, 2007. Alden-Biesen, Belgium. Epilepsia. 2009;50(Suppl7):1–82
Panayiotopoulos CP. A Clinical Guide to Epileptic Syndromes and Their Treatment: Based on the ILAE Classifications and Practice Parameter Guidelines. 2nd ed. London, UK: Springer; 2007:249–254

Langerhans cell histiocytosis (LCH)

Histiocytosis X

This rare granulomatous disorder has a broad clinical phenotype, ranging from solitary eosinophilic granuloma of bone to aggressive multisystem disease (Letterer–Siwe disease); Hand–Schüller–Christian disease is a form intermediate between these extremes. Lesions may be solitary, multiple, or systemic, affecting bone, parenchymatous organs, lymph nodes, or skin. Pathophysiologically, there is a clonal (nonmalignant) proliferation of a subgroup of histiocytes bearing the Langerhans cell phenotype, most convincingly demonstrated by the presence on electron microscopy of Birbeck (Langerhans cell) granules. LCH is generally a disease of childhood, but the neurological manifestations afflict an older age group, of juveniles and young adults.

Clinical features

* Neurological features may affect:
  – Hypothalamic-hypophyseal axis: *diabetes insipidus*, endocrine dysfunction.
  – Extrahypothalamic lesions are rare, but may manifest as epileptic seizures, focal signs, or raised intracranial pressure either from mass lesion or dural involvement leading to venous sinus thrombosis.

Investigation

Neuroimaging (MR) may show tumor-like parenchymal or dural masses or diffuse infiltration; intense enhancement with gadolinium. Tissue biopsy of bone, skin, and brain is diagnostic.

Differential diagnosis

Other causes of hypothalamic-hypophyseal disease, e.g., *neurosarcoidosis*, *Erdheim–Chester disease*

Treatment and prognosis

Very variable, dependent on extent of disease. Solitary lesions may be treated with surgery, +/– radiation; multiple lesions require chemotherapy +/– radiation.

Reference

Hund E, Steiner HH, Jansen O, Sieverts H, Sohl G, Essig M. Treatment of cerebral Langerhans cell histiocytosis. J Neurol Sci. 1999;171:145–152

Lathyrism

Lathyrism is a nonprogressive spastic paraparesis of acute, subacute, or, rarely, chronic insidious onset with or without pain and cramps in lumbosacral, waist, and thigh area. Sensory and autonomic features may occur but are unusual. Lathyrism is endemic in Ethiopia, India, Bangladesh, Nepal, and China, believed to be a result of consumption of the chickling pea, *Lathyrus sativus*. The toxin was initially thought to be the non-protein amino acid β-oxalyl-amino-L-alanine (BOAA). Unlike the irreversible clinical syndrome, BOAA administration produces a reversible anterior horn cell syndrome in monkeys. There is no specific treatment. Neurological deficits are permanent; muscle atrophy and contractures may develop.

Lead and the nervous system: Overview

Plumbism

Lead may have a variety of effects on the nervous system. Ingestion may be occupational (metalworkers) or in children following consumption of lead-based paints. Organic lead exposure is usually related to tetraethyl lead, the anti-knock compound in petrol.

Clinical features

- Inorganic lead:
  - Adults: motor peripheral neuropathy (especially wrist drop from radial nerve palsy; foot drop)
  - Children: subacute encephalopathy +/– anemia; seizures, ataxia, raised intracranial pressure
- Organic lead:
  - Irritability, confusion, psychosis (hallucinations), myoclonus, ataxia (peripheral neuropathy not reported)

Other possible consequences include toxic optic neuropathy, auditory, and vestibular symptoms. Low-level lead exposure in children may produce developmental cognitive and behavioral problems; the safe level of lead exposure remains a subject of debate.

Investigation

Index of clinical suspicion is probably the most important factor in establishing the diagnosis.

- Bloods: anemia, basophilic stippling of erythrocytes on blood film; serum lead concentration may be measured to assess recent exposure, but the best measure of chronic exposure is free erythrocyte protoporphyrin level.
- Imaging: lead lines in the epiphyseal plates of the long bones may be seen in children.
- Neurophysiology: EMG/NCS may show motor nerve conduction velocities slowed in those with neuropathic presentation.
- Nerve biopsy: loss of large myelinated axons, paranodal demyelination.

Differential diagnosis

Of neuropathy: *porphyria*. Other causes of subacute encephalopathy

Treatment and prognosis

Removal from source of lead. Chelation therapy. Neurobehavioral features persist.

Reference

Rubens O, Logina I, Kravale I et al. Peripheral neuropathy in chronic occupational inorganic lead exposure: a clinical and electrophysiological study. J Neurol Neurosurg Psychiatry. 2001;71:200–204

Leber's hereditary optic neuropathy (LHON)

Leber's hereditary optic neuropathy is one of the phenotypic syndromes resulting from *mitochondrial disease*, characterized by subacute blindness due to retinal ganglion cell degeneration. Around 95% of cases are associated with one of three mutations of the mitochondrial genome encoding proteins of complex I, but clinical expression shows incomplete penetrance and marked gender bias (80–90% male).

Clinical features

- Onset usually in adolescence, early adulthood.
- Bilateral subacute loss of central vision (central scotoma) due to focal degeneration of the retinal ganglion cell layer and optic nerve; telangiectatic microangiopathy and swelling of nerve fiber layer around optic disc may be evident on fundoscopy acutely. Some recovery of vision may occur.
- +/– Cardiac conduction defects.

Investigation

Neurogenetics: Most usual associated mutations are point mutations in mitochondrial DNA: G3460A, G11778A, and T14484C.

Differential diagnosis

Optic neuritis, ischemic optic neuropathy.

Treatment and prognosis

No specific treatment. Low vision aids. Some patients with the typical LHON mutation G11778A evolve to a multiple sclerosis-like clinical picture (*Harding's syndrome*).

Reference

Man PY, Turnbull DM, Chinnery PF. Leber hereditary optic neuropathy. J Med Genet. 2002;39:162–169

Legionnaires' disease

The organism *Legionella pneumophila* lives in water and is transmitted to humans via airborne droplets. It may be found in air conditioning systems and often causes small epidemics of disease. It causes an "atypical pneumonia," so called because of the prominent extrapulmonary symptoms, including neurological features.

Clinical features

- Incubation period 2–10 days
- Symptoms:
  - Respiratory: cough, often nonproductive
  - Systemic: fever, myalgia

- Gastrointestinal: frequent; nausea, vomiting, diarrhea (25–50%)
- Neurological (ca. 50% of patients):
  - Encephalopathy: greater than expected on the basis of metabolic disturbance; ranges from mild confusion to coma
  - Ataxia.
  - Peripheral neuropathy: predominantly a motor axonopathy
  - Cranial neuritis: especially sixth cranial nerve

Investigation

Bloods: leukocytosis, raised ESR, hyponatremia, hypophosphatemia; serology for *L. pneumophila*. Urine: antigen test. Imaging: CXR: pneumonia; lobar infiltrates may be diffuse or interstitial; pleural effusion; CT/ MRI no focal lesion. CSF may show elevated protein (5%), pleocytosis (20%).

Differential diagnosis

Other "atypical pneumonias": watery diarrhea, hyponatremia point to Legionnaires' disease.

Treatment and prognosis

Supportive treatment. Antibiotics: erythromycin 1 g qds for 10 days then 500 mg qds for a further 10 days; alternatives are doxycycline, ciprofloxacin, cotrimoxazole, clarithromycin. Seven percent die despite appropriate treatment and apparent immunocompetence.

References

Johnson JD, Raff MJ, Van Arsdall JA. Neurologic manifestations of Legionnaires' disease. Medicine (Baltimore). 1984;63:303–310
Stout JE, Yu VL. Legionellosis. N Engl J Med. 1997;337:682–687

Leigh's syndrome

Subacute necrotizing encephalomyelopathy

Leigh's syndrome is one of the classical syndromes of *mitochondrial disease*, characterized by subacute relapsing encephalopathy with cerebellar and brainstem signs presenting in infancy, with the neuroradiological correlate of basal ganglia lucencies. However, the clinical phenotype is heterogeneous with seizures, nystagmus, ophthalmoparesis, optic atrophy, ataxia, dystonia, and respiratory failure, and less commonly peripheral neuropathy, myopathy, and non-neurological features such as diabetes mellitus, short stature, vomiting, and diarrhea (Leigh-like syndrome). Most cases are of childhood onset, but occasionally the presentation is in adulthood. There is also marked genetic heterogeneity, with cases resulting from dysfunction in respiratory chain complexes, coenzyme Q, pyruvate dehydrogenase complex, or mutations in the mitochondrial or nuclear genome.

Clinical features

Heterogeneous: onset in infancy, childhood, or adulthood.

- Feeding difficulties (poor sucking), failure to thrive: first or second year of life
- Recurrent episodes of apnea, ataxic breathing, tachypnea
- Oculomotor abnormalities: ophthalmoplegia, retinitis pigmentosa
- Relapsing acute encephalopathy
- Epileptic seizures
- Psychomotor retardation, regression: progressive cerebral degeneration
- Early hypotonia, later spasticity
- Ataxia
- Peripheral neuropathy
- *NARP syndrome*
- +/− cardiomyopathy
- +/− multifocal myoclonus

Investigation

Bloods: persistent *lactic acidosis*, although sometimes it is difficult to know whether this reflects a primary defect in lactic acid metabolism or the consequence of uncontrolled seizure activity. Glucose, ammonia usually normal. Urine organic acids are usually normal. Neuroimaging shows destructive lesions in brainstem, basal ganglia, thalamus, usually symmetrical; white matter T_2 signal hyperintensity (may suggest leukodystrophy). CSF shows raised lactate; less likely to be spuriously elevated than plasma lactate. EEG shows background slowing, typical of encephalopathy. Muscle biopsy may be required for mitochondrial features, mtDNA analysis. Maternally inherited Leigh's syndrome is associated with point mutations in the mitochondrial ATP6 gene (as in NARP syndrome). Autosomal recessive Leigh's syndrome is due to mutations in nuclear DNA encoding respiratory chain subunits.

Differential diagnosis

Other causes of lactic acidosis with seizures: Alpers disease, mitochondrial encephalomyopathies, metabolic encephalopathies, hepatic failure.

Treatment and prognosis

No effective treatment. Supportive care: ventilation, feeding, treatment of infection, antiepileptic drugs when appropriate. Biotin, thiamine, coenzyme Q10 may be tried. The disease pursues a variable course, with periods of partial recovery and acute deterioration, but is inevitably fatal.

Reference

Finsterer J. Leigh and Leigh-like syndrome in children and adults. Pediatr Neurol. 2008;39:223–235

Lemierre's syndrome

Fusobacterium infection of the head and neck may cause fever, rigors, oropharyngeal and neck pain and swelling, headache, thrombophlebitis of the internal jugular vein, and metastatic abscesses.

Reference

Tan NCK, Tan DYL, Tan LCS. An unusual headache: Lemierre's syndrome. J Neurol. 2003;250:245–246

Lemieux–Neemeh syndrome

This name has been used for a syndrome of hereditary hearing loss, possibly autosomal recessive, with chronic sensorimotor polyneuropathy (of *Charcot–Marie–Tooth disease* type) with associated nephritis.

Reference

Lemieux G, Neemeh JA. Charcot-Marie-Tooth disease and nephritis. Can Med Assoc J. 1967;97:1193–1198

Leprosy

Hansen's disease

Infection with the acid-fast bacillus *Mycobacterium leprae* remains a common cause of morbidity and mortality globally, and the most common cause of *neuropathy* worldwide, though rarely seen in the West. Spread is by aerosol or skin-to-skin transmission. A spectrum of disease is recognized dependent upon the degree of host immunological/inflammatory reaction to the bacilli, ranging from tuberculoid (paucibacillary) through borderline to lepromatous (multibacillary). Neurological features may be seen at either end of the disease spectrum, and in association with reversal reactions encountered during treatment.

Clinical features

Neurological features include:

- Tuberculoid leprosy (vigorous tissue-mediated immune response to *M. leprae*):
  - Anesthetic skin lesions: erythematous or hypopigmented macular skin lesions, clearly demarcated, are often the earliest sign of disease, and generally show impairment of light touch and pin prick sensation and anhidrosis; nerve damage due to local epithelioid granulomata. Tend to self-heal. Local major nerves may demonstrate nerve thickening, especially ulnar, peroneal, with sensorimotor deficits in the area innervated by the thickened nerve.
- Lepromatous leprosy (little evidence of tissue-mediated immune response to *M. leprae*):
  - Organisms proliferate in cool body parts, leading to widespread symmetrical involvement of skin reminiscent of a distal sensory neuropathy (although palms of hands and soles of feet may be spared); other sites (anterior chamber of eye, tip of nose, ears, malar area) also involved; moreover, tendon reflexes are preserved.
- Borderline leprosy: features fall somewhere between tuberculoid and lepromatous.

Change in immunity, either occurring spontaneously or, more commonly, in response to treatment may cause acute deterioration in neurological features (erythema nodosum leprosum), with neuritis, iritis, and orchitis.

Investigation

The diagnostic test is the demonstration of acid-fast bacilli in skin smears; however, most disease is paucibacillary in which case skin smears are negative. Lepromin skin testing: positive in tuberculoid, negative in lepromatous leprosy.

Differential diagnosis

Painless injury may also be seen in *syringomyelia, neurosyphilis* (tabes dorsalis), and *congenital insensitivity to pain* (probably a form of hereditary sensory neuropathy).

Treatment and prognosis

Prevention: vaccination with BCG. Drug treatment to eradicate *M. leprae*: dapsone, rifampicin +/– clofazimine. Treatment of leprosy reactions, which may be more devastating than the disease itself: steroids, thalidomide, clofazimine. Rehabilitation: cosmetic surgery.

References

Gunatilake SB, Settinayake S. Leprosy. Pract Neurol. 2004;4:194–203

Jardin MR, Antunes SLG, Santos AR et al. Criteria for diagnosis of pure neural leprosy. J Neurol. 2003;250:806–809

Lockwood DNJ, Reid AJC. The diagnosis of leprosy is delayed in the United Kingdom. Q J Med. 2001;94:207–212

Leptospirosis

Weil's disease

Zoonotic infection with Gram-negative spirochaetes of the genus *Leptospira*, from direct or indirect exposure to urine of infected rodents or domestic animals, may cause a biphasic illness, initially with pyrexia, myalgia, meningism, and headache. Disease is often subclinical or mild, but an aseptic *meningitis* may be found, or the organism may be recovered from CSF (or blood). Jaundice and renal failure may also occur (Weil's disease). Following the acute illness, there may rarely be neurological complications such as encephalitis, myelitis, optic neuritis, or peripheral neuritis, thought to be immune mediated since the organism can no longer be isolated. Treatment is with penicillin or tetracyclines.

Reference

Russell RW. Neurological aspects of leptospirosis. J Neurol Neurosurg Psychiatry. 1959;22:143–148

Lesch-Nyhan disease

X-linked hypoxanthine phosphoribosyltransferase (HPRT) deficiency

This syndrome of severe learning disability and self-mutilation results from deficiency of the purine salvage enzyme hypoxanthine phosphoribosyltransferase (HPRT), an X-linked disorder due to mutations in the HPRT gene on

chromosome Xq26. The phenotype is variable, with a milder condition resulting from partial HPRT deficiency. Genotype:phenotype correlations provide
no indication that specific disease features associate with specific mutations.

Clinical features

- Motor disorder: severe action dystonia, baseline hypotonia, +/– extrapyra-
  midal and pyramidal signs
- Psychomotor retardation
- Compulsive self-mutilation: biting lips, cheeks, fingers
- Partial deficiency: gouty arthritis, nephrolithiasis; neurological features in
  20%: cerebellar ataxia, mild learning disability, no self-mutilation

Investigation

Blood and urine show increased uric acid; specific enzyme assay may be performed with leukocytes, fibroblasts.

Differential diagnosis

Cerebral palsy, glutaric aciduria type I, *neuroacanthocytosis*.

Treatment and prognosis

Allopurinol may help the arthritis and nephrolithiasis, but there is no specific
treatment for the neurological features.

References

Jinnah HA, De Gregorio L, Harris JC, Nyhan WL, O'Neill JP. The spectrum of inherited mutations causing HPRT deficiency: 75 new cases and a review of 196 previously
reported cases. Mutat Res. 2000;463:309–326
Jinnah HA, Visser JE, Harris JC et al. Delineation of the motor disorder of Lesch-
Nyhan disease. Brain. 2006;129:1201–1217

Leucoencephalopathy with neuroaxonal spheroids (LENAS)

Leucoencephalopathy with neuroaxonal spheroids (LENAS) is a rare disease
of cerebral and cerebellar white matter characterized clinically by cognitive
decline, behavioral features, cerebellar ataxia, and gait dysfunction. The white

matter changes are evident on MR imaging, and axonal spheroids are seen at biopsy or autopsy. Differential diagnosis includes the cerebellar subtype of *multiple system atrophy*.

Reference

Mayer B, Oelschlaeger C, Keyvani K, Niederstadt T. Two cases of LENAS: diagnosis by MRI and biopsy. J Neurol. 2007;254:1453–1454

Leukodystrophies: overview

The leukodystrophies are a heterogeneous group of disorders, having in common a noninflammatory demyelinating neuropathology. The advent of neuroimaging has perhaps made these conditions easier to recognize, yet they remain rare. They are most often diseases of childhood, but occasionally may be diagnosed in young adults. Peripheral nerve involvement may also occur. The specific biochemical defects causing some of these conditions are known.

Classification may be according to inheritance pattern:

- Autosomal recessive:
  - *Metachromatic leukodystrophy* (*MLD*)
  - Austin disease (juvenile sulfatidosis, multiple sulfatase deficiency)
  - *Krabbe's disease* (globoid cell leukodystrophy)
  - Canavan disease (aspartoacylase deficiency [OMIM#271900])
- Sex-linked:
  - *Adrenoleukodystrophy* (*X-ALD*)
  - Pelizaeus–Merzbacher disease (PMD)
- Others:
  - *Alexander's disease*
  - *Eighteen q deletion syndrome*
  - Cockayne syndrome
  - *Schilder's disease*

Leukodystrophies may also be described as orthochromatic or sudanophilic, an ill-defined group including PMD.

Differential diagnosis

- Vascular encephalopathies: CADASIL, Homocystinuria
- Some *mitochondrial diseases*

- Vanishing white matter disease
- Others: *cerebrotendinous xanthomatosis* (*CTX*); *Refsum's disease*, phenylketonuria (PKU)

References

Baumann N, Turpin J-C. Adult-onset leukodystrophies. J Neurol. 2000;247:751–759
Berger J, Moser HW, Forss-Petter S. Leukodystrophies: recent developments in genetics, molecular biology, pathogenesis and treatment. Curr Opin Neurol. 2001; 14:305–312
Gordon N. Canavan disease: a review of recent developments. Eur J Paediatr Neurol. 2001;5:65–69
Ozdirim E, Topcu M, Ozon A et al. Cockayne syndrome: review of 25 cases. Pediatr Neurol. 1996;15:312–316

Lewis Sumner syndrome

MADSAM, Multifocal CIDP

Lewis Sumner syndrome is a *m*ultifocal *a*cquired *d*emyelinating *s*ensory *a*nd *m*otor neuropathy (hence MADSAM) that is steroid responsive. It may be classified as one of the variants of *chronic inflammatory demyelinating polyradiculoneuropathy* (*CIDP*). It is characterized clinically by asymmetric weakness and sensory loss, more usually in the upper limbs and distal more than proximal. Neurophysiology shows asymmetrical multifocal demyelinating features with frequent conduction block. CSF protein is elevated. It responds to both steroids and IVIg.

References

Lewis RA, Sumner AJ, Brown MJ, Asbury AK. Multifocal demyelinating neuropathy with persistent conduction block. Neurology. 1982;32:958–964
Rajabally YA, Chavada G. Lewis-Sumner syndrome of pure upper-limb onset: diagnostic, prognostic, and therapeutic features. Muscle Nerve. 2009;39:206–220

Lhermitte–Duclos disease

Dysplastic cerebellar gangliocytoma

Lhermitte–Duclos disease is a slowly evolving mass lesion of the cerebellum of uncertain pathogenesis, which may be associated with macrocephaly, raised intracranial pressure, learning disability, and developmental delay.

Pathologically, the lesion contains granule, Purkinje, and glial elements. It has been variously labeled as a hamartoma (possibly related to Cowden disease), a dysplastic gangliocytoma, a neoplasm, or a malformation. The growth potential is small, and the prognosis good.

Li–Fraumeni syndrome (LFS) [OMIM#161523]

The Li–Fraumeni syndrome is a rare hereditary (autosomal dominant) disorder of familial and intraindividual clustering of malignancies, specifically:

- Sarcoma before the age of 45 years, +/– premenopausal breast carcinoma, brain tumors (e.g., *glioma*), leukemias, adrenocortical carcinoma (in children), epithelial or mesenchymal tumors
- A first degree relative with carcinoma before the age of 45 years
- A first or second degree relative with carcinoma before the age of 45 years or sarcoma at any age

Hence the condition is heterogeneous with respect to clinical features and age at onset.

Germline mutations in the coding region of the tumor suppressor gene p53 are found in 50–70% of cases (LFS1), but there are other forms, LFS2 which is caused by mutation in the CHEK2 gene, and LFS3 which maps to a locus on chromosome 1q23.

References

Chompret A. The Li-Fraumeni syndrome. Biochimie. 2002;84:75–82
Li FP, Fraumeni JF Jr. Prospective study of a family cancer syndrome. JAMA. 1982;247:2692–2694

Limb-girdle muscular dystrophies (LGMD): overview

Limb-girdle muscular dystrophies (LGMD) form the most heterogeneous group of *muscular dystrophies*, with over 20 genetic types defined to date, both autosomal recessive conditions, which tend to be clinically more severe and more common, and autosomal dominant. Cardiac involvement is prominent in some. Inter- and intrafamilial heterogeneity may be seen.

The following LGMD types are recognized:

LGMD Type	Chromosome linkage	Abnormal protein	Clinical complications	Allelic disorders
Autosomal dominant				
1A	5q31	Myotilin	Myofibrillar myopathies, cardiac and respiratory complications	Myofibrillar myopathies, spheroid body myopathy
1B	1q11-21	Lamin A/C	Arrhythmia, cardiomyopathy, respiratory failure	Emery–Dreifuss muscular dystrophy, dilated cardiomyopathy
1C	3p25	Caveolin 3		Rippling muscle disease, hyperCKemia, hypertrophic cardiomyopathy
1D	7q	??		
1E	6q23	??		Cardiomyopathy
1F	7q32	??		
1G	4p21	??		
Autosomal recessive				
2A	15q15.1	Calpain-3		
2B	2p13	Dysferlin		Miyoshi myopathy
2C	13q12	γ-Sarcoglycan	Cardiomyopathy and respiratory features	
2D	17q21	α-Sarcoglycan	Cardiomyopathy and respiratory features	

2E	4q12	β-Sarcoglycan	Cardiomyopathy and respiratory features	
2F	5q33	δ-Sarcoglycan	Cardiomyopathy and respiratory features	
2G	17q12	Telethonin		
2H	9q31	TRIM32		Sarcotubular myopathy
2I	19q	FKRP	Cardiomyopathy and respiratory features	Congenital muscular dystrophy type 1C
2J	2q24.2	Titin		Autosomal dominant *tibial muscular dystrophy*
2K	9q34	POMT1		Walker–Warburg syndrome
2L	11p13	??		
2M	9q31	Fukutin		Fukuyama muscular dystrophy
2N	14q24	POMT2		Walker–Warburg syndrome

Clinical features

- Wasting and weakness of limb girdle musculature; no facial weakness; cognitive function normal
- Cardiac involvement: types 1B, 1D, 2C, 2E, 2F, 2I
- +/– respiratory muscle involvement

Investigation

Blood creatine kinase of around 1,000 IU/L or more. EMG shows myopathic features. Neurogenetic testing has helped with the classification of LGMD, but about 25% of patients presenting with this clinical phenotype still currently elude molecular diagnosis. Cardiac evaluation (ECG, echocardiography) may be indicated.

Differential diagnosis

Other causes of proximal limb weakness:

- X-linked dystrophies (Duchenne, Becker)
- Facioscapulohumeral (FSH) dystrophy
- Pompe disease (acid-maltase deficiency), other metabolic myopathy
- Bethlem myopathy

Treatment and prognosis

No specific treatment. Treatment of cardiac and respiratory complications.

Reference

Bushby K. Diagnosis and management of the limb girdle muscular dystrophies. Pract Neurol. 2009;9:314–323

Limbic encephalitis

Limbic encephalitis is a syndrome of impairment of recent memory (amnesia), often accompanied by anxiety and depression, which may be subacute or chronic in its onset. In addition, there may be other neurological features such as epileptic seizures, hypersomnia, and hallucinations. CSF may show pleocytosis and raised protein. Brain imaging may be normal or there may be medial temporal lobe abnormalities.

Limbic encephalitis may be classified as:

- Viral.
- Paraneoplastic: a complication of underlying malignancy, hence a *paraneoplastic syndrome*, particularly associated with small-cell lung cancer but also reported with other carcinomas and Hodgkin's disease. Antibodies directed against intracellular or classic paraneoplastic antigens may be present, such as Hu, Ma2, CV2/CRMP5, amphiphysin. Limited response to treatment.
- Non-paraneoplastic: with serum antibodies directed against cell membrane antigens such as voltage-gated potassium channels (VGKC) and *N*-methyl-D-aspartate receptor, often associated with hyponatremia; responds to immunotherapy, for example, with steroids, IVIg, and plasma exchange.

References

Schott J. Limbic encephalitis: a clinician's guide. Pract Neurol. 2006;6:143–153
Tüzün E, Dalmau J. Limbic encephalitis and variants: classification, diagnosis and treatment. Neurologist. 2007;13:261–271

Limb shaking

"Limb shaking" episodes are recurrent, involuntary, irregular movements described by patients as shaking, trembling, twitching, or flapping. They are associated with severe *carotid artery disease*, stenosis, or occlusion of the contralateral artery with exhausted intracranial vasomotor reactivity; hence, these are *transient ischemic attacks* in the carotid territory reflecting hemodynamic failure (hypoperfusion rather than embolism). They may be precipitated by exercise, and usually last less than 5 min. These episodes may be mistaken for simple partial epileptic seizures. The differential diagnosis of unilateral limb shaking also includes Parkinson's disease.

Reference

Persoon S, Kappelle LJ, Klijn CJ. Limb-shaking transient ischaemic attacks in patients with internal carotid artery occlusion: case-control study. Brain. 2010;133;915–922

Locked-in syndrome

De-efferented state, Pseudocoma

Locked-in syndrome refers to a condition in which a patient is mute and motionless yet awake, alert, aware of self, and able to perceive sensory stimuli. This most often results from basilar artery thrombosis, sometimes heralded by laughter (*fou rire prodromique*) causing bilateral ventral pontine infarction or hemorrhage, but may also occur with pontine tumors, and central pontine myelinolysis; rare causes include tentorial herniation, Guillain–Barré syndrome, botulism, and myasthenia gravis. These lesions interrupt descending motor pathways, resulting in a state of de-efferentation, but spare the reticular formation, hence wakefulness is preserved.

Clinical history

- Usually acute onset: brainstem infarct, hemorrhage.
- Awake, alert; mute, motionless.
- Able to cooperate with examination, i.e., can blink to command, and answer yes/no (e.g., two blinks/one blink) if instructed.
- Horizontal eye movements often impaired > vertical eye movements, eyelid movements.
- Cognition is typically preserved, in as far as it can be tested.

Investigation

Neuroimaging (MRI) demonstrates ventral pontine lesion; if infarction, angiography may be undertaken to see if basilar artery thrombosed. Catheter angiography also presents an opportunity for local thrombolysis.

Differential diagnosis

- Abulia
- Akinetic mutism
- Catatonia
- *Coma*
- *Vegetative state*
- Minimally conscious state

Treatment and prognosis

Of cause, where identified. If ischemia/infarction is identified early, attempts to recanalize the basilar artery with local or systemic thrombolysis have been undertaken, with variable outcome in terms of degree of recovery; the risk is that ventral pontine infarction will be converted to hemorrhage. Once established, the deficits are permanent; the anguish of survivors, alert but unable to move and able to communicate only with blinking or eye movements, cannot be imagined. One survivor has "written" an account.

References

Bauby J-D. The Diving-Bell and the Butterfly. London, UK: Fourth Estate; 1997
Smith E, Delargy M. Locked-in syndrome. BMJ. 2005;330:406–409

Long QT syndromes (LQTS)

Prolonged QT syndromes

Long QT syndromes (LQTS) are characterized by prolongation of the Q-T interval on the ECG. They may present with *syncope* or *epilepsy*, consequent upon impaired cerebral perfusion. Correction of the arrhythmia may abolish the episodes of loss of consciousness. Some of the inherited syndromes are genetic *channelopathies*.

Causes include:

- Inherited:
  - Jervell–Lange-Nielsen syndrome: autosomal recessive, + deafness
  - Romano–Ward syndrome: autosomal dominant, no hearing deficit
  - *Andersen's syndrome*
- Acquired:
  - Coronary artery disease
  - Cardiomyopathy
  - Drugs (tricyclic antidepressants, antiarrhythmics)
  - Metabolic (hypocalcemia, hypomagnesemia, hypokalemia)

Several genes have been linked to the inherited long QT syndromes:

- LQT1 locus = KCNQ1 K" channel gene [OMIM#192500] may be associated with either Jervell–Lange-Nielsen type 1 [OMIM#220400] or Romano–Ward phenotype.
- LQT2 locus = KCNL2 K" channel gene [OMIM#152427].
- LQT3 locus = SCN5A Na" channel gene [OMIM#603830].
- LQT4 locus = ankyrin-2 gene [OMIM#600919].
- LQT5 locus = KCNE1 K^+ channel gene.
- LQT6 locus = KCNE2 K^+ channel gene.
- LQT7 (Andersen's syndrome) = KCNJ2 K^+ channel gene.
- LQT8 (Timothy syndrome) = CACNA1C calcium channel gene.
- LQT9 = CAV3 gene (allelic with *limb girdle muscular dystrophy* type 1c, *rippling muscle disease, idiopathic hyperCKemia*).
- LQT10 = SCN4B Na^+ channel gene.
- LQT11 = AKAP9 gene.
- LQT12 = SNTA1 gene.

Clinical features

- Ventricular tachyarrhythmias
- Family history of sudden death, deafness
- Epileptic seizures: may be preceded by syncopal symptoms or palpitations
- Periodic paralysis (Andersen's syndrome)

Investigation

ECG shows prolonged QT interval after correction for heart rate (QTc). EEG and neuroimaging are typically normal.

Differential diagnosis

Other etiologies of seizure. Certain drugs may produce a prolongation of QT interval on ECG, e.g., pimozide.

Treatment and prognosis

Untreated, there is a risk of sudden death due to malignant ventricular arrhythmias. Treatment with beta-blockers, or with a pacemaker or implantable defibrillator, reduces risks and should abolish epileptic seizures.

References

Pacia SV, Devinsky O, Luciano DJ, Vazquez B. The prolonged QT syndrome presenting as epilepsy: a report of two cases and literature review. Neurology. 1994;44:1408–1410
Roden DM. Long-QT syndrome. N Engl J Med. 2008;358:169–176

Long thoracic nerve palsy

The long thoracic nerve of Bell originates from the motor roots of C5, C6, and often C7, descends through the medial scalenus muscle and dorsal to the brachial plexus, and along the medial axillary wall to innervate the serratus anterior muscle. Long thoracic nerve palsy results in weakness of serratus anterior, manifests as winging of the scapula (scapula alata), either at rest or when elevating the upper arm (e.g., pushing against a wall with arms slightly flexed at elbows). The absence of other symptoms (sensory) and signs differentiates it from C6 and C7 root lesions. The most common causes are *neuralgic amyotrophy* and trauma (e.g., *rucksack paralysis*, chest wall surgery), and it has also been reported with *neuroborreliosis*. Spontaneous recovery is the rule.

Reference

Staal A, Van Gijn J, Spaans F. Mononeuropathies: Examination, Diagnosis and Treatment. London, UK: WB Saunders; 1999:19–21

Low back pain: overview

Low back pain, with or without radiation to the leg(s), is an extremely common clinical problem; in most instances, degenerative disease of the bony and ligamentous spinal column is to blame. For the neurologist referred a patient with low back pain, the issue is to determine whether compromise of the spinal cord and/or spinal roots is contributing, i.e., lumbosacral radiculopathy, lumbar canal stenosis.

Clinical features

Features which suggest a cause other than mechanical for low back pain include:

- No history of trauma.
- Pain at night.
- Fever: consider infection.
- Leg pain, weakness, sensory disturbance.
- Sphincteric symptoms.

Symptoms and signs correlating with radiological (MR) evidence of lumbosacral nerve root compression include:

- Leg pain > back pain
- Dermatomal pain
- Pain exacerbated by coughing, sneezing, straining at stool
- Paroxysmal pain
- Pain on straight leg raising
- Limb paresis, reflex loss
- Finger–floor distance >25 cm on bending to touch floor with fingers

Investigation

- Neuroimaging:
  - Plain radiology may disclose mechanical factors (fracture, tumor, ankylosing spondylitis); but degenerative osteoarthritic change is increasingly frequent with age even without symptoms, so of doubtful diagnostic value, especially in the older age group.
  - MR: definitive investigation for lumbar spinal cord and lumbosacral nerve root compression; myelography +/– CT may still be required if patient intolerant of MR.
  - Bone scan may be undertaken if malignant disease is suspected.
- Neurophysiology (EMG/NCS): may show evidence of radiculopathy.
- CSF: seldom required, unless malignant root infiltration suspected on clinical +/– radiological grounds (cytology).

Differential diagnosis

- Musculoskeletal problems:
  - Posttraumatic, fracture
  - Osteoarthritis
  - Spondylolisthesis (slippage of one vertebral body over another)
  - Scoliosis
  - *Ankylosing spondylitis*
  - Bony tumors: primary, metastatic
  - Infection: epidural space, *discitis*
- Cord/root tumors: ependymoma, chordoma, neurofibroma
- Vascular insufficiency (claudication) more likely to cause exercise-related leg pain, not back pain

Treatment and prognosis

Of cause where identified. Low back pain without neurological features requires analgesia. Lumbar cord compression, lumbosacral nerve root compression, and lumbar canal stenosis may all require surgical intervention. "Failed back syndrome" refers to the situation where surgery for such conditions fails to alleviate symptoms and indeed the patient may have more severe chronic pain than preoperatively. Symptoms most often relate to progression of spinal degenerative disease, postoperative arachnoiditis, or inappropriate initial indication for surgery. Re-imaging may assist reevaluation. Further surgery is seldom indicated, rather appropriate pain management.

Reference

Leach JP. Spinal symptoms: neck pain and backache. In: Greene J, Bone I. Understanding Neurology: A Problem-Oriented Approach. London, UK: Manson Publishing; 2007:204–213

Luft disease

Euthyroid hypermetabolism

An extremely rare *mitochondrial disease* with defective coupling of oxidation and phosphorylation, characterized clinically by early childhood onset of heat intolerance, hyperthermia, excessive sweating, polyphagia, polydipsia, and mild generalized fatiguable weakness. Basal metabolic rate is elevated, but thyroid function tests are normal. ECG shows sinus tachycardia; EMG shows features of myopathy. Muscle biopsy shows ragged red fibers, increased oxidative enzymes, and accumulations of mitochondria which may have enlarged and tightly packed cristae. Isolated mitochondria show a maximal respiratory rate, even in the absence of ADP, indicating a loss of respiratory control. Chloramphenicol has been reported of benefit in one patient.

References

DiMauro S, Bonilla E, Zeviani M, Nakagawa M, DeVivo DC. Mitochondrial myopathy. Ann Neurol. 1985;17:521–538
Luft R, Ikkos D, Palmieri G et al. A case of severe hypermetabolism of nonthyroid origin with a defect in the maintenance of mitochondrial respiratory control: a correlated clinical, biochemical and morphological study. J Clin Invest. 1962;41:1776–1804

Lumbar cord and root disease: overview

Lumbar myelopathy, Lumbar radiculopathy

Although only a small percentage of patients with *low back pain* have compromise of spinal cord or nerve roots, nonetheless these conditions are common and need to be considered in all patients presenting with low back pain.

Clinical features

- Myelopathy:
  - History:
    - Pain may or may not be a feature.
    - Complaint of limb weakness, giving way, dragging, tripping.
    - May be sphincter involvement, especially if intramedullary lesion.
  - Examination: Upper motor neurone signs: spasticity, pyramidal pattern of weakness (flexors > extensors), hyperreflexia, Babinski sign.
- Radiculopathy:
  - History:
    - Leg pain usually > back pain.
    - Dermatomal pain.
    - Paroxysmal pain, increased by coughing, sneezing, straining at stool.

- Examination: Pain on straight leg raising (Lasègue's sign).
  - ○ Paresis appropriate to root(s) involved.
  - ○ Reflex loss appropriate to root(s) involved.
  - ○ Finger–floor distance on bending to touch floor with fingers >25 cm

Specific roots:

- L1 (rare): inguinal sensory symptoms +/− lower abdominal paresis (internal oblique, transverse muscles).
- L2: sensory symptoms over anterior thigh; +/− weak thigh adduction, flexion, eversion, leg extension; depressed cremasteric reflex.
- L3: sensory symptoms over lower anterior thigh and medial knee; +/− weak thigh adduction, flexion, eversion, leg extension; +/− depressed (patellar) knee reflex.
- L4: low back, buttock, anterior thigh and leg pain; sensory disturbance on knee and medial leg; +/− weak leg extension, foot dorsiflexion and inversion; +/− depressed (patellar) knee reflex.
- L5 (common): low back, buttock, lateral thigh and anterolateral calf pain; sensory disturbance on lateral leg, dorsomedial foot, hallux; weak glutei, knee flexion, foot dorsiflexion, and plantarflexion, inversion (cf. common peroneal nerve palsy) and eversion; knee and ankle reflexes spared.
- S1 (common): low back, buttock, lateral thigh and calf pain; sensory disturbance on little toe, lateral foot, sole of foot; +/− weak hip extension, knee flexion, foot plantarflexion; depressed ankle (Achilles) reflex.
- S2–S5: sensory disturbances on calf, posterior thigh, buttocks, perianal region; +/− sphincteric control impaired.

More than 80% of lumbar disc herniations involve L5 or S1.

Investigation

Neuroimaging (MR) to identify lumbar cord and root lesions, compression. Neurophysiology (EMG/NCS) may confirm presence of radiculopathy.

Differential diagnosis

- Other causes of low back pain
- Peripheral mononeuropathies may be confused, e.g., common peroneal nerve palsy with L5 radiculopathy
- *Lumbosacral plexopathies* with multiple radiculopathies

Treatment and prognosis

Surgical decompression may be required to prevent further neurological deterioration; reversal of neurological deficits already present cannot be guaranteed.

References

Coster S, de Bruijn SFTM, Tavy DLJ. Diagnostic value of history, physical examination and needle electromyography in diagnosing lumbosacral radiculopathy. J Neurol. 2010;257:332–337

Nelson PB. Approach to the patient with low back pain, lumbosacral radiculopathy, and lumbar stenosis. In: Biller J, ed. Practical Neurology. 2nd ed. Philadelphia, PA: Lippincott Williams & Wilkins; 2002:282–288

Patel N. Surgical disorders of the thoracic and lumbar spine: a guide for neurologists. J Neurol Neurosurg Psychiatry. 2002;73(SupplI): i42–i48

Vroomen PCAJ, de Krom MCTFM, Wilmink JT, Kester ADM, Knottnerus JA. Diagnostic value of history and physical examination in patients suspected of lumbosacral nerve root compression. J Neurol Neurosurg Psychiatry. 2002;72:630–634

Lumbosacral plexopathies

Various causes of lumbosacral plexopathy are recognized, as for *brachial plexopathy*. These include:

- Idiopathic
- Infection: influenza, varicella zoster; anogenital herpes simplex type 2 infection
- Drug abuse: heroin
- Vasculitis
- Tumor infiltration
- Compression: pelvic fracture, surgery; psoas hematoma in bleeding diathesis
- *Hereditary neuropathy with liability to pressure palsies (HNLPP)*
- Radiation plexopathy

Clinical features

- Pain, often of abrupt onset and severe; anterior thigh with upper plexus lesions; buttock, posterior thigh with lower plexus involvement. Pain not aggravated by movement (cf. radiculopathy)
- Muscle weakness; pattern dependent on level and extent of plexus involvement; reflex diminution, loss
- Limb paraesthesia

Some causes may be obvious from history.

Investigation

Bloods may give clues to etiology (FBC, ESR; glucose, electrolytes, LFTs, syphilis serology, autoantibodies). Imaging (CT/MRI) of lumbar spine and plexus may be undertaken.

CSF should be examined (cell count, protein, glucose, oligoclonal bands, cytology). Neurophysiology (EMG/NCS) changes are often diffuse and patchy which may assist in differentiation from radiculopathy; paraspinal muscles are normal with plexopathy (cf. radiculopathy); lower limb sensory nerve action potentials are spared in radiculopathy.

Differential diagnosis

- Radiculopathy: acute disc prolapse, diabetic
- *Mononeuritis multiplex*
- Sacral myeloradiculitis (*Elsberg syndrome*)
- Mononeuropathies of lower limbs

Treatment and prognosis

Of cause, where possible. Idiopathic lumbosacral plexopathy may be responsive to steroids or other immunosuppressive therapy. Prognosis is thought poorer than for brachial plexopathy, especially if there is distal weakness.

Reference

Planner AC, Donaghy M, Moore NR. Causes of lumbosacral plexopathy. Clin Radiol. 2006;61:987–995

Lymphocytic hypophysitis

Lymphocytic hypophysitis is a rare inflammatory, probably autoimmune, *pituitary disease*, affecting particularly women in the peripartum period.

Clinical features

- Prolactin hypersecretion.
- Anterior pituitary hormone failure.
- *Diabetes insipidus* is unusual ("infundibulohypophysitis").
- Pathology may extend to the suprasellar region, cavernous sinus, causing neuro-ophthalmological signs
- +/– coexisting autoimmune disorders.

Investigation

Bloods: prolactin, thyroid function, LH, FSH. Neuroimaging (MRI) shows pituitary mass lesion; thickened stalk; peripheral enhancement. Pathology shows lymphocytic (T and B cells) infiltrate of anterior pituitary tissue with foci of infarction and necrosis, cavitation; no granulomata, no caseation. Surrounding interstitial reactive fibrosis.

Differential diagnosis

Nonfunctioning pituitary adenoma: may be impossible to distinguish on clinical and radiological grounds. Other pituitary masses: *craniopharyngioma*, Rathke's pouch remnant, metastasis.

Treatment and prognosis

Spontaneous recovery may occur; hormone replacement may be required. Expanding lesion with visual signs may require surgery.

References

De Bellis A, Ruocco G, Battaglia M et al. Immunological and clinical aspects of lymphocytic hypophysitis. Clin Sci. 2008;114:413–421

Lymphoma

Primary lymphoma of the central nervous system accounts for around 1% of all CNS tumors, but its incidence has increased in recent years, both among immunosuppressed (e.g., post-transplantation, *HIV/AIDS*) and apparently immunocompetent individuals, the latter for reasons that are not clear. Most lymphomas are of B cell lineage. Neurological features may occur with systemic and/or localized lymphomatous deposits of Hodgkin's or non-Hodgkin's types. *Intravascular lymphoma* may also occur.

Clinical features

- Parenchymal: headache, disturbance of higher cortical function, focal signs such as cranial nerve palsies
- CSF: lumbosacral radiculitis, *cauda equina syndrome*
- Subacute motor neuronopathy
- Sensory neuropathy, presumed *paraneoplastic syndrome*
- Ocular: vitreous lymphoma

Recognized predisposing immunodeficiency states/disease associations of lymphoma:

- HIV/AIDS
- Organ transplantation

- Wiskott–Aldrich syndrome
- Systemic lupus erythematosus
- Sarcoidosis
- Sjögren's syndrome
- Primary CNS angiitis
- Idiopathic thrombocytopenic purpura
- Ataxia telangiectasia
- Coeliac disease (gluten-sensitive enteropathy)
- Immunosuppressive therapy for a range of autoimmune disorders

Investigation

Bloods may show monoclonal gammopathy. Neuroimaging (CT/MRI) typically shows space-occupying lesion(s), which may be central in location (basal ganglia, corpus callosum) or in paraventricular sites, abutting ependymal surfaces; the latter are characteristic and may explain the capacity for CSF spread. Supratentorial lesions are more common than infratentorial, and may be symmetrical. Focal meningeal deposits may occur. Lymphomatous lesions usually enhance homogeneously with contrast. Lesions may shrink with steroids. Imaging features may be suggestive but are not diagnostic. CSF cytology/immunocytochemistry for lymphoma cells; CSF may have raised protein, reduced glucose. Biopsy is the diagnostic test. Consider HIV test if risk factors (following appropriate counseling).

Differential diagnosis

Other CNS mass lesions: *glioma, abscess, toxoplasmosis*, inflammatory mass lesions (e.g., *neurosarcoidosis*).

Treatment and prognosis

Lymphomatous mass lesions may shrink with empirical steroid therapy, giving a false sense of security ("inflammatory lesion"), for which reason biopsy of all mass lesions is advocated by some. Current therapy is usually methotrexate-based chemotherapy with or without whole brain radiotherapy, but the optimal treatment regimen remains undecided.

References

Abrey LE. Primary central nervous system lymphoma. Curr Opin Neurol. 2009;22: 675–680
Morris PG. Abrey LE. Therapeutic challenges in primary CNS lymphoma. Lancet Neurol. 2009;8:581–592
Peak S, DeAngelis L. Primary central nervous system lymphoma. In: Bernstein M, Berger MS eds. Neuro-Oncology. The Essentials. 2nd ed. New York: Thieme; 2008:359–366

Lysosomal storage disorders: overview

Conditions resulting from lysosomal enzyme disorders may be classified as follows:

- Mucopolysaccharidoses:
  - The mucopolysaccharidoses are hereditary lysosomal storage diseases in which enzyme deficiencies lead to pathological accumulation and urinary excretion of mucopolysaccharides. All varieties exhibit a period of normal development followed by regression of mental and motor function. The mucopolysaccharidoses may be classified as follows:

Type I:	Hurler's syndrome (I-H), Scheie's syndrome (I-S), and an overlap syndrome (I-H/S)
Type II:	Hunter's syndrome
Type III:	Sanfilippo disease (types A, B, C, D)
Type IV:	Morquio disease (types A and B)
Type VI:	Maroteaux–Lamy disease
Type VII:	Sly disease
Type VIII:	De Ferrante syndrome

  - Multiple sulfatase deficiency (Austin disease) may be included in the mucopolysaccharidosis group. Clinical phenotype is supplemented by enzymatic assay on cultured fibroblasts or white cells; urine analysis for mucopolysaccharides by thin layer chromatography may also be required: dermatan sulfate (Types I-H, I-S, II, VI, VII); heparan sulfate (Types I-H, I-S, II, III, IVB, VII); and keratan sulfate (Types IVA, IVB).
- Mucolipidoses:
  - Uncommon lysosomal storage diseases, inherited as autosomal recessive traits, in which both mucopolysaccharides and lipids accumulate in lysosomes, giving a clinical picture akin to both the mucopolysaccharidoses and the GM1 gangliosidoses. The four mucolipidoses may be classified as follows:

Type I:	Infantile sialidosis
Type II:	I-cell disease
Type III:	Pseudo-Hurler polydystrophy
Type IV:	Berman's mucolipidosis

  - Diagnosis is confirmed by enzymatic analysis of fibroblasts.
- Glycoproteinoses:
  - Galactosialidosis
  - *Fucosidosis*
  - α-, β-Mannosidosis
  - Aspartylglycosaminuria
  - Pycnodysostosis

- Sphingolipidoses:
  - GM1 gangliosidosis
  - GM2 gangliosidosis: Tay–Sachs, Sandhoff
  - *Metachromatic leukodystrophy*; Multiple sulfatase deficiency (Austin syndrome)
  - *Krabbe's disease*
  - *Fabry's disease*
  - *Niemann–Pick disease*, types A-C
  - Schindler's disease
  - Farber lipogranulomatosis
  - *Gaucher disease*, type I
- Neuronal ceroid lipofuscinoses:
  - Infantile: Santavuori–Haltia
  - Late infantile: Jansky–Bielschowsky
  - Juvenile: Vogt–Spielmeyer
  - Adult: *Kufs disease*
- Other lysosomal enzyme disorders:
  - Acid lipase deficiency (Wolman's disease, cholesterol ester storage disease)
  - Glycogenosis II (*Pompe's disease*)
  - Sialic acid storage disease (infantile form, Salla disease)
- *Aminoacidopathies*:
  - Cystinosis

Many of these are childhood disorders, but some may present in adult life.

References

Krivit W, Peters C, Shapiro EG et al. Bone marrow transplantation as effective treatment of central nervous system disease in globoid cell leukodystrophy, metachromatic leukodystrophy, adrenoleukodystrophy, mannosidosis, fucosidosis, aspartylglucosaminuria, Hurler, Maroteaux-Lamy, and Sly syndromes, and Gaucher disease type III. Curr Opin Neurol. 1999;12:167–176

Levade T, Graber D, Flurin V et al. Human β-mannosidase deficiency associated with peripheral neuropathy. Ann Neurol. 1994;35:116–119

Lyon G, Adams RD, Kolodny EH. Neurology of Hereditary Metabolic Diseases of Children. 2nd ed. New York: McGraw-Hill; 1996:151–165

Maertens P, Dyken PR. Storage diseases: neuronal ceroid-lipofuscinoses, lipidoses, glycogenoses, and leukodystrophies. In: Goetz CG, ed. Textbook of Clinical Neurology. 2nd ed. Philadelphia, PA: Saunders; 2003:601–628

Niemann S, Beck M, Seidel G, Spranger J, Vieregge P. Neurology of adult α-mannosidosis. J Neurol Neurosurg Psychiatry. 1996;61:116–117

Pastores GM, Kolodny EH. Lysosomal storage disorders. In: Noseworthy JH, ed. Neurological Therapeutics: Principles and Practice. London, UK: Dunitz; 2003:1484–1498

Platt FM, Walkley SU eds. Lysosomal Disorders of the Brain. Oxford, UK: Oxford University Press; 2004

Wraith JE. The mucopolysaccharidoses: a clinical review and guide to management. Arch Dis Childhood. 1995;72:263–267

M

Machado–Joseph disease (MJD) [OMIM#109150]

Azorean disease, spinocerebellar ataxia type 3

This autosomal dominant condition, which is common among those of Portuguese or Azorean descent, is characterized by progressive cerebellar ataxia, parkinsonism, dystonia, eyelid retraction with bulging eyes, and bulbar fasciculation. Considerable variation within and between families is noted. Classified phenotypically within the category of *autosomal dominant cerebellar ataxia (ADCA)* type I, its genetic basis has been shown to be mutation of a gene, ATXN3, at chromosome 14q32.1, with a trinucleotide (CAG) expansion (normal 13–44; abnormal 65–84 repeats) affecting expression of the ataxin 3 protein. Hence, Machado–Joseph disease is now classified as *spinocerebellar ataxia* (SCA) type 3, and one of the *trinucleotide repeat diseases*. This is the most common of the SCAs.

Reference

Rüb U, Brunt ER, Deller T. New insights into the pathoanatomy of spinocerebellar ataxia type 3 (Machado-Joseph disease). Curr Opin Neurol. 2008;21:111–116

Malaria

A diffuse encephalopathy, termed cerebral malaria, occurs in 0.5–1% of cases of infection with the protozoan parasite *Plasmodium falciparum*. The pathophysiology of cerebral malaria is uncertain, and is probably multifactorial, related to sequestration of parasitized erythrocytes in cerebral vessels, with cerebral ischemia, immune-mediated damage, intravascular thrombosis, cerebral hypoxia, and hypoglycemia. The role of raised intracranial pressure from cerebral edema is uncertain, since steroids have a detrimental effect on outcome.

Clinical features

- Prodromal systemic illness: fever, arthralgia, abdominal and muscle pain, tachypnea (duration hours to weeks).
- *Encephalopathy*: coma, fever, convulsions.
- *Headache*, meningism, delirium.
- Focal signs: aphasia, hemiparesis, ataxia, ophthalmoplegia.
- Chorea, tremor, rigidity.
- Bruxism.
- Postmalaria neurological syndromes (delayed or late neurological complications of malaria):
  - Relapse of cerebral malaria, 1–2 days after recovery: coma, with raised CSF protein +/– pleocytosis. Recovery may range from complete to poor.
  - Psychosis, encephalopathy, epileptic seizures, tremor, cerebellar ataxia following uncomplicated *P. vivax* or mixed infections, lasting days to weeks. Complete recovery is usual.

Investigation

Blood films, thick and thin, to look for parasites. Neuroimaging (CT/MRI) may show brain swelling, or be normal. CSF is often normal, but may show raised pressure, pleocytosis, raised protein, and raised lactate.

Differential diagnosis

- Bacterial *meningitis*.
- Viral encephalitides.
- *Heat stroke*.
- Babesiosis is a malaria-like illness caused by a protozoan parasite and transmitted by tick bite, occurring in northeastern and western USA.

Treatment and prognosis

Untreated, cerebral malaria is uniformly fatal within 72 h.

Treatment: IV quinine (high dose) or artemeter; 50% dextrose for hypoglycemia +/– anticonvulsants (phenobarbitone); steroids are not helpful, in fact deleterious. Prevention is by chemoprophylaxis during travel to endemic areas. Sequelae include hemiplegia, aphasia, cerebellar ataxia, cortical blindness, and psychosis.

References

Newton CRJC, Hien TT, White N. Cerebral malaria. J Neurol Neurosurg Psychiatry. 2000;69:433–441

White NJ. Cerebral malaria. Pract Neurol. 2004;4:20–29

Malignant hyperthermia [OMIM#145600]

King–Denborough syndrome

Malignant hyperthermia is a syndrome characterized by hyperthermia, *rhabdomyolysis*, and high mortality, reflecting an autosomal dominant inherited susceptibility to the effects of general anesthetic agents. Uncontrolled skeletal muscle metabolism related to malfunction of the sarcoplasmic reticulum calcium channel, or ryanodine receptor, is the ultimate cause in many cases, although other susceptibility loci have been defined.

Clinical features

During/following general anesthesia, especially with agents such as halothane, succinylcholine:

- Hyperthermia (hyperpyrexia), up to 43°C
- Metabolic acidosis
- Tachycardia
- Muscle rigidity, e.g., trismus
- Disseminated intravascular coagulation
- Coma, death

A family history of adverse reactions to general anesthetic agents may be discovered. Patients with *Duchenne muscular dystrophy* and *central core disease* (allelic with malignant hyperthermia) may be predisposed to develop malignant hyperthermia.

Investigation

Bloods show very high creatine kinase + other muscle enzymes; hyperkalemia, metabolic acidosis, renal failure. Urine may show myoglobinuria. Neurogenetic testing may show mutations in the ryanodine receptor gene on chromosome 19 (the central core disease phenotype, characterized by myopathy, is also associated with mutations in this gene).

Differential diagnosis

Neuroleptic malignant syndrome has similar clinical features but a slower onset.

Treatment and prognosis

Discontinue anesthesia. Supportive care: correction of acid-base disorder, ventilation if necessary, intravenous fluids, +/- steroids. Dantrolene is specific therapy since it uncouples excitation and contraction by preventing calcium release from the sarcoplasmic reticulum. Fatality may occur despite full supportive care. Screening of relatives of patients suffering malignant hyperthermia may be undertaken.

References

Carpenter D, Robinson RL, Quinnell RJ, et al. Genetic variation in RYR1 and malignant hyperthermia phenotypes. Br J Anaesth. 2009;103:538–548
Quane KA, Healy JM, Keating KE, et al. Mutations in the ryanodine receptor gene in central core disease and malignant hyperthermia. Nat Genet. 1993;5:51–55

Malingering

Malingering may be defined as the false and fraudulent simulation or exaggeration of physical or mental disease or defect, performed in order to obtain money or drugs, or to evade duty or criminal responsibility, or for other reasons that may be readily understood by an objective observer from the individual's circumstances, rather than from learning the individual's psychology. The last rider is included to preclude the need to establish whether or not the patient has insight into what is happening (i.e., are actions wilful, or involuntary). The exaggeration of neurological symptoms, or at least a lack of correlation between reported symptoms and what is observed clinically, is not uncommon in the neurology clinic. However, it may be better to label such phenomena as "neurologically unexplained symptoms" rather than use such a charged term as malingering.

Reference

Halligan PW, Bass C, Oakley DA. Malingering and Illness Deception. Oxford: Oxford University Press; 2003

Manganese poisoning, manganism

Manganese poisoning (manganism) was first described in miners of manganese ore who inhaled and ingested manganese particles, causing an early confusional–hallucinatory state with psychomotor excitement ("manganese madness"), or a later symmetrical *parkinsonian syndrome*, action tremor, impaired postural reflexes, with or without limb dystonia, corticobulbar (dysarthria) and corticospinal signs, and psychiatric features. Axial rigidity and dystonia similar to *Wilson's disease* may occur. Dystonic symptoms may respond to levodopa, but parkinsonian signs generally do not. On MR T_1-weighted imaging, high signal may be seen in the medial segment of the globus pallidus. Similar features may also occur following treatment with total parenteral nutrition or intravenous drugs contaminated with manganese. The neurotoxic effects of manganese have prompted speculations that this metal might be implicated in *non-Wilsonian hepatocerebral degeneration*.

References

Huang C-C, Chu N-S, Lu C-S, et al. Long-term progression in chronic manganism. Neurology. 1998;50:698–700
Pal PK, Samii A, Calne DB. Manganese neurotoxicity: a review of clinical features, imaging and pathology. Neurotoxicology. 1999;20:227–238

Marburg disease

Marburg described an acute monophasic demyelinating encephalitis leading to death within weeks to months. This may reflect a malignant monophasic presentation of *multiple sclerosis* or, possibly, the acute hemorrhagic leukoencephalitic subtype (Hurst's disease) of *acute disseminated encephalomyelitis (ADEM)*.

Reference

Marburg O. Die sogenannte "akute multiple sklerose" (encephalomyelitis periaxialis scleroticans). Jahrb Psychiat Neurol. 1906;27:211–312

Marchiafava–Bignami syndrome

Marchiafava–Bignami syndrome or disease is a rare neurological complication of chronic alcoholism characterized by lesions in the corpus callosum (and sometimes elsewhere, such as the putamen) causing an interhemispheric *disconnection syndrome* with combinations of apraxia, agraphia, and Balint's syndrome. Based on a literature review of reported cases, two clinicoradiological subtypes have been suggested: in type A, patients may present with coma or major impairment of consciousness, T_2-hyperintense swelling of the entire corpus callosum and have a poor prognosis; in type B, there is slight or no impairment of consciousness, partial callosal lesions on MRI, and favorable outcome. The role of thiamine treatment is controversial, concurrent thiamine deficiency is not uncommon in chronic alcoholics but whether this plays a pathogenetic role in the callosal lesions is not known. Recovery with or without thiamine supplements is recorded.

Reference

Heinrich A, Runge U, Khaw AV. Clinicoradiologic subtypes of Marchiafava-Bignami disease. J Neurol. 2004;251:1050–1059

Marfan syndrome [OMIM#154700]

Marfan syndrome is an autosomal dominant disorder of connective tissue producing a typical body habitus, first described by the French pediatrician Antonin Marfan in 1896. Abraham Lincoln and Sergei Rachmaninov are claimed as famous sufferers. Linkage to chromosome 15q21.1 led to the identification of the mutant gene encoding fibrillin-1. More than 100 mutations have now been identified.

Clinical features

- Neurological: young stroke (secondary to cardiac problems); arachnoid diverticula; *spontaneous intracranial hypotension* (low-pressure headache); subarachnoid hemorrhage.
- Family history of similarly affected relatives (although ca. 25% of cases result from new spontaneous mutations).
- Skeletal: tall stature; high-arched palate; arachnodactyly; scoliosis, chest wall deformity, acetabular protrusion, joint hypermobility, dural ectasia.
- Cardiac: aortic dilatation, aortic dissection; aortic regurgitation, mitral valve prolapsed.
- Ophthalmological: myopia, ectopia lentis.

Investigation

Diagnosis usually possible on clinical picture and family history. ECG, echocardiogram for cardiac status. Ophthalmology opinion, slit lamp examination for lens abnormalities. Neurogenetic testing for mutation in the fibrillin gene on chromosome 15.

Differential diagnosis

- Homocystinuria: may produce a similar body habitus but ectopia lentis does not occur; mental retardation would also be more suggestive of homocystinuria.

- Stickler's syndromes (hereditary arthro-ophthalmopathy), a multisystem disorder characterized by ocular features (retinal detachment, myopia, vitreoretinal degeneration), skeletal findings (craniofacial dysmorphology, such as midfacial hypoplasia, micrognathia, cleft palate), and cardiac features (mitral valve prolapse); at least three types, associated with mutations encoding collagen genes COL2A1, COL11A1, and COL11A2.

Treatment and prognosis

No specific treatment. Attention to cardiovascular status may reduce risk of cerebrovascular events.

References

Aburawi EH, O'Sullivan J, Hasan A. Marfan's syndrome: a review. Hosp Med. 2001; 62:153–157
Robinson PN, Arteaga-Solis E, Baldock C, et al. The molecular genetics of Marfan syndrome and related disorders. J Med Genet. 2006;43:769–787

Marin-Amat syndrome

Inverse Marcus Gunn phenomenon

This synkinetic syndrome consists of involuntary eyelid closure on jaw opening (cf. jaw winking, or the Marcus Gunn phenomenon, in which congenital ptosis improves with jaw opening, chewing, or swallowing). The Marin-Amat syndrome is thought to result from aberrant regeneration of the facial (VII) nerve, e.g., after a *Bell's palsy*.

Reference

Rana PVS, Wadia RS. The Marin-Amat syndrome: an unusual facial synkinesia. J Neurol Neurosurg Psychiatry. 1985;48:939–941

MASA syndrome [OMIM#303350]

This rare syndrome of mental retardation, aphasia, spastic paraplegia, and adducted thumbs results from mutations in the gene encoding the neural cell adhesion molecule L1, hence is allelic with one form of *hereditary spastic paraplegia* (SPG1).

Reference

Jouet M, Rosenthal A, Armstrong G, et al. X-linked spastic paraplegia (SPG1), MASA syndrome and X-linked hydrocephalus result from mutations in the L1 gene. Nat Genet. 1994;7: 402–407

Mast syndrome [OMIM#248900]

Hereditary spastic paraplegia (HSP) type 21

An autosomal recessive disorder observed in the Amish community, with onset in the second decade of life, consisting of spastic paraplegia, dysarthria, dementia, and athetosis, now categorized as a form of *hereditary spastic paraplegia* (SPG21) related to mutations in the ACP33 gene.

Reference

Cross HE, McKusick VA. The Mast syndrome: a recessively inherited form of presenile dementia with motor disturbances. Arch Neurol. 1967;16:1–13

McArdle's disease [OMIM#232600]

Glycogen storage disease (GSD) type V, myophosphorylase deficiency

Myophosphorylase deficiency is an inborn error of metabolism, one of the *glycogen storage disorders*, which typically presents in early adulthood with muscle cramps induced by intense exercise, reflecting a defect in the glycolytic pathway. With brief periods of rest, moderate levels of activity can be resumed without pain, the "second wind phenomenon," presumably due to a metabolic switch to fatty acid oxidation to provide muscle energy. Most cases are autosomal recessive but autosomal dominant transmission has been reported in a few families.

Clinical features

- Intense exercise induces muscle cramps, causing exercise intolerance, and sometimes leading to *rhabdomyolysis*, myoglobinuria, and acute renal failure.
- Permanent proximal muscle weakness may develop.

Investigation

Bloods show marked creatine kinase elevation during cramps, may also be elevated at rest; urea and creatinine to look for renal failure. Ischemic forearm exercise test: no accumulation of lactic acid as in normals; exaggerated increase in plasma ammonium. Urine may appear pink (wine-colored), due to presence of myoglobin. Neurogenetic testing of the gene encoding myophosphorylase: R49X is the most common mutation found. Phosphorus magnetic resonance spectroscopy: absence of normal fall in intramuscular pH with exercise, due to impaired lactate production. Muscle biopsy shows accumulation of glycogen, absence of phosphorylase staining.

Differential diagnosis

- Muscle phosphofructokinase deficiency (glycogen storage disease type VII, Tarui disease)
- Myoadenylate deaminase deficiency
- Carnitine palmitoyltransferase type II (CPT II) deficiency
- Lactate dehydrogenase (LDH) deficiency (glycogen storage disease type XI)
- Phosphoglycerate kinase deficiency (Bresolin's disease, glycogen storage disease type IX)
- Phosphoglycerate mutase deficiency (Tonin's disease, glycogen storage disease type X)

Treatment and prognosis

No specific treatment. Branched chain amino acid supplements have been advocated but there is no controlled evidence for efficacy.

References

Hilton-Jones D. McArdle's disease. Pract Neurol. 2001;1:122–125
McArdle B. Myopathy due to a defect in muscle glycogen breakdown. Clin Sci. 1951;10:13–33

McLeod's syndrome

Benign X-linked myopathy with acanthocytes

This form of *neuroacanthocytosis* is an X-linked condition in which there is a weak expression of the immunogenic Kell antigens on erythrocytes in the absence of the otherwise ubiquitous surface antigen Kx. Clinically this may occur in asymptomatic individuals (first detected in blood donors), but may also be associated with similar neurological features to choreoacanthocytosis, although lip-biting, dystonia and parkinsonism, and epileptic seizures are uncommon. There may be a myopathy, amyotrophy, cardiomyopathy (60%) with atrial fibrillation, and peripheral neuropathy. Acanthocytes may be found in a blood film, and there may be raised levels of serum creatine kinase. Female heterozygotes may develop CNS symptoms.

Reference

Danek A, Rubio JP, Rampoldi L, et al. McLeod neuroacanthocytosis: genotype and phenotype. Ann Neurol. 2001;50:755–764

Median neuropathy

The median nerve may be compressed or damaged in *carpal tunnel syndrome*, the most common example of the *entrapment neuropathies*, and between the heads of the pronator teres muscle (*pronator teres syndrome*); the *anterior interosseous syndrome* ensues when this branch is selectively compressed.

Clinical features

- Motor: Weakness of median innervated muscles: lateral lumbricals, opponens pollicis, abductor pollicis brevis, flexor pollicis brevis; long finger and wrist flexors, with the exception of flexor carpi ulnaris and third and fourth flexor digitorum profundis (innervated by the ulnar nerve); weak pronator teres, pronator quadratus; no reflex changes expected.
- Sensory: Loss on ventral aspect of hand, thumb, index, middle, and half of ring finger (palmar cutaneous branch); tips of dorsal aspects of thumb, index, middle, and half of ring finger (digital nerves).

Tinel and Phalen's signs may be evident in carpal tunnel compression of the median nerve

Investigation

Neurophysiology (EMG/NCS) may identify reduced amplitude CMAP in median innervated muscles and reduced or absent SNAPs. Local slowing of nerve conduction, with or without evidence of denervation and/or reinnervation in EMG of abductor pollicis brevis, are found in carpal tunnel syndrome. Abnormalities beyond median nerve territory may refute a diagnosis of mononeuropathy.

Differential diagnosis

Radiculopathy, *brachial plexopathy*: clinical features unlikely to be mistaken.

Treatment and prognosis

Of cause where possible.

References

McNamara B. Clinical anatomy of the median nerve. Adv Clin Neurosci Rehabil. 2003;2(6):19–20
Staal A, Van Gijn J, Spaans F. Mononeuropathies: Examination, Diagnosis and Treatment. London: W.B. Saunders; 1999:49–68

Medication-overuse headache

Analgesia-induced headache, medication-maintained headache

A number of medications prescribed for tension-type or *migraine* headache may, if used repeatedly, exacerbate or maintain *headache*, having previously been helpful. Examples include ergotamine and sumatriptan for migraine, narcotic analgesics, and probably most commonly mild analgesics (aspirin or paracetamol plus narcotic, caffeine, benzodiazepine, barbiturate) given for tension-type headache. The result is constant headache of waxing and waning severity, often causing nocturnal waking, briefly relieved by further doses of medication, hence creating a vicious cycle. Weaning from medication may be difficult since headache will inevitably worsen on cessation of medication; withdrawal may necessitate hospitalization.

References

Evers S, Marziniak M. Clinical features, pathophysiology, and treatment of medication-overuse headache. Lancet Neurol. 2010;9:391–401
Larner AJ. Not all morning headaches are due to brain tumours. Pract Neurol. 2009;9:80–84

Medulloblastoma

Medulloblastoma is the most commonly diagnosed primitive neuroectodermal tumor, typically occurring in the posterior fossa, in the pediatric age group, with slight male preponderance. It may be one feature of *incontinentia pigmenti*, of *nevoid basal cell carcinoma syndrome*, and of Turcot syndrome, a familial (autosomal dominant or recessive) polyposis coli syndrome associated with malignant neuroepithelial tumors such as glioblastoma and medulloblastoma.

Presentation of medulloblastoma is with raised intracranial pressure, with or without focal brainstem signs. Metastasis may occur throughout the craniospinal axis, and to sites outside the neuraxis such as bone, lymph nodes, lung, pleura, liver, and breast (poor prognostic feature). Treatment is by maximal surgical resection and radiotherapy, both local and to the rest of the neuraxis, with around 50% 10-year survival. Recurrences may be treated with multidrug chemotherapy regimes.

Reference

Garton GR, Schomberg PJ, Scheithauer BW, et al. Medulloblastoma: prognostic factors and outcome of treatment – review of Mayo Clinic experience. Mayo Clin Proc. 1990;65:1077–1086

Meige's syndrome

Meige's syndrome is an involuntary movement disorder affecting the face with *blepharospasm* and oromandibular dystonia, characterized as a cranial focal or segmental *dystonia*. Incomplete syndromes may occur.

Clinical features

- Blepharospasm
- Oromandibular dystonia: involuntary mouth opening, jaw clenching, tongue protrusion, dysarthria, dysphagia
- +/– Spasmodic dysphonia
- +/– Cervical dystonia

Investigation

Usually idiopathic: investigations may be undertaken to exclude other, secondary, causes of dystonia. Condition may sometimes be drug induced.

Differential diagnosis

Neuroacanthocytosis, Lesch–Nyhan syndrome, may produce involuntary facial dyskinesia, as may *tardive dyskinesia* syndromes.

Treatment and prognosis

Botulinum toxin injections may be used to control symptoms.

Reference

Tolosa ES, Klawans HL. Meige's disease: clinical form of facial convulsion, bilateral and medial. Arch Neurol. 1979;36:635–637

Melanoma

This tumor originating from neural crest tissues, most commonly skin, is usually malignant and may give rise to cerebral metastases, even when a primary origin may not be evident. Metastases are often multiple and may be associated with significant edema on neuroimaging. Familial cases of melanoma occur, and may be associated with cerebral or optic gliomas.

MELAS syndrome

The syndrome of mitochondrial encephalomyopathy, lactic acidosis, and stroke-like episodes (MELAS) is one of the classic phenotypes of *mitochondrial disease*, usually presenting in middle to late childhood although cases presenting in the fifth or sixth decade have been reported. Clinical heterogeneity is the norm. Various mutations of the mitochondrial genome have been associated with this clinical syndrome, with a particular "hot spot" at nucleotide 3243; the mitochondrial complex I ND5 gene may be another.

Clinical features

- Psychomotor delay, growth failure, short stature.
- Headaches (*migraine*), vomiting (sometimes exercise induced).
- Epileptic seizures: many types, including recurrent episodes of epilepsia partialis continua and generalized convulsive *status epilepticus*; nonconvulsive status has also been described
- Hemiparesis: may be alternating.
- Visual field defects: hemianopia, cortical blindness.
- Muscle weakness.
- +/− Sensorineural deafness.
- +/− Movement disorders: jaw tremor.
- +/− Renal tubular dysfunction.
- +/− Diabetes mellitus.

- +/− Cardiomyopathy.
- No ophthalmoplegia, retinal degeneration, cerebellar dysfunction, or myoclonus is reported in "pure" MELAS, but some overlap with the typical phenotypic features of *Kearns–Sayre syndrome* and *chronic progressive external ophthalmoplegia (CPEO)* may occur.

Investigation

Bloods: lactic acidosis, especially during periods of acute encephalopathy, but may be normal between episodes of decompensation; lactate/pyruvate (L/P) ratio may be helpful. Neuroimaging: CT/MRI brain shows patchy cortical abnormalities of ischemic origin, but not conforming to the boundaries of arterial territories; these changes may therefore represent focal areas of metabolic disorder. CSF may show elevated protein, lactate, lactate/pyruvate (L/P) ratio. Neurophysiology: EEG may show various abnormalities, but seldom focal changes. Muscle biopsy: histochemical studies for ragged red fibers (not always seen); electron microscopy; biochemical studies. Neurogenetics: most commonly associated with mutation at nucleotide 3243 (A3243G) of the mitochondrial genome (although mutations at this nucleotide may be associated with other phenotypes such as CPEO, *MERRF syndrome*, myopathy alone). Mutations at nucleotides 3250, 3271 also reported.

Differential diagnosis

- Childhood acute encephalopathy, seizures: Alpers disease, *Leigh's syndrome*
- Other mitochondrial multisystem disorders
- Adult: progressive, relapsing disorders, e.g., *multiple sclerosis.*

Treatment and prognosis

There is currently no specific treatment for MELAS: coenzyme Q10, idebenone may be tried. Acute deteriorations merit full supportive care, since marked recovery may occur. However, overall prognosis is poor.

References

Montagna P, Gallassi R, Medori R, et al. MELAS syndrome: characteristic migrainous and epileptic features and maternal transmission. Neurology. 1988;38:751–754
Pavlakis SG, Phillips PC, DiMauro S, DeVivo DC, Rowland LP. Mitochondrial myopathy, encephalopathy, lactic acidosis and strokelike episodes: a distinctive clinical syndrome. Ann Neurol. 1984;16:481–488

Sproule DM, Kaufmann P. Mitochondrial encephalopathy, lactic acidosis, and strokelike episodes: basic concepts, clinical phenotype, and therapeutic management of MELAS syndrome. Ann N Y Acad Sci. 2008;1142:133–158

Melioidosis

Infection with the Gram-negative organism *Buckholderia pseudomallei* is a common cause of sepsis in east Asia and northern Australia, to which individuals with diabetes mellitus are peculiarly susceptible. The cardinal clinical feature is abscess formation in the lung, liver, spleen, and skeletal muscle, but about 4% of Australian patients present with brainstem encephalitis.

Reference

White NJ. Melioidosis. Lancet. 2003;361:1715–1722

Melkersson–Rosenthal syndrome

Classical Melkersson–Rosenthal syndrome consists of the triad of:

- Recurrent facial palsy
- Orofacial swelling/edema
- Fissured tongue (lingua plicata)

Monosymptomatic presentations of this syndrome are common, e.g., as cheilitis granulomatosa. The condition is characterized histologically by noncaseating granulomata. No controlled trials have been performed in this rare syndrome, but steroids may be of benefit for the neurological features. Surgical intervention (facial nerve decompression) has also been reported.

Meningeal carcinomatosis

Carcinomatous meningitis, Leptomeningeal metastasis, Malignant meningitis

Dissemination of tumor cells throughout the leptomeninges may occur with metastatic spread of many different tumors but breast, lung, and gastrointestinal adenocarcinomas, melanoma, and leukemias are the most common causes. Clinically the condition may resemble infective meningitis.

Clinical features

- Headache, may reflect meningism and/or the development of hydrocephalus.
- Backache.
- Cranial nerve palsies, may be multiple: III, IV, VI, V, VII, VIII.
- Radiculopathy, especially of cauda equina.
- Confusional state.

Investigation

CSF is almost always abnormal: lymphocytic pleocytosis; cytology may show malignant cells (may need to repeat CSF analysis if clinical suspicion high but cytology initially negative); hypoglycorrhachia; raised pressure; elevated protein concentration; may also look for tumor markers in CSF, such as lactate dehydrogenase, β_2-microglobulin, and carcinoembryonic antigen. Neuroimaging (CT/MRI) may show hydrocephalus; MRI with gadolinium may show enhancement on surface of nerve roots, spinal cord; may be abnormal despite nondiagnostic CSF.

Differential diagnosis

Infective meningitis, particularly bacterial or fungal.

Treatment and prognosis

Systemic disease status should be considered in treatment decisions. Craniospinal irradiation, focused on most symptomatic areas may be appropriate, or intrathecal chemotherapy; e.g., methotrexate; ventricular catheter with subcutaneous (Ommaya) reservoir may be used for drug delivery. Combination therapy may be tried. Better response of leukemia/lymphoma as opposed to other solid tumors. Prognosis is generally poor.

Reference

Fischer-Williams M, Bosanquet FD, Daniel PM. Carcinomatosis of the meninges. Brain. 1955;78:42–58

Meningioma

Meningioma is a common tumor of the central nervous system, with a predilection for certain sites that determines the clinical features: olfactory groove, falx, parasagittal region, sphenoid bone, and spinal cord. They are more common in women, especially cord tumors, and may grow rapidly during pregnancy. Meningiomas may occur in the context of inherited syndromes, such as *neurofibromatosis*. Imaging studies generally show a well-circumscribed lesion, with a dural attachment, with usually uniform post-contrast enhancement. Generally, they are slow growing and benign tumors, amenable to complete resection with excellent prognosis, although recurrence may occur. Occasionally malignant meningioma with anaplastic features occurs, necessitating closer follow up. Similar clinical and radiological appearances may be reported with CNS lymphoma, *neurosarcoidosis* ("sarcoid tumor"), *Erdheim–Chester disease*, and *Rosai–Dorfman disease*.

Reference

Pamir MN, Black PM, Fahlbusch R. Meningiomas. A Comprehensive Text. Philadelphia, PA: W.B. Saunders; 2010

Meningitis: overview

Meningitis is inflammation of the meninges. This may have various etiologies, including:

- Infective:
  - Bacterial:
    - Meningococcus
    - Hemophilus influenza
    - Pneumococcus
    - Gram-negative organisms
    - Streptococcus
    - Listeria
    - *Tuberculosis*
    - Leptospirosis
  - Viral:
    - Enterovirus
    - Coxsackie
    - *HIV*
    - HSV (probably includes *Mollaret's meningitis*)
  - Fungal:
    - Cryptococcus
    - Coccidiodomycosis
    - Histoplasmosis
  - Parasitic:
    - Amoebae: *Naegleria, Acanthamoeba*
    - *Angiostrongyliasis* (eosinophilic meningitis)
- *Aseptic meningitis*
- Infiltrative: neoplastic, carcinomatous (malignant meningitis)
- Chemical: e.g., blood from *subarachnoid hemorrhage*, leak from epidermoid cysts, rupture of parasitic cysts (e.g., *echinococcosis*)

Clinical features

- Pace of onset may vary from acute to subacute; occasionally chronic.
- Clinical features are common to all types, but of variable severity, including:
  - Fever, malaise, irritability
  - Headache
  - Photophobia
  - Neck stiffness (nuchal rigidity): Kernig's sign, Brudzinski's sign
  - Vomiting
  - Confusion
  - +/− Epileptic seizures
  - +/− Systemic infection
  - +/− Focal signs: hemiparesis, aphasia

The typical signs may be absent in:
  - Very young and very old patients
  - Immunocompromised patients
  - Overwhelming infection

Index of clinical suspicion must be accordingly raised in these groups.

Investigation

Neuroimaging: to exclude subarachnoid hemorrhage, focal lesions (e.g., *abscess*, *subdural empyema*). CSF for opening pressure, cell count, protein, glucose, Gram stain, Ziehl–Nielsen stain, culture; Indian ink stain, cryptococcal antigen may be appropriate in some situations. CSF PCR for viral agents.

Differential diagnosis

- Infective:
  - *Encephalitis* (may coexist with meningitis as meningoencephalitis)
  - Cerebral abscess
  - Subdural empyema
  - Septicemia
- Noninfective:
  - Inflammatory disorders: Systemic lupus erythematosus, Behçet's disease, neurosarcoidosis, primary angiitis of the CNS (PACNS), Vogt–Koyanagi–Harada syndrome
  - Subarachnoid hemorrhage
  - Migraine
  - Drug-induced meningitis
  - Brain tumor

Treatment and prognosis

Of cause, when possible. However, prompt administration of "best guess" antibiotics before a microbiological diagnosis is made may be life-saving in some forms of bacterial meningitis (e.g., meningococcal). Antimicrobial therapy appropriate for viruses, fungi, and parasites. Supportive care; hydration, ventilation. Antiepileptic drugs if seizures occur; prophylaxis may be appropriate in some forms of bacterial meningitis. Steroids also recommended in certain instances. Mortality highest in infants and elderly.

References

Anderson M. Meningitis. In: Donaghy M, ed. Brain's Diseases of the Nervous System. 11th ed. Oxford: OUP; 2001:1097–1116

Logan SAE, MacMahon E. Viral meningitis. BMJ. 2008;336:36–40

Tunkel AR. Bacterial Meningitis. Philadelphia, PA: Lippincott Williams & Wilkins; 2001

Tunkel AR, Hartman BJ, Kaplan SL, et al. Practical guidelines for the management of bacterial meningitis. Clin Infect Dis. 2004;39:1267–1284

Meningococcal disease

The Gram-negative aerobic diplococci of *Neisseria meningitidis* may be classified into several serogroups according to immunological reactivity of capsular polysaccharides (e.g., A, B, C, W, Y). The human nasopharynx is the only natural reservoir, from which organisms are transmitted by aerosol or secretions. Recognized risk factors for developing disease include:

- Immunodeficiency (of antibody-dependent, complement-mediated immune lysis), e.g., asplenia, properdin deficiency, terminal complement component deficiency; possibly HIV infection.
- Low socioeconomic status (possibly related to crowding).
- Exposure (active or passive) to tobacco smoke.
- Crowded living conditions, e.g., military recruits, university students.

Clinical features

Infection with *N. meningitidis* may produce various clinical syndromes:

- Meningococcal meningitis
- Meningococcal bacteremia
- Meningococcemia: purpura fulminans, Waterhouse–Friederichsen syndrome

- Respiratory tract infection:
  - Pneumonia
  - Epiglottitis
  - Otitis media
- Focal infection (uncommon):
  - Conjunctivitis
  - Septic arthritis
  - Urethritis
  - Purulent pericarditis
- Chronic meningococcemia: intermittent fever, rash, arthralgia, headache

Investigation

Bloods: serology with ELISA. CSF: Gram-negative diplococci; PCR. Culture of the organism from blood, CSF; culture from the nasopharynx is nonspecific since many individuals harbor the organism as a commensal.

Differential diagnosis

Other causes of *meningitis* (e.g., *Streptococcus pneumoniae*), pneumonia.

Treatment and prognosis

Antibiotics: most strains are sensitive to penicillin, but because the differential diagnosis of meningitis includes *Streptococcus pneumoniae*, which is often penicillin-resistant, cephalosporins and vancomycin are often used. In epidemics in developing countries, treatment with a single intramuscular dose of chloramphenicol in an oily suspension has been effective. Treatment should be initiated early: if the index of clinical suspicion for meningococcal meningitis is high (e.g., child with fever and purpuric rash), then "best guess" antibiotics should be administered immediately, prior to hospital transfer and further investigations. Household contacts of index cases are those at highest additional risk of developing disease, and should receive chemoprophylaxis as soon as possible, e.g., with rifampicin, ciprofloxacin. Despite treatment with appropriate antibiotics and optimal medical care, there is still a substantial mortality (ca. 10%). Up to 20% of survivors have sequelae such as hearing loss, neurological disability, or loss of limb(s). Vaccines with efficacy against various serogroups are available for at-risk populations.

Reference

Rosenstein NE, Perkins BA, Stephens DS, Popovic T, Hughes JM. Meningococcal disease. N Engl J Med. 2001;344:1378–1388

Meralgia paresthetica

Bernhardt–Roth syndrome, lateral femoral cutaneous neuropathy

Sensory impairment in the distribution of the lateral cutaneous nerve of the thigh, or lateral femoral cutaneous nerve, is one of the most common forms of *entrapment neuropathy*, producing the syndrome of meralgia paresthetica. Arising from the L2–3 spinal nerves, this cutaneous nerve passes under the lateral border of the inguinal ligament and supplies a variable area on the anterolateral thigh. Entrapment is most commonly at the level of the inguinal ligament although occasionally retroperitoneal pathology may injure the nerve. Surgical trauma is the most common identified precipitant, although most cases are idiopathic. Obesity may be a risk factor.

Clinical features

- Sensory: pain, numbness, crawling sensation, over anterolateral thigh. Usually unilateral but on occasion symptoms are bilateral.
- Motor: no features.

Investigation

Diagnosis is clinical. EMG/NCS may be used in atypical cases to detect involvement of muscles which would refute the diagnosis of meralgia paresthetica. Conduction studies may be useful in diagnosis, more so than SNAP amplitudes.

Differential diagnosis

Femoral neuropathy, lumbosacral plexopathy, L2 radiculopathy.

Treatment and prognosis

Reassurance is often sufficient. No specific treatment; symptomatic treatment of sensory features (e.g., pregabalin, lidocaine patch, TENS) may be tried.

References

Larner AJ. Meralgia paraesthetica in the general neurology clinic: 7-year survey [Abstract P1527]. Eur J Neurol. 2008;15(suppl 3):167–168
Seror P, Seror R. Meralgia paraesthetica: clinical and electrophysiological diagnosis in 120 cases. Muscle Nerve. 2006;33:650–654

MERRF syndrome

Fukuhara syndrome

The syndrome of myoclonic epilepsy and ragged red fibers (MERRF) is one of the classic phenotypes of *mitochondrial disease*, with onset usually in childhood or adolescence (before 20 years of age). It results from point mutations in the mitochondrial genome, most commonly at nucleotide 8344 (hence allelic with *NARP syndrome*).

Clinical features

- Epileptic seizures: myoclonic
- Cerebellar dysfunction
- Action-induced polymyoclonus
- Psychomotor delay, growth failure, short stature
- +/− Sensorineural deafness
- +/− Weakness, hypotonia (myopathy)
- No ophthalmoplegia, retinal degeneration, cortical blindness, hemiparesis, renal tubular dysfunction, diabetes mellitus

Investigation

Bloods: lactic acidosis, especially during periods of acute encephalopathy, but may be normal between episodes of decompensation; lactate/pyruvate (L/P) ratio may be helpful. Neuroimaging (CT/MRI) brain shows patchy cortical abnormalities of ischemic origin, not conforming to the boundaries of arterial territories; leukoencephalopathy. CSF: elevated protein, lactate; lactate/pyruvate (L/P) ratio. Muscle biopsy: histochemical studies for ragged red fibers; electron microscopy; biochemical studies. Neurogenetics: most commonly associated with mutation at nucleotide 8344 (A8344G) of the mitochondrial genome.

Differential diagnosis

Other causes of *progressive myoclonus epilepsy*, mitochondrial disease

Treatment and prognosis

No specific treatment; symptomatic treatment of seizures (valproate, clonazepam). Coenzyme Q10, riboflavin may be tried.

Reference

DiMauro S, Hirano M, Kaufmann P, et al. Clinical features and genetics of myoclonic epilepsy with ragged red fibres. Adv Neurol. 2002;89:217–229

Metabolic storage disorders: overview

With increasingly sophisticated definition of the metabolic disturbance lead-ing to substrate accumulation, this categorization is less used nowadays. A common consequence of inborn errors of metabolism is dysmorphism, with characteristic ("storage") facies, organomegaly (especially hepatosplenom-egaly), and sometimes bone changes (dysostosis multiplex). Within the cate-gory of metabolic storage diseases may be included:

- *Lysosomal storage disorders*:
  - Mucopolysaccharidoses
  - Mucolipidoses
  - Glycoproteinoses
  - Sphingolipidoses
  - Neuronal ceroid lipofuscinoses
  - Other lysosomal enzyme disorders: Wolman's disease, Pompe's disease
- Peroxisomal disorders:
  - Zellweger syndrome
  - Pseudo–Zellweger syndrome
  - Neonatal adrenoleukodystrophy
  - Infantile *Refsum's disease*
  - Rhizomelic chondrodysplasia punctata
- *Mitochondrial disease*:
  - Electron transport chain defects
  - Pyruvate dehydrogenase (PDH) deficiency
  - *Glutaric aciduria* type II
- Other biosynthetic defects:
  - Smith–Lemli–Opitz syndrome
  - *Homocystinuria*
  - Menkes' disease
  - Sjögren–Larsson syndrome

Because of the lack of dysmorphic features, *glycogen storage disorders* are not typically included in this rubric.

Metachromatic leukodystrophy (MLD)

Arylsulfatase A deficiency

An autosomal recessive disease characterized biochemically by an accumula-tion of sulfatides (sulfogalactosylceramides), classically due to deficiency of the lysosomal hydrolase arylsulfatase A (also known as cerebroside sulfate sulfatase) associated with mutations in the arylsulfatase A gene on chromo-some 22q13.31 [OMIM#250100]. The normal catalytic function of arylsulfatase A requires a sphingolipid activator protein saposin B, deficiency of which may be associated with mutations in the prosaposin gene on chromosome 10q21

[OMIM#249900]. Genetic and clinical heterogeneity (age of onset, phenotype) is a feature of MLD, but CNS and PNS demyelination is invariable.

Clinical features

Different forms are recognized according to age at onset, itself inversely correlated with residual enzyme activity:

- Late infantile, classical, MLD (Greenfield's disease): onset 12–30 months
  - Difficulty walking; flaccid paresis with absent tendon reflexes (neuropathy).
  - Mental regression, dysarthria.
  - Bulbar, pseudobulbar palsy; optic atrophy, quadriparesis.
  - Epileptic seizures (late).
- Juvenile MLD (Scholz's disease): onset 3–10 years
  - Similar to late infantile MLD, but emotional disturbance or dementia (e.g., declining school performance) may be initial symptom; gait disorder, tremor, nystagmus (cerebellar, upper motor neurone).
- Adult MLD: onset around 30 years
  - Psychiatric disorder that may be misdiagnosed as schizophrenia or manic-depressive disease; progressive dementia; truncal ataxia, hyperreflexia, epileptic seizures; no clinical signs of peripheral neuropathy.

If there are additional sulfatase deficiencies (as in Austin disease), symptoms relevant to them may be evident, e.g., ichthyosis, mucopolysaccharidosis.

Investigation

Bloods: standard hematology and biochemistry are normal. Reduced arylsulfatase A activity in leukocytes or fibroblasts found in the classical form; pseudodeficiency is an autosomal recessive trait in which enzyme activity is diminished in the absence of neurological disease. Normal activity may be seen in some cases of MLD in which there is a genetic deficiency of sulfatide activator protein (sphingolipid activator protein B, saposin B). Neuroimaging (CT/MRI) shows diffuse demyelination, bilateral, symmetrical; may temporarily be limited to periventricular regions. Urine shows sulfatiduria. CSF may show elevated protein. Neurophysiology: EMG/NCS shows slowed nerve conduction velocities; VER and SSEP may be delayed in adult form. Pathology: metachromasia of stored substances = sulfatides: brain, peripheral nerve (segmental demyelination and remyelination), liver, kidney, spleen. Neurogenetic testing: numerous mutations in the arylsulfatase A gene on chromosome 22 are described (hence biochemical studies remain important for diagnosis); prosaposin mutations in patients with normal arylsulfatase A activity (allelic to saposin C deficiency causing *Gaucher's disease*).

Differential diagnosis

- Psychiatric features may resemble schizophrenia.
- Neuroimaging features: other *leukodystrophies*.
- Adult onset disease may be mistaken for *multiple sclerosis* if ataxia prominent.

Treatment and prognosis

No specific treatment; bone marrow transplantation has been tried without conspicuous success. Natural history is of slow but relentless progression to death: infantile form within about 5 years, juvenile form may live 20 years or more.

References

Gieselmann V. Metachromatic leukodystrophy: genetics, pathogenesis and therapeutic options. Acta Paediatr Suppl. 2008;97:15–21
Polten A, Fluharty AL, Fluharty CB, et al. Molecular basis of different forms of metachromatic leukodystrophy. N Engl J Med. 1991;324:18–22

Metastatic disease and the nervous system: overview

Metastasis must be considered in any patient with known malignancy developing new neurological symptoms and in the differential diagnosis of any cerebral mass lesion or spinal root or cord compression; metastasis to vertebral column, with resultant spinal root or cord compression, is more common than metastasis to the spinal cord per se.

- Common sources of brain metastases include:
  - Lung
  - Breast
  - Melanoma
  - Unknown
- Common sources of vertebral metastases include:
  - Lung
  - Breast
  - Thyroid
  - Prostate

Spread of malignancy along CSF pathways may present with malignant meningitis (*meningeal carcinomatosis*) or root infiltration

Clinical features

- Cerebral metastasis may present with
  - Epileptic seizures: focal +/− secondary generalization
  - Focal signs: weakness, ataxia, sensory features, behavioral change
  - Headache: if raised intracranial pressure
- Vertebral column metastasis may present with
  - Focal signs: weakness, sensory features suggestive of intramedullary myelopathy; acute cord compression

Investigation

Neuroimaging (CT/MRI) may be diagnostic. Biopsy may sometimes be required for brain lesions, especially if isolated with no known primary. Search for a primary tumor may be necessary, often with a focus on the lungs.

Differential diagnosis

- Other cranial/spinal mass lesions: *tumor, abscess, hematoma, cysts, lymphoma*
- Other causes of spinal root/cord compression: especially spondylotic radiculopathy, myelopathy

Treatment and prognosis

Short-term symptomatic treatment with steroids may be indicated, +/− symptomatic treatment for headache, emesis. Local radiotherapy, especially in context of cord compression, single brain metastasis. Whole brain irradiation for multiple metastases. Systemic chemotherapy for multiple metastases of chemoresponsive tumor (e.g., breast, small-cell lung tumor, germ cell tumors). Surgery probably not indicated if active cancer elsewhere; no improvement in survival.

Reference

DeAngelsi LM, Posner JB. Neurologic Complications of Cancer. 2nd ed. New York: Oxford University Press; 2009

Methanol poisoning

Methanol (methyl alcohol) poisoning produces drowsiness, headache, nausea, vomiting, visual blurring, dyspnea, and cyanosis; it may progress to delirium and coma. Blindness is the most common symptom and may persist after recovery from acute intoxication: there is reduced visual acuity, central scotoma, and constriction of the peripheral fields. Methanol may produce a toxic parkinsonism. Treatment of acute poisoning is by means of gastric lavage, administration of alkali, and ethanol (antagonizes oxidation of methanol to formaldehyde and formic acid in the liver).

Reference

Henderson WR, Brubacher J. Methanol and ethylene glycol poisoning: a case study and review of current literature. Can J Emer Med Care. 2002;4:34–40

Migraine

The precise pathophysiology of migraine is still debated, but probably involves an alteration of blood flow in the cerebral vessels, such that intracranial vessels are constricted and extracranial vessels are dilated; a wave of spreading electrical depression over the cortex, first observed in animals by Leao in 1944, may be significant in the genesis of the progressive focal neurological signs. A family history of migraine is common, suggesting genetic risk factors, and in one variant (familial hemiplegic migraine) deterministic mutant genes have been identified. Migraine is more common in women, suggesting a role for hormonal factors.

Clinical features

A number of clinical variants of migraine are described. Generally, migraine is characterized by an episodic headache, usually severe, often but not exclusively unilateral (cf. *cluster headache*), throbbing or pulsating in character, often accompanied by nausea and vomiting, such that the patient wishes to lie still (cf. cluster headache) and rest, avoiding light (photophobia) and noise (phonophobia) and smells (osmophobia). Headache often improves with sleep.

- Migraine with aura: preceded by visual disturbances: flashing spots, lines, jagged edges (fortification spectra, teichopsia), for perhaps 20–30 min; followed by headache, with gradual build up in intensity. Tingling, sensory complaints, or heaviness on one side of the face or body are not uncommon; this is not the same as familial hemiplegic migraine.
- Migraine without aura: no preceding visual disturbance.
- Migraine aura without headache (= migraine equivalent, acephalgic migraine): an aura not followed by headache.
- Familial hemiplegic migraine (FHM), cerebellar migraine: transient hemiparesis associated with migraine headache; associated mutations have been defined, in brain-specific neuronal voltage-gated calcium channel α_1-subunit gene (CACNA1A) at 19q13.1 [OMIM#141500] (hence one of the *channelopathies*, allelic with *spinocerebellar ataxia* type 6 and *episodic ataxia* type 2), in ATP1A2 at 1q23 [OMIM#602481], and in the SCN1A gene at 2q24 [OMIM#609634] allelic with one form of *generalized epilepsy with febrile seizures* plus (GEFS+).

- Basilar (artery) migraine: bilateral visual disturbances followed by paresthesia of lips, hands, and feet, dysarthria and diplopia, occipital headache, +/− impairment of consciousness. Features thought suggestive of posterior circulation ischemia.
- Status migrainosus: recurrent episodes of migraine headache without recovery from previous episode; rare.
- Abdominal migraine: cyclical vomiting of childhood may be a migraine equivalent.
- Retinal migraine: occurrence of photopsia, monocular field defects (altitudinal) and blindness, occurring with migraine headache.
- Facial migraine: sometimes referred to as lower half migraine, Sluder's neuralgia, sphenopalatine (ganglion) neuralgia, carotidynia: episodic pain of ear, nose, neck.
- Migrainous infarction, migrainous stroke: may be defined as a stroke occurring in a patient with a past medical history of migraine; no other identified cause for stroke; cortical infarction, stroke occurring in the context of a migraine headache; or an aura lasting >7 days. Migraine per se may be a risk factor for stroke, but not of as a great a magnitude as other modifiable factors: smoking and oral contraceptive pill use.

Ophthalmoplegic migraine is now better characterized as a focal variant of demyelinating neuropathy.

Migraine may sometimes occur in the context of another neurological disorder such as *CADASIL* or *mitochondrial disease*, or with an underlying disorder of blood clotting.

Investigation

Diagnosis is essentially clinical, i.e., based on history and examination. Neuroimaging (CT/MRI) has no diagnostic role, but may be used to rule out other possibilities in the differential, e.g., *subarachnoid hemorrhage*. Previous suggestions that consistently unilateral headaches might be associated with an underlying *arteriovenous malformation* have not been borne out by systematic studies. CSF may be performed on occasion to exclude *meningitis*. Neurogenetic testing in familial hemiplegic migraine may be indicated.

Differential diagnosis

- Other types of *headache*: cluster headache, episodic tension-type headache, *medication overuse headache*; subarachnoid hemorrhage, meningitis.
- Migraine without headache may be erroneously labeled as *transient ischemic attack* (*TIA*).

Treatment and prognosis

- Identify/avoid trigger factors: sleep deprivation, dietary triggers; stop smoking.
- Acute therapy: triptans (contraindicated in basilar migraine), aspirin, non-steroidal anti-inflammatory agents may be used. There is potential for excess triptan consumption to lead to medication overuse headache. Vomiting and impaired gastrointestinal motility may reduce absorption of oral medication; concurrent use of an antiemetic, or administration by parenteral route (nasal spray, injection) may be required.
- Prophylactic therapy: options include propranolol, topiramate, amitriptyline, sodium valproate, pizotifen, cyproheptadine, methysergide (6 months only, monitor for pleuroperitoneal fibrosis).
- In women, headaches may be more evident at times of hormonal change, e.g., menarche, menopause, oral contraceptive pill use; may improve or remit during pregnancy.
- Rarely a permanent hemiparesis develops in FHM, or as a consequence of migrainous stroke.

References

Antonaci F, Dumitrache C, De Cillis I, Allena M. A review of current European treatment guidelines for migraine. J Headache Pain. 2010;11:13–19

De Vries B, Frants RR, Ferrari MD, van den Maagdenberg AM. Molecular genetics of migraine. Hum Genet. 2009;126:115–132

Evers S, Afra J, Frese A, et al. EFNS guideline on the drug treatment of migraine – revised report of an EFNS task force. Eur J Neurol. 2009;16:968–981

Lane R, Davies P. Migraine. New York: Taylor & Francis; 2006

Snow V, Weiss K, Wall EM, et al. Pharmacologic management of acute attacks of migraine and prevention of migraine headache. Ann Intern Med. 2002;137:840–849

Migralepsy

This term has sometimes been used to describe the phenomenon of *migraine* with aura triggering epileptic seizures. Although migraine and *epilepsy* are associated (i.e., comorbid), a definite temporal association between seizures and migraine aura is rare.

Reference

Marks DA, Ehrenberg BL. Migraine-related seizures in adults with epilepsy, with EEG correlation. Neurology. 1993;43:2476–2483

Mild cognitive impairment (MCI)

In the continuum between normal and abnormal cognitive function, there are individuals with cognitive impairment with respect to others matched for age and education, who are destined to develop *dementia* but are not yet demented; these individuals may be labeled as having mild cognitive impairment (MCI). Intervention at this stage of illness might prevent progression to dementia. However, modern diagnostic criteria for *Alzheimer's disease (AD)* discard the category of MCI in favor of an earlier, biologically based, diagnosis of AD. The annual conversion rate of MCI to dementia may be less than previously thought.

Clinical features

Suggested clinical criteria for MCI are:

- Memory complaint (preferably corroborated by an informant)
- Objective memory impairment
- Intact general cognition
- Essentially preserved activities of daily living
- Not demented

MCI is heterogeneous. Distinctions may be drawn between:

- Amnestic MCI, thought to be a harbinger of AD.
- Multiple domain MCI: may reflect AD, *vascular dementia*, or normal aging.
- Single non-memory domain MCI: may reflect vascular dementia, *dementia with Lewy bodies, frontotemporal lobar degeneration* (e.g., *progressive nonfluent aphasia*).

Investigation

As for dementia syndromes, MCI destined to become AD may show selective hippocampal shrinkage.

Differential diagnosis

Besides dementia syndromes, MCI patients may have affective disorder (e.g., depression) or normal aging.

Treatment and prognosis

No specific treatment yet known. Cholinesterase inhibitors do not appreciably slow conversion rate. Risk factors for known dementia syndromes may be addressed.

References

Mitchell AJ, Shiri-Feshki M. Rate of progression of mild cognitive impairment to dementia – meta-analysis of 41 robust inception cohort studies. Acta Psychiatr Scand. 2009;119:252–265
Petersen RC, ed. Mild Cognitive Impairment. Aging to Alzheimer's disease. Oxford: Oxford University Press; 2003
Portet F, Ousset PJ, Visser PJ, et al. Mild cognitive impairment (MCI) in medical practice: a critical review of the concept and new diagnostic procedure. Report of the MCI Working Group of the European Consortium on Alzheimer's disease. J Neurol Neurosurg Psychiatry. 2006;77:714–718

Miller Fisher syndrome (MFS)

Miller Fisher syndrome is a monophasic inflammatory disorder, thought to be a variant of *Guillain–Barré syndrome (GBS)*, which may be associated with the presence of antibodies directed against the ganglioside GQ1b. There may be preceding respiratory or gastrointestinal (*Campylobacter*) infection. Whether the disorder has a central, peripheral or combined origin has been debated. It may form a clinical continuum with *Bickerstaff's brainstem encephalitis*.

Clinical features

- Ophthalmoplegia, causing diplopia; may progress to complete immobilization of the eyes; +/− ptosis, pupillary sphincter paralysis.
- Ataxia: gait > limb clumsiness.
- Areflexia.
- +/− Peripheral neuropathy; paresthesia; oropharyngeal, facial weakness; dysautonomia.

Investigation

Bloods: Anti-GQ1b antibody seems to correlate with the presence of ophthalmoplegia. CSF protein is elevated in the majority of cases. Neurophysiology (EMG/NCS): most studies show demyelinating peripheral neuropathy, with reduced sensory nerve action potential amplitudes and lesser degrees of slowing. Neuroimaging: cases with CT/MRI evidence of central lesions occur, but whether these are necessary for the clinical signs is less certain.

Differential diagnosis

- Guillain–Barré syndrome.
- Bickerstaff's brainstem encephalitis (BBE): exact relationship uncertain, both may be associated with anti-GQ1b antibody. Purists would say that BBE presents with drowsiness, which is never a feature of MFS.

- *Botulism.*
- Diphtheritic neuropathy.

Treatment and prognosis

By analogy with GBS, treatment with plasma exchange or intravenous immunoglobulin is often given. Most patients recover, although relapsing cases have been described.

References

Fisher M. An unusual variant of acute idiopathic polyneuritis (syndrome of ophthalmoplegia, ataxia, and areflexia). N Engl J Med. 1956;255:57–65
Lo YL. Clinical and immunological spectrum of the Miller Fisher syndrome. Muscle Nerve. 2007;36:615–627
Schabet M. Miller Fisher syndrome. Pract Neurol. 2009;9:289–291

Mills' syndrome, Mills' variant

Mills (1900) described a slowly progressive ascending or descending hemiplegia, which was ascribed to a primary degeneration of the corticospinal pyramidal pathways. The entity has remained controversial, since other disease processes might produce a similar clinical picture, e.g., brain tumor, cervical spine, or cervico-occipital abnormalities, pontine lesions, small lacunar infarcts, and multiple sclerosis. In more recent times, it has been suggested that Mills' syndrome is in fact a variant of *primary lateral sclerosis*, itself a form of *motor neurone disease*, characterized by upper motor neurone signs only. Concurrent *frontotemporal lobar degeneration* has been described, supporting this conceptualization.

References

Gastaut J-L, Bartolomei F. Mills' syndrome: ascending (or descending) progressive hemiplegia: a hemiplegic form of primary lateral sclerosis? J Neurol Neurosurg Psychiatry. 1994;57:1280–1281
Larner AJ, Gardner-Thorpe C. Mills syndrome with dementia. Eur Neurol J. 2011:in press.

Mitochondrial disease: overview

Mitochondrial cytopathies, mitochondriopathies

Diseases due to defects in the function of the mitochondrial electron transport chain show marked clinical heterogeneity. Their inheritance may be autosomal recessive, autosomal dominant, X-linked, or mitochondrial (matrilineal), depending on whether they result from mutations in nuclear genes that encode mitochondrial respiratory chain proteins, or in the small mitochondrial DNA (mtDNA) genome. They may manifest as multisystem diseases, affecting both central and peripheral nervous systems. Whether these should be "lumped" or "split" is still a subject of debate; certain it is that overlap between syndromes occurs. Despite this heterogeneity, some reasonably distinct syndromes have been described:

- *Chronic progressive external ophthalmoplegia (CPEO)*
- *Kearns–Sayre syndrome (KSS)*
- *Leber's hereditary optic neuropathy (LHON)*
- Leigh's disease, Leigh's syndrome
- *MELAS syndrome*
- *MERRF syndrome*
- *NARP syndrome*

Mitochondrial dysfunction has also been implicated in other neurodegenerative diseases such as Parkinson's disease, Alzheimer's disease, Huntington's disease, and motor neurone disease. A number of conditions have now been shown to be due to mutations in nuclear encoded mitochondrial non-respiratory chain proteins, e.g., Friedreich's ataxia, Wilson's disease, hereditary spastic paraplegia linked to chromosome 16 (paraplegin mutations), Mohr–Tranebjaerg syndrome. These disorders could also legitimately be labeled "mitochondrial diseases." To these might also be added:

- Launois-Bensaude disease (Madelung's disease, *multiple symmetric lipomatosis*)
- Luft disease
- Mitochondrial neurogastrointestinal encephalopathy (MNGIE) syndrome
- Wolfram syndrome

Clinical features

The clinical phenotype is very heterogeneous, but features that should alert the clinician to the possibility of mitochondrial disease include the following.

- Common features:
  - Persistent lactic acidosis
  - Myopathy (weakness, hypotonia)
  - Failure to thrive, short stature
  - Psychomotor retardation, dementia
  - Epileptic seizures
- Other neurological features often encountered:
  - Ophthalmoplegia
  - Retinal pigmentary degeneration
  - Cerebellar ataxia
  - Myoclonus
  - Sensorineural hearing loss

- Stroke-like episodes
- Peripheral neuropathy
- Cognitive impairment
- Raised CSF protein
• Other non-neurological features often encountered:
  - Cardiomyopathy
  - Diabetes mellitus
  - Renal tubular dysfunction, Fanconi syndrome
  - Respiratory abnormalities (tachypnea, periodic apnea)
  - Gastrointestinal hypomotility, pseudo-obstruction
  - Hypoparathyroidism
  - Lipomatosis

Investigation

Bloods: persistent lactic acidosis (but beware of false positives with this test; CSF is more reliable). Neuroimaging: MR may show cerebellar atrophy, strokes not conforming to vascular territories. Neurophysiology: EEG may show a range of abnormalities; SSEP may show cortical hyperexcitability; abnormal ERGs. CSF may show increased protein, lactate. Muscle biopsy: histochemical studies with the Gomori trichrome stain may show subsarcolemmal aggregations of mitochondria as ragged red fibers (although these may occur in some other myopathies, and with normal aging); fibers deficient in cytochrome oxidase staining may also be seen. Electron microscopy may show abnormal mitochondrial cristae with paracrystalline inclusions of variable morphology. Extraction of mitochondria may allow biochemical studies showing deficient respiratory chain function. Neurogenetic testing for deletions and point mutations of mitochondrial DNA may be performed according to phenotype; if negative but suspicion for a mitochondrial disease is high, muscle mtDNA analysis may be performed.

Differential diagnosis

Although the gestalt may make diagnosis obvious, it may be necessary, dependent upon the clinical presentation, to consider other causes of young stroke, myopathy, ophthalmoplegia, and seizures. Other hereditary metabolic disorders may be considered.

Treatment and prognosis

There is currently no specific treatment for mitochondrial diseases. Symptomatic and supportive care (e.g., for seizures, diabetes, cardiac involvement) is the mainstay of management.

References

Andreu AL, DiMauro S. Current classification of mitochondrial disorders. J Neurol. 2003;250:1403–1406

Chinnery PF. Could it be mitochondrial? When and how to investigate. Pract Neurol. 2006;6:90–101

DiMauro S, Schon EA. Mitochondrial respiratory-chain diseases. N Engl J Med. 2003;348:2656–2668

Schmiedel J, Jackson S, Schäfer J, Reichmann H. Mitochondrial cytopathies. J Neurol. 2003;250:267–277

Zeviani M, Di Donato S. Mitochondrial disorders Brain. 2004;127:2153–2172

Mixed connective tissue disease (MCTD)

Sharp's syndrome

A disorder in which there is overlap of features from more than one collagen vascular or rheumatic disorder, such as systemic sclerosis, systemic lupus erythematosus, Sjögren's syndrome, and polymyositis. Antinuclear antibody is positive with a speckled pattern, high levels of antibodies directed against extractable nuclear antigens (ENA) are found, particularly nuclear ribonucleoprotein (nRNP), and rheumatoid factor (RhF) may be positive. As with other collagen vascular disorders, neurological features may occur, affecting > 50% of patients in one series, including:

- Aseptic meningitis
- Epileptic seizures
- Psychosis
- Trigeminal neuralgia
- Sensory neuropathy
- Stroke (small vessel vasculitis)

References

Bennett RM, Bong DM, Spargo BH. Neuropsychiatric problems in mixed connective tissue disease. Am J Med. 1978;65:955–962

Hoffman RW, Maldonado ME. Immune pathogenesis of mixed connective tissue disease: a short analytical review. Clin Immunol. 2008;128:8–17

Miyoshi myopathy [OMIM#254130]

An autosomal recessive distal muscular dystrophy usually of early-onset (<30 years), common in Japan, characterized by muscle wasting and weakness in a predominantly distal distribution (e.g., the posterior compartment of the legs), although intrafamilial phenotypic variation does occur. Creatine kinase is elevated (>10 times normal). Muscle biopsy pathology shows dystrophic changes without rimmed vacuoles (cf. *Nonaka myopathy*). Linkage is to chromosome 2p, and mutations within the gene encoding dysferlin have been identified. Hence this is a *dysferlinopathy*, and allelic with *limb-girdle muscular dystrophy* type 2B.

Reference

Nakagawa M, Matsuzaki T, Suehara M, et al. Phenotypic variation in a large Japanese family with Miyoshi myopathy with nonsense mutation in exon 19 of dysferlin gene. J Neurol Sci. 2001;184:15–19

MNGIE syndrome

Mitochondrial encephalomyopathy with polyneuropathy, ophthalmoplegia and pseduo-obstruction (MEPOP); Mitochondrial neurogastrointestinal encephalopathy syndrome; Myoneurogastrointestinal encephalopathy

A rare *mitochondrial disease*, generally beginning in childhood. The clinical features include:

- Gastrointestinal dysmotility: diarrhea, intestinal pseudo-obstruction (may prompt inappropriate laparotomy), malabsorption
- Ophthalmoplegia: almost invariant; +/− ptosis
- Progressive leukodystrophy: cognitive impairment, dementia
- Myopathy
- Peripheral neuropathy: sensorimotor polyneuropathy

Ragged red fibers are prominent on muscle biopsy. The pattern of inheritance may be maternal, autosomal recessive, or autosomal dominant. Depletion and/or multiple deletions of mitochondrial DNA have been observed in some families; defective electron transport chain activity affecting complex IV (cytochrome c oxidase) has also been observed. Autosomal recessive disease is associated with mutations in the gene encoding thymidine phosphorylase (TP), and there is reduced leukocyte TP activity. The differential diagnosis includes abetalipoproteinemia, but there is no retinopathy or acanthocytosis in MNGIE. There is no specific treatment, only supportive care. Death usually occurs in the fourth decade.

References

Lara MC, Valentino ML, Torres-Torronteras J, Hirano M, Marti R. Mitochondrial neurogastrointestinal encephalomyopathy (MNGIE): biochemical features and therapeutic approaches. Biosci Rep. 2007;27:151–163

Nishino I, Spinazzola A, Papadimitriou A, et al. Mitochondrial neurogastrointestinal encephalomyopathy: an autosomal recessive disorder due to thymidine phosphorylase mutations. Ann Neurol. 2000;47:792–800

Möbius syndrome

Congenital facial diplegia

The clinical features of this syndrome are:

- Congenital facial diplegia
- Bilateral sixth nerve (abducens) palsies
- +/− Dysarthria, dysphagia, hearing loss
- +/− Mental retardation

The syndrome may be evident in the neonatal period as poor sucking and lack of facial expression, but if the facial paralysis is incomplete diagnosis may not be made until later. Unlike other causes of facial paralysis, the lower face is often less severely affected than the upper face, with more difficulty closing the eyes than moving the lips. The syndrome may have more than one cause, including agenesis of brainstem motor neurones or aplasia of ocular muscles. The differential diagnosis includes congenital myotonic muscular dystrophy or facioscapulohumeral dystrophy. Other anomalies may coexist, e.g., Poland anomaly. Möbius syndrome is now classified as one of the *congenital cranial dysinnervation disorders*.

Reference

Verzijl HT, Padberg GW, Zwarts MJ. The spectrum of Möbius syndrome: an electrophysiological study. Brain. 2005;128:1728–1736

Mohr–Tranebjaerg syndrome [OMIM#304700]

A sex-linked syndrome of sensorineural deafness and *dystonia*, sometimes accompanied by blindness, fractures, and mental retardation. Linkage to chromosome Xq21.3-Xq22 was followed by identification of mutations in a gene named deafness/dystonia peptide (DDP) gene. Mutations in the same gene have been identified in Jensen syndrome (opticoacoustic nerve atrophy and dementia), hence the conditions are allelic. In one mutation, female carriers may show dystonic features.

Reference

Swerdlow RH, Wooten GF. A novel deafness/dystonia peptide gene mutation that causes dystonia in female carriers of Mohr-Tranebjaerg syndrome. Ann Neurol. 2001;50:537–540

Mollaret meningitis

A rare syndrome of recurrent, apparently aseptic, *meningitis*, originally described with a distinctive CSF cytology featuring large mononuclear (Mollaret) cells. For long classified as idiopathic, in recent years use of the polymerase chain reaction has identified herpes simplex virus type 2 (HSV-2) in CSF of many cases, without necessarily a prior history of genital herpes. These findings suggest that antiviral therapy such as aciclovir might be appropriate. A similar syndrome of recurrent *aseptic meningitis* may be caused by rupture of a *dermoid* or *epidermoid* into the CSF.

Reference

Ellerin TB, Walsh SR, Hooper DC. Recurrent meningitis of unknown aetiology. Lancet. 2004;363:1772

Monoclonal gammopathies

Paraproteins are present in about 1% of the general population, often without clinical correlate, but in a much greater percentage of patients with a peripheral neuropathy, perhaps 10%. In a few of these, there is an underlying malignancy (myeloma, lymphoma) or amyloidosis, but most have a "monoclonal gammopathy of undetermined significance" (MGUS). Follow up to see whether a malignancy emerges is suggested. *Paraproteinemic demyelinating neuropathy* enters the differential diagnosis. The neuropathy associated with MGUS is typically sensory, affecting lower limbs more than upper, and slowly progressive over years. Neurophysiological studies show features of both axonal and demyelinating involvement. Neuropathies associated with IgM, IgG, and IgA may be heterogeneous, since IgM has been reported not to respond to plasma exchange. Other immunosuppressive agents such as prednisolone, azathioprine, cyclophosphamide, and ciclosporin have been tried in these cases, sometimes with success.

References

Dyck PJ, Low PA, Windebank AJ, et al. Plasma exchange in polyneuropathy associated with monoclonal gammopathy of undetermined significance. N Engl J Med. 1991;325:1482–1486
Notermans NC, Fransses H, Eurelings M, et al. Diagnostic criteria for demyelinating polyneuropathy associated with monoclonal gammopathy. Muscle Nerve. 2000;23:73–79

Monomelic amyotrophy

Chronic asymmetric spinal muscular atrophy (CASMA), Hirayama disease, Sobue disease

Monomelic amyotrophy is a syndrome of neurogenic muscular wasting, affecting a single limb (arm > leg), more common in men, usually occurring in the second to fourth decades. Wasting progresses for a year or two, then seems to arrest. EMG/NCS shows chronic partial denervation, MRI may show asymmetry of the spinal cord. This is thought to be a localized form of *spinal muscular atrophy*, but it may also sometimes be the presenting feature of *motor neurone disease*.

References

Kiernan MC, Lethlean AK, Blum PW. Monomelic amyotrophy: non progressive atrophy of the upper limb. J Clin Neurosci. 1999;6:353–355
Talbot K. Monomelic amyotrophy or Hirayama's disease. Pract Neurol. 2004;4: 362–365

Mononeuritis multiplex: overview

Mononeuropathy multiplex, multiple mononeuropathy

Involvement of several peripheral (and cranial) nerves over a period of days to weeks, causing patchy sensorimotor deficits and pain, is the characteristic of mononeuritis multiplex, or mononeuropathy multiplex since the etiology is not always inflammatory. Neurophysiological studies confirm the patchy nature of the process, which may progress to become more like polyneuropathy. Recognized causes include:

- Vasculitis:
  - Polyarteritis nodosa
  - Churg–Strauss syndrome
  - Rheumatoid arthritis
  - Systemic lupus erythematosus
  - Wegener's granulomatosis
  - Giant cell arteritis
  - Behçet's disease
- Infections:
  - Meningococcal septicemia
  - Infective endocarditis
- Diabetes

- Neurosarcoidosis
- Neurofibromatosis
- Hematological disorders:
  - Leukemia, lymphoma
  - Paraproteinemia

Treatment and prognosis are related to cause, where established.

Reference

Staal A, Van Gijn J, Spaans F. Mononeuropathies: Examination, Diagnosis and Treatment. London: W.B. Saunders; 1999:169–173

Morton's metatarsalgia

Morton's metatarsalgia describes pain in the sole of the foot, constant aching plus paroxysms of lancinating pain, due to compression of a digital nerve neuroma between the heads of the metatarsals (second/third, third/fourth). Pressure over the neuroma on the sole of the foot may reproduce the symptoms. Ultrasonography is the radiological investigation of choice. The neuroma may be amenable to surgical resection.

Reference

Hassouna H, Singh D. Morton's metatarsalgia: pathogenesis, aetiology and current management. Acta Orthop Belg. 2005;71:646–655

Morvan's syndrome

Morvan's fibrillary chorea

This syndrome is characterized by myokymia, muscle pain, hyperhidrosis, severe insomnia (agrypnia), and hallucinations, initially described by Morvan in 1890. As myokymia, perhaps more appropriately termed neuromyotonia (Isaacs' syndrome, *peripheral nerve hyperexcitability*), has been shown to be associated with autoantibodies directed against presynaptic voltage-gated potassium channels (VGKC), it was logical to look for these antibodies in Morvan's syndrome, which may be classified as neuromyotonia with CNS involvement. Other features reported in cases with high titers of VGKC antibodies include CSF oligoclonal bands and a neurohormonal profile showing elevated noradrenaline and cortisol with absent circadian rhythms of melatonin and prolactin (as seen in the prion disorder *fatal familial insomnia*). Clinical improvement with plasma exchange has been reported. There may be an underlying neoplasm (i.e., this may be one of the *paraneoplastic syndromes*). Not all cases of Morvan's syndrome show VGKC antibodies.

References

Barber PA, Anderson NE, Vincent A. Morvan's syndrome associated with voltage-gated K+ channel antibodies. Neurology. 2000; 54:771–772
Loscher WN, Wanschitz J, Reiners K, Quasthoff S. Morvan's syndrome: clinical, laboratory and in vitro electrophysiological studies. Muscle Nerve. 2004;30:157–163

Motor neurone disease (MND)

Amyotrophic lateral sclerosis (ALS), Charcot's disease, Lou Gehrig's disease

Motor neurone disease (MND) may be used to describe a disorder of both upper and lower motor neurones causing muscle wasting and weakness, with gradual and inexorable decline of function leading to death (equivalent in the USA to amyotrophic lateral sclerosis), or a broader use encompassing disorders affecting either or both upper and lower motor neurones (e.g., *progressive lateral sclerosis*).

MND remains one of the most feared diagnoses in neurological practice because of its dismal prognosis, although some patients do survive many years. Etiology remains uncertain, although deterministic genes have been identified in some of the 10% of cases in which the disease is inherited as an autosomal dominant condition. Mutations in the copper-zinc superoxide dismutase (Cu/Zn-SOD) gene suggested a possible pathophysiological role for oxidative stress.

Clinical features

Diagnostic criteria exist, but essentially the diagnosis requires:

- Evidence (clinical, electrophysiological, neuropathological) of lower motor neurone degeneration.
- Evidence (clinical) of upper motor neurone degeneration.
- Progressive spread of symptoms and signs.
- Absence of electrophysiological, pathological, or neuroimaging evidence of other disease process(es) that might better explain the observed signs.
- Sensory loss and early sphincter dysfunction would argue against the diagnosis.

The criteria propose a number of diagnostic categories (Clinically definite, Clinically probable, Clinically probable-laboratory supported, Clinically possible) that are helpful for clinical trials. Clinically definite MND is defined by UMN and LMN signs in three regions. Older clinical classifications enumerated variants such as progressive bulbar palsy, progressive muscular atrophy, indicating where the brunt of the initial clinical problem was, but it is recognized that these all reflect the same underlying disease. Symmetrical wasting and weakness of the arms without, or with only minimal, leg and bulbar involvement has been labeled the flail arm syndrome, and may correspond to what was previously called Vulpian–Bernhardt syndrome. Recognized types and patterns of MND may be listed as sporadic MND, genetically determined MND, and MND plus syndromes, e.g., with parkinsonism, frontal-type dementia (*frontotemporal lobar degeneration* with motor neurone disease, some cases of NIFID). About 5–10% of MND patients have a family history of the condition. More than ten loci for familial ALS have been defined, and a number of genes characterized, including SOD1, TARDBP, FUS, senataxin, VAPB, and dynactin-1.

Investigation

Bloods: creatine kinase may be modestly elevated; depending upon the patients age, additional tests may be undertaken to exclude other cause of a motor neurone disease, e.g., hexosaminidase deficiency (white cell enzymatic assays), and *spinal muscular atrophy* (SMN gene mutations). If there is a family history suggesting autosomal dominant inheritance, mutations for causative genes may be sought. Neurophysiology: EMG/NCS shows evidence of denervation, particularly significant if found in clinically normal muscles, distant from clinically symptomatic areas. Neuroimaging: MRI of the cervical spine may be undertaken to exclude multiple compressive radiculopathies as a cause for upper limb wasting, weakness, and fasciculation. CSF may be analyzed to look for evidence of inflammatory change (oligoclonal bands); very rarely, motor neurone diseases responding to immunosuppression have been reported. Muscle biopsy is now seldom performed to confirm neurogenic change, and/or exclude inflammatory (and potentially treatable) myopathy. Neurogenetic testing may be available for familial ALS.

Differential diagnosis

- Other *motor neurone diseases*
- Multiple radiculopathies
- Motor neuropathies, e.g., *multifocal motor neuropathy*

Treatment and prognosis

No curative treatment. Natural history is one of progressive decline, often leading to respiratory failure, aspiration, and death. Occasional long-term survivors, sometimes > 15 years. Riluzole may prolong life for 3–6 months, and is licensed for the treatment of MND. Supportive therapy is of the greatest importance: physiotherapy, occupational therapy (including home modifications such as grab rails, banisters, stair-lift, bed hoist, walk-in shower, downstairs bedroom), speech therapy. Access to appropriate financial benefits. The issues of respiratory support (nasal CPAP, nocturnal intermittent positive pressure ventilation) and assisted feeding (percutaneous endoscopic gastrostomy or jejunostomy) should be addressed, preferably sometime before their institution becomes necessary, particularly before respiratory failure requires urgent intervention. Some patients and families will want such interventions, others not.

Diagnostic criteria

Brooks BR, Miller RG, Swash M, Munsat TL. El Escorial revisited: revised criteria for the diagnosis of amyotrophic lateral sclerosis. Amyotrop Lateral Scler Other Motor Neuron Disord. 2000;1:293–299
www.wfnals.org for El Escorial criteria

References

Dion PA, Daoud H, Rouleau GA. Genetics of motor neuron disorders: new insights into pathogenic mechanisms. Nat Rev Genet. 2009;10:769–782
The Amyotrophic Lateral Sclerosis Online Database, ALSOD. www.alsod.iop.kcl.ac.uk
Traynor BJ, Codd MB, Corr B, Forde C, Frost E, Hardiman OM. Clinical features of amyotrophic lateral sclerosis according to the El Escorial and Airlie House diagnostic criteria: a population-based study. Arch Neurol. 2000;57:1171–1176

Motor neurone diseases: overview

Motor neurone diseases may be classified clinically on the basis of whether disease is localized to the upper motor neurones, lower motor neurones, or both.

- Combined upper and lower motor neurone involvement:
  - Motor neurone disease (MND)/amyotrophic lateral sclerosis (ALS)
    - Sporadic
    - Familial (adult onset; juvenile onset)

- Pure upper motor neurone involvement:
  - Primary lateral sclerosis (PLS)
  - Hereditary spastic paraplegia (HSP)
  - Lathyrism
  - Konzo
- Pure lower motor neurone involvement:
  - *Spinal muscular atrophy (SMA)*:
    ○ Proximal hereditary motor neuronopathy, e.g., Werdnig–Hoffmann, Kugelberg–Welander types
    ○ Hereditary bulbar palsy, e.g., Fazio–Londe, Brown–Vialetto–Van Laere
    ○ Focal/segmental variants: monomelic amyotrophy (Hirayam disease), O'Sullivan-McLeod syndrome
  - Spinal and bulbar atrophy (Kennedy's syndrome)
  - Hexosaminidase deficiency
  - Multifocal motor neuropathies
  - Poliomyelitis, postpolio syndrome
  - Postirradiation syndrome

References

Donaghy M. The motor neuron diseases. In: Donaghy M, ed. Brain's Diseases of the Nervous System. 11th ed. Oxford: Oxford University Press; 2001:443–460
World Federation of Neurology Classification Subcommittee. Classification of neuromuscular diseases. J Neurol Sci. 1988;86:333–360

Moyamoya

Moyamoya is an occlusive vasculopathy of uncertain etiology, most commonly seen in the Japanese. It may present in childhood as a syndrome of recurrent cerebral ischemia and infarction, associated with cognitive impairment, headache, and epileptic seizures; or in adulthood with recurrent *intracerebral hemorrhage* or *subarachnoid hemorrhage*. Radiologically there is severe stenosis or occlusion of one or both distal internal carotid arteries, sometimes extending to the circle of Willis, with fine anastomotic (telangiectatic) collateral vessels developing from perforating and pial arteries at the base of the brain (basal cerebral *rete mirabile*), orbital and ethmoidal branches of the external carotid artery, and leptomeningeal vessels. These vessels are the source of hemorrhage in cases presenting in adulthood, and may be visualized at angiography as a "puff of smoke" or "haze," from the Japanese term for which the syndrome takes its name. Although often idiopathic, recognized associations and symptomatic causes of moyamoya include:

- Basal meningeal/nasopharyngeal infection
- *Vasculitis*
- Irradiation

- Trauma
- *Fibromuscular dysplasia*
- *Sickle cell disease*
- *Neurofibromatosis*

Atheromatous disease very rarely produces a moyamoya picture; presumably the extensive collateralization can only develop during childhood. Treatment is uncertain. Drug treatment with steroids, calcium channel blockers, and anti-platelet drugs has produced variable results; anticoagulation is not helpful. Surgical revascularization is advocated by some authorities, e.g., with superficial temporal artery to middle cerebral artery anastomosis, or simply by apposition of the temporalis muscle to the surface of the brain (arterial myosynangiosis).

Reference

Kuroda S, Houkin K. Moyamoya disease: current concepts and future perspectives. Lancet Neurol. 2008;7:1056–1066

Mucormycosis

Phycomycosis, zygomycosis

Infection with the fungus *Mucorales* spreads from the nasal turbinates and paranasal sinuses to the retro-orbital space, causing proptosis, ophthalmoplegia, and periorbital edema, and to the brain causing hemorrhagic infarction; vasculitis has also been reported. Infection is a complication of poorly controlled *diabetes mellitus* or diabetic acidosis, drug abuse, and may also occur in the context of leukemia and lymphoma. Necrotic eschar replacing the nasal mucosa is a highly suggestive sign. Malignant invasive infection is often rapidly fatal, although recovery may occur with correction of risk factors and administration of intravenous amphotericin.

Reference

Brotman D, Taege A, Ruggieri P, Kinkel PR. Acute ophthalmoplegia. Lancet. 2003;361:930

Multifocal motor neuropathy (MMN)

Multifocal motor neuropathy with conduction block (MMNCB)

Originally described in 1986, this neuropathy of probable autoimmune pathogenesis is characterized electrophysiologically by conduction block, runs a chronic course and is more common in women (M:F = 1:3), with onset generally in the second to fifth decades. It is important to identify MMN since the condition does respond to intravenous immunoglobulin (IVIg), and if untreated may progress to tetraplegia.

Clinical features

- Early: gradually evolving weakness in territory of single peripheral nerve (e.g., radial, median, ulnar), hence asymmetric, with little or no wasting.
- Progression: involvement of other sites in upper and lower limbs, such that confluent involvement may develop; denervation atrophy frequent.
- Muscle cramp, fatigue, twitching/fasciculation; occasionally true muscle hypertrophy.
- Tendon reflexes variable: lost, normal, or brisk!
- Although sensory nerves are classically spared, sensory symptoms and signs may sometimes occur (differential diagnosis = *Lewis Sumner syndrome*, MADSAM).

Investigation

Bloods: creatine kinase, serum IgM may be slightly elevated; anti-GM1 antiganglioside antibodies present in 50% of cases (absence unhelpful). Neurophysiology (EMG/NCS) hallmark is the finding of conduction block away from usual sites of nerve entrapment; block is variably defined but suggests a reduction in CMAP amplitude (>10%) and increase in duration (<20%) when stimulating from adjacent sites; chronic neurogenic change with fasciculation may be seen in the later stages. CSF may show elevated protein in one third of cases; cell count normal. Neuroimaging: MRI may show increased signal intensity on T_2-weighted images in parts of the brachial plexus. Nerve biopsy is rarely required, to differentiate MMN from nerve tumor or vasculitis; must biopsy a motor or mixed nerve, which may show demyelination, onion bulb formation, and axonal atrophy.

Differential diagnosis

- Early: solitary or multiple mononeuropathy, entrapment neuropathy
- Late:
    - *Chronic inflammatory demyelinating polyradiculoneuropathy (CIDP)*
    - Motor neurone disease
    - Spinal muscular atrophy
    - Other motor neuropathies: lead, hereditary neuropathy with liability to pressure palsies

Treatment and prognosis

Mild cases may require no treatment. Benefit has been clearly demonstrated with IVIg (e.g., 2 g/kg over 3–5 days) but the effect wanes over a few months such that repeated courses may be necessary. Neither steroids nor plasma exchange are helpful; steroids may on occasion worsen the condition.

References

European Federation of Neurological Societies, Peripheral Nerve Society, Schaik IN, et al. European Federation of Neurological Societies/Peripheral Nerve Society guideline on management of multifocal motor neuropathy. Eur Neurol. 2006;13:802–808
Roth G, Rohr J, Magistris MR, Ochsner F. Motor neuropathy with proximal multifocal persistent conduction block, fasciculations and myokymia. Evolution to tetraplegia. Eur Neurol. 1986;25:416–423
Slee M, Selvan A, Donaghy M. Multifocal motor neuropathy: the diagnostic spectrum and response to treatment. Neurology. 2007;69:1680–1687
Willison H, Mills K. Multifocal motor neuropathy. Pract Neurol. 2002;2:298–301

Multi-minicore disease

This congenital myopathy, usually with perinatal onset but sometimes adult onset, is characterized by multiple small areas of myofibrillar disruption (cores). A number of categories are recognized, the most common type being associated with recessive mutations in the SEPN1 gene, hence overlapping with *rigid spine syndrome* [OMIM#602771]. Others show clinical and histological overlap with *central core disease* with recessive mutations in the ryanodine receptor gene RYR1 [OMIM#255320].

Reference

Ferreiro A, Estournet B, Chateau D, et al. Multi-minicore disease – searching for boundaries: phenotype analysis of 38 cases. Ann Neurol. 2000;48:745–757

Multiple sclerosis (MS)

Disseminated sclerosis

Multiple sclerosis (MS) is a common inflammatory demyelinating disorder of CNS white matter, believed to reflect immune attack on the myelin–oligodendrocyte complex. The ultimate causes of this process are unknown, but may include nonspecific viral infection, and possibly, trauma (controversial).

Genetic predisposition is related to HLA types and possibly other genes relating to immune function. Epidemiology confirms greater risk further from the equator.

Clinical features

Phenotype is very diverse. The old requirement for episodes of demyelination disseminated in space and time has been superseded with the advent of MRI, which may demonstrate spatial dissemination at time of single (initial) attack. Typical presentations include:

- Clinically isolated syndromes:
  - *Optic neuritis*
  - *Transverse myelitis*/myelopathy (usually partial rather than complete)
  - Brainstem syndrome
  - *Acute disseminated encephalomyelitis* (*ADEM*) and variants
- Cerebellar ataxia

However, virtually any focal sensory and/or motor presentation may occur. Internuclear ophthalmoplegia (INO) in a young patient is highly suggestive. Pattern of disease varies with time:

- Relapsing–remitting (RRMS) disease: common in early stages, relapses followed by full or almost full recovery.
- Secondary progressive: RRMS often evolves with time into a slowly progressive disorder, with or without superimposed acute relapses.
- Primary progressive: occasionally disease is unremitting from the outset.

Variants are recognized:

- *Balò's concentric sclerosis*
- *Marburg disease*, Marburg syndrome
- *Schilder's disease*

Investigation

Neuroimaging: MRI is modality of choice to display multiple white matter lesions, both clinically relevant and clinically silent; most usually periventricular in location, lesions often oriented away from axis of ventricles; brainstem lesions, especially cerebellar white matter; spinal cord lesions (usually only one vertebra in longitudinal extent). Enhancement with gadolinium, indicative of blood–brain barrier breakdown, in newer lesions, other (older) lesions non-enhancing. Interval scan (6 months) may show development and regression of lesions. Various MR criteria for the diagnosis of MS have been suggested. Neurophysiology: VERs typically showed delayed waveform after optic neuritis, even in clinically silent cases. CSF: oligoclonal bands found in the majority (>95%), although nonspecific, may occur in other inflammatory CNS diseases.

Differential diagnosis

- Monophasic illness: clinically isolated syndromes, ADEM
- Other relapsing–remitting disorders: inflammatory (e.g., *neurosarcoidosis, Behçet's disease*); structural (cavernous hemangioma, meningioma)
- Primary progressive disease: other causes of *myelopathy*

Treatment and prognosis

Benign disease (single relapse, or relapses separated by years or decades), without acquisition of neurological disability, requires no specific treatment.

Treatment, when required, remains largely symptomatic: intravenous methylprednisolone probably hastens recovery from an acute relapse, oral steroids possibly so.

So-called disease-modifying drugs (interferons, glatiramer) have been shown to reduce relapse rate by one third (as have other immunosuppressive agents such as azathioprine), but whether this translates into longer-term prevention of disability remains an open question, trials to date having been inconclusive. Interferons may reduce the risk of conversion of clinically isolated syndrome to MS. Other immunomodulatory drugs such as CAMPATH-1H may modify disease but at risk of other immune-mediated disorders (Graves' disease). Oral agents are now becoming available (cladribine, fingolimod). With the development of fixed disability, such as limb spasticity or bladder dysfunction, symptomatic treatments may be appropriate: baclofen, tizanidine for spasticity, oxybutynin, clean intermittent self-catheterization for bladder dysfunction. Physiotherapy, occupational therapy, and speech therapy may have much to offer at this stage of the disease. Cognitive decline ("white matter" or subcortical type dementia) may develop, likewise epileptic seizures.

Diagnostic criteria

Polman CH, Reingold SC, Edan G, et al. Diagnostic criteria for multiple sclerosis: 2005 revisions to the "McDonald criteria." Ann Neurol. 2005;58:840–846

References

Compston A, Coles A. Multiple sclerosis. Lancet. 2008;372:1502–1517
Compston A, Confavreux C, Lassmann H, McDonald I, Miller D, Noseworthy J, Smith K, Wekerle H. McAlpine's Multiple Sclerosis. 4th ed. London: Churchill Livingstone; 2005

Multiple symmetric lipomatosis

Launois–Bensaude disease, Madelung's disease

This syndrome of symmetrical lipomata of the neck and shoulders, with sparing of the buttocks and legs, is associated in up to 80% of patients with axonal sensorimotor polyneuropathy, and sometimes deafness. It may be classified as a *mitochondrial disease* since abnormalities of complex IV and multiple mitochondrial DNA deletions have been observed, including that responsible for *MERRF syndrome* (A8344G).

References

Klopstock T, Naumann M, Schalke B, et al. Multiple symmetric lipomatosis: abnormalities in complex IV and multiple deletions in mitochondrial DNA. Neurology. 1994;44:862–866
Naumann M, Schalke B, Klopstock T, et al. Neurological multisystem manifestation in multiple symmetric lipomatosis: a clinical and electrophysiological study. Muscle Nerve. 1995;18:693–698

Multiple system atrophy (MSA)

Multiple system atrophy (MSA) is a sporadic neurodegenerative disorder characterized by autonomic, parkinsonian, cerebellar, and pyramidal features that may occur in any combination. For this reason, subtypes have been defined according to the presenting neurological feature:

- MSA-P: parkinsonism
- MSA-C: cerebellar (includes cases previously labeled olivopontocerebellar atrophy, OPCA)
- MSA-M: mixed, combination of neurological features (includes striatonigral degeneration)

Autonomic features are integral to the diagnosis; Shy–Drager syndrome was once used to label such patients. Some patients diagnosed with isolated autonomic failure evolve to MSA; likewise, some idiopathic late-onset cerebellar ataxias (ILOCA) eventually prove to be MSA-C. It may be difficult to differentiate MSA-P from idiopathic *Parkinson's disease* in the early stages but clues come from early bladder symptoms and lack of response to levodopa. Oligodendroglial intracytoplasmic argyrophilic inclusions (GCI) containing α-synuclein are the specific pathological feature; hence, MSA may be considered a *synucleinopathy*. There is neuronal loss and gliosis in the striatum, substantia nigra, locus ceruleus, pontine nuclei, cerebellum (Purkinje cells), and inferior olivary nuclei; and in the spinal cord intermediolateral columns and Onuf's nucleus. The condition is slightly more common in males; its prevalence is less than that of *progressive supranuclear palsy* (*PSP*). In Europe, the parkinsonian form predominates; the reverse is true in Japan.

Clinical features

- Dysautonomia:
  - Erectile failure (early).
  - Urinary incontinence (neurogenic bladder, urge incontinence early).
  - *Syncope*, presyncope.
  - Urinary retention.
  - Fecal incontinence (rare).
- Parkinsonism:
  - Akinetic-rigid syndrome.
  - Tremor: postural > rest > action; postural tremor is often jerky and irregular, exaggerated by tapping the hand (i.e., stimulus sensitive myoclonus); pill-rolling rest tremor rare.
- Cerebellar syndrome:
  - Limb ataxia > gait; intention tremor.
  - Dysarthria: atypical, "strangled," dystonic.
  - Dysphagia.
  - Stridor.
  - Antecollis.

Some cases have early anosmia and *REM sleep behavior disorder*. Cognition is generally believed to be preserved, but occasional cases with cognitive dysfunction akin to PSP have been presented. Some MSA presentations have "evolved" to *dementia with Lewy Bodies*.

Investigation

Diagnosis is essentially clinical. Neuroimaging: MRI hypointensity in putamen, +/− juxtaposed slit-like T_2 hyperintensity; velar atrophy ("hot cross bun sign") is suggestive but may occur in other conditions; it is thought to be due to loss of pontine neurones and myelinated transverse pontocerebellar fibers with preservation of corticospinal tracts. Sphincter EMG: denervation previously thought to be diagnostic of MSA but may also be seen in advanced PD and PSP. Clonidine test: administration of clonidine fails to elicit the rise in growth hormone levels seen in normals, PD, and PAF (peripheral autonomic involvement); claimed to be sensitive and specific, but not all authorities agree. Otorhinolaryngology consult for vocal cord visualization may be helpful.

Differential diagnosis

- Autonomic features: may be difficult to separate MSA from *pure autonomic failure (PAF)*.
- MSA-P: very difficult to differentiate from Parkinson's disease in early stages.
- MSA-C: idiopathic late-onset cerebellar ataxias (ILOCA).

Treatment and prognosis

Progressive disease; tends to progress more quickly than PD. MSA-P: there is poor or no response to levodopa; if the latter, then the medication should be withdrawn, since it may exacerbate orthostatic hypotension. Levodopa-induced dyskinesias may occur in MSA, as in PD. Dopamine agonists, amantadine may also be tried. Focal dystonias may be treated with botulinum toxin, but not antecollis (may cause or exacerbate dysphagia).

Dysautonomia:
Orthostatic hypotension: Head-up bed tilt; elastic stockings; increase salt intake; fludrocrtisone, ephedrine, midodrine.
Postprandial hypotension: octreotide.
Bladder: oxybutinin for detrusor hyperreflexia; desmopressin for nocturnal polyuria; intermittent self-catheterization for retention, increase residual volume.
Erectile failure: sildenafil (Viagra), intracavernosal papaverine, penile prosthesis.

Diagnostic criteria

Gilman S, Wenning GK, Low PA, et al. Second consensus statement on the diagnosis of multiple system atrophy. Neurology. 2008;71:670–676

Reference

Stefanova N, Bücke P, Duerr S, Wenning GK. Multiple system atrophy: an update. Lancet Neurol. 2009;8:1172–1178

Muscular dystrophies: overview

Muscular dystrophies are myogenic disorders causing progressive muscle wasting and weakness of variable distribution (generally symmetrical) and severity. They are hereditary degenerative diseases of muscle, without neuropathic abnormality.

The following conditions may be classified as muscular dystrophies:

- *Duchenne muscular dystrophy (DMD), Becker muscular dystrophy (BMD)* = dystrophinopathies
- *Emery–Dreifuss muscular dystrophy (EDMD)*
- *Facioscapulohumeral (FSH) muscular dystrophy*
- Scapuloperoneal muscular dystrophy
- *Limb girdle muscular dystrophy (LGMD)*
- Distal muscular dystrophies
- *Oculopharyngeal muscular dystrophy (OPMD)*
- *Congenital muscular dystrophies (CMD)*

Investigation

Bloods: many of these conditions are associated with raised creatine kinase, DMD from birth.

Neurophysiology (EMG) myopathic; excludes neurogenic cause for weakness.

Muscle biopsy: variation in fiber size, fiber necrosis, macrophage invasion; inflammatory changes may be prominent (e.g., FSH, LGMD type 2B) sufficient to cause confusion with polymyositis; rimmed vacuoles may be seen (e.g., OPMD, some distal myopathies) as may nuclear inclusions (OPMD). Immunohistochemistry may show absence or deficiency of certain proteins, e.g., dystrophin, sarcoglycans, and dysferlin.

Neurogenetic testing: certain diseases are allelic:

- Dystrophin: DMD, BMD
- Lamin A: EDMD (autosomal dominant, autosomal recessive), LGMD type 1B, Dunnigan partial lipodystrophy, progeria
- Dysferlin: LGMD type 2B, Miyoshi-type distal myopathy
- Caveolin 3: LGMD type 1C, rippling muscle disease, idiopathic hyperCKemia

References

Emery AEH, ed. The Muscular Dystrophies. Oxford, UK: Oxford University Press; 2002
Emery AEH. The muscular dystrophies. Lancet. 2002;359:687–695

Musculocutaneous neuropathy

Mononeuropathy of the musculocutaneous nerve, which arises from the lateral cord of the brachial plexus is uncommon. It may follow shoulder dislocation or trauma.

Clinical features

- Motor: weak arm flexion due to involvement of biceps and brachialis muscles; biceps reflex may be reduced or normal.
- Sensory: loss over lateral forearm (lateral cutaneous nerve of the forearm).

Investigation

Neurophysiology (EMG/NCS) shows reduced lateral cutaneous nerve of the forearm SNAP; EMG changes are confined to muscles innervated by musculocutaneous nerve.

Differential diagnosis

C5 radiculopathy.

Myasthenia gravis (MG)

Erb–Goldflam disease

Although probably first described by Thomas Willis in the seventeenth century, myasthenia gravis was so named by Jolly in 1895. It is characterized by fatigable weakness of striated muscles, with a predilection for the extraocular, bulbar, and proximal limb musculature. The autoimmune nature of MG was postulated in the 1960s, borne out by the strong association with thymic hyperplasia and thymoma, other autoimmune disorders, especially thyrotoxicosis but also rheumatoid arthritis, systemic lupus erythematosus and polymyositis, and the identification of autoantibodies directed against nicotinic acetylcholine receptors in a large percentage of cases. Both symptomatic treatment with anticholinesterases and disease-modifying treatment with immunomodulatory therapies and thymectomy are possible.

Clinical features

- Onset is usually insidious; most common age of presentation is 10–30 years old in women and 50–70 years old in men.
- The typical presentation is with ocular symptoms and signs: variable ptosis and diplopia, worse at the end of the day and better after sleep, with asymmetric involvement of extraocular muscles on examination, with ptosis, frontalis overactivity, and bilateral weakness of orbicularis oculi (which is almost pathognomonic for this condition). Test for fatigability of both eye

movements (e.g., ask patient to fixate in a non-primary position) and ptosis (i.e., looking up). In ca. 10% of patients, MG remains clinically restricted to ocular muscles.

- Other cranial musculature may be involved, commonly the facial and bulbar muscles, causing fatigable dysarthria and dysphagia. It is always advisable to check swallowing function in patients with MG, as they are at risk of aspiration.
- Proximal weakness is common in MG and again needs to be tested after exercise (e.g., lifting the arms up and down 20 times, "wing flaps"). The neck flexors are especially vulnerable to the disease process. Occasionally predominantly distal limb weakness may occur.
- Sensory loss, sphincter disturbance and loss of reflexes are not features of MG; muscle atrophy is rarely seen.

Certain drugs may interfere with neurotransmission at the neuromuscular junction and worsen, or even induce, the clinical features of, MG. Examples include:

- Antibiotics: streptomycin, neomycin, gentamicin, tetracyclines, ciprofloxacin.
- Cardiovascular drugs: lidocaine, procainamide, quinine, quinidine, propranolol, oxprenolol.
- Antirheumatic drugs: chloroquine, D-penicillamine.
- Psychotropic drugs: lithium, chlorpromazine.
- Antiepileptic drugs: phenytoin.
- Others: corticosteroids, interferon-α, succinylcholine, d-tubocurarine; anticholinergics?

Investigation

Bloods: routine hematology and biochemistry usually all normal; need to check thyroid function tests. Acetylcholine receptor (AChR) antibodies are found in 85% of patients with generalized MG and 60% of patients with purely ocular involvement. The titer is not correlated with disease severity, but very high levels may be suggestive of an underlying thymoma. In addition, anti-striated muscle (or anti-myosin) antibodies are found in some patients with MG, and when present suggest an underlying thymoma. AChR antibodies are only occasionally seen in other conditions (e.g., SLE, primary biliary cirrhosis, Satoyoshi syndrome). Pathogenic antibodies directed against muscle specific tyrosine kinase (MuSK) are seen in some AChR negative patients. Neurophysiology: EMG/NCS routine studies show a decremental response to repetitive nerve stimulation in 60% of cases. Single fiber studies (SFEMG) demonstrate increase jitter and intermittent block in 99% of cases, although the technique is operator dependent. These abnormal findings are not normally affected by acetylcholinesterase medication. Tensilon test: undertaken with the patient lying down with full resuscitation facilities to hand. A clear endpoint needs to be established (e.g., degree of ptosis, strength of particular muscle group). Failure to define accurately the endpoint will produce an equivocal test response. The procedure varies slightly from one neurologist to another, but one method is

- Give the patient 0.6 mg atropine iv.
- Give test dose of 2 mg tensilon iv and monitor for any response.
- If no adverse reaction, give remaining 8 mg of tensilon; a positive response is usually evident within a minute and lasts for 3–4 min.
- Confirmation that the drug has produced an effect may be forthcoming if fasciculations are seen, especially in the periorbital musculature, and if there is watering of the eyes.
- If a negative result is obtained and the suspicion of MG is strong, a double dose (20 mg) tensilon test can be given with care, or alternatively a neostigmine test.

Ice test: for ptosis, holding an ice cube over the eyelid aponeurosis for 2–5 min may produce objective improvement, consistent with the clinical observation that some myasthenic patients improve in the cold. Sleep test: the clinical observation that ptosis improves with rest or sleep has been operationalized into a test for MG. Neuroimaging: CT or MRI of the chest is necessary, in order to assess whether there is thymic enlargement or tumor. Spirometry: vital capacity should be checked, since symptoms of impending respiratory failure may be few. If the vital capacity is less than 1 L in a weak patient, elective ventilation should be contemplated.

Differential diagnosis

There is usually no difficulty in diagnosing cases of generalized MG. In cases with restricted ocular involvement, *mitochondrial disease* and *thyroid disease* should be considered; posterior fossa mass lesions have also been reported to mimic the ocular features of MG. Other conditions that can occasionally cause confusion are *polymyositis*, *Lambert–Eaton myasthenic syndrome* (*LEMS*), *oculopharyngeal muscular dystrophy* (*OPMD*), *botulism*, polyneuritis cranialis, and motor neuropathies.

Treatment and prognosis

- Symptomatic:
  - Anticholinesterase drugs: e.g., pyridostigmine (Mestinon); enhance the efficacy of endogenous acetylcholine by inhibiting its enzymatic breakdown. Usually start at a low dose (e.g., pyridostigmine 30 mg tds) and titrate upward according to efficacy and side effects (maximum ~ 90 mg six times a day). Side effects include blurred vision and gastrointestinal upset; the latter may be treated with buscopan. Overdosage can produce cholinergic crisis, which can resemble a myasthenic crisis, but in the former the pupils are classically small. If in doubt a tensilon test can

be done in the ITU, the tensilon will improve a myasthenic crisis but will worsen a cholinergic crisis.

* Disease-modifying:
  - Immunosuppressive therapy; various options, of which steroids are most often used. Prednisolone is introduced at a low dose and increased slowly, since some patients initially deteriorate on high-dose steroid therapy (some neurologists pursue a policy of hospitalization for introduction of steroids). A standard regime would be 10 mg on alternate days, increasing by 10 mg a week to a maintenance dose of between 60 and 80 mg of prednisolone every other day. Around 75% of patients will improve markedly with this therapy and a further 15% will have a moderate improvement in their condition. Once the patient has been stabilized the prednisolone dose may be slowly reduced to a level that controls the disease process. If long-term steroid use is required, osteoporosis prophylaxis should be started. Ocular disease may be completely controlled with alternate-day steroids. If rapid introduction of high-dose steroids is required this should be done in hospital, often in conjunction with plasma exchange. Azathioprine may be used as a steroid sparing agent, but it may take 6 months or more before it takes effect. The usual starting dose is 50 mg/day, increasing to a maintenance dose of 150 mg/day. FBC and LFTs should be monitored, weekly for 8 weeks and thereafter every 3 months. Dose reduction or discontinuation may be required if the WCC drops below 3.5×10^9 or a lymphocyte count of less than 0.5×10^9, or if LFTs become abnormal. Mycophenylate mofetil may also have a place. Plasma exchange may be used acutely in MG patients with threatened respiratory failure. It is highly effective, but repeated use may catalyze the production of AChR antibodies. Intravenous immunoglobulin appears to have a similar clinical effect. Other treatments that have been tried include methotrexate, cyclophosphamide, and ciclosporin. Thymectomy was pioneered before the autoimmune nature of MG was understood. It is mandatory in patients with thymoma, and strongly recommended in patients <50 years old with positive AChR antibodies. In these cases, a third are cured, a third improve, and a third are unchanged. The greatest risk of morbidity and mortality from MG is during the first year. 10–15% of cases of MG improve spontaneously. Younger onset patients tend to run a more benign course. If MG remains confined to the eyes for >2 years, there is only a 15% chance of it becoming generalized.

References

Hart I. Myasthenia Gravis – The Essentials. 2nd ed. Barnham, UK: Eurocommunica, 2006
Jaretzki A, Barohn RJ, Ernstoff RM, et al. Myasthenia gravis: recommendations for clinical research standards. Task Force of the Medical Scientific Advisory Board of the Myasthenia Gravis Foundation of America. Neurology. 2000;55:16–23
Kaeser HE. Drug-induced myasthenic syndromes. Acta Neurol Scand. 1984;70 (suppl 100):39–47

Sathasivam S, Larner AJ. Disorders of the neuromuscular junction. In: Sinclair A, Morley JE, Vellas B, eds. Pathy's Principles and Practice of Geriatric Medicine. 5th ed. Chichester, UK: Wiley, 2011:in press.
Skeie GO, Apostolski S, Evoli A, et al. Guidelines for the treatment of autoimmune neuromuscular transmission disorders. Eur J Neurol. 2006;13:691–699

Mycoplasma

Infection with *Mycoplasma pneumoniae* causes an *"atypical pneumonia"* which may be complicated by constitutional symptoms including a variety of neurological features.

Clinical features

Mycoplasma tends to affect young adults, often occurring in epidemics although sporadic cases are recognized. Symptoms include:

- Respiratory: pneumonia, tracheobronchitis or pharyngitis, with persistent cough
- Systemic: fever, headache, myalgia
- Neurological (ca. 10% of patients):
  - Encephalitis, meningitis, or meningoencephalitis
  - Ataxia
  - Peripheral neuropathy
  - Transverse myelitis +/– ADEM; multiple sclerosis-like presentation
  - Bullous myringitis (5%)

Investigation

Bloods: leukocytosis, raised ESR, +/– cold agglutinins; positive serology for *M. pneumoniae*. Imaging: CXR shows pneumonia; CT/MRI may show white matter changes suggestive of ADEM or MS.

Differential diagnosis

- Other causes of pneumonia with associated neurological features
- Other causes of meningoencephalitis

Treatment and prognosis

Supportive treatment. Antibiotics: erythromycin 0.5 g tds for 14–21 days, or doxycyline 100 mg bd for 14–21 days. Recovery is often complete but occasional patients with transverse myelitis or CNS involvement fail to recover. The suggestion that mycoplasma infection was a cause of multiple sclerosis seems to have been disproved.

Reference

Sotgiu S, Pugliatti M, Rosati G, Deiana GA, Sechi GP. Neurological disorders associated with Mycoplasma pneumonia infection. Eur J Neurol. 2003;10:165–168

Myelopathy: overview

Myelopathy is a disorder of the spinal cord. Myelopathies may be characterized as intrinsic or intramedullary (lesions are always intradural), or extrinsic or extramedullary (lesions may be intradural or extradural). It may be possible to differentiate intramedullary from extramedullary lesions on clinical grounds, although this distinction is never absolute because of clinical overlap. Pathologies recognized to cause myelopathy include:

- Intrinsic:
  - Inflammatory disease: myelitis.
    - Primary/Idiopathic: clinically isolated syndrome ("transverse myelitis"), may be harbinger of *multiple sclerosis.*
    - Secondary: Post-infectious, e.g., varicella, EBV, *mycoplasma,* Brucella.
    - Postvaccination (e.g., influenza).
    - Multiple sclerosis, *neuromyelitis optica* (Devic's syndrome).
    - *Neurosarcoidosis.*
    - Collagen vascular diseases: *Systemic lupus erythematosus, Sjögren's syndrome, antiphospholipid syndrome, giant cell arteritis.*
  - Infection: HTLV-1 infection, HIV-related vacuolar myelopathy (often discovered incidentally at postmortem), tabes dorsalis.
  - Tumor: primary, secondary.
  - Syringomyelia.
  - Infarction, e.g., *anterior spinal artery syndrome.*
  - Metabolic causes: vitamin B_{12} deficiency producing *subacute combined degeneration of the cord, adrenoleukodystrophy* (adrenomyeloneuropathy).
- Extrinsic:
  - Prolapsed disc, osteophyte bar.
  - Tumor (primary, secondary).
  - *Arteriovenous malformation, dural arteriovenous fistula, hematoma.*
  - *Abscess.*

Clinical features

- Intrinsic/intramedullary myelopathy: dependent on the extent to which the cord is involved, the following features may occur: some pathologies have a predilection for posterior columns, central cord, etc.
  - Motor: lower motor neurone signs may be prominent and diffuse; upper motor neurone signs tend to occur late (spastic paraparesis below level of lesion). A combination of upper and lower motor neurone signs is much more likely to reflect intrinsic than extrinsic pathology.
  - Sensory: symptoms of central (funicular) pain may occur; dissociated sensory loss (spinothalamic > dorsal column involvement, or *vice versa*), suspended sensory loss, and sacral sparing are characteristic of intramedullary lesions; a Brown-Séquard syndrome may occur. Vibratory sensibility is more often affected than proprioception.
  - Sphincters: bladder involvement common, often early and slow to recover.
- Extrinsic/extramedullary myelopathy:
  - Motor: sequential spastic paraparesis below the level of the lesion; upper motor neurone signs occur early; lower motor neurone signs are unusual and have a segmental (radicular) distribution if present.
  - Sensory: symptoms of pain may be radicular (e.g., secondary to a neurofibroma) or vertebral (e.g., secondary to neoplastic or inflammatory processes); sensory signs are not usually marked until the later stages, and all modalities are often involved. A Brown-Séquard syndrome may be more common in extrinsic than intrinsic myelopathies.
  - Sphincters: may have bladder urgency, impotence.

Investigation

Bloods: dependent upon context, may require FBC, vitamin B_{12}, autoantibodies, very long-chain fatty acids; serology for HIV, HTLV-1, syphilis, and EBV. Neuroimaging with MR is often helpful in defining the cause of myelopathy. CSF: may be required, for cell count, protein, glucose, oligoclonal bands, and serology.

References

Andersen O. Myelitis. Curr Opin Neurol. 2000;13:311–316
Larner AJ. Diseases of the spinal cord. In: Cox TM, et al., eds. Oxford Textbook of Medicine. 5th ed. Oxford: Oxford University Press; 2010:5039–5045
Wong SH, Boggild M, Enevoldson TP, Fletcher NA. Myelopathy but normal MRI: where next? Pract Neurol. 2008;8:90–102

Myoadenylate deaminase deficiency (MADD)

Myoadenylate deaminase deficiency (MADD) is a common inherited metabolic defect, resulting from mutations in the AMPD1 gene, with heterogeneous clinical phenotype, ranging from asymptomatic to mild exercise-induced myalgia and cramps (which enters the differential diagnosis of *McArdle's disease*). In the ischemic forearm exercise test, creatine kinase may be elevated, there is a normal lactate response but no increase in ammonium. Distinctions have been drawn between primary MADD, resulting from homozygous mutation of the AMPD1 gene, and secondary or acquired MADD in which nongenetic factors, such as the presence of another neuromuscular disease, lead to discovery of MADD, perhaps due to the carrier state; heterozygous mutations of AMPD1 are present in 20% of Westerners.

References

Fishbein WN. Primary, secondary, and coincidental types of myoadenylate deaminase deficiency. Ann Neurol. 1999;45:547–548
Sabina RL. Myoadenylate deaminase deficiency. A common inherited defect with heterogeneous clinical presentation. Neurol Clin. 2000;18:185–194

Myoclonus-dystonia syndrome (MDS)

DYT11

This autosomal dominant condition is characterized by:

- Brief, alcohol-responsive, myoclonic jerks: neck and arms affected more than legs, gait
- +/− Cervical/brachial *dystonia*, writer's cramp
- +/− Psychiatric features: obsessive-compulsive disorder, panic attacks, alcohol dependence

Imaging (MRI) is normal. Mutations in a gene on chromosome 7 encoding ε-sarcoglycan have been demonstrated (all other *sarcoglycanopathies* cause *limb girdle muscular dystrophies*).

References

Asmus F, Zimprich A, Tezenas du Montcel S, et al. Myoclonus-dystonia syndrome: ε-sarcoglycan mutations and phenotype. Ann Neurol. 2002;52:489–492
Wong SH, Steiger MJ, Larner AJ, Fletcher NA. Hereditary myoclonus dystonia (DYT11): a novel SGCE gene mutation with intrafamilial phenotypic heterogeneity. Mov Disord. 2010;25:956–957

Myopathy: overview

Myopathy is a disease of muscle. Myopathies may be classified according to location (proximal vs distal), but more usually they are classified according to etiology:

- Inflammatory: polymyositis, dermatomyositis
- Muscular dystrophies
- Myotonic dystrophy (types 1 and 2)
- Non-dystrophic myotonias, periodic paralysis
- Congential myopathies (central core, nemaline, myotubular)
- Metabolic myopathies:
  Carbohydrate metabolism, e.g., McArdle's disease;
  Lipid metabolism, e.g., carnitine palmitoyltransferase deficiency;
  Mitochondrial myopathy;
  Malignant hyperthermia
- Endocrine myopathies: Steroid myopathy, thyroid myopathies
- Toxin/drug-induced myopathies: ethanol, statins

Clinical features

- History: look for evidence of muscle pain, weakness; distribution, diurnal pattern; myotonia
- Preceding illness, drug exposure
- Family history of muscle disease
- Examination: muscle wasting, tone, power (distribution of weakness); reflexes
- Other systems: especially skin, heart (concurrent cardiomyopathy)

Investigation

Bloods: muscle-related enzymes: creatine kinase +/− aldolase, LDH. Neurophysiology (EMG/NCS): myopathic change. Muscle biopsy: often diagnostic: weak but not atrophic muscle is probably best target. For specific diagnoses, additional investigations may be required, e.g., other blood tests, lumbar puncture. Neurogenetics is increasingly useful as loci and mutations are defined.

Differential diagnosis

- Neuromuscular junction disease, e.g., *myasthenia gravis*
- Motor neuropathies, e.g., *multifocal motor neuropathy* (*MMN*) with conduction block
- Motor neuronopathy, e.g., *motor neurone disease*
- Other causes of weakness: neuropathy, radiculopathy

Reference

Karpati G, Hilton-Jones D, Bushby K, Griggs RC, eds. Disorders of Voluntary Muscle. 8th ed. Cambridge: Cambridge Univesrity Press; 2010

Myositis: overview

The myositides are inflammatory disorders of muscle. These may be classified as:

- Infective:
    - Bacterial:
        ○ Pyomyositis: muscle abscess due to *Staphylococcus aureus*.
        ○ Neuroborreliosis (Lyme disease).
        ○ *Clostridia perfringens*.
        ○ *Mycobacteriae*: *tuberculosis*, *leprae*.
    - Viral:
        ○ Influenza.
        ○ HIV.
        ○ HTLV1.
        ○ Coxsackievirus B: pleurodynia (devil's grip, Bornholm disease) may be accompanied by an inflammatory myopathy.
    - Parasitic:
        ○ Trichinosis.
        ○ Toxoplasmosis (may be more severe in context of AIDS).
        ○ Cysticercosis.
        ○ Echinococcosis.
    - Fungal:
        ○ Candida (rare).
- Idiopathic:
    - Polymyositis.
    - Dermatomyositis.
    - Inclusion body myositis.
    - Polymyalgia rheumatica.
- Other:
    - Eosinophilic myositis.
    - Sarcoid myositis.

Inflammatory changes may be seen in muscle biopsies in conditions not typically thought inflammatory, e.g., *facioscapulohumeral* (*FSH*) *dystrophy*, metabolic myopathies, and in normals following vigorous exertion.

Reference

Mandler RN. Myopathy. In: Biller J, ed. Practical Neurology. 2nd ed. Philadelphia, PA: Lippincott Williams & Wilkins; 2002:623–641

Myositis ossificans [OMIM#135100]

Fibrodysplasia ossificans progressiva

An extremely rare autosomal dominant disorder characterized by progressive ossification of muscle tissue, beginning in childhood and affecting the muscles of the neck, back, shoulder, and pelvic girdles, caused by mutation in the ACVR1 gene on chromosome 2q23. Muscles are painful, tender to touch, and become progressively stiffer and restricted in their range of movement. Although the diaphragm is not affected by ossification, restriction of thoracic movement may lead to respiratory compromise and death. Heterotopic ossification of muscle occurs more commonly in the context of trauma (myositis ossificans traumatica), sometimes associated with repeated minor (occupational) trauma, such as thigh adductors (horse riding) and pectoralis and deltoid (drilling).

Reference

Kaplan FS, Delatycki M, Gannon FH, et al. Fibrodysplasia ossificans progressiva. In: Emery AEH, ed. Neuromuscular Disorders: Clinical and Molecular Genetics. New York: Wiley; 1998:289–321

Myotonia congenita

Hereditary myotonic syndromes may be either autosomal dominant or recessive:

- Thomsen disease: autosomal dominant [OMIM#160800], mutation in skeletal muscle chloride channel-1 (CLCN1) gene
- Becker disease: autosomal recessive [OMIM#255700], also caused by mutation in skeletal muscle chloride channel-1 (CLCN1) gene
- Myotonia levior: autosomal dominant [OMIM#160800]

Hence, these disorders are allelic *channelopathies*, all linked to chromosome 7q32.

Clinical features

- Myotonia: severe (Thomsen, Becker), mild (levior); appears after exercise, sometimes with emotional stress or pregnancy; warm-up phenomenon may be evident (i.e., better after repeated contractions).
- Pain in muscle may occur after prolonged activity but spasm per se is painless.
- Weakness not evident.
- Percussion myotonia.
- Muscle hypertrophy (especially Becker).

- No other features of myotonic dystrophy (e.g., frontal balding, cataracts, endocrine changes).
- No cardiac involvement.

Investigation

Bloods: mild increase in creatine kinase may be observed during attacks; serum K^+ during and between attacks is normal. Neurogenetic testing for mutations in chloride ion channel (CLCN1) gene at chromosome 7q32.

Differential diagnosis

- Myotonic dystrophy.
- Autosomal dominant myotonia congenita may be confused with potassium-aggravated myotonia (indeed some cases reported as Thomsen's disease have been shown to harbor sodium channel gene mutations typical of potassium-aggravated myotonia); myotonia fluctuates in the latter.
- Bruck–de Lange syndrome: congenital muscle hypertrophy.

Treatment and prognosis

Myotonia may be treated with mexiletine, quinidine sulfate, procainamide, or phenytoin.

Reference

Lossin C, George AL Jr. Myotonia congenita. Adv Genet. 2008;63:25–55

Myotonic dystrophy type 1 (DM1) [OMIM#160900]

Dystrophia myotonica, Steinert's disease

Myotonic dystrophy type 1 (DM1) is an autosomal dominant disorder caused by a trinucleotide repeat expansion in the myotonin protein kinase gene, a serine/threonine protein kinase which is expressed in muscle >>> heart and brain, encoded on chromosome 19. It is the most common inherited myopathy seen in adulthood, occurring in 1:8,000 live births. As in other *trinucleotide repeat diseases*, disease severity is proportional to the number of repeats, although the mechanism by which trinucleotide repeats cause disease is still unknown. At its most severe (>2,000 repeats), disease presents in the neonatal period; mild disease with adult onset occurs with 50–80 repeats. The clinical phenotype is variable, features including frontal baldness, cataracts, myopathic facies, weakness (usually distal > proximal), myotonia, a cardiomyopathy, diabetes mellitus, and testicular atrophy.

Clinical features

- Neonatal disease (very large repeats):
  - Extreme hypotonia with facial paralysis.
  - Feeding difficulties and failure to thrive.
  - Clubfeet and mental retardation are common.
  - Prone to URTI, pneumonia, and death.
- Adult disease:
  - Muscle:
    - Myotonia: difficulty in relaxing contracted muscle, manifest as difficulty letting go of objects, especially in cold weather. Myotonia may be induced clinically by voluntary contraction or percussion of muscle. It tends to disappear with advancing disease and loss of muscle.
    - Wasting and weakness, typically involves the distal limb muscles, the neck muscles (especially sternocleidomastoid), and facial muscles (especially masseter and temporalis). This produces a "hollowed" face with hooded eyes (ptosis), and a tented or slack mouth that can cause dislocation of the jaw. In advanced cases, there is proximal muscle involvement, including the respiratory musculature, as well as involvement of the palate and pharynx causing dysphagia and dysarthria.
    - Somnolence +/− respiratory depression may occur due to respiratory muscle involvement and an abnormal central ventilatory response to carbon dioxide.
    - Smooth muscle involvement may account for dysphagia and aspiration, constipation, symptoms akin to irritable bowel syndrome, fecal soiling; and impaired uterine contraction.
  - Cardiac:
    - Cardiomyopathy occurs with advanced disease, causing conduction abnormalities, arrhythmias, heart failure, and sudden death.
  - Ophthalmological:
    - Cataracts are very common.
  - Endocrine:
    - Testicular atrophy with infertility; ovarian dysfunction with infertility; diabetes mellitus; frontal balding.

Investigation

Detailed family history; check for cataracts in other family members. Bloods: creatine kinase is usually normal; check glucose for diabetes mellitus.

Arterial blood gases may be useful if respiratory depression is suspected, contributing to somnolence and/or heart failure.

Imaging: CXR for cardiomyopathy. Neurophysiology: EMG/NCS shows myopathic changes and myotonic discharges. Muscle biopsy is seldom necessary with the advent of genetic testing; it shows random variability in size of fibers with fibrosis, along with numerous ring fibers in which small bundles of myofibrils are oriented at 90° to majority. Neurogenetic testing for the trinucleotide CTG repeat in the 3′ untranslated region of myotonin protein kinase (DMPK) gene on chromosome 19q13.3 is definitive: normal = 5–40 repeats; abnormal = 44–3,000. Prenatal diagnosis can now be made using genetic test with tissue samples from chorionic villous biopsy. ECG/24 h ECG: for conduction abnormalities.

Differential diagnosis

- *Myotonic dystrophy type 2 (DM2)*
- Other *myotonic syndromes*

Treatment and prognosis

There is no curative treatment and the condition is progressive. Supportive treatment involves the use of:

- Prostheses: foot and/or wrist splints.
- Symptomatic treatment of myotonia: phenytoin; quinine; procainamide or acetazolamide (but need to watch for respiratory depression with phenytoin).
- Cardiac and respiratory treatment may involve pacemakers or respiratory support (e.g., CPAP). Symptomatic treatment of diabetes mellitus.
- Ophthalmologists may need to do cataract extraction.
- Genetic counseling may be required.

Reference

Harper PS, van Engelen B, Eymard B, Wilcox DE, eds. Myotonic Dystrophy: Present Management, Future Therapy. Oxford: Oxford University Press; 2004

Myotonic dystrophy type 2 (DM2) [OMIM#602668]

Proximal myotonic myopathy (PROMM), Ricker's disease, Thornton–Griggs–Moxley disease

Myotonic dystrophy type 2 (DM2) is an autosomal dominant disorder characterized by myotonia, proximal myopathy, and cataracts, with onset between the ages of 20 and 40 years. Clinically it seems to be more benign than classical *myotonic dystrophy type 1 (DM1)*. It has been linked to chromosome 3q and is associated with a CCTG repeat expansion in intron 1 of the zinc finger protein 9 (ZNF9) gene, with repeats of unprecedented size, up to 5,000.

Clinical features

- Myotonia: intermittent, affecting hands, proximal legs
- Proximal limb weakness: mild, slowly progressive, without atrophy; normal face; muscle pain is prominent. No distal weakness (cf. DM1)
- +/– Calf hypertrophy
- Cataracts
- ?Cardiac arrhythmias (rare)

Investigation

Bloods: creatine kinase normal. Neurophysiology (EMG) shows myotonic discharges. Neurogenetics shows an expansion of a nucleotide quadruplet $[CCTG]_n$ repeats in the gene encoding zinc finger protein 9 (ZNF9) on chromosome 3q.

Differential diagnosis

Myotonic dystrophy type 1, but no distal weakness, facial weakness, ptosis.

Treatment and prognosis

No specific treatment.

References

Day JW, Ricker K, Jacobsen JF, et al. Myotonic dystrophy type 2. Molecular, diagnostic and clinical spectrum. Neurology. 2003;60: 657–664
Ricker J. Myotonic dystrophy and proximal myotonic myopathy. J Neurol. 1999;246:334–338

Myotonic syndromes: overview

Myotonia is a stiffness of muscle, with difficulty in relaxing following voluntary contraction. This may give rise to symptoms of cramp or stiffness. Typically this improves with repeated muscle use ("warm up phenomenon");

in paramyotonia, a related condition, stiffness is precipitated and exacerabted by exercise and cold. Such stiffness may have various causes:

- Myogenic:
  - Dystrophic myotonias:
    - ○ *Myotonic dystrophy type 1* (dystrophia myotonica, DM1)
    - ○ *Myotonic dystrophy type 2* (proximal myotonic myopathy, PROMM, Ricker's disease, Thornton–Griggs–Moxley disease; DM2)
  - Non-dystrophic myotonias:
    - ○ Channelopathies:
    - ○ *Myotonia congenita*: Thomsen (autosomal dominant)
    - ○ Becker (autosomal recessive)
    - ○ *Myotonia fluctuans*
    - ○ *Periodic paralysis*: hypokalemic, hyperkalemic, thyrotoxic
    - ○ Paramyotonia congenita
    - ○ *Potassium-aggravated myotonia*
    - ○ *Schwartz–Jampel syndrome* (chondrodystrophic myotonia)
    - ○ *Andersen–Tawil syndrome*
- Neurogenic:
  - Neuromyotonia (Isaacs syndrome, *peripheral nerve hyperexcitability*)

Investigation

EMG reveals myotonic discharges with prolonged twitch relaxation phase; discharges typically wax and wane, producing a characteristic "dive bomber" effect on the audio recording.

Differential diagnosis

Myotonias need to be differentiated from pseudomyotonia, slow muscle relaxation not accompanied by myotonic EMG discharges, e.g., in hypothyroidism with "hung up" tendon reflexes (Woltman's sign), *Brody disease*. Muscle rigidity is also a feature of *malignant hyperthermia*.

References

Cannon SC. Myotonia and periodic paralysis: disorders of voltage-gated ion channels. In: Noseworthy JH, ed. Neurological Therapeutics: Principles and Practice. London: Dunitz; 2003:2365–2377
Mankodi A, Thornton CA. Myotonic syndromes. Curr Opin Neurol. 2002;15:545–552
Trip J, Drost G, Ginjaar HB, et al. Redefining the clinical phenotypes of non-dystrophic myotonic syndromes. J Neurol Neurosurg Psychiatry. 2009;80:647–652

Myotubular/Centronuclear myopathies

The myotubular/centronuclear myopathies are forms of congenital myopathy characterized by the histological appearance of central nuclei surrounded by an area devoid of myofibrils with mitochondrial aggregates in small rounded muscle fibers. The most common form is an X-linked disorder (MTM1) presenting in boys at birth with hypotonia, ventilatory insufficiency, feeding difficulties, and ophthalmoplegia (an unusual feature in other congenital myopathies). This is caused by mutations in the myotubularin gene [OMIM#310400]. Autosomal dominant and recessive forms are also described, with a later onset, in childhood or early adulthood, with facial weakness, ophthalmoplegia, ptosis, and proximal limb weakness. Epileptic seizures may be a feature.

Creatine kinase may be normal or slightly elevated. Neurophysiology shows a nonspecific myopathy.

All variants show the histological feature of centrally placed internal nuclei in small muscle fibers, in addition to the normal peripherally located nuclei. Three genes have been identified: dynamin 2 [OMIM#160150] (allelic with *Charcot–Marie–Tooth disease* type 2B), amphiphysin 2 [OMIM#255200], and ryanodine receptor (RYR1). There is no specific treatment.

Reference

Wallgren-Pettersson C, Clarke A, Samson F, et al. The myotubular myopathies: differential diagnosis of the X-linked recessive, autosomal dominant, and autosomal recessive forms and present state of DNA studies. J Med Genet. 1995;32:673–679

N

Naegleria

Along with *Acanthamoeba*, this protozoan, *Naegleria fowleri*, is one of the causes of primary amoebic meningoencephalitis, most often affecting children who have been swimming in infected water; the presentation mimics that of acute bacterial *meningitis*. Examination of CSF may reveal motile trophozoites. Prognosis is poor, with death within 1 week the norm. Amphotericin (systemic, intrathecal) is the treatment most usually given, although miconazole, rifampicin, doxycycline, or chloramphenicol may be tried.

Reference

Kaushal V, Chhina DK, Ram S, Singh G, Kaushal RK, Kumar R. Primary amoebic meningoencephalitis due to Naegleria fowleri. J Assoc Phys India. 2008;56:459–462

Nevoid basal cell carcinoma syndrome

Basal cell nevus syndrome, Gorlin-Goltz syndrome

This condition of uncertain inheritance (autosomal dominant, autosomal recessive) is characterized by skin, bone, and CNS abnormalities, with a tendency to develop neoplastic change. The skin shows increased sensitivity to X-irradiation. Features include:

- CNS:
  - Posterior fossa tumors, e.g., *medulloblastoma*; falx calcification, agenesis of the corpus callosum, occasionally mental retardation.
- Skin:
  - Basal cell carcinoma, affecting head, neck, upper trunk; 15% develop before puberty.
  - Small epidermal depressions (pits) in the palms and soles, which may undergo malignant change.

- Bone:
  - Odontogenic cysts of the jaw, which are usually asymptomatic.
  - Frontoparietal bossing.
- Kyphoscoliosis.

Mutations in the PTCH gene have been identified in some familial cases.

Reference

Gorlin RJ. Nevoid basal cell carcinoma (Gorlin) syndrome. In: Roach ES, Miller VS, eds. Neurocutaneous Disorders. Cambridge: Cambridge University Press;2004:77–87

Narcolepsy

Gélineau's syndrome, Narcoleptic syndrome

Narcolepsy is a disorder of excessive daytime sleepiness with "sleep attacks," usually beginning in adolescence or young adulthood. Some authors require features in addition to narcolepsy to establish the diagnosis, specifically cataplexy, sleep paralysis, and hypnagogic (and/or hypnapompic) hallucinations. The syndrome or complex is closely associated with certain HLA antigens, and has been linked with mutations in a gene encoding the protein orexin or hypocretin, lower levels of which are found in CSF of narcoleptics compared to normals. Disturbed aminergic mechanisms in REM sleep seem to be the underlying pathogenesis.

Clinical features

The core clinical tetrad of the narcoleptic syndrome consists of:

- Excessive daytime sleepiness, sleep attacks: irresistible desire to fall asleep, often in inappropriate circumstances, such as when driving, eating, talking; brief naps (10–20 min) which refresh the patient (cf. *obstructive sleep apnea-hypopnea syndrome (OSAHS)*). May present with poor school performance. Variable frequency, persist throughout life.
- Cataplexy: transient episodes of weakness or even frank paralysis (atonia), causing falls, often precipitated by strong emotion (laughter, anger).
- Sleep paralysis: a sensation of paralysis during the transition between sleep and waking, often with inability to speak; frightening.
- Hypnagogic/hypnapompic hallucinations: frightening visual, auditory or movement perceptions which reflect dreaming whilst awake.

Additional features which may occur include:

- Insomnia (with the preceding four, may constitute the narcoleptic pentad)
- Complaints of poor memory
- Depression
- Automatic behaviors

Investigation

Bloods: strong HLA linkage, to DR2, DQw15. CSF: low levels of the hypothalamic peptide hypocretin (orexin). Polysomnography: short sleep latency; early-onset of REM sleep; reduced sleep efficiency. Multiple sleep latency test (MLST), usually performed the day after overnight polysomnography, should show excessive sleepiness with at least two REM-onset sleep periods; a labor-intensive investigation, essentially requires an observer to be with the patient for a whole day. Neurogenetic testing for mutations in the hypocretin/orexin gene is available in specialist centers; eventually may obviate the need for MLST.

Differential diagnosis

Other causes of excessive daytime somnolence, e.g., OSAHS; this is more common than narcolepsy, generally has a later age at onset, and results in sleep episodes which are not refreshing; idiopathic CNS hypersomnolence, *Kleine-Levin syndrome*. Episodes of loss of consciousness, e.g., epilepsy.

Treatment and prognosis

For narcolepsy, options include:

- Modafinil (200–800 mg/day), armodafinil
- Sodium oxybate
- Mazindol (2–8 mg/day)
- Methylphenidate
- Dexamphetamine (5–60 mg/day; NB abuse potential)

For cataplexy, fluoxetine (20–60 mg/day), clomipramine, and other antidepressants may be tried.

Diagnostic criteria

Silber MH, Krahn LE, Olson EJ. Diagnosing narcolepsy: validity and reliability of new diagnostic criteria. Sleep Med. 2002;3:109–113

References

Billiard M, Bassetti C, Dauvilliers Y, et al. EFNS guidelines on management of narcolepsy. Eur J Neurol. 2006;13:1035–1048
Keam S, Walker MC. Therapies for narcolepsy with or without cataplexy: evidence-based review. Curr Opin Neurol. 2007;20:699–703
Scammell TE. The neurobiology, diagnosis, and treatment of narcolepsy. Ann Neurol. 2003;53:154–166
Taheri S, Zeitzer JM, Mignot E. The role of hypocretins (orexins) in sleep regulation and narcolepsy. Annu Rev Neurosci. 2002;25:283–313

NARP syndrome

NARP syndrome, an acronym for *n*eurogenic weakness, *a*taxia, and *r*etinitis *p*igmentosa, is a *mitochondrial disorder* most commonly resulting from a point mutation at base pair 8993 (T8993C or T8993G) of the mitochondrial genome. Besides the clinical features encapsulated in the name, there may also be psychomotor regression (it may enter the differential diagnosis of *cerebral palsy*), epileptic seizures, diabetes mellitus, cardiomyopathy, and lactic acidosis. Mutations at the same position may also cause maternally inherited *Leigh's syndrome* (MILS).

Reference

Holt IJ, Harding AE, Petty RK, et al. A new mitochondrial disease associated with mitochondrial DNA heteroplasmy. *Am J Hum Genet.* 1990;46:428–433

Nasu-Hakola disease

Membranous lipodystrophy, Polycystic lipomembranous osteodysplasia with sclerosing leukoencephalopathy (PLOSL), Presenile dementia with bone cysts

Nasu-Hakola disease is an autosomal recessive disorder characterized by large-scale destruction of cancellous bone and presenile *dementia*. In the 20s, bone cysts filled with triglycerides cause pain and swelling of wrists and ankles, and fractures may occur. In the 30s, cognitive decline and epileptic seizures develop. MR imaging reveals frontal myelin loss and massive gliosis ("sclerosing leukoencephalopathy"). Death in the fifth decade is common. The combination of neurological and radiological features is said to be unique, precluding the necessity for brain biopsy to make the diagnosis. Families have been identified with deletions of chromosome 19q13.1 which partially encompass the *DAP12* gene; point mutations and single base deletions have been identified in this gene in other families, but not in all, indicating genetic heterogeneity. Mutations have also been identified in the TREM2 gene.

References

Bianchin MM, Capella HM, Chaves DL, et al. Nasu-Hakola disease (polycystic lipomembranous osteodysplasia with sclerosing leukoencephalopathy – PLOSL): a dementia associated with bone cystic lesions. From clinical to genetic and molecular aspects. Cell Mol Neurobiol. 2004;24:1–24
Madry H, Prudlo J, Grqic A, Freyschmidt J. Nasu-Hakola disease (PLOSL): report of five cases and review of the literature. Clin Orthop Relat Res. 2007;454:262–269

Nathalie syndrome

Nathalie syndrome is characterized by deafness, cataract, muscular dystrophy, skeletal abnormalities, growth retardation, underdeveloped secondary sexual characteristics, and ECG abnormalities. It enters the differential diagnosis of the *Brown-Vialetto-Van Laere syndrome.*

References

Cremers CW, Ter Haar BG, Van Rens TJ. The Nathalie syndrome. A new hereditary syndrome. Clin Genet. 1975;8:330–340

Sathasivam S. Brown-Vialetto-Van Laere syndrome. Orphanet J Rare Dis. 2008;Apr 17;3:9

Neck-tongue syndrome

The neck-tongue syndrome is characterized by pain in the upper neck and occiput accompanied by numbness of the ipsilateral half of the tongue on sudden turning of the head. Lingual pseudoathetosis may also occur. It is thought to be due to irritation of the second cervical dorsal nerve root, which carries proprioceptive fibers from the tongue via the hypoglossal nerve. Pseudoathetosis may reflect lingual deafferentation.

References

Orrell RW, Marsden CD. The neck-tongue syndrome. J Neurol Neurosurg Psychiatry. 1994;57:348–352

Sjaastad O, Bakketeig LS. Neck-tongue syndrome and related (?) conditions. Cephalalgia. 2006;26:233–240

Necrotizing myelopathy

Diseases of the spinal cord which can cause tissue necrosis, with or without secondary cavity (syrinx) formation, include:

- Spinal dural arteriovenous fistula (Foix-Alajouanine syndrome)
- Malignancy: primary, metastatic
- Paraneoplasia
- *Neuromyelitis optica* (Devic's disease); *Vernant's disease*
- Post vaccination syndrome
- Idiopathic disease

Reference

Kim RC. Necrotizing myelopathy. Am J Neuroradiol. 1991;12: 1084–1086

Nemaline myopathy

Nemaline myopathy is an inherited myopathy with both autosomal dominant and, more commonly, autosomal recessive forms, with variable clinical phenotype but typical histological findings of granules or rods of filamentous material (*nema* = thread, in Greek). Mutations in a number of genes have been associated with nemaline myopathy; hence, routine genetic testing is not possible.

Clinical features

Variable phenotype:

- Birth: floppy infant, feeding difficulty, +/– respiratory muscle involvement
- Childhood: delayed motor milestones; weak face, tent-shaped mouth, high-arched palate, nasal voice, diffuse limb weakness, usually proximal > distal
- Adult: facial and proximal weakness, *dropped head syndrome*, respiratory involvement

+/– Cardiomyopathy
+/– Kyphoscoliosis
Once diagnosis is made, respiratory function should be monitored for insidious onset of hypoventilation.

Investigation

Bloods: normal or only slightly elevated creatine kinase. EMG/NCS: nonspecific myopathic EMG. Muscle biopsy hallmark is nemaline rods in the subsarcolemmal region, staining red with the Gomori trichrome method. Nemaline rods can be secondary phenomena in other disorders. Type 1 fiber predominance, selective atrophy of type 1 fibers, deficiency of type 2b fibers. Neurogenetic testing may show deterministic mutations in genes encoding the proteins nebulin (NEB), α-actin (ACTA1), α-tropomyosin 3 (TPM3), slow skeletal muscle troponin T (TNNT1), β-tropomyosin (TPM2), and muscle-specific cofilin (CFL2). Other genes may be discovered.

Differential diagnosis

Other *congenital myopathies*

Treatment and prognosis

Progression of weakness is typically slow. Hypoventilation may require nocturnal positive pressure ventilation. Scoliosis may require surgery.

Reference

Wallgren-Pettersson C, Laing NG. Report of the 70th ENMC international workshop: nemaline myopathy, 11–13 June 1999, Naarden, the Netherlands. Neuromuscul Disord. 2000;10:299–306

Neuralgic amyotrophy

Brachial plexus neuritis, Idiopathic brachial plexopathy, Parsonage Turner syndrome

Neuralgic amyotrophy is a syndrome of painful brachial plexopathy, often following an upper respiratory tract infection or immunization and thought to be immune mediated. Exercise, such as carrying a heavy rucksack, may also be a precipitating factor. Familial forms are also described: Hereditary neuralgic amyotrophy (HNA) is linked to chromosome 17q25 due to mutations in the SEPT9 gene [OMIM#162100] (i.e., distinct from *hereditary neuropathy with liability to pressure palsies*, which may also manifest with isolated *brachial plexopathy*); these patients may have mild dysmorphic features (epicanthic folds, hypertelorism).

Clinical features

- Abrupt onset of severe arm pain, usually unilateral, worse with movement; may be confused with cardiac ischemia if left sided
- Followed by weakness of the arm, more usually proximal than distal, involving selectively or in combination muscles innervated by the axillary, suprascapular, long thoracic, radial, musculocutaneous, and anterior interosseous nerves.
- Wasting may be marked and extremely focal.
- Reflexes may be lost.
- Sensory loss or paraesthesia may occur, but these are minor features in comparison to the motor deficit.
- Diaphragmatic weakness may occur, with possible respiratory compromise.
- Bilateral symptoms occur in ~25% of cases, with the involvement being sequential rather than simultaneous in onset.
- Neuralgic amyotrophy may be recurrent in perhaps 5% of cases.

Investigation

Neurophysiology (EMG/NCS) may show no abnormalities early in the course, but 7–10 days after the onset of weakness axonal injury is evident in the distribution of the specific nerves affected and fibrillation potentials are seen in weak muscles and even in some clinically normal muscles.

Differential diagnosis

Pain may mimic a musculoskeletal disorder, acute cervical disc prolapse, or ischemic cardiac pain. Focal onset may be confused with mononeuropathy, radiculopathy. Other causes of brachial plexopathy may be considered, although none are associated with such an acute onset of pain. (Metastatic infiltration of the plexus has a slower onset.)

Treatment and prognosis

Natural history is improvement but very slowly, up to 2–3 years. Wasting, weakness, and reflex loss may persist. No effective treatment is known.

References

Chance PF. Inherited focal, episodic neuropathies: hereditary neuropathy with liability to pressure palsies and hereditary neuralgic amyotrophy. NeuroMolecular Med. 2006;8:159–174

Sathasivam S, Lecky B, Manohar R, Selvan A. Neuralgic amyotrophy. J Bone Joint Surg Br. 2008;90:550–553

Tsairis P, Dyck PJ, Mulder DW. Natural history of brachial plexus neuropathy. Report on 99 patients. Arch Neurol. 1972;27:109–117

Van Alfen N. The trouble with neuralgic amyotrophy. Pract Neurol. 2006;6:298–307

Neuroacanthocytosis

Chorea-acanthocytosis, Levine–Critchley syndrome

Acanthocytes are red blood cells with a crenellated, spiky membrane, which are found in a number of conditions, including systemic diseases which may have neurological features, lipoprotein disorders (including *abetalipoproteinemia* and familial hypobetalipoproteinemia), and the neuroacanthocytosis syndromes which are genetically defined disorders causing progressive neurodegeneration of the basal ganglia. These include autosomal recessive chorea-acanthocytosis, X-linked McLeod syndrome, Huntington's disease-like 2, and pantothenate kinase-associated neurodegeneration. The clinical entity of a hereditary movement disorder associated with acanthocytes and no biochemical abnormality was first reported in the 1960s, most notably by Critchley and Levine.

Clinical features

Chorea-acanthocytosis (ChAc):

- Autosomal recessive inheritance, symptoms onset usually in 20s.
- Movement disorder: especially orofacial dyskinesias, feeding dystonia, involuntary vocalizations, mutilating injuries to the lips and tongue.
- Generalized chorea akin to that seen in *Huntington's disease*.
- Seizures, typically generalized, in about one-third of patients.
- Parkinsonism (minority).
- Cognitive disorder: tends to be progressive, may ultimately lead to dementia. However, the extent and progression of cognitive deficits is very variable.
- Psychiatric symptoms: schizophrenia-like psychosis, obsessive-compulsive disorder.
- Sensory-motor neuropathy with amyotrophy, reduced tendon jerks.
- Autonomic involvement.

McLeod syndrome (MLS):

- X-linked. Female heterozygotes may develop CNS symptoms.
- Similar neurological features, but lip-biting, dystonia, and parkinsonism exceptional. Most have a degree of muscle weakness and atrophy.
- Sixty percent develop cardiomyopathy, atrial fibrillation.
- Contiguous gene syndrome with MLS, Duchenne muscular dystrophy, chronic granulomatous disease, +/– X-linked retinitis pigmentosa is described.

Huntington's disease-like 2 (HDL2):

- Autosomal dominant, all of African ancestry
- Psychiatric symptoms usually precede movement disorder, usually chorea but also dystonia and parkinsonism
- No peripheral nerve or muscle abnormalities, no seizures

Pantothenate kinase-associated neurodegneration: See *Neurodegeneration with brain iron accumulation*.

Investigation

Bloods: Detecting acanthocytes is difficult to standardize and not obligatory for the diagnosis of a neuroacanthocytosis syndrome. Creatine kinase raised in almost all (MLS) or most (ChAc) patients, normal in HDL2. In MLS, Kx antigen is absent and Kell antigens reduced on erythrocytes in males. ChAc patients have absent chorein expression in erythrocytes on Western blot. Neuroimaging (CT/MRI) shows striatal atrophy (head of caudate) and striatal hypometabolism (PET). CSF is usually normal. Neurophysiology

(EMG/NCS) may show a predominantly axonal neuropathy with or without myopathy. Neuropsychology is often impaired, especially on tests sensitive to frontal lobe function. Neurogenetic testing shows mutations in the following genes: chorein (VPS13A) gene on chromosome 9 in ChAc; in the XK gene encoding the XK protein in MLS; expanded trinucleotide repeat (CTG/CAG) in the junctophilin 3 gene in HDL2. Trinucleotide repeat disorders, HD and DRPLA, may be excluded on genetic testing.

Neuropathological findings are severe neuronal loss and gliosis in the head of the caudate and to a lesser extent in the putamen, globus pallidus, and substantia nigra.

Differential diagnosis

- On clinical features: Huntington's disease, *dentatorubral-pallidoluysian atrophy (DRPLA)*, *Tourette syndrome*, cerebral vasculitis
- On hematological features: abetalipoproteinaemia, hypobetalipoproteinemia; severe malnutrition, thyroid disorders, splenectomy, liver cirrhosis, MELAS

Treatment and prognosis

There is no curative or disease-modifying treatment at present. Treatment of abnormal movements and epileptic fits is symptomatic. Dopamine antagonists or tetrabenazine may help chorea. Enteral feeding may be required if swallowing is impaired or there is nutritional compromise. The disease tends to run a progressive course, but the speed of progression is very variable (~5–30 years).

References

Danek A, ed. Neuroacanthocytosis Syndromes. Dordrecht, The Netherlands: Springer, 2004
Jung HH, Danek A, Walker RH. Neuroacanthocytosis. Adv Clin Neurosci Rehabil. 2009;9(5):16,18,20
Storch A, Kornhass M, Schwarz J. Testing for acanthocytosis. A prospective reader-blinded study in movement disorder patients. J Neurol. 2005;252:84–90
Zeman A, Shenton G. Neuroacanthocytosis. Pract Neurol. 2004;4:298–301

Neuroblastoma

Neuroblastoma is a tumor of neural elements, a CNS primitive neuroectodermal tumor (PNET), and one of the most common solid tumors seen in children. It is consistently associated with deletion of the short arm of chromosome 1; a possible tumor suppressor gene may be located at 1p36.1.

Adrenal medulla and sympathetic ganglia are the most common locations, but cerebral and olfactory (esthesioneuroblastoma) tumors may also occur. Differentiated neuroblastoma or neurocytoma is a variant, usually found in the lateral ventricles, with a good prognosis.

A small proportion of children with neuroblastoma develop the opsoclo-nus-myoclonus syndrome (Kinsbourne's syndrome), one of the *paraneoplastic syndromes*. An underlying neuroblastoma is found in about 50% of children with opsoclonus-myoclonus syndrome: those with a tumor have a better prognosis because it is a benign tumor. In cases with tumor, which may be demonstrated by CT of thorax and abdomen, there may be elevated urinary catecholamines.

Reference

Faragalla H, Weinreb I. Olfactory neuroblastoma: a review and update. Adv Anat Pathol. 2009;16:322–331

Neuroborreliosis

Bannwarth's syndrome, Garin-Bujadoux meningopolyneuritis, Lyme disease

Infection with the spirochaete *Borrelia burgdorferi*, transmitted by the bite of infected *Ixodes* ticks, is the cause of borreliosis, a condition endemic in various areas (coastal northeastern USA, New Forest UK, Germany). Sequelae of infection may be dermatological, cardiological, and neurological; the latter may include aseptic meningitis +/− multiple radicular or peripheral nerve lesions (Garin-Bujadoux meningopolyneuritis), myelitis, cranial neuropathy (especially facial nerve) +/− meningoradiculitis of the cauda equina (Bannwarth's syndrome).

Clinical features

Early local infection produces a rash (erythema migrans chronicum) as the first recognizable manifestation, occurring 3–30 days after tick bite, but this may be missed. Influenza-type symptoms such as fatigue, malaise, fever, polyarthralgia (large joints > distal), myalgia, lymphadenopathy and headache may occur.

- Early neuroborreliosis:
  - Lymphocytic meningitis and meningoradiculitis: one or multiple nerve roots and/or cranial (facial nerve in half, often bilateral, cf. *Bell's palsy*) or peripheral nerve roots (Bannwarth's syndrome)
  - Multiple mononeuropathy without meningitis (rare)
  - Lyme myositis (rare)

- Late neuroborrelisosis:
  - Persistent chronic meningitis, radiculomyelitis, encephalomyelitis
  - Chronic mononeuropathy, asymmetrical polyneuropathy
  - Subacute encephalopathy
  - Axonal peripheral neuropathy

A syndrome of fatigue, myalgia, paraesthesia, memory complaints, and depression following treatment of Lyme disease has been described as "chronic Lyme disease" or "post-Lyme disease syndrome" (PLDS), but the exact nature of this syndrome is uncertain. Some patients with these symptoms present to neurologists as (self-diagnosed) cases of PLDS but with no evidence of prior infection with Borrelia.

Investigation

Blood serology for antibodies to *B. burgdorferi*, if positive, indicates exposure (may be positive in asymptomatic individuals in endemic areas). Tests usually remain positive after treatment. Neurophysiology (EMG/NCS) in appropriate cases may show neuropathy or radiculopathy. CSF may show a lymphocytic pleocytosis, elevated protein, but normal glucose.

Differential diagnosis

Facial palsy: Bell's palsy, other causes of facial weakness. Differential diagnosis of radiculopathy, meningitis, encephalopathy.

Treatment and prognosis

Most cases respond to antibiotics. Oral doxycycline and intravenous ceftriaxone are equally effective in patients with symptoms confined to the peripheral nervous system, and in meningitis. CNS parenchymal disease requires intravenous ceftriaxone for 2–3 weeks. With appropriate treatment, improvement of neurological features should be expected in days to weeks, although encephalopathy may not improve. An inverse correlation between time to diagnosis and treatment, and degree of clinical improvement has been noted. PLDS does not respond to antibiotics.

References

Lipsker D, Jaulhac B, eds. Lyme Borreliosis. Biological and Clinical Aspects. Basel: Karger; 2009
Mygland A, Ljøstad U, Fingerle V, Rupprecht T, Schmutzhard E, Steiner I. EFNS guidelines on the diagnosis and management of European Lyme neuroborreliosis. Eur J Neurol. 2010;17:8–16

Steere AC, Sikand VK. The presenting manifestations of Lyme disease and the out-comes of treatment. N Engl J Med. 2003;348: 2472–2474
Wokke JHJ, Vanneste JAL. Neuroborreliosis. Pract Neurol. 2004;4:152–161

Neurobrucellosis

Brucella melitensis, a Gram-negative coccobacillus, is the most common of the *Brucella* species to cause human disease. *B. abortus, B. suis,* and *B. canis* (natu-rally found in goats/sheep/camels; cattle; pig and dog, respectively) may also cause human disease. Acquisition of this zoonosis is often through consump-tion of contaminated (unpasteurized) milk or its products, or contact with infected animals. Spread is from gastrointestinal tract to bloodstream, organs particularly affected being bone, spleen, lungs, as well as brain. Chronic relaps-ing illness, often involving the nervous system, is typical. Brucellosis is diag-nosed by serological testing and when treated early has a good prognosis.

Clinical features

- Acute:
  - Meningoencephalitis (headache, fever, sweating, weight loss, back pain; meningeal irritation, confusion, hepatosplenomegaly)
- Chronic:
  - Lymphocytic *meningitis*
  - Demyelination, e.g., retrobulbar neuritis
  - Polyneuropathy; radiculopathy, especially lumbar
  - Cranial nerve mononeuritis, particularly VIII
  - Cerebral arteritis, subarachnoid hemorrhage: stroke
  - Spinal cord compression by granuloma: paraplegia
  - Extrapyramidal syndrome
  - Abscess formation
  - Depression

Investigation

Culture of organism from blood, CSF, lymph node, or bone marrow. Serology: Rose-Bengal/agglutination tests may be positive in endemic areas without active disease; ELISA is more sensitive and specific. Neuroimaging (CT/MRI) may show periventricular change; spinal MRI may identify extradural compressive granulomatous disease. CSF may show raised protein, lymphocytic pleocytosis, low glucose in 20%; may have oligoclonal bands. Elevated adenine deaminase (ADA) is nonspecific. PCR for *Brucella* may be helpful. Neurophysiology: EEG: in meningoencephalitis shows slowing and sometimes epileptiform fea-tures; may be helpful to differentiate other causes of encephalopathy. EMG: in cases of radiculopathy. Other investigations: plain radiology, bone scan for sacroiliitis, lumbar spine involvement. ECG, echocardiogram for *endocarditis*.

Differential diagnosis

Broad neurological differential diagnosis:

- *Tuberculosis*
- *Neurosyphilis*
- *Neuroborreliosis*
- *Neurosarcoidosis*
- *Behçet's disease*
- CNS lymphoma
- CNS vasculitis
- Extradural spinal cord compression

Treatment and prognosis

A combination of rifampicin (e.g., 600–900 mg/day) and doxycycline (e.g., 100–200 mg/day) may be given, with ceftriaxone or co-trimoxazole; streptomycin is now discouraged because of poor CSF penetration and neurotoxicity. In chronic disease, a drug cocktail should be given for 3–6 months, with rechecking of CSF to look for resolution of infection.

Recovery is the norm for acute episodes. In chronic disease, the outlook is good for cord compression if recognized and treated early, but less good for radiculopathy and meningoencephalitis.

References

Gul HC, Erdem H, Bek S. Overview of neurobrucellosis: a pooled analysis of 187 cases. Int J Infect Dis. 2009;13:e339–e343
Pappas G, Akritidis N, Christou L. Treatment of neurobrucellosis: what is known and what remains to be answered. Expert Rev Anti Infect Ther. 2007;5:983–990

Neurocutaneous syndromes

Congenital ectodermosis, phakomatosis

Neurocutaneous syndromes are hereditary disorders involving ectodermal structures (CNS, eyes, skin), which evolve slowly during childhood and adolescence, and show a tendency to formation of hamartomas, benign tumorlike developmental lesions which may undergo malignant transformation.

The disorders encompassed by this category include:

- *Neurofibromatosis*
- *Tuberous sclerosis*

A number of conditions characterized by cutaneous angiomatosis with CNS abnormalities, including:

- *Sturge-Weber syndrome*
- *Von Hippel Lindau disease*
- *Ataxia telangiectasia* (Louis-Bar syndrome)
- *Fabry's disease*
- *Hereditary hemorrhagic telangiectasia* (Osler–Weber–Rendu syndrome)

These conditions are usually set apart from other diseases involving skin and brain in which ectodermal malformations (often hemangiomas) develop *in utero* rather than in childhood and adolescence, although both may be encompassed under the rubric of "neurocutaneous syndrome." Within the latter group are conditions such as:

- Bloch-Sulzberger syndrome (incontinentia pigmenti)
- Blue rubber bleb nevus syndrome
- Epidermal nevus syndrome
- Sjögren-Larsson syndrome
- Rothmund-Thomson syndrome
- Xeroderma pigmentosum

Other conditions with neurological and non-hemangiomatous dermatological features may also be labeled as neurocutaneous syndromes, e.g., *cerebrotendinous xanthomatosis*, Cowden's disease, Ehlers–Danlos syndrome, kinky hair syndrome, Leopard syndrome, Lesch–Nyhan syndrome, *Parry–Romberg syndrome*, pseudoxanthoma elasticum, Sweet's syndrome, Weber–Christian disease, Wyburn–Mason syndrome.

Neurofibromatosis, tuberous sclerosis, and von Hippel Lindau disease probably result from mutations in tumor suppressor genes, as in retinoblastoma. A loss of heterozygosity in tumor cells suggests a "two-hit" mechanism in tumor pathogenesis.

References

Islam MP, Roach ES. Neurocutaneous syndromes. In: Bradley WG, Daroff RB, Fenichel GM, Jankovic J, eds. Nz, 5th ed. Philadelphia, PA: Butterworth-Heinemann Elsevier; 2008:1821–1853

Miller VS, Roach ES eds. Neurocutaneous Disorders. Cambridge: Cambridge University Press; 2004

Neurocysticercosis

Infection with the larval stage (cysticercus) of the helminth cestode *Taenia solium*, the pork tapeworm, usually results from eating undercooked pork, and may lead to diverse neurological syndromes when cysticerci reach the CNS; muscle, eye, and subcutaneous tissues may also be involved.

In some tropical countries, it is the most common cause of *epilepsy*, and hence probably the most common cause of epilepsy worldwide.

Clinical features

- Focal or generalized epilepsy.
- Focal neurological deficits, e.g., episodic ataxia (nausea, projectile vomiting, fever, malaise).
- Raised intracranial pressure.
- Cognitive decline.
- Meningitis (acute, chronic).
- Myelopathy, spinal epidural abscess.
- Fulminant encephalitis (rare).
- Focal or generalized muscle enlargement: Examine subcutaneous tissues for calcified cysts.

Investigation

Bloods: eosinophilia (not often helpful); ELISA (high false positive rate). Stool to look for ova (not often helpful). Neuroimaging: CT for granuloma, calcified cysts; MRI for cysts; may see lesions at different stages of development. CSF may show a mononuclear or lymphocytic pleocytosis, raised pressure. Brain biopsy may be required for definitive diagnosis.

Differential diagnosis

- *Echinococcosis*
- *Cryptococcosis*
- *Paragonimiasis*
- Cystic astrocytoma
- *Epidermoid*
- *Episodic ataxias* of genetic etiology
- Other symptomatic causes of epilepsy

Treatment and prognosis

Symptomatic treatment of epileptic seizures, raised intracranial pressure (e.g., shunting for *hydrocephalus*). Role of antiparasitic drugs remains a subject of debate: Single granulomatous lesions may not require such treatment whereas viable cysts and enhancing lesions may be treated with agents such as albendazole and praziquantel, with or without steroid (dexamethasone) cover. Surgery may be required for single big cysts causing mass effect.

Reference

Garcia HH, Gonzalez AE, Tsang VCW, et al. Neurocysticercosis: some of the essentials. Pract Neurol. 2006;6:288–297

Neurodegeneration with brain iron accumulation (NBIA)

Pantothenate kinase-associated neurodegeneration

Neurodegeneration with brain iron accumulation-1 (NBIA-1) is an autosomal recessive disorder associated with mutations in the pantothenate kinase 2 (PANK2) gene on chromosome 20p13.

Clinical features

- Early-onset, typically in childhood, with progressive dystonia, choreoathetosis, spasticity, pigmentary retinopathy, cognitive impairment.
- Late-onset is reported with parkinsonian syndrome and dementia.

Investigation

Bloods: About 8% are said to have acanthocytosis, so this condition may be classified as one of the *neuroacanthocytosis* syndromes. Neuroimaging with MRI shows the "eye-of-the-tiger" sign on T_2-weighted scans, decreased signal intensity in the pallidal nuclei with central hyperintensity due to iron deposition; this sign is highly suggestive although not entirely specific for NBIA-1. CSF, neurophysiology are normal. Neurogenetic testing shows mutations in the PANK2 gene: Truncating mutations are responsible for the majority of cases, but atypical cases with late-onset usually harbor missense mutations and have greater residual enzyme activity. Neuropsychology may show frontal-subcortical type deficits with bradyphrenia, reduced verbal fluency, judgment difficulties, attentional impairment but relative preservation of memory.

Differential diagnosis

Other neuroacanthocytosis syndromes, *neuroferritinopathy*, *Wilson's disease*.

Treatment and prognosis

No specific treatment. Symptomatic treatment of dystonia. Death usually occurs after 5–20 years of disease.

References

Thomas M, Hayflick SJ, Jankovic J. Clinical heterogeneity of neurodegeneration with brain iron accumulation (Hallervorden-Spatz syndrome) and pantothenate kinase-associated neurodegeneration. Mov Disord. 2004;19:36–42
Zhou B, Westaway SK, Levinson B, Johnson MA, Gischier J, Hayflick SJ. A novel pantothenate kinase gene is defective in Hallervorden-Spatz syndrome. Nat Genet. 2001;28:345–349

Neuroferritinopathy

Neuroferritinopathy is an adult-onset movement disorder caused by mutations in the gene encoding ferritin light polypeptide or ferritin light chain (FTL); the phenotype is heterogeneous with movement disorders including dystonia, chorea, and akinetic-rigid syndrome. The differential diagnosis includes idiopathic torsion dystonia, *Parkinson's disease*, and *Huntington's disease*. Disease progresses to aphonia, dysphagia, motor disability, and subcortical/frontal cognitive dysfunction. There is usually a low serum ferritin with brain aggregates of ferritin and iron, particularly the globus pallidus, with associated cystic degeneration of the caudate and lentiform nuclei.

References

Chinnery PF, Crompton DE, Birchall D, et al. Clinical features and natural history of neuroferritinopathy caused by the FTL1 460InsA mutation. Brain. 2007;130:110–119
Curtis AR, Fey C, Morris CM, et al. Mutation in the gene encoding ferritin light polypeptide causes dominant adult-onset basal ganglia disease. Nat Genet. 2001;28:350–4

Neurofibromatosis (NF)

Von Recklinghausen's disease

Neurofibromatosis is a common, autosomal dominant, neurocutaneous syndrome characterized by tumors arising from nerves (neurofibroma, neuroma) and café-au-lait spots, with a wide spectrum of severity. A clinical and neurogenetic distinction is made between:

- Neurofibromatosis type 1 (NF1) = peripheral type (von Recklinghausen's disease)
- Neurofibromatosis type 2 (NF2) = central type (much rarer than NF1)
- Localized NF: segmental, gastrointestinal, spinal, multiple café-au-lait spots

Whether "mixed NF," a phenotype with features of both NF1 and NF2, is a specific entity remains an open question, likewise whether related forms such as Noonan/NF1 are more than chance concurrence. NF1 is one of the most common monogenic Mendelian disorders seen in general neurology clinics.

Clinical features

- Diagnostic criteria for NF1 require two or more of:
  - Café-au-lait macules (Café-au-lait "spots"), ≥6
  - Axillary or inguinal freckling
  - Two or more dermal fibromas
  - A plexiform neurofibroma
  - First degree relative with NF1
  - Optic nerve glioma
  - Two or more Lisch nodules (= melanocytic, brown, hamartomas of the iris; 100% of patients)
  - Distinctive osseous lesion such as sphenoid dysplasia or thinning of the long bone cortex, with or without pseudoarthrosis
- Diagnostic criteria for NF2:
  - Bilateral acoustic neuromas (= *vestibular schwannoma*)
  - First degree relative with NF2
  - Unilateral acoustic neuroma, neurofibroma, glioma, meningioma, schwannoma, early lens opacity
- Segmental neurofibromatosis:
  - Neurofibromas, café-au-lait spots, limited to one segment of the body; there may be underlying intra-thoracic or intra-abdominal neurofibromas.

+/– Kyphoscoliosis
+/– Macrocephaly
+/– Hypertension (1% pheochromocytoma; renal artery stenosis)
+/– Epilepsy
+/– Thoracic, abdominal pain from neurofibromas
Risk factor for subarachnoid hemorrhage.

Investigation

Diagnosis is essentially clinical. Neurogenetic testing may be available (NF1: mutations in neurofibromin gene, chromosome 17q11.2; NF2: mutations in the merlin or schwannomin gene, chromosome 22q12; tumor suppressor gene; may also be mutated in cases of sporadic acoustic neuroma, meningioma). Neuroimaging (MRI) for identification and monitoring of intracranial tumors; increased incidence of aqueduct stenosis in NF1.

Differential diagnosis

NF1 is unlikely to be mistaken; some overlap with Proteus syndrome. Café-au-lait spots may be seen in Noonan syndrome, Watson syndrome.

Treatment and prognosis

No specific treatment. Monitoring for intracranial tumors, optic nerve tumors, with surgical intervention if appropriate. Shunting of aqueduct stenosis only if symptomatic. Symptomatic treatment of epilepsy, pain. Monitor blood pressure: Screen for pheochromocytoma, renal artery stenosis if hypertensive. Malignant brain tumors may reduce life expectancy.

Diagnostic criteria

NIH Consensus Development Conference Statement. Neurofibromatosis. Arch Neurol. 1988; 45:575–578

References

Evans DGR. Neurofibromatosis type 2. In: Roach ES, Miller VS, eds. Neurocutaneous Disorders. Cambridge: Cambridge University Press; 2004:50–59
Ferner RE. The neurofibromatoses. Pract Neurol 2010;10:82–93
Huson SM, Hughes RAC eds. The Neurofibromatoses. A Pathogenetic and Clinical Overview. London: Chapman & Hall; 1994
Korf BR, Rubenstein AE. Neurofibromatosis: A Handbook for Patients, Families, and Health Care Professionals, 2nd ed. New York: Thieme; 2005
Ward BA, Gutmann DH. Neurofibromatosis 1: from lab bench to clinic. Pediatr Neurol 2005;32:221–228

Neuroleptic malignant syndrome (NMS)

Malignant catatonia

Neuroleptic malignant syndrome is characterized by hyperpyrexia, hypertonia, fluctuating consciousness and autonomic instability associated, in most cases, with the use of neuroleptic drugs. A similar phenomenon may be seen with sudden withdrawal of levodopa in patients with *Parkinson's disease*, and descriptions of "lethal catatonia" from the pre-neuroleptic era seem similar. Loss of dopaminergic drive in the basal ganglia has been suggested as a mechanism, although other neurotransmitters may also be implicated. Some authorities classify this syndrome as a malignant form of catatonia, responsive to the same treatments as catatonia. It is the syndrome, not the neuroleptic, which is malignant.

Clinical features

- Development of severe muscular rigidity and elevated temperature associated with the use of neuroleptic drugs (major criterion)
- Two or more of the following (minor criteria):
  - Diaphoresis
  - Dysphagia
  - Tremor
  - Incontinence
  - Changes in level of consciousness ranging from confusion to coma
  - Mutism
  - Tachycardia (autonomic disturbance)
  - Elevated or labile blood pressure (autonomic disturbance)
  - Leucocytosis
  - Laboratory evidence of muscular injury, such as elevated creatine kinase

History of neuroleptic drug use may in fact be optional, as in Parkinson's disease, so-called non-neuroleptic malignant syndrome.

Investigation

Bloods typically show raised creatine kinase and lactate dehydrogenase. Neuroimaging shows no diagnostic features, but preexisting or concurrent organic brain disease (e.g., vascular change) is recognized to be a predisposing factor. CSF is normal.

Differential diagnosis

Hypertonia may suggest an akinetic-rigid syndrome but the acute onset is against this. NMS shares features with the *serotonin syndrome*.

Treatment and prognosis

Full supportive treatment is required: hydration, sometimes sedation, intubation, and ventilation. Dopamine agonists (e.g., bromocriptine) are sometimes tried. Lorazepam, ECT, as used for catatonia, may also be helpful in NMS.

References

Guze BH, Baxter LR. Neuroleptic malignant syndrome. N Engl J Med. 1985;313:163–166

Larner AJ, Smith SC, Farmer SF. "Non-neuroleptic malignant" syndrome. J Neurol Neurosurg Psychiatry. 1998;65:613

Mann SC, Caroff SN, Keck PE, Lazarus A. Neuroleptic Malignant Syndrome and Related Conditions, 2nd ed. Washington, DC: American Psychiatric Association; 2003

Neuromuscular junction (NMJ) diseases: overview

Defects of neurotransmission at the neuromuscular junction underlie the pathogenesis of a variety of disorders:

- *Myasthenia gravis*:
    - Juvenile and adult forms
    - Neonatal myasthenia
    - *Congenital myasthenic syndromes*
    - Drug-induced myasthenia (e.g., following penicillamine therapy)
- *Lambert–Eaton myasthenic syndrome (LEMS)*
- *Neuromyotonia*
- *Botulism*
- Antibiotic-induced neuromuscular blockade: aminoglycosides, polypeptide antibiotics

Reference

Sathasivam S, Larner AJ. Disorders of the neuromuscular junction. In: Sinclair A, Morley JE, Vellas B, eds. Pathy's Principles and Practice of Geriatric Medicine, 5th ed. Chichester, UK: Wiley, 2011: in press

Neuromyelitis optica (NMO)

Devic's disease

In 1894, Eugene Devic described a distinct syndrome characterized by acute or subacute onset of optic neuropathy with visual impairment in one or both eyes, associated with a severe transverse myelitis. This syndrome may be seen in a number of conditions including *multiple sclerosis* (MS), *acute demyelinating encephalomyelitis (ADEM)*, connective tissue disorders such as *systemic lupus erythematosus (SLE)*, and tuberculosis, but it is often an isolated condition with distinctive MRI appearances: neuromyelitis optica.

The idiopathic syndrome may occur more frequently in Japan. The precise relationship of NMO to MS was a subject of debate until relatively recently, with the discovery of a specific NMO IgG with antibodies directed against aquaporin-4. Despite this evidence for an autoimmune etiology, IgG oligoclonal bands are frequently not found in the CSF (cf. MS) and patients respond poorly to immunotherapy with steroids and so may be left with severe disability.

Clinical features

Acute severe transverse myelitis, causing paraparesis or quadriparesis +/– sphincter involvement.

Acute unilateral or bilateral optic neuropathy, often with poor recovery (typically blind or counting fingers only).

Typically a mono- or multiphasic illness with little in the way of relapsing-remitting symptoms.

There is no clinical evidence for involvement of other cranial nerves or other parts of the nervous system.

Aquaporin-4 antibody positive individuals with optic neuritis only (including *CRION*) or myelitis only forms of disease have been reported.

Investigation

NMO-IgG antibodies to aquaporin-4 are diagnostic. Bloods are otherwise usually normal, although some patients may have raised markers of inflammation and/or positive serology to indicate an underlying infection or connective tissue disorder. Neuroimaging (MRI) reveals a diffuse abnormality of the cord (typically cervical and thoracic) with a long high signal lesion associated with edema. Brain MRI is normal in about 50% of cases; in the other 50%, there are nonspecific scattered and clinically silent white matter lesions. CSF is usually normal with only about 20% of cases having a raised white cell count and evidence of intrathecal IgG production (i.e., oligoclonal bands). Neurophysiology is not usually necessary, but SSEPs and VEPs are abnormal. Pathology shows demyelination, gliosis, and sometimes necrosis and cavitation of the spinal cord and optic nerve.

Differential diagnosis

- Multiple sclerosis
- Acute disseminated encephalomyelitis (ADEM)
- *Neurosarcoidosis*
- Vasculitis
- *Leber's hereditary optic neuropathy*
- Vitamin B_{12} deficiency (*subacute combined degeneration of the spinal cord*)

Treatment and prognosis

The syndrome responds poorly to steroid therapy, including intravenous methylprednisolone, and patients may be left with permanent and severe neurological deficits. However, there is increasing evidence that patients respond best to plasma exchange in the acute situation. The drug(s) of choice for the more long-term immunosuppression of these patients is currently unresolved.

Rituximab and mycophenolate mofetil may reduce attack frequency and stabilize or improve disability.

Diagnostic criteria

Wingerchuk DM, Lennon VA, Pittock SJ, Lucchinetti CF, Weinshenker BG. Revised diagnostic criteria for neuromyelitis optica. Neurology. 2006;66:1485–1489

References

Devic E. Myelite subaigue compliquee de nevrite optique. Bull Med. 1894;8:1033–1034
Jacob A, Boggild M. Neuromyelitis optica. Pract Neurol. 2006;6: 180–184

Neuronal ceroid lipofuscinosis (NCL): overview

The neuronal ceroid lipofuscinoses are a group of *lysosomal storage diseases* characterized by the accumulation of autofluorescent inclusion bodies in neurones and other tissues. A number of forms are recognized. Initially these were characterized according to age of onset, e.g.,:

- Infantile (INCL)/Santavuori-Haltia disease/Finnish type.
- Late-infantile (LINCL)/early childhood/Jansky-Bielschowsky type.
- Juvenile (JNCL)/Vogt–Spielmeyer or Spielmeyer-Sjögren type.
- Adult/*Kufs' disease*.

Inheritance is autosomal recessive, with the exception of the adult form which may show autosomal dominant inheritance. At least ten genetic loci (CLN1–10) have currently been mapped and mutant genes identified encoding lysosomal enzymes or putative membrane proteins. With the increasing understanding of the genetic basis of these conditions, a revised classification based on linkage and mutant enzyme has been suggested, with Kufs' disease being NCL4.

Tissue biopsy (rectal mucosa, skin, endothelial cells, blood lymphocytes, conjunctival cells) may show typical inclusion bodies/cytosomes, including fingerprint inclusions (NCL 3, 4, 5, 6, 7), curvilinear inclusion bodies (NCL 2; atypical in NCL 5, 6, 7, 8), granular osmiophilic deposit (GROD; NCL1; may be seen in NCL4), and rectilinear bodies (NCL 4, 5, 6, 7, 8). Lipofuscin bodies are not diagnostic. Neurogenetic testing is available for mutations in genes encoding lysosomal enzyme palmitoyl-protein thioesterase (PPT1; NCL1) and lysosomal enzyme tripeptidyl peptidase (TPP1; NCL2).

No specific treatment is currently available. Bone marrow transplantation has been attempted, without conspicuous success. Symptomatic control of seizures (valproate), dystonia, and myoclonus may be possible. Prognosis is generally poor.

References

Bennett MJ, Hofmann SL. The neuronal ceroid-lipofuscinoses (Batten disease): a new class of lysosomal storage diseases. J Inherit Metab Dis. 1999;22:535–544
Wisniewski KE, Kida E, Golabek AA, Kaczmarski W, Connell F, Zhong N. Neuronal ceroid lipofuscinoses: classification and diagnosis. Adv Genet. 2001;45:1–34

Neuropathies: overview

Pathological processes affecting the peripheral nerves may be classified in various ways:

- Course: time course of evolution: acute, subacute, chronic
- Anatomy:
  - principal locus of pathology within the nerve trunk: axon, myelin sheath
  - Principal fiber type affected: motor, sensory, autonomic; mixed
  - Distribution: mononeuropathy, mononeuritis multiplex, polyneuropathy
- Inherited or acquired

Examples may be given for each of these classifications:

- Course:
  - Acute:
    - Guillain-Barré syndrome (GBS)
    - Acute sensory ataxic neuropathy (ASAN)
    - Acute motor axonal neuropathy (AMAN) = axonal variant of GBS
    - Acute post-infectious axonal polyradiculoneuropathy (AMSAN, axonal GBS)
  - Subacute: Subacute inflammatory demyelinating polyneuropathy.
  - Chronic:
    - Chronic inflammatory demyelinating polyneuropathy (CIDP).
    - Many cryptogenic neuropathies of later life.
- Anatomy: axonal/demyelinating
  - Axonal:
    - Trauma.
    - Malignancy
    - Critical illness polyneuropathy
    - Toxins: especially thallium, organophosphates
    - Acute axonal form of GBS = AMAN
    - Cryptogenic sensory neuropathy of late life
  - Demyelinating:
    - GBS.
    - CIDP
    - Paraproteinemic demyelinating neuropathy (PDN)
    - Post-immunization neuropathy
    - Diphtheritic neuropathy
    - Infectious mononucleosis; hepatitis; HIV
- Anatomy: motor/sensory/autonomic
  - Motor: Multifocal motor neuropathy (MMN) with conduction block
  - Sensory:
    - Acute sensory ataxic neuropathy (ASAN)
    - Cryptogenic sensory neuropathy of elderly patients
    - Hereditary sensory (and autonomic) neuropathies
    - Pure sensory variant of CIDP (rare)
  - Autonomic:
    - GBS may be predominantly or exclusively autonomic
    - Amyloid neuropathy
  - Mixed:
    - Hereditary motor and sensory neuropathies
    - Diabetic polyneuropathy

- Anatomy: mononeuropathy, mononeuritis multiplex, polyneuropathy
  - Mononeuropathy: Arm and trunk:
    - Dorsal scapular nerve
    - Long thoracic nerve
    - Suprascapular nerve
    - Axillary nerve
    - Musculocutaneous nerve
    - Radial nerve
    - Median nerve
    - Ulnar nerve
  - Leg:
    - Iliohypogastric, ilioinguinal nerves
    - Genitofemoral nerve
    - Lateral cutaneous nerve of thigh
    - Posterior cutaneous nerve of thigh
    - Femoral nerve
    - Obturator nerve
    - Gluteal nerve
    - Sciatic nerve
    - Tibial nerve
    - Peroneal nerve
    - Sural nerve
  - Neuronopathy:
    - Motor: Anterior horn cell disease
    - Sensory (= ganglionopathy): Paraneoplastic sensory neuronopathy (with or without anti-Hu antibodies); Sjögren's syndrome
  - Mononeuritis multiplex, Mononeuropathy multiplex
  - Polyneuropathy: e.g., diabetes mellitus, vitamin B_{12} deficiency, drug/toxin induced
- Inherited/Hereditary:
  - Inherited neuropathies:
    - Hereditary motor and sensory neuropathies (HMSN); Charcot-Marie-Tooth (CMT) disease
    - Hereditary sensory and autonomic neuropathies (HSAN)
    - Familial amyloid neuropathies (FAP)
    - Spinocerebellar syndromes, e.g., Friedreich's ataxia
    - Fabry's disease
    - Some leukodystrophies (X-linked *adrenoleukodystrophy*)
- Acquired:
  - Inflammatory: Vasculitic, e.g., polyarteritis nodosa (PAN); rheumatoid arthritis; systemic lupus erythematosus (SLE); Wegener's granulomatosis, Sjögren's syndrome, non-systemic vasculitic neuropathy
  - Metabolic/nutritional: diabetes, uremia, vitamin B_{12} deficiency, porphyria, amyloidosis
  - Infective: leprosy, neuroborreliosis (Lyme disease), neurosyphilis, HIV
  - Drug/toxin induced: alcohol-induced, cisplatin, pyridoxine, lead, nitrofurantoin, isoniazid, arsenic, mercury, thallium

    – Granulomatous: neurosarcoidosis
    – Infiltrative: amyloid; malignancy
    – Cryptogenic sensory neuropathy of elderly patients

Clinical features

- Pace of onset: acute, subacute, chronic
- Predisposing/precipitating factors: diabetes, drug use, recent infection (especially gastrointestinal infection)
- Careful family history, with examination of other family members if possible
- Motor:
    - Weakness appropriate to single nerve (mononeuropathy)
    - Patchy weakness appropriate to several nerves (mononeuropathy multiplex)
    - Distal > proximal weakness +/– distal reflex loss (polyneuropathy)
- Sensory:
    - Focal sensory loss appropriate to a single nerve (mononeuropathy)
    - Patchy loss suggestive of involvement of several different cutaneous nerve territiories (mononeuropathy multiplex).
    - Distal "glove and stocking" loss (polyneuropathy).
    - Predominantly pain and temperature sensory loss in some neuropathies (e.g., Tangier disease); ganglionopathies may have marked proprioceptive loss leading to sensory ataxia (which may be mistaken for a cerebellar syndrome).
- Autonomic: Vomiting, diarrhea, impotence; cardiac arrhythmia

Other features of specific diseases, e.g., ataxia in spinocerebellar ataxias, sicca syndrome in Sjögren's syndrome.

Investigation

Many investigations may be performed in an attempt to discover the cause of a peripheral neuropathy. Not all are required in every case; particular circumstances may dictate the most appropriate. The importance of diabetes mellitus cannot be overestimated. Despite extensive investigation, an etiological cause remains elusive in many cases, often more than 50% of cases although some centers claim a better rate of diagnosis.

- Bloods:
    - Hematology: FBC, ESR, vitamin B_{12}, cryoglobulins.
    - Biochemistry: glucose (fasting, +/– HbA_{1c}, oral glucose tolerance test), urea and electrolytes, liver function tests, CRP, immunoglobulins, serum angiotensin converting enzyme (ACE), porphyria screen, serum lead.
    - Serology: autoantibody profile including ANA, ANCA, ENA, rheumatoid factor, *Borrelia* serology, hepatitic serology, antiganglioside antibodies

(GD1b in acute sensory axonal neuropathy [ASAN], GQ1b in Miller Fisher syndrome), anti-neuronal antibodies (anti-Hu antibodies in paraneoplastic neuronopathy).
- Urine:
  - Microscopy: for active sediment.
  - Biochemistry: porphyrins, ALA and phorphobilinogen; 24 h urine for heavy metals.
- Feces:
  - Biochemistry: fecal porphyrins.
  - Culture: for *Campylobacter jejuni* infection.

Neurophysiology: EMG/NCS: often unhelpful in the early stages of an acute neuropathy, but generally reliable for differentiating established axonal from demyelinating neuropathy, and mononeuropathy from mononeuritis multiplex and polyneuropathy. Changes may be confined to sensory evaluation (e.g., reduced or absent sensory nerve action potentials) in pure sensory neuropathy, or to motor evaluation (e.g., reduced CMAP amplitude) in pure motor neuropathy. Conduction block should be sought in a purely motor neuropathy.

Imaging: may include CXR, chest/abdominal/pelvic CT/MRI, as well as cranial and spinal cord imaging, looking for amyloid, malignancy and CNS lesions.

CSF: cell count, protein (may be very high in GBS, CIDP), glucose, oligoclonal bands, ACE, cytology.

Nerve biopsy: may need to be considered if diagnosis not forthcoming from other investigations, especially if the patient is deteriorating rapidly and/or vasculitis is a possible diagnosis. Selective fiber loss may suggest diagnosis (e.g., reduction of unmyelinated fibers in HSAN type IV, or of small myelinated fibers in HSAN types II, V). Amyloid infiltration.

Skin biopsy: may be useful for small fiber and autonomic neuropathies.

Differential diagnosis

Neuropathies should be differentiated from plexopathies and radiculopathies (may sometimes coexist, as in acute inflammatory radiculoneuropathies)

Acute peripheral weakness mimicking neuropathy may occur in:

- Hypokalemia.
- "Spinal shock" or extensive spinal cord damage with areflexia and hypotonia; this may also be seen in vascular events involving the lower brainstem.
- Neuromuscular junction dysfunction (e.g., botulism).

Treatment and prognosis

Dependent on cause, where identified. Cryptogenic neuropathies in the elderly tend not to progress rapidly and seldom take people off their legs.

References

Dyck PJ, Thomas PK eds. Peripheral Neuropathy, 4th ed. Philadelphia, PA: W.B. Saunders; 2005

Ginsberg L, King R, Orrell R. Nerve biopsy. Pract Neurol. 2003;3:306–312

Hughes RA. Peripheral neuropathy. BMJ. 2002;324:466–469

Kuhlenbäumer G, Young P, Hünermund G, Ringelstein B, Stögbauer F. Clinical features and molecular genetics of hereditary peripheral neuropathies. J Neurol. 2002;249:1629–1650

Lauria G, Lombardi R. Skin biopsy: a new tool for diagnosing peripheral neuropathy. BMJ. 2007;334:1159–1162

Mumenthaler M, Schliack H, Mumenthaler M, Goerke H. Peripheral Nerve Lesions: Diagnosis and Treatment. New York: Thieme; 1990

Pareyson D. Diagnosis of hereditary neuropathies in adult patients. J Neurol. 2003;250:148–160

Russell SM. Examination of Peripheral Nerve Injuries. An Anatomical Approach. New York: Thieme; 2006

Staal A, Van Gijn J, Spaans F. Mononeuropathies: Examination, Diagnosis and Treatment. London: W.B. Saunders; 1999

Stewart JD. Focal Peripheral Neuropathies, 4th ed. Vancouver: JBJ Publishing, 2010

Willison HJ, Winer JB. Clinical evaluation and investigation of neuropathy. J Neurol Neurosurg Psychiatry. 2003;74(Suppl 2):ii3–ii8

Neurosarcoidosis

Sarcoidosis is a sporadic systemic disease characterized pathologically by non-caseating epithelioid cell granulomata. The organs most commonly affected are the lymph nodes, lungs, liver, spleen, skin, and eyes, but no system is exempt (with the possible exception of the adrenal glands), including the nervous system in approximately 5% of cases. The majority of these patients are known to have systemic sarcoidosis and then develop neurological signs; a small group have systemic disease presenting with neurological signs; but very rarely, sarcoidosis may be confined exclusively to the nervous system. Prevalence rates for sarcoidosis vary but the condition is much commoner in Afro-Caribbeans compared to whites, and is slightly more common in women. The cause remains unknown, although the condition is clearly immunologically mediated; whether or not cryptic infection underlies the disorder is not clear.

Clinical features

- Neurosarcoidosis:
  - Meningeal infiltration (granulomatous):
    - Cranial nerve palsies: especially VII, but optic neuritis and VIII lesions are also well recognized; Heerfordt syndrome is facial nerve palsy of sarcoid origin with parotid enlargement and uveitis (uveoparotid fever).

  o Hypothalamo-pituitary effects: diabetes insipidus, hypopituitarism, hypothalamic sarcoid (hypersomnia, obesity, personality change), +/− optic chiasm involvement causing visual disturbances.
- Vasculitis may occur (uncommon).
- Peripheral nerve involvement: mononeuropathy multiplex; plexopathy; polyneuropathy, *cauda equina syndrome* (rare).
- Muscle: sarcoid myopathy: proximal muscle atrophy, palpable nodules in muscle, may be present.
- Spinal cord: inflammatory (sarcoid) myelopathy.
- Intraparenchymal (hemisphere) mass lesions of brain and spinal cord ("sarcoid tumor").
- Intracerebral/intraretinal hemorrhage due to sarcoid-related thrombo-cytopenia (rare).
- Infarction? (reported in some series).
• Almost any other organ system can be affected, but the most common presentations are:
  - Reticuloendothelial: lymphadenopathy; epitrochlear nodes said to be particularly suggestive of diagnosis.
  - Respiratory: bilateral hilar lymphadenopathy (asymptomatic); restrictive lung disease.
  - Gastrointestinal: hepatosplenomegaly.
  - Dermatological: erythema nodosum; lupus pernio.
  - Ophthalmological: uveitis (anterior > posterior); optic neuritis (occasionally bilateral).
  - Hematological: lymphopenia, thrombocytopenia.
  - *Progressive multifocal leukoencephalopathy* (*PML*) can develop in patients with neurosarcoidosis.
  - +/− Systemic features: fever, weight loss, lethargy.

Investigation

No specific test. Bloods may show lymphopenia, thrombocytopenia, hyper-calcaemia, polyclonal hypergammaglobulinemia, raised serum angiotensin-converting enzyme (ACE). CSF may show increased protein, pleocytosis; oligoclonal bands in acute disease, but not in stable chronic disease (cf. multiple sclerosis), raised ACE (nonspecific); glucose may be low. Imaging: Chest X-ray may show bilateral hilar lymphadenopathy; fine cut CT thorax is more sensitive. Gallium scan may show typical uptake in lymphoid tissues of nasopharynx (Waldeyer's ring), plus lacrimal and salivary glands, mediastinum. For neurosarcoidosis, MRI with gadolinium is particularly helpful in showing widespread meningeal enhancement and focal uptake in hypothalamic region; intraparenchymal mass lesions may be indistinguishable from tumors (glioma, meningioma). Bone marrow aspirate, liver biospy, bronchial biopsy, lymph node biopsy, muscle biopsy may show characteristic epithelioid non-caseating granulomata if relevant organ is involved. Occasionally neurosarcoidosis is diagnosed on brain biopsy with changes in meninges or, less commonly, mass lesion. The Kveim test is no longer in use.

Differential diagnosis

Broad! *Multiple sclerosis*, vasculitides, especially Wegener's granulomatosis, other autoimmune and inflammatory conditions such as SLE, rheumatoid arthritis, Behçet's disease. *Neurosyphilis, tuberculosis*. Brain tumors, lymphoma (sarcoid tumor).

Treatment and prognosis

There are no randomized controlled trials of treatment options in sarcoidosis. The mainstay of treatment, when required, is with tapering doses of steroids and, if needed, steroid-sparing immunosuppressive agents such as azathioprine, methotrexate, or cyclophosphamide. Prolonged treatment may be required; early cessation may lead to relapse. Ciclosporin has been used in patients intolerant of or unresponsive to these treatments. Total body irradiation has been used as a last resort. There are no longitudinal studies examining course of disease and prognosis in neurosarcoidosis. It seems likely that around 65% of patients have an acute and monophasic illness, the remainder have a chronic relapsing condition (especially those with hemisphere and cord lesions).

Diagnostic criteria

Zajicek JP, Scolding NJ, Foster O, et al. Central nervous system sarcoidosis - diagnosis and management. Q J Med. 1999;92:103–117

References

Hoitsma E, Faber CG, Drent M, Sharma OP. Neurosarcoidosis: a clinical dilemma. Lancet Neurol. 2004;3:397–403

Joseph FG, Scolding NJ. Sarcoidosis of the nervous system. Pract Neurol. 2007;7:234–244

Larner AJ, Ball JA, Howard RS. Sarcoid tumour: continuing diagnostic problems in the MRI era. J Neurol Neurosurg Psychiatry. 1999;66:510–512

Nowak DA, Widenka DC. Neurosarcoidosis: a review of its intracranial manifestation. J Neurol. 2001;248:363–372

Neurosyphilis

Following infection, the spirochaete *Treponema pallidum* may invade the nervous system (neurosyphilis), usually within 18 months of inoculation, producing a meningitic picture (asymptomatic or clinically apparent) which may regress spontaneously or progress to parenchymal disease, which also involves the blood vessels. The clinical syndromes often show more widespread pathological evidence of chronic meningitis. In meningovascular syphilis, inflammation and fibrosis of arteries may be found (Heubner's arteritis). A resurgence of neurosyphilis cases was seen in the context of *HIV/AIDS* infection.

Clinical features

Neurological features of treponemal infection are protean and include:

- Asymptomatic meningitis (based entirely on CSF findings)
- Meningeal: headache, stiff neck, cranial nerve palsies, no fever; +/− raised intracranial pressure
- Parenchymal disease:
    - Meningovascular: cerebrovascular events (e.g., in a young person) causing hemiplegia, aphasia, visual disturbances, sensory loss.
    - Tabes dorsalis, tabetic neurosyphilis: sensory (locomotor) ataxia, absent lower limb tendon reflexes, lightning pains in the legs, Charcot joints, urinary incontinence, Argyll Robertson pupils, ptosis, ophthalmoplegia, optic atrophy; pathologically, there is degeneration of the posterior columns of the spinal cord.
    - General paralysis/paresis (of the insane, GPI), dementia paralytica: dementia, myoclonus, seizures, hyperreflexia, Argyll Robertson pupils.
    - Syphilitic optic atrophy: often coexists with tabes dorsalis.
    - Spinal syphilis (other than tabes): meningomyelitis, meningovascular disease.
    - Syphilitic nerve deafness.
- Gummatous disease (may mimic mass lesions)
- Osteitis of skull and spine

Investigation

Blood serological tests include: Venereal Disease Research Laboratory (VDRL) test: flocculation technique: this may be negative in neurosyphilis. Fluorescent treponemal antibody absorption (FTA-ABS) test: for antibodies specifically directed against treponemal antigens. CSF is the key investigation in suspected neurosyphilis: raised cell count, mostly lymphocytes; raised protein; increased gammaglobulins with oligoclonal bands; normal glucose; positive serology. Consider checking HIV status dependent on clinical circumstances. Neuroimaging may show consequences of infection such as brain atrophy, cerebrovascular changes.

Differential diagnosis

Other chronic meningitides: tuberculosis, neurobrucellosis, fungal infections. Other causes of stroke in the young: vasculitis, dissection. Other causes of sensory ataxia (peripheral neuropathy, cervical myelopathy). Other causes of cognitive decline. Other causes of positive VDRL: yaws, SLE (false positive).

Treatment and prognosis

Penicillin or erythromycin or tetracycline. Monitor CSF after 6 months to see if alterations have reversed (positive VDRL may persist); if not, further courses of antibiotics may be given.

References

Marra CM. Update on neurosyphilis. Curr Infect Dis Rep. 2009;11:127–134
Merrit H, Adams R, Solomon H. Neurosyphilis. Oxford: Oxford University Press, 1946
National guideline for the management of early syphilis. Clinical Effectiveness Group (Association of Genitourinary Medicine and the Medical Society for the Study of Venereal Diseases). Sex Trans Infect. 1999;75(Suppl 1):S29–S33
National guideline for the management of late syphilis. Clinical Effectiveness Group (Association of Genitourinary Medicine and the Medical Society for the Study of Venereal Diseases). Sex Trans Infect. 1999;75(Suppl 1):S34–S37

Neurovascular compression syndromes: overview

Several disorders are postulated to result from compression of cranial nerves by vascular loops, causing aberrant transmission of nerve impulses as a result of local demyelination. Possible examples include:
- Trigeminal neuralgia (Vth cranial nerve)
- Hemifacial spasm (VIth cranial nerve)
- Superior oblique myokymia (IVth cranial nerve)
- Vascular cross compression of the eighth cranial nerve (= disabling positional vertigo, vestibular paroxysmia)

Niemann–Pick disease (NPD) type C [OMIM#257220]

Juvenile dystonic lipidosis

Niemann–Pick disease type C (NP-C) is a lysosomal storage disease characterized by clumsiness, limb and gait ataxia, dysarthria, dysphagia, and cognitive deterioration (dementia). Pathophysiology is impaired intracellular lipid
trafficking leading to excessive storage of cholesterol and glycosphingolipids
in brain and other tissues. Treatment was solely supportive until recent
reports on the efficacy of miglustat as a disease stabilizer.

Clinical features

- Type C:
  - Autosomal recessive: type NPC1 linked to mutations on chromosome
    18q11 (NPC1 gene), type NPC2 to chromosome 14q24 (HE1 gene)
  - May present in infancy or early childhood as a hepatic syndrome, or in
    later childhood as a progressive neurodegenerative disease with:
    o Progressive gait disturbance, dystonia
    o Dysarthria
    o Emotional lability
    o Intellectual regression
    o Supranuclear gaze palsy with impaired vertical saccadic eye movements
    o Ataxia
    o Extrapyramidal signs
    o Seizures
    o Cataplexy
    o Mild hepatosplenomegaly
- Type D (Nova Scotia variant):
  - Allelic variant of NPC1
  - Early-onset hepatosplenomegaly
  - Neurological features as for type C
  - Protracted course, survival into adulthood

Investigation

Standard bloods are usually unremarkable although liver-related blood tests
may be mildly abnormal. On neuroimaging, skeletal radiographs are usually
normal; chest radiograph commonly shows diffuse reticular infiltration. Bone
marrow biopsy smears show foamy storage histiocytes (suggestive but not
pathognomonic, since they also occur in sialidosis) and sea-blue histiocytes in
type C (but may be absent). Measurement of sphingomyelinase enzyme
activity in leukocytes or fibroblasts is almost absent in type A. Filipin staining
of cultured skin fibroblasts may be seen in type C. On brain biopsy, neurofibrillary tangles may be seen in the hippocampus in type C.

Differential diagnosis

Gaucher disease, but neurological involvement is later in NPD.

Treatment and prognosis

Miglustat has been reported to stabilize disease over a 12-month period.

Reference

Fink JK, Filling-Katz MR, Sokol J, et al. Clinical spectrum of Niemann-Pick disease type C. Neurology. 1989;39:1040–1049

NIFID

FTLD-FUS, FTLD-IF, Neuronal intermediate filament inclusion disease

Neuronal intermediate filament inclusion disease (NIFID) is a neurodegenerative disorder characterized pathologically by intraneuronal cytoplasmic inclusions of variable morphology which immunostain for all class IV intermediate filament (IF) proteins, namely NF-H, NF-M, NF-L, and alpha-internexin. More recently, these inclusions have been shown to be immunoreactive for the fused in sarcoma (FUS) protein. The clinical phenotype is heterogeneous, encompassing behavioral changes, language impairment, perseveration, executive dysfunction with or without early-onset dementia, extrapyramidal features, and subclinical or clinical involvement of upper and lower motor neurones. The diagnosis of NIFID merits consideration in any patient with an extrapyramidal syndrome and evidence of *motor neurone disease*.

Reference

Cairns NJ, Grossman M, Arnold SE, et al. Clinical and neuropathologic variation in neuronal intermediate filament inclusion disease. Neurology. 2004;63:1376–1384

NMDA-receptor encephalitis

NMDA-receptor encephalitis is a severe form of encephalitis associated with antibodies directed against NR1–NR2 heteromers of the NMDA receptor. Affected patients are usually young women; there is an association with underlying ovarian teratoma in some, but not all, cases.

Clinical features

- Psychiatric symptoms
- Memory problems
- Epileptic seizures
- Unresponsiveness
- Dyskinesias
- Autonomic instability
- Hypoventilation

Investigation

The presence of antibodies directed against NMDA receptors is diagnostic.

Differential diagnosis

Other forms of acute encephalitis, infective or immune mediated.

Treatment and prognosis

Tumor immunotherapy and decrease of serum antibody titers are associated with better outcome, only a quarter of patients are left with severe deficits or die. In non-tumor associated cases, treatment with steroids and plasma exchange is useful.

Reference

Dalmau J, Gleichman AJ, Hughes EG, et al. Anti-NMDA-receptor encephalitis: case series and analysis of the effects of antibodies. Lancet Neurol. 2008;7:1091–1098

Nocardiosis

Nocardia species are aerobic actinomycetes; filamentous, weakly Gram positive, bacteria, spread from soil by inhalation, which cause localized (cutaneous, pulmonary) or disseminated infections, the latter often involving the CNS, most particularly in immunocompromised individuals such as *HIV/AIDS*. Pulmonary disease may seed via the bloodstream to the brain as multiple abscesses, often multiloculated, causing space occupation, raised intracranial pressure, focal deficits, and epilepsy. The abscesses are clincally and radiologically identical to abscesses of different etiology, diagnosis relying on identification of the organism in pus from a stereotactic biopsy. Meningitis may also occur. Treatment is with sulfonamides and trimethoprim, minocycline, imipenem or an aminoglycoside, despite which mortality remains high (30–60%).

Reference

Minero MV, Marin M, Cercenado E, Rabadan PM, Bouza E, Munoz P. Nocardiosis at the turn of the century. Medicine (Baltimore). 2009;88:250–261

Nonaka myopathy [OMIM#605820]

Distal myopathy with rimmed vacuoles

Nonaka myopathy is an autosomal recessive *distal myopathy* usually of early-onset characterized by muscle wasting and weakness in a predominantly distal distribution, e.g., the anterior compartment of the legs, causing foot drop and steppage gait; hand and finger weakness may also be present. Creatine kinase is elevated (<10 times normal). Muscle biopsy shows a vacuolar myopathy (cf. *Miyoshi myopathy*); vacuoles are rimmed and have nuclear or cytoplasmic inclusions (15–18 nm filaments). Linkage is to chromosome 9p. Mutations in the (UDP-N-acetyl)-2-epimerase/*N*-acetylmannosamine kinase gene (GNE) have been identified.

References

Kayashima T, Matsuo H, Saitoh A et al. Nonaka myopathy is caused by mutations in the UDP-N-acetylglucosamine-2-epimerase/N-acetylmannosamine kinase gene (GNE). J Hum Genet. 2002;47:77–79
Nonaka I, Sunohara N, Ishiura S, Satoyoshi E. Familial distal myopathy with rimmed vacuole and lamellar (myeloid) body formation. J Neurol Sci. 1981;51:141–155

Non-epileptic attack disorder (NEAD)

Dissociative seizures, Pseudoseizures, Psychogenic seizures

Non-epileptic attack disorder (NEAD) is characterized by seizure-like attacks which arise for reasons other than *epilepsy*, often as a sign of emotional difficulties such as anxiety or depression. There is often a prior history of physical or sexual abuse. Attacks may coexist with true epileptic seizures. They are more common in women.

Clinical features

- Convulsive movements, often not typical of epileptic attacks, e.g., head shaking from side to side; resistance to eye opening, no deviation of eyes, increased amplitude of movements with time and audience, "thrashing" movements.

- Forced eye closure, distractibility, other evidence of responsiveness may be present.
- Pelvic thrusting is a common manifestation (although may be seen in some types of epileptic seizure).
- Attacks may be prolonged: "Pseudostatus epilepticus" is described, often in individuals with a history of non-epileptic seizures, multiple episodes of "status," unexplained illness, and deliberate self-poisoning.
- No cyanosis, post-ictal confusion; urinary incontinence, tongue-biting rare (may be on tip, rather than sides, of tongue).
- Self-injury absent or minimal (e.g., confined to carpet burns).
- No focal neurological signs, no pathological reflexes.
- No elevation in serum prolactin post-event.
- Increasing attack frequency despite increasing dose and number of anti-epileptic drugs being given is suggestive.

Investigation

Diagnosis is often based on suggestive clinical history. Ideally, investigations should be kept to a minimum. Witnessing an attack, or seeing a video if possible (need patient's permission beforehand) may be very helpful. Neurophysiology (EEG, telemetry) may show an absence of typical epileptic EEG changes during a typical attack, although movement artifact may obscure EEG changes. Neuroimaging (CT/MRI) is normal, unless there is concurrent or incidental pathology.

Differential diagnosis

Epileptic seizures.

Treatment and prognosis

Patient education with appropriate literature, counseling, support groups, cognitive behavior therapy. Withdraw inappropriate antiepileptic medication if possible. Treat any underlying anxiety or depression.

References

Mellers JDC. The approach to patients with "non-epileptic seizures". Postgrad Med J. 2005;81:498–504
Plug L, Reuber M. Making the diagnosis in patients with blackouts: it's all in the history. Pract Neurol. 2009;9:4–15
Schachter SC, LaFrance WC Jr eds. Gates and Rowan's Nonepileptic Seizures. 3rd ed. Cambridge: Cambridge University Press, 2010

Non-Wilsonian hepatocerebral degeneration (NWHCD)

Acquired hepatocerebral degeneration

This condition is characterized clinically by heterogeneous fixed or progressive neurological deficits, including orobuccolingual dyskinesias, reminiscent of *tardive dyskinesia*, with dysarthria, bilateral symmetrical *parkinsonism* largely unresponsive to dopaminergic medication, gait ataxia, intention tremor, choreoathetosis, cognitive impairments (apathy, bradyphrenia, impaired attention with relatively preserved language, memory and praxis), and myelopathy akin to *subacute combined degeneration of the spinal cord*. The symptoms and signs are thought to reflect cerebral degeneration in the context of repeated episodes of hepatic encephalopathy, since portosystemic shunting seems to be a sine qua non for the occurrence of the condition, which may be seen in many forms of liver disease. Individually such episodes may be reversible but there seems to be a cumulative effect on neural tissue. MR imaging may show increased signal on T1-weighted images in the pallidal nuclei, sometimes extending to other parts of the basal ganglia and thalamus. Pathologically the brain shows microcavitary degenerative changes in layers V and VI of the cortex, underlying white matter, basal ganglia, and cerebellum. Intranuclear PAS + ve inclusions may be seen, as well as abnormalities in spinal cord tracts. Some authors have doubted the existence of this condition as a separate entity. An overlap with extrapontine myelinolysis has been reported, suggesting that there may be factors common to both disorders, and similarities (and differences) with manganism have been noted. Differential diagnosis includes *Wilson's disease*, toxic-metabolic encephalopathy, Wernicke's encephalopathy, and *central pontine myelinolysis*. Dopamine antagonists and tetrabenazine may be tried for chorea, dopaminergic agents for parkinsonism. Liver transplantation may produce a gradual improvement in symptoms.

References

Ferrara J, Jankovic J. Acquired hepatocerebral degeneration. J Neurol. 2009;256:320–332
Victor M, Adams RD, Cole M. The acquired (non-Wilsonian) type of chronic hepatocerebral degeneration. Medicine (Baltimore). 1965;44:345–395

Normal pressure hydrocephalus (NPH)

Chronic hydrocephalus, Hakim-Adams syndrome

Although the term "normal pressure hydrocephalus" was coined by Adams and colleagues in 1965, it is likely that similar cases had been described prior to this. The classical picture is the clinical triad of gait difficulty, urinary symptoms, and dementia (cognitive decline) in association with communicating hydrocephalus. Normal pressure hydrocephalus may be primary or idiopathic (iNPH), or secondary to some defined disease process, such as subarachnoid hemorrhage, basal meningitis, or a disorder causing raised CSF protein concentration. The exact incidence of the primary condition, its pathogenesis, and the optimal treatment still remain subjects of debate, but it does seem to be more common in the elderly. Some authors advocate abolition of the term "normal pressure hydrocephalus" in favor of "chronic hydrocephalus."

Clinical features

Clinical triad:

- Gait difficulty, sometimes labeled "apraxia" or "magnetic gait."
- Urinary symptoms.
- Cognitive decline: although described as "dementia" in the original accounts, the more common picture is of subcortical deficits (increased forgetfulness, inertia, reduced attention, mental slowness); NPH may not in fact be a true cause of "reversible dementia."

No rest tremor; no clinical benefit from levodopa.

Investigation

Neuroimaging (CT/MRI) shows the hydrocephalus to be communicating in type; the presence of normal sized Sylvian fissures and cortical sulci may increase the suspicion of NPH (cf. *ex vacuo* atrophy). Evans index (= maximum width of frontal horns/maximum width to inner tables of the skull) >0.3 is in keeping with the diagnosis of NPH. Proton-density MR imaging may show periventricular hyperintensity suggesting transependymal flow. Isotope cisternography has been used to demonstrate impaired CSF absorption but is not a reliable predictor of response to shunting. CSF may show raised protein, oligoclonal bands; single pressure measurements are typically normal, but prolonged intracranial pressure monitoring may show mild elevations or episodic appearance of high-pressure beta waves. The place of CSF infusion studies remains to be clarified. The CSF tap test or Fisher's test requires the removal of 20–30 mL of CSF, with assessment of gait +/- cognitive function before and after puncture. This may be helpful, since clinical improvement may suggest that shunting will be beneficial, although both false positive and false negative results are well recognized. Pathological studies in NPH are very rare, and may disclose underlying neurodegenerative disease such as Alzheimer's disease or progressive supranuclear palsy, both of which have been reported to respond temporarily to shunting procedures.

Differential diagnosis

Cerebrovascular disease may produce a similar clinical picture, and in elderly patients, there may be incidental atrophy causing *ex vacuo* ventricular dilatation; however, cortical sulci and the Sylvian fissures are usually widened too. Subdural hematoma and degenerative dementias may produce a similar picture.

Treatment and prognosis

Ventriculoperitoneal shunting (not ventriculo-atrial, or lumboperitoneal) in carefully selected cases can be beneficial. Good response occurs in those with:

- Identified etiology
- Predominantly gait abnormalities with little or no cognitive deficit
- Substantial improvement with the CSF tap test
- Normal sized Sylvian fissures, cortical sulci
- Minimal white matter change

If there are contraindications to surgery, medical therapy with acetazolamide or repeated lumbar punctures may be undertaken.

References

Adams RD, Fisher CM, Hakim S, et al. Symptomatic occult hydrocephalus with "normal" cerebrospinal fluid pressure. N Engl J Med. 1965;273:117–126
Bret P, Guyotat J, Chazal J. Is normal pressure hydrocephalus a valid concept in 2002? A reappraisal in five questions and proposal for a new designation of the syndrome as "chronic hydrocephalus". J Neurol Neurosurg Psychiatry. 2002;73:9–12
Malm J, Eklund A. Idiopathic normal pressure hydrocephalus. Pract Neurol. 2006;6:14–27

Notalgia paresthetica

Notalgia paresthetica is a condition of unknown etiology characterized by burning, paraesthesia, and itching over an area at the medial edge of scapula. It is entirely benign and may wax and wane over the years. The territory involved encompasses the dorsal branches of roots T2–T6.

References

Knight R. Notalgia paraesthetica. Pract Neurol. 2001;1:56–57
Pleet AB, Massey EW. Notalgia paresthetica. Neurology. 1978;28:1310–1312

"Numb and clumsy hands" syndrome

A syndrome of "numb and clumsy hands" has been described with midline cervical disc protrusions at the C3/C4 level, hence well above the segments supplying the hand and so a false-localizing sign. Concurrent with numbness of fingertips and palms, there may be a tightening sensation at midthoracic level. With the availability of MR imaging of the cervical cord, the responsible lesion is unlikely to be overlooked.

Reference

Nakajima M, Hirayama K. Midcervical central cord syndrome: numb and clumsy hands due to midline cervical disc protrusion at the C3–4 intervertebral level. J Neurol Neurosurg Psychiatry. 1995;58:607–613

Numb cheek syndrome, Numb chin syndrome

Numb chin syndrome (Roger's sign) is an isolated neuropathy affecting the mental branch of the mandibular division of the trigeminal (V) nerve, causing pain, swelling, and numbness of the lower lip, chin, and mucous membrane inside the lip. This is usually a sign of metastatic spread of cancer to the jaw, although has also been described as a complication of treatment with bisphosphonates.

Numb cheek syndrome, involving the cheek, upper lip, upper incisors, and gingiva, is due to involvement of the infraorbital portion of the maxillary division of the trigeminal nerve, usually by an infiltrating malignancy.

Both these presentations require investigation for underlying malignancy.

References

Campbell WW Jr. The numb cheek syndrome: a sign of infraorbital neuropathy. Neurology. 1986;36:421–423
Evans RW, Kirby S, Purdy RA. Numb chin syndrome. Headache. 2008;48:1520–1524

O

Obsessional slowness

Obsessional slowness is a feature in some patients with obsessive–compulsive disorder, characterized by difficulty initiating goal-directed action and suppressing intrusive or perseverative behavior. Washing and eating may be extremely slow because of rituals, checking behavior, and compulsions. These patients may have subtle neurological signs such as cogwheel rigidity and tics, such that the condition may be confused with other *parkinsonian syndromes* with akinetic rigidity. Dysfunction in a frontal–basal ganglia loop is implicated in pathogenesis, and PET scanning has demonstrated hypermetabolism in orbital frontal, premotor, and mid-frontal cortex.

Reference

Hymas N, Lees A, Bolton D, Epps K, Head D. The neurology of obsessional slowness. Brain. 1991;114:2203–2233

Obstructive sleep apnea-hypopnea syndrome (OSAHS)

Obesity-hypoventilation syndrome, Pickwickian syndrome

Critical narrowing of the upper airway during sleep, due to reduced muscle tone, leads to increased resistance to the flow of air, and partial airway obstruction results in apnea, hypopnea, and loud snoring. A gradation exists between the normal sleep-related increase in upper airway resistance, through upper airway resistance syndrome (UARS; subtle airflow limitation with nocturnal arousals), to obstructive sleep apnea-hypopnea syndrome (OSAHS). Sleep is restless due to successive episodes of apnea, which are relieved by brief arousals from sleep, with excessive daytime somnolence in consequence. Risk factors for the development of OSAHS include narrow anteroposterior pharyngeal diameter, obesity, high alcohol intake, and male sex. The condition is associated with increased cardiovascular and cerebrovascular morbidity and mortality and an increased risk of road traffic accidents. De novo presentation to neurological services is rare.

Clinical features

- Excessive daytime somnolence. History from a bed partner, regarding snoring, apneas, and daytime sleepiness may be helpful in establishing the diagnosis.
- Neurological features:
  - "Loss of consciousness" (falling asleep in inappropriate circumstances)
  - Personality change
  - Cognitive decline
  - Morning headache with features of raised intracranial pressure; may simulate *idiopathic intracranial hypertension*
  - Peripheral neuropathy

Examination may reveal obesity (increased body mass index, collar size), stridor at rest, narrow pharyngeal anteroposterior diameter, short thick neck, enlarged tonsils (ENT referral may be appropriate), asterixis, and hypertension. Papilledema may occur. History of alcohol intake, road traffic accidents.

Investigation

Bloods may show raised hemocrit as a consequence of nocturnal hypoxemia; arterial blood gases during the night may confirm hypoxemia, although this is intermittent. Sleep studies, either formal nocturnal polysomnography or overnight oximetry (which may be done at home), to look for dips in oxygen saturation associated with heart rate rise. Severity of OSAHS may be measured by apnea/hypopnea index (AHI), or respiratory disturbance index (RDI), calculated as the number of apneas/hypopneas per hour of sleep on polysomnography: AHI or RDI of 10–20 = mild, 20–50 = moderate, and >50 = severe disease. With pulse oximetry, a desaturation index (DI) may be calculated as the number of desaturations (decrease in oxygen saturation by $\geq 4\%$) per hour of sleep or, if the recording is unattended, per time of recording; $DI \geq 5$ may be used to define sleep-disordered breathing.

Other measures (subjective rating scales) may be used including the Epworth Sleepiness Scale, Stanford Sleepiness Scale, and the Sleep–Wake Activity Inventory.

Differential diagnosis

Other causes of excessive daytime somnolence; *narcolepsy* generally occurs in a younger age group than OSAHS and is less common; the absence of associated features of the narcoleptic syndrome (cataplexy, hypnagogic hallucinations, sleep paralysis) may assist in differential diagnosis. Narcoleptics usually feel refreshed after waking from a sleep attack, whereas OSAHS

- Visual field defect, typically a central scotoma, but other patterns may occur, includingly rarely an altitudinal field defect, although this is more suggestive of *ischemic optic neuropathy*, likewise hemorrhage and swelling of the disc.
- Fundus normal with retrobulbar neuritis (perhaps two thirds of cases).
- Natural history is of gradual improvement (if no onset of recovery by 4 weeks diagnosis of optic neuritis may be questioned), although full recovery may not occur; impairment of color vision, as tested with pseudoisochromatic (Ishihara) plates, may remain.
- Other clinical features of underlying neurological disease: multiple sclerosis, *neurosarcoidosis*.
- Recurrence occurs in up to one-fourth of cases, and carries increased risk for development of MS.

Investigation

Neurophysiology: Visual evoked potentials/responses (VEPs/VERs) showing increased latency with relatively preserved waveform are highly suggestive of optic neuritis. Imaging with MRI can visualize optic nerves, and show swelling and focal increased signal, especially in optic neuritis; MRI may also show inflammatory lesions elsewhere, which if periventricular may suggest a diagnosis of MS. CSF may show oligoclonal bands; if so, there is increased risk of progression to MS. If clinically appropriate, investigations may be undertaken to confirm or refute the diagnosis of neurosarcoidosis.

Differential diagnosis

- Structural lesions of optic nerve (usually more gradual onset).
- Ischemic optic neuropathy usually has a more acute onset.
- Neuromyelitis optica (Devic's syndrome).
- *Leber's hereditary optic neuropathy (LHON)*.
- Toxic amblyopia.
- Acute disseminated encephalomyelitis: especially if bilateral, in young person, with other neurological features.

Treatment and prognosis

Acute use of intravenous steroids (e.g., intravenous methylprednisolone, 1 g/day for 3–5 consecutive days) is recommended, and may hasten recovery, without impacting on the natural history of any underlying disease. About 40% of patients with optic neuritis have converted to MS by 10 years, especially if the initial MR brain scan shows demyelinating lesions; although 20% of those with a normal scan will also have progressed to MS by 10 years. β-Interferons may reduce the rate of conversion of clinically isolated lesions to multiple sclerosis.

References

Balcer LJ. Clinical practice. Optic neuritis. N Engl J Med. 2006;354:1273–1280
Hess RF, Plant GT, eds. Optic Neuritis. Cambridge: Cambridge University Press; 1986
Hickman SJ, Dalton CM, Miller DH, Plant GT. Management of acute optic neuritis. Lancet. 2002;360:1953–1962

Orbital apex syndrome

Superior orbital fissure syndrome

A lesion at the orbital apex may involve several cranial nerves, causing:

• External ophthalmoplegia: III, IV, VI
• Sensory deficit in face: V, ophthalmic division
• Visual deficit: II (peripheral, central field defects, papilledema, optic atrophy)

Clearly, there is clinical overlap with the syndrome resulting from *cavernous sinus disease*.

Reference

Bone I, Hadley DM. Syndromes of the orbital fissure, cavernous sinus, cerebello-pontine angle, and skull base. J Neurol Neurosurg Psychiatry. 2005;76(SupplIII):iii29–iii38.

Orbital tumors: overview

Mass lesions within the orbit may be divided into:

• Intraconal: within the cone of the extraocular muscles
• Extraconal

This division provides some clue as to underlying pathology. Periorbital lesions may also sometimes impinge on orbital structures.

Clinical features

• Intraconal: forward displacement of the globe (proptosis), +/– impairment of visual acuity, diplopia, optic disc swelling. Scirrhous breast tumor metastases may cause tethering and enophthalmos.
• Extraconal: upward or downward displacement of the globe.

Investigation

Imaging: MR is modality of choice, +/− fat suppression sequences; angiography may be required if a vascular lesion is suspected. Biopsy may be undertaken if a histological diagnosis is required to facilitate planning of appropriate treatment, but a vascular lesion must be excluded before biopsy.

Differential diagnosis

- Intraconal:
  - Tumor:
    o Primary: Optic nerve sheath meningioma, optic nerve glioma, lymphoma
    o Secondary: metastasis (breast, lung, prostate)
  - Vascular: cavernous hemangioma, varices
- Extraconal:
  - Tumor: Primary: orbital rhabdomyosarcoma; *dermoid*, mucocele
  - Inflammatory: orbital pseudotumor: *Wegener's granulomatosis,* "*Tolosa–Hunt syndrome*."

Treatment and prognosis

Of specific cause: some may be amenable to resection (e.g., cavernous hemangioma); others may be left (e.g., varices). Steroids are treatment of choice for inflammatory masses. Resection plus enucleation of the eye may be necessary in some cases.

Ornithine transcarbamoylase (OTC) deficiency

Ornithine transcarbamoylase (OTC), encoded by a gene on the short arm of the X-chromosome, catalyzes the condensation of intramitochondrial ornithine, an analog of the amino acid lysine, with carbamoylphosphate to produce citrulline. OTC deficiency, the commonest of the *urea cycle enzyme defects (UCED)*, presents in boys in the newborn period with an acute encephalopathy; stroke-like episodes may occur. OTC deficiency is characterized biochemically by severe hyperammonemia and accumulation of carbamoylphosphate. The latter diffuses to the cytosol where orotic acid and orotidine are produced, increased concentrations of which are found in the urine. Citrulline biosynthesis is defective resulting in low plasma levels of citrulline.

Female carriers of OTC deficiency may be symptomatic: feeding problems, failure to thrive, intermittent ataxia, intermittent encephalopathy; may precede an acute (and sometimes) fatal encephalopathy. It may present in adults with *coma* or acute liver failure, sometimes associated with fasting.

Oromandibular dystonia

Lingual dystonia

Oromandibular dystonia is a focal *dystonia* involving the lower face and tongue, and may manifest as jaw clenching, forced jaw opening (gaping), or involuntary tongue protrusions, with or without dysphagia and dysarthria. It is often exacerbated by talking and eating. The combination of oromandibular dystonia with blepharospasm is termed *Meige's syndrome*. Like other forms of cranial dystonia, such as blepharospasm, oromandibular dystonia may respond to botulinum toxin injections, although such treatment is not recommended for isolated lingual dystonia because of the risk of inducing bulbar weakness. The differential diagnosis of these movements includes tardive dyskinesia and *neuroacanthocytosis*.

Ortner syndrome

Cardiovocal syndrome

In the Ortner syndrome, dysphonia due to left recurrent laryngeal nerve dysfunction is caused by enlargement of the left atrium of the heart.

Ossification of the posterior longitudinal ligament (OPLL)

Ossification of the posterior longitudinal ligament (OPLL) of the spine has been recognized as a cause of myelopathy in Japan for many years, but only in more recent times has a similar condition been identified in the West. It is more common in men, the peak age of onset is in the sixth decade, and its cause remains unknown although it may occur in association with diffuse idiopathic skeletal hyperostosis (DISH), spondylosis, and *ankylosing spondylitis*.

Clinical features

- May be asymptomatic
- Most commonly affects the cervical spine causing a spastic quadriparesis; may be progressive or acute, may cause quadriplegia

Investigation

Imaging: ossification of the posterior longitudinal ligament may be evident with plain radiography of the cervical spine, myelography, or MRI.

Differential diagnosis

Other causes of spastic quadriplegia, especially compressive cervical spondy-lotic myelopathy.

Treatment and prognosis

Some cases progress, others improve spontaneously or with surgical intervention.

Reference

Mochizuki M, Aiba A, Hashimoto M, Fujiyoshi T, Yamazaki M. Cervical myelopathy in patients with ossification of the posterior longitudinal ligament. J Neurosurg Spine. 2009;10:122–128

Osteogenesis imperfecta

This group of inherited connective tissue disorders results from quantitative or qualitative defects in collagen synthesis resulting in bone fragility. There is clinical heterogeneity with respect to age at onset and number of fractures, which in turn influences walking ability and prognosis. In addition to cardiac and respiratory consequences of bone fractures and deformity, a number of neurological features have been reported:

- Spinal deformity
- Basilar impression/invagination
- Impaired hearing (sensorineural)
- Cerebrovascular associations (occasional)
  - Carotico-cavernous fistula (CCF)
  - Moyamoya disease
  - Cerebral aneurysms

Differential diagnosis may include *Ehlers–Danlos syndrome, Marfan syndrome*, and *pseudoxanthoma elasticum (PXE)*.

Treatment of the underlying bone disease with growth hormone and bis-phosphonates has been attempted. The latter may improve bone density, reduce fracture rate, and enhance growth. Symptomatic treatment of neuro-logical complications may be required.

Reference

Ibrahim AG, Crockard HA. Basilar impression and osteogenesis imperfecta: a 21-year retrospective review of outcomes in 20 patients. J Neurosurg Spine. 2007;7:594–600

Osteomalacia

Osteomalacia may be associated with proximal *myopathy* as well as bone pain and skeletal problems. Creatine kinase level is usually normal, EMG and muscle biopsy are myopathic.

O'Sullivan–McLeod syndrome

A rare form of distal *spinal muscular atrophy* (*SMA*), of autosomal recessive or autosomal dominant inheritance, causing slowly progressive wasting of the hands. Electrophysiological studies may confirm anterior horn cell disease, and focal changes have on occasion been seen on MR imaging of the anterior horns of the spinal cord at a level appropriate to the wasting.

Reference

Petiot P, Gonon V, Froment JC, Vial C, Vighetto A. Slowly progressive spinal muscular atrophy of the hands (O'Sullivan-McLeod syndrome): clinical and magnetic resonance imaging presentation. J Neurol. 2000;247:654–655

Overlap syndrome

The term overlap syndrome is given to the concurrence of an inflammatory myopathy (*polymyositis*, *dermatomyositis*) with a connective tissue disease (*Sjögren's syndrome*, *systemic sclerosis*, *systemic lupus erythematosus*).

P

Paget's disease

Osteitis deformans

Paget's disease is a disorder of bone characterized by increased bone turn-over with excessive osteoclastic resorption and disorganized new bone for-mation, predominantly affecting the older population. Bone pain is often the major symptom although the condition is frequently asymptomatic, coming to light as the explanation for an elevated blood level of alkaline phosphatase. There is a predilection for the skull and vertebral column, resulting in a vari-ety of neurological complications secondary to the bony pathology.

Clinical features

- Cranial nerve palsies, due to foraminal entrapment by pathological bone: VIII (deafness), II (optic atrophy), V, VII, I; IV, VI.
- Basilar invagination: lower cranial nerve palsies (IX, X, XI, XII).
- Hydrocephalus: gait disorder, sphincter incontinence, frontal-subcortical type of cognitive decline, apathy, hypersomnia.
- Extradural myelopathy, secondary to disease in several adjacent vertebrae affecting bodies, pedicles, and laminae: quadriparesis, paraparesis.
- Radiculopathy: cauda equina syndrome.
- Syringomyelia: secondary to skull base Paget's.
- A syndrome of *inclusion body myositis* with early-onset Paget's disease and frontotemporal dementia (IBMPFD) due to mutations in the valosin-containing protein (VCP) has been described [OMIM#167320].

Investigation

Raised blood alkaline phosphatase reflects disease activity; calcium, phos-phate normal unless the patient has been immobile. Urinary hydroxyproline levels reflect osteoclastic activity.

Imaging: plain radiology (skull, spine) for typical bone changes: irregular bone thickening, areas of resorption; widening of diploic spaces in skull with osteolytic and osteosclerotic areas giving "cotton wool" like appearance. Neuroimaging (CT/MRI) for hydrocephalus, skull base changes; MRI for cord compression. Radioisotope scanning (Tc^{99m}) may be helpful in determining extent and activity of disease.

Differential diagnosis

Other causes of isolated or combined cranial nerve palsies, myelopathy; normal pressure hydrocephalus.

Treatment and prognosis

Treatment of Paget's: diphosphonates (e.g., etidronate) reduce osteoclastic activity; calcitonin inhibits bone resorption. Symptomatic treatment: decompression for cord compression; repeated lumbar puncture or shunting for hydrocephalus; analgesia (e.g., NSAIDs) for pain.

References

Hamdy RC. Clinical features and pharmacologic treatment of Paget's disease. Endocrinol Metab Clin North Am. 1995;24:421–436
Klein RM, Norman A. Diagnostic procedures for Paget's disease. Radiologic, pathologic and laboratory testing. Endocrinol Metab Clin North Am. 1995;24:437–450

Painful legs and moving toes (PLMT)

Painful legs and moving toes (PLMT) is a condition of unknown etiology manifesting as deep, chronic, poorly localized pain, usually within the feet or legs, with involuntary writhing movements of the digits. Pain predates movements, sometimes by years. The syndrome may on occasion be associated with nerve root or spinal cord lesions.

Clinical features

- Gnawing, aching, twisting pain, deep in an extremity (usually lower leg and foot, maybe toes); bilateral > unilateral, sometimes relieved by activity. A similar syndrome has been described in the upper limbs ("painful arms and moving fingers").
- Involuntary writhing movements of toes (1–2 Hz); may be temporarily suppressed by voluntary effort.

- Absence of abnormal sensory or motor neurological signs.
- A painless variant ("painless legs and moving toes") has also been described.

Investigation

EMG/NCS to exclude a nerve root lesion; MRI of spinal cord to exclude intrinsic lesions.

Differential diagnosis

Restless legs syndrome.

Treatment and prognosis

There is no specific treatment. Symptomatic treatment with agents useful for dysesthesia (gabapentin, amitriptyline, carbamazepine, TENS, lumbar sympathetic blockade) may be tried. Symptoms usually continue indefinitely.

References

Alvarez MV, Driver-Dunckley EE, Caviness JN, Adler CH, Evidente VG. Case series of painful legs and moving toes: clinical and electrophysiologic observations. Mov Disord. 2008;23:2062–2066
Spillane JD, Nathan PW, Kelly RE, Marsden CD. Painful legs and moving toes. Brain. 1971;94:541–556

Pallido-pyramidal syndrome

This rare entity, first described in 1954, comprises:

- Extrapyramidal features: bradykinesia, cogwheel rigidity, +/– pill-rolling tremor, hypomimia, hypophonia, stooped posture, striatal toes, equino-varus deformity, blepharospasm
- Pyramidal features: paraparesis, gait scissoring, pseudobulbar affect, hyperreflexia, Babinski sign
- +/– Cerebellar features

Unlike the related *Kufor-Rakeb syndrome*, supranuclear upgaze paresis and dementia do not occur. The syndrome presents in young adulthood. Structural brain imaging may be normal, although basal ganglia calcification has been reported. Functional imaging (PET) indicates dopaminergic denervation of the striatum. Neuropathology shows pallidal, pyramidal, and nigral degeneration without inclusions. The parkinsonian features are sometimes levodopa-responsive.

References

Davidson C. Pallido-pyramidal disease. J Neuropathol Exp Neurol. 1954;13:50–59
Srivastava T, Goyal V, Singh S, Shukla G, Behari M. Pallido-pyramidal syndrome with blepharospasm and good response to levodopa. J Neurol. 2005;252:1537–1538

Pancoast syndrome

Tumor in the lung apex or superior sulcus, usually a squamous cell carcinoma, may involve the lower cervical and upper thoracic spinal nerves, producing a *brachial plexopathy*, the sympathetic chain, and in the later stages, may invade the spinal cord causing compression. This may occur in the absence of pulmonary symptoms.

Clinical features

- Pain in the arm (inner aspect), behind the upper part of the scapula
- Numb hand, inner arm (T1, T2)
- Weakness of hand muscles, +/– triceps
- Horner's syndrome +/– warm dry ipsilateral hand if stellate ganglion involved (stellate ganglion syndrome)
- Other features occasionally seen: spinal cord compression, paraplegia; recurrent laryngeal nerve palsy, unilateral vocal cord paresis, weak ("bovine") cough; superior vena cava syndrome
- Late features: cough, hemoptysis, dyspnea

Investigation

Imaging: Chest X-ray, CT, MRI: Neurological symptoms may predate radiological evidence of tumor. Cytology: sputum, bronchoscopic washings, fine needle aspiration. EMG/NCS may confirm root, brachial plexus lesion.

Differential diagnosis

Cervical radiculopathy, spinal cord metastasis.

Treatment and prognosis

Treatment of tumor; symptomatic treatment of arm pain.

References

Attar S, Krasna MJ, Sonett JR, et al. Superior sulcus (Pancoast) tumor: experience with 105 patients. Ann Thorac Surg. 1998;66:193–198

Pancoast HK. Superior pulmonary sulcus tumor: tumor characterized by pain, Horner's syndrome, destruction of bone and atrophy of hand muscles. J Am Med Assoc. 1932;99:1391–1396

Paragonimiasis

Infection with trematodes of the *Paragonimus* species (Oriental lung fluke), following ingestion of larval metacercaria in raw or undercooked freshwater crustaceans or water plants, may lead to pulmonary disease or, with aberrant fluke migration, cerebral disease. Cyst, abscess, and granuloma formation may occur as a consequence of host reaction to worms and eggs, manifesting clinically as acute or chronic encephalitis with seizures and focal neurological signs. Brain hemorrhage, infarction, space-occupying lesions, raised intracranial pressure, papilledema, and optic atrophy may occur. Oral praziquantel is the treatment of choice.

Reference

Kusner DJ, King CH. Cerebral paragonimiasis. Semin Neurol. 1993;13:201–208

Paraneoplastic syndromes: overview

Paraneoplastic disorders are a heterogeneous group of neurological disorders, usually subacute and progressive, which are the indirect (non-metastatic) effect of a tumor, the symptoms of which usually precede those of the underlying malignancy. Paraneoplastic syndromes are thought to be autoimmune phenomena, in which neurological dysfunction is triggered by immune responses directed against antigens on distant tumor cells. Devastating though the neurological syndromes may be (they are often rapidly progressive), the autoimmune responses may hold the tumor in check. Detection of the underlying tumor may be difficult with conventional imaging techniques, and it may be several years before a tumor is located, sometimes only at postmortem. In some circumstances, primary treatment is directed against the underlying neoplasm, but in others, immunotherapy is helpful.

Clinical features

A number of paraneoplastic neurological syndromes are described, more than one of which may occur concurrently. These include:

• Cerebral:	Encephalomyelitis (+/– sensory neuronopathy)
	Limbic encephalitis (+/– sensory neuronopathy)
• Basal ganglia:	Chorea, complex movement disorders
• Cerebellar/brain stem:	Cerebellar degeneration
	Opsoclonus/myoclonus ("dancing eyes, dancing feet," Kinsbourne's syndrome)
	Brain stem encephalitis
• Eye:	Cancer-associated retinopathy
• Spinal cord:	Amyotrophic lateral sclerosis-like syndromes
• Peripheral nerves:	Paraneoplastic sensory neuropathy/neuronopathy
	Paraneoplastic motor neuropathy
• Neuromuscular junction:	*Lambert–Eaton myasthenic syndrome (LEMS)*
	Thymoma-associated *myasthenia gravis*
• Muscle:	*Dermatomyositis*

Investigation

Antineuronal (onconeural) antibodies define disease as being tumor-related (paraneoplastic) and prompt the search for a tumor, although onconeural antibodies are found in only around 60% of paraneoplastic syndromes. The antibodies may be epiphenomenal rather than pathogenetic, since passive transfer of antibodies does not induce disease and immunotherapy is not always effective. Moreover, since false positives and negatives may occur, referral to a specialist laboratory is required.

Paraneoplastic clinical syndrome	Most common associated tumors	Onconeuronal antibodies
Limbic encephalitis	Small cell lung cancer (SCLC), non-SCLC, testicular tumors, thymoma, ovary, breast, prostate	Hu, Ma2, CV2, amphiphysin, Voltage-gated potassium channel (VGKC)
Cerebellar degeneration	Ovary, breast, SCLC, non-SCLC, Hodgkin's disease	Yo, Hu, Tr, CV2, amphiphysin, Ma

(continued)

Paraneoplastic clinical syndrome	Most common associated tumors	Onconeuronal antibodies
Panencephalomyelitis	SCLC, non-SCLC, breast, thymoma	Hu, CV2, amphiphysin
Encephalitis, movement disorder	Ovarian teratoma	NMDA receptor
Sensory neuronopathy	SCLC, non-SCLC, prostate	Hu, CV2, amphiphysin, Ma2
Opsoclonus/myoclonus	SCLC, non-SCLC, breast	Hu, Ri
Retinopathy	SCLC	Anti-CAR
LEMS	SCLC, non-SCLC	Voltage-gated calcium channels (VGCC), Hu, amphiphysin, Yo, Ri, CV2, Tr
Myasthenia gravis	Thymoma	AChR
Peripheral nerve hyperexcitability	Thymoma, SCLC, non-SCLC, Hodgkin's disease	VGKC
Dermatomyositis	SCLC, non-SCLC, ovary, breast, prostate	None

Depending upon the exact clinical syndrome, investigations may include MRI, EEG, EMG/NCS, CSF analysis, electroretinogram, muscle biopsy.

Investigation for underlying tumor is partially dependent upon the clinical syndrome which may suggest the most likely tumor type (e.g., CT thorax, abdomen; bronchoscopy), although none of the onconeural antibodies are 100% organ-specific. Re-investigation every 6 months is recommended if no tumor is found. A search for occult malignancy may be required: [18F] fluoro-2-deoxyglucose positron emission tomography (FDG-PET) scanning may be helpful in these circumstances, due to its excellent spatial resolution (of the order of 6–8 mm) and the fact that small tumors may be more easily seen by their metabolic activity than size per se.

Differential diagnosis

Typical antineuronal antibodies are extremely rare in patients without tumors. However, non-paraneoplastic cases of some paraneoplastic syndromes occur, often in association with autoimmune responses to ion channels, for example, myasthenia gravis, Lambert–Eaton myasthenic syndrome, and limbic encephalitis with serum voltage-gated potassium channel (VGKC) antibodies.

Treatment and prognosis

Treatment of the underlying tumor may bring a halt to neurological disease progression. Immunotherapy is also indicated, more particularly in association with ion channel autoantibodies, with steroids, IVIg, and plasma exchange forming the mainstay of treatment, although there is currently little high-grade evidence to support this. Syndromes associated with typical anti-neuronal antibodies generally respond poorly to immunotherapy, exceptions being Ma2 antibody–associated paraneoplastic syndromes associated with testicular tumor, and limbic encephalitis associated with NMDA receptor autoantibodies and ovarian teratoma.

Diagnostic criteria

Graus F, Delattre JY, Antoine JC, et al. Recommended diagnostic criteria for paraneoplastic neurological syndromes. J Neurol Neurosurg Psychiatry. 2004;75:1135–1140

References

Dalmau J, Rosenfeld MR. Paraneoplastic syndromes of the CNS. Lancet Neurol. 2008;7:327–340
Vedeler CA, Antoine JC, Giometto B, et al. Management of paraneoplastic neurological syndromes: report of an EFNS Task Force. Eur J Neurol. 2006;13:682–690

Paraproteinemic demyelinating neuropathy (PDN)

A paraprotein associated with a *peripheral neuropathy* may be of pathogenetic relevance, as is believed to be the case in paraproteinemic demyelinating neuropathy (PDN); or a marker for an underlying process such as malignancy as in myeloma or Waldenström's macroglobulinemia, or an inflammatory process such as vasculitis or amyloidosis, or of uncertain relevance as in monoclonal gammopathy of undetermined significance (MGUS); or entirely incidental to the neuropathy. Clinical phenotype may vary with immunoglobulin class. Antibodies directed against myelin-associated glycoprotein (MAG) are found in 50% of IgM PDN and probably have a causal relationship. PDN may respond to immunosuppressive therapies.

Clinical features

- IgM: commonly a distal acquired demyelinating symmetrical (DADS) clinical phenotype, with slowly progressive symmetrical sensory impairment (especially vibration, joint position sense) with ataxia, mild or no weakness, and often *tremor* of action and/or postural type (3.5–6.5 Hz), +/– fasciculation

- IgG, IgA: often clinically indistinguishable from *chronic inflammatory demyelinating polyradiculoneuropathy* (*CIDP*), but sometimes the DADS phenotype

Investigation

Paraproteins may be detected by serum electrophoresis, serum immuno-electrophoresis, or serum immunofixation, and characterized quantitatively and in terms of heavy (M,G,A) and light chains (λ or κ). There may also be raised ESR, CRP, and viscosity. Urinary analysis may show Bence-Jones protein, although this is absent or small in amount in MGUS. CSF may show increased protein (70% in PDN) with matched monoclonal band in the CSF and serum. Imaging with a skeletal survey to look for myeloma (osteolytic, osteosclerotic) is advised. Bone marrow examination is needed to diagnose myeloma, Waldenström's macroglobulinemia, and MGUS. Neurophysiology (EMG/NCS) most commonly shows slowing of nerve conduction velocities suggesting a demyelinating process (IgM usually demyelinating), but axonal changes are also reported (IgA, IgG may be demyelinating or axonal). Nerve biopsy usually shows demyelination and loss of myelinated fibers; immunocytochemistry may demonstrate IgM deposits on myelin; EM shows widely spaced myelin outer lamellae. Characterization of the specificity of autoantibodies may only be available in specialist centers, e.g., MAG, sulfatide, SGPG, GM1 (especially *multifocal motor neuropathy* with conduction block). Around 50% of IgM PDN cases are anti-MAG + ve, yet paradoxically response to plasma exchange is better with IgA and IgG.

Differential diagnosis

Myeloma, especially osteosclerotic type (plasmacytoma); Waldenström's macroglobulinemia; MGUS; *POEMS syndrome*; other demyelinating neuropathies: genetic (*hereditary motor and sensory neuropathy*), CIDP, vasculitic neuropathy.

Treatment and prognosis

Evidence to recommend any particular immunotherapy is lacking. In IgM PDN with anti-MAG antibodies, antibody titers may be reduced with treatments such as plasma exchange, IvIg, steroids (ineffective alone), chlorambucil, cyclophosphamide, interferon-alpha, or rituximab. IgG and IgA PDN are treated as for CIDP (plasma exchange, IvIg, steroids). Rarely, irradiation of isolated osteosclerotic myelomatous bone lesions may be curative.

References

Hadden RD, Nobile-Orazio E, Sommer C, et al. European Federation of Neurological Societies/Peripheral Nerve Society guideline on management of paraproteinaemic demyelinating neuropathies: report of a joint task force of the European Federation of Neurological Societies and the Peripheral Nerve Society. Eur J Neurol. 2006;13:809–818

Lunn MP, Nobile-Orazio E. Immunotherapy for IgM anti-myelin-associated glycoprotein paraprotein-associated peripheral neuropathies. Cochrane Database Syst Rev. April 19, 2006;(2):CD002827

Parasomnias

Parasomnias are non-epileptic phenomena associated with sleep. Most are benign and more common in childhood. Their recognition, usually based on clinical history, is important in order to avoid inappropriate investigation and to reassure patients (and parents).

Clinical features

Classification relates to sleep stage:

- Non-REM: (1) wake-sleep transition disorders: hypnic jerks (sleep starts), sensory starts (including *exploding head syndrome*), head banging, proprio-spinal myoclonus; (2) abnormal movements in light non-REM sleep (stage II): periodic limb movements of sleep; (3) disorders of arousal from deep non-REM sleep (stage III and IV): night terrors (pavor nocturnus), confusional arousals, sleepwalking (somnambulism), sleep-related eating disorder
- REM: nightmares, sleep paralysis, *REM sleep behavior disorder* (*REMBD*)
- Non-state dependent: bruxism, catathrenia, rhythmic movement disorder

History from a bed partner or witness may be crucial in making a diagnosis.

Investigation

Polysomnography may be undertaken in specialist centers to determine whether events occur during rapid eye movement (REM) sleep (e.g., nightmares, sleep paralysis) or non-REM sleep (e.g., sleep walking, night terrors, talking in sleep). Such monitoring may also confirm the presence of myoclonus (hypnic/pompic jerks).

Differential diagnosis

Periodic movements of sleep as a feature of *restless legs syndrome*. *Epilepsy* syndromes with nocturnal seizures. Isolated sleep paralysis may be mistaken as an indication of *narcolepsy*.

Treatment and prognosis

Explanation is often sufficient. Prognosis is very good, although sleepwalking can lead to self-injury. Evidence base for pharmacotherapy is almost nonexistent: Clomipramine has been tried in sleep paralysis. Serotonin reuptake inhibitors may be helpful. Benzodiazepines are largely unsuccessful, other than clonazepam in REMBD.

Reference

Reading P. Parasomnias: the spectrum of things that go bump in the night. Pract Neurol. 2007;7:6–15

Parkinsonian syndromes, parkinsonism

Extrapyramidal syndromes

A number of syndromes characterized by parkinsonism (akinesia with or without rigidity, tremor, postural disturbance) have been described, sometimes under the rubric of "Parkinson's plus syndromes" due to additional clinical features not evident in idiopathic *Parkinson's disease* (PD), which is by far the most common cause of parkinsonism. These syndromes are poorly, if at all, responsive to levodopa preparations, unlike PD, and they tend to progress more quickly. Although most parkinsonian syndromes reflect an underlying neurodegenerative disease process, parkinsonism resulting from remediable CNS structural, inflammatory, or metabolic disease does occur.

Clinical features

- Akinesia, rigidity present, but tremor less common than in idiopathic PD.
- Supranuclear gaze palsy, early falls, may suggest *progressive supranuclear palsy* (PSP).
- Marked unilateral apraxia, pyramidal signs may suggest *corticobasal degeneration* (CBD).
- Early visual hallucinations, fluctuations, and dementia suggest *dementia with Lewy bodies* (DLB); dementia may be the presenting feature of CBD.
- Autonomic features (orthostatic hypotension), cerebellar syndrome may suggest *multiple system atrophy* (MSA).
- Pyramidal signs: *pallido-pyramidal syndrome, Kufor-Rakeb syndrome.*

Investigation

See individual entries. Since *Wilson's disease* is potentially treatable, this diagnosis must not be missed and hence it is advisable to check copper and ceruloplasmin levels and perform slit lamp examination of the eye for Kayser-Fleischer rings in all patients presenting with parkinsonism below the age of 50 years.

Differential diagnosis

- Idiopathic Parkinson's disease.
- Progressive supranuclear palsy.
- Multiple system atrophy with predominant parkinsonism (MSA-P).
- Corticobasal degeneration, corticobasal degeneration syndrome.
- Drug/toxin-induced parkinsonism, especially related to use of some anti-emetics and neuroleptics; *neuroleptic malignant syndrome*; manganese poisoning, carbon disulphide, carbon monoxide, cyanide; MPTP. Other drugs that can induce parkinsonism include sodium valproate and lithium.
- Wilson's disease.
- Dementia with Lewy bodies.
- Post-encephalitic parkinsonism: *encephalitis lethargica*, Von Economo's disease.
- *Huntington's disease*, especially juvenile onset form (Westphal variant).
- Subcortical cerebrovascular disease ("arteriosclerotic parkinsonism").
- *Normal pressure hydrocephalus.*
- Posttraumatic parkinsonism, dementia pugilistica.
- Pallido-pyramidal syndrome, *Kufor-Rakeb disease.*
- Guam parkinsonism-dementia complex.
- Systemic lupus erythematosus, Sjögren's syndrome.
- Hypoparathyroidism.
- Tumor-associated parkinsonism: a debatable entity: a cerebral tumor and PD may be coincidental, although some reports of parkinsonism "responding" to tumor removal have been published.
- Perry syndrome: very rare autosomal dominant parkinsonian syndrome, which may be levodopa-responsive, with associated mental depression, apathy, central hypoventilation, and weight loss.

Treatment and prognosis

See under individual entries for appropriate symptomatic treatments. These conditions are largely unresponsive to levodopa preparations. Wilson's disease mandates chelation therapy.

Reference

Oertel WH, Quinn NP. Parkinsonism. In: Brandt T, Caplan LR, Dichgans J, Diener HC, Kennard C, eds. Neurological Disorders: Course and Treatment. San Diego, CA: Academic; 1996:715–772

Parkinson's disease (PD)

Paralysis agitans

Parkinson's disease (PD) is an idiopathic disorder characterized by slowness in the initiation and performance of movement (hypokinesia, akinesia, bradykinesia) with limb resistance to passive movement (rigidity) and sometimes tremor, most usually more evident at rest. The condition was first described by James Parkinson in 1817 as "paralysis agitans" (a misnomer). PD is caused, at least in part, by depletion of dopamine in the striatum due to death of nigral dopaminergic neurones with loss of the nigrostriatal pathway. A number of genetic loci have been defined associated with autosomal dominant or autosomal recessive Parkinson's disease, and a number of genes identified. Interruption of normal proteosomal function may be the pathway through which these mutations exert their effects. Most patients respond well to dopamine replacement therapy but response fluctuations become troublesome as the disease progresses. Dementia may develop, with features akin to those seen in *dementia with Lewy bodies* (DLB).

Clinical features

The classical triad of PD features, not all of which need be present at onset, comprises:

- Akinesia/hypokinesia: slowness or inability to initiate voluntary movement; bradykinesia, slowness in the performance of voluntary movement, is also present.
- Rigidity: involuntary resistance to passive limb movement which is consistent throughout the range of joint movement (cf. spasticity) and for this reason sometimes known as "leadpipe rigidity"; a jerky quality ("cogwheeling") may be evident due to superimposed tremor.
- Tremor: typically a 4–6 Hz "pill-rolling" rest tremor of the hand, although a postural tremor (especially with walking) may predate this.

Other features which may be seen include:

- Postural instability, which may also be considered a key feature (hence a tetrad)
- Stooped posture; reduced arm swing on walking; difficulty turning; falls only occur in later stages (cf. *progressive supranuclear palsy*)

- Pain in rigid muscles
- Micrographia, progressively more evident as writing continues ("slow micrographia")
- Hypomimia, poverty of facial expression, "mask-like" facies
- Hypophonia, monotonic voice
- Sialorrhea
- Seborrhea
- Hypometric saccadic eye movements
- Impaired olfactory sense
- Limb dystonia (late)
- Cognitive impairments (late): "Parkinson's disease dementia" (PD-D)

Symptoms and signs are typically unilateral at onset, gradually spreading to involve the other side. Staging of disease based on symptoms and signs may be performed using the modified Hoehn & Yahr staging or the Unified Parkinson's Disease Rating Scale.

A number of genetic loci and mutations underpinning autosomal dominant and recessive forms of PD have been described, permitting a genetic classification:

Gene	Locus	Clinical classification	Protein/gene
PARK1	4q21	Autosomal dominant, early onset, less likely to have tremor	α-Synuclein
PARK2	6q25.2–q27	Autosomal recessive, early onset, more dystonia, Lewy bodies absent	Parkin
PARK3	2p13	Autosomal dominant, late onset.	
PARK4	4q21 = PARK1	Autosomal dominant, autonomic dysfunction, dementia	α-Synuclein expression doubled
PARK5		Possibly autosomal dominant, only reported in 2 German siblings.	UCH-L1
PARK6	1p35–p36	Autosomal recessive, early onset.	PINK1
PARK7	1p36	Autosomal recessive, early onset, psychiatric disturbance, dystonia.	DJ-1
PARK8	12p11.2–q13.1	Autosomal dominant, signs similar to those of idiopathic PD.	LRRK2
PARK9	1p36	*Kufor-Rakeb disease.*	ATP13A2
PARK10	Unknown	Late onset, reported in Icelandic families.	
PARK11	Unknown	Similar to idiopathic PD.	

Investigation

Diagnosis of PD remains clinical, but problematic: postmortem studies indicate that only around 90% of patients diagnosed with PD in life by experienced neurologists have the typical pathological features. Atypical features should prompt consideration of other parkinsonian syndromes, e.g., early falls consider progressive supranuclear palsy. In patients under 50 years of age, checking blood copper and ceruloplasmin to exclude Wilson's disease is appropriate, since there is specific treatment for this condition which, if missed, produces irreversible effects. Prompt and satisfactory response to levodopa preparations is suggestive of the diagnosis of Parkinson's disease, but may also be seen in some other parkinsonian syndromes.

Rare families with autosomal dominant PD may be screened for mutations following appropriate genetic counseling.

Postmortem pathology shows macroscopic depigmentation of the substantia nigra, and microscopic depletion of dopaminergic cells with eosinophilic inclusions (Lewy bodies) in those remaining.

Differential diagnosis

Other parkinsonian syndromes: progressive supranuclear palsy, multiple system atrophy with predominant parkinsonism, corticobasal degeneration, drug-induced parkinsonism, Wilson's disease, dementia with Lewy bodies, post-encephalitic parkinsonism, Huntington's disease in its juvenile onset form, subcortical cerebrovascular disease ("arteriosclerotic parkinsonism"), normal pressure hydrocephalus, posttraumatic parkinsonism.

Treatment and prognosis

Levodopa preparations, in combination with peripheral dopa-decarboxylase inhibitors, currently remain the "gold standard" for the treatment of Parkinson's disease. They are the most reliable medications to produce motor benefit (especially for the akinesia and rigidity, less reliably for tremor), but their prolonged use is associated with development of motor fluctuations (dyskinesias) which can become intrusive and disabling. For this reason, deferring their use is recommended, particularly in young patients (i.e., those judged likely to survive more than 10 years with the disease), in favor of dopamine agonists. Monotherapy with dopamine agonists in newly diagnosed patients results in fewer dyskinesias at the cost of slightly less good motor improvement. Other options for early monotherapy include selegiline and rasagiline, monoamine oxidase B inhibitors. Anticholinergics such as benzhexol may be helpful for tremor, but their use is increasingly not advised, particularly in patients with confusion (likewise dopamine agonists). The role of surgery in disease management remains to be defined.

When response fluctuations with levodopa set in, they are initially predictable (end of dose or wearing-off effects, peak dose dyskinesias) and may be ameliorated by fractionation of levodopa doses or intraduodenal administration. The catechol-*O*-methyl transferase (COMT) inhibitor entacapone prolongs the action of levodopa by inhibiting inappropriate metabolism, and is useful for the treatment of wearing-off effects. Addition of dopamine agonists to a levodopa regime may enhance motor benefit and allow reduction of total levodopa dose with reduction in dyskinesias. When response fluctuations become unpredictable (on-off phenomenon, yo-yoing), treatment is difficult and the patient may have to choose between mobility with dyskinesia or immobility: Most prefer the former. The dopamine agonist apomorphine, given as an intermittent or continuous subcutaneous injection, may help in this situation. Amantadine is sometimes helpful for dyskinesias. Stereotactic surgery, once popular for tremor, is increasingly used, with deep brain stimulators being applied to the subthalamic nucleus and pedunculopontine nucleus. A prior positive response to dopaminergic therapy is necessary for functional neurosurgery to be beneficial. Epidemiological studies suggest that the prevalence of dementia increases with increased survival, perhaps 80% of patients eventually developing cognitive impairment.

Diagnostic criteria

Gelb DJ, Oliver E, Gilman S. Diagnostic criteria for Parkinson disease. Arch Neurol. 1999;56:33–39
Gibb WR, Lees AJ. The relevance of the Lewy body to the pathogenesis of idiopathic Parkinson's disease. J Neurol Neurosurg Psychiatry. 1988;51:745–752 [UK Parkinson's Disease Society Brain Bank criteria]

References

Clarke C. Parkinson's Disease in Practice. 2nd ed. London: Royal Society of Medicine; 2007
Foltynie T, Lewis S, Barker RA. Parkinson's Disease: Your Questions Answered. Edinburgh, UK: Churchill Livingstone; 2003
Gardner-Thorpe C. James Parkinson 1755–1824. Exeter: A Wheaton & Co. Ltd, 1987 [includes facsimile of Parkinson's book on the shaking palsy]
Horstink M, Tolosa E, Bonuccelli U, et al. Review of the therapeutic management of Parkinson's disease. Report of a joint task force of the European Federation of Neurological Societies and the Movement Disorder Society-European Section. Part I: early (uncomplicated) Parkinson's disease. Eur J Neurol. 2006;13:1170–1185
Horstink M, Tolosa E, Bonuccelli U, et al. Review of the therapeutic management of Parkinson's disease. Report of a joint task force of the European Federation of Neurological Societies (EFNS) and the Movement Disorder Society-European Section (MDS-ES). Part II: late (complicated) Parkinson's disease. Eur J Neurol. 2006;13:1186–1202
National Collaborating Centre for Chronic Conditions. Parkinson's Disease: National Clinical Guideline for Diagnosis and Management in Primary and Secondary Care. London: Royal College of Physicians; 2006

Parkinson's syndrome

Parkinson's syndrome of unilateral abducens (VI) nerve palsy and ipsilateral Horner's syndrome suggests *cavernous sinus disease*, localizing pathology to that part of the cavernous sinus where the sympathetic fibers to the eye briefly join the abducens nerve as they pass from the pericarotid plexus to the ophthalmic branch of the trigeminal nerve.

References

Silva MN, Saeki N, Hirai S, Yamaura A. Unusual cranial nerve palsy caused by cavernous sinus aneurysms. Clinical and anatomical considerations reviewed. Surg Neurol. 1999;52:148–149

Paroxysmal dyskinesias

Paroxysmal dystonias

The paroxysmal dyskinesias are a group of involuntary movement disorders characterized by brief bursts of painless choreiform and/or dystonic movements lasting seconds to hours with a normal neurological examination between attacks. Some movements are provoked by movement (kinesigenic). In familial forms, genetic loci are located near ion channel genes, giving rise to the possibility that these may be *channelopathies*, as in *episodic ataxias* and some autosomal dominant *epilepsy* syndromes.

Clinical features

- Paroxysmal kinesigenic dyskinesia/Paroxysmal kinesigenic choreoathetosis:
  - Chorea, ballismus, dystonic postures, unilateral or bilateral, attacks last seconds to 5 min
  - Triggered by sudden movement, startle, hyperventilation, anxiety, stress
  - Frequency of attacks: up to 20 per day
  - No alteration of consciousness
  - Sensitive to anticonvulsants: carbamazepine, phenytoin, benzodiazepines
  - Associated conditions: past history of febrile fits, migraine, writer's cramp, essential tremor
  - Inheritance: autosomal dominant, linked to 16q

- Paroxysmal non-kinesigenic dyskinesia/Paroxysmal dystonic chore-oathetosis:
  - Chorea, ballismus, dystonia, plus speech involvement, attacks last 2 min to 12 h
  - Not triggered by movement, but may be by alcohol, caffeine, stress; aborted by sleep
  - Frequency of attacks: one per week
  - Not sensitive to anticonvulsants, but respond to benzodiazepines
  - Associated conditions: migraine
  - Inheritance: autosomal dominant, myofibrillogenesis regulator-1 (MR-1) gene mutation on chromosome 2q35 in some cases
- Paroxysmal exercised-induced dyskinesia/Paroxysmal exercised-induced dystonia:
  - Mainly dystonia of the legs, attacks last 10–15 min
  - Triggered by 10–15 min of continuous exercise
  - No alteration of consciousness
  - Sensitive to acetazolamide, L-dopa
  - Associated conditions: migraine, writer's cramp
  - Inheritance: linkages to chromosomes 16 and 1p
- Paroxysmal hypnogenic dyskinesia: = *autosomal dominant nocturnal frontal lobe epilepsy.*

Investigation

Video attack if possible. Keep attack diary to look for triggers, precipitants, as well as record attack frequency and duration. Investigate for symptomatic causes, e.g., endocrine tests, brain imaging, +/− EEG, polysomnography for nocturnal episodes.

Differential diagnosis

Other involuntary movement disorders which are both paroxysmal/episodic and dyskinetic are not usually considered under this rubric (e.g., *hyperekplexia*, tics, stereotypies, Sandifer's syndrome).

- Paroxysmal dystonic features may occur in some symptomatic dystonias:
  - Metabolic disorders: hypoparathyroidism, thyrotoxicosis, Hartnup's disease, pyruvate decarboxylase deficiency, D-glyceric acidemia
  - Degenerative conditions (rarely): Parkinson's disease, progressive supranuclear palsy
  - Cerebral palsy
  - Drug-induced dystonia

- Other conditions which may masquerade as paroxysmal dystonia include:
  - Focal epilepsy
  - Hyperekplexia
  - Tetany
  - Hysteria
  - Transient ischemic attacks
  - Tonic spasms of multiple sclerosis

Treatment and prognosis

Kinesigenic dyskinesia is sensitive to anticonvulsants, e.g., carbamazepine, non-kinesigenic dyskinesia to benzodiazepines, and exercise-induced dystonia may respond to acetazolamide or L-dopa.

References

Houser MK, Soland VK, Bhatia KP, Quinn NP, Marsden CD. Paroxysmal kinesigenic choreoathetosis: a report of 26 patients. J Neurol. 1999;246:120–126
Van Rootselaar A-F, Schade van Westrum S, Velis DN, Tijssen MA. The paroxysmal dyskinesias. Pract Neurol. 2009;9:102–109

Paroxysmal hemicrania

Episodic hemicrania, Sjaastad syndrome

This rare primary *headache* syndrome is categorized with the *trigeminal autonomic cephalalgia* group, sharing similarities with *cluster headache* and *SUNCT* but also differences. It is characterized by repeated attacks of strictly unilateral pain (orbital, frontal, occipital), of short duration (around 15 min), with autonomic features (lacrimation, conjunctival injection, rhinorrhea, nasal congestion), and exquisitely sensitive to indomethacin. The indomethacin test or Indotest (positive placebo control response to 100–200 mg indomethacin given intramuscularly) may be diagnostic.

References

Cittadini E, Matharu MS, Goadsby PJ. Paroxysmal hemicranias: a prospective clinical study of 31 cases. Brain. 2008;131:1142–1155
Sjaastad O, Dale I. A new (?) headache entity "chronic paroxysmal hemicrania." Acta Neurol Scand. 1976;54:140–159

Parry-Romberg syndrome

Facial hemiatrophy, Hemifacial atrophy

Parry-Romberg syndrome is a clinically and etiologically heterogeneous syndrome characterized by hemifacial atrophy, sometimes with ipsilateral intracerebral abnormalities producing neurological features. It may be classified with the *neurocutaneous syndromes*. Usually, it begins in adolescence or early adult life, but late-onset cases are also reported. Pathophysiology may be maldevelopment of autonomic innervation or vascular supply, or an acquired feature following trauma, or a consequence of linear *systemic sclerosis* (scleroderma; morphea). A genetic basis has been suggested, but discordance in monozygotic twins has been observed.

Clinical features

- Hemifacial atrophy, especially subcutaneous tissues; may involve bone, brain +/− ipsilateral limb/trunk atrophy.
- Neurological manifestations: migraine/facial pain (45%); focal seizures (10%); hemiparesis, hemianopia, cognitive impairment.
- Dermatological manifestations: *Coup de sabre*, circumscribed alopecia, achromia/hyperchromia of hair, telangiectatic nevus.
- In its most advanced state, the face is gaunt, the skin thin and wrinkled, the hair white or absent, and the sebaceous glands atrophic while the muscles are unaffected.

Investigation

Examination of old photographs may confirm acquired change in facial appearance. Bloods may be positive for markers for scleroderma (e.g., SCL70, anti-ds DNA, anti-centromere). In the presence of neurological features, neuroimaging may reveal ipsilateral cerebral atrophy; EEG may show focal epileptiform abnormalities. Autonomic function testing may show abnormalities, e.g., of pupil, facial sweating.

Differential diagnosis

Congenital hemiatrophy (usually of whole body) secondary to *in utero* insult or birth injury.

Treatment and prognosis

No specific treatment; symptomatic treatment of seizures. In extreme cases, cosmetic surgery may be appropriate.

References

Larner AJ, Bennison DP. Some observations on the aetiology of progressive hemifacial atrophy ("Parry-Romberg syndrome"). J Neurol Neurosurg Psychiatry. 1993;56:1035–1036
Stone J. Parry-Romberg syndrome. Pract Neurol. 2006;6:185–188

Patent foramen ovale (PFO)

Patent foramen ovale (PFO) may be associated with neurological disease:

- Stroke: due to paradoxical embolism. Divers are at particular risk. Isolated PFO does not seem to increase the risk of recurrent stroke unless it is associated with an atrial septal aneurysm.
- Migraine: there is undoubtedly an increased incidence of PFO in *migraine with aura*, but whether PFO closure improves headache frequency or severity remains uncertain and controversial.

An association has also been reported between PFO and *transient global amnesia* but remains to be corroborated.

References

Dowson A, Mullen MJ, Peatfield R, et al. Migraine Intervention with STARFlex Technology (MIST) trial: a prospective, multi-center, double-blind, sham-controlled trial to evaluate the effectiveness of patent foramen ovale closure with STARFLex septal repair implant to resolve refractory migraine headache. Circulation. 2008;117:1397–1404 [Erratum: Circulation. 2009;120:e71–72]
Horton SC, Bunch TJ. Patent foramen ovale and stroke. Mayo Clin Proc. 2004;79:79–88
Mas JL, Arquizan C, Lamy C, Zuber M, Cabanes L, Derumeaux G, Coste J. Recurrent cerebrovascular events associated with patent foramen ovale, atrial septal aneurysm, or both. N Engl J Med. 2001;345:1740–1746

Pavor nocturnus

Night terrors, Sleep terrors

This common *parasomnia* of non-REM slow-wave sleep begins in childhood and may persist into adulthood. There is abrupt arousal in the first part of the night, with intense autonomic and motor symptoms, including loud piercing screams, and the patient appears confused and frightened. In the morning, the patient has no recollection of the event. Many patients have concurrent sleep walking (somnambulism) and a positive family history. Pharmacotherapy is of limited efficacy, options including hypnotics (e.g., zopiclone), benzodiazepines (e.g., clonazepam), SSRIs (e.g., fluoxetine), and neuroleptics.

Payne syndrome

Rowland-Payne syndrome

Metastatic disease to the neck, usually from breast carcinoma, may involve the phrenic nerve, sympathetic chain, and recurrent laryngeal nerve, producing a syndrome comprising:

- Phrenic nerve palsy
- Ipsilateral Horner's syndrome
- Ipsilateral vocal cord paresis

Reference

Payne CME. Newly recognized syndrome in the neck: Horner's syndrome with ipsilateral vocal cord and phrenic nerve palsies. J R Soc Med. 1981;74:814–818

Pelizaeus-Merzbacher disease (PMD) [OMIM#312080]

Sudanophilic leukodystrophy, Tigroid leukoencephalopathy

An X-linked recessive disorder of myelin due to deficiency of proteolipid protein (PLP) usually presenting in the first months of life with a combination of a movement disorder and intellectual decline. Various forms have been described (connatal, classic, transitional, late onset). More than 60 point mutations in the PLP gene have been identified, accounting for 15–20% of cases; duplication of a portion of the X chromosome containing the PLP gene may account for another 50–75% of cases. Deletion mutations have also been reported. One of the X-linked forms of *hereditary spastic paraplegia* (SPG2) is allelic. Patients with the clinical phenotype of PMD but normal PLP gene have been identified, suggesting that other regulatory genes may also be involved in disease pathogenesis.

Clinical features

Variable:

- Eye movement disorder: nystagmus (pendular, rotatory, chaotic)
- Head tremor
- Laryngeal stridor
- Choreoathetosis
- Pyramidal signs
- Intellectual decline
- Microcephaly
- Cerebellar ataxia

- Epileptic seizures (occasional)
- Optic atrophy (late)
- +/– Pes cavus, kyphoscoliosis

An adult form of PMD known as Lowenberg-Hill syndrome has been described, with autosomal dominant inheritance.

Investigation

Bloods are usually normal. Neuroimaging (MRI) may show diffuse symmetrical white matter abnormalities (low intensity on T_1, high intensity on T_2) reflecting dysmyelination. Neurophysiology may show abnormal evoked potentials (BSAEP, SSEP, sometimes VEP); EEG is nonspecifically abnormal. Brain biopsy shows patchy dysmyelination, reduced numbers of oligodendrocytes, and an absence of myelin in some (Seitelberger variant, neonatal onset). Neurogenetic testing may show point mutations or duplications in PLP gene.

Differential diagnosis

Other *leukodystrophies*

Treatment and prognosis

No specific treatment. Prognosis is uniformly fatal, although survival into the third decade is recorded.

References

Garbern J, Cambi F, Shy M, Kamholz J. The molecular pathogenesis of Pelizaeus-Merzbacher disease. Arch Neurol. 1999;56:1210–1214
Seitelberger F. Neuropathology and genetics of Pelizaeus-Merzbacher disease. Brain Pathol 1995;5:267–273

Pellagra

The syndrome of pellagra is often remembered as "dermatitis, diarrhea, and dementia," although not all these features need be present. It has been thought that pellagra results from a deficiency of niacin (nicotinic acid and nicotinamide). Niacin is found in many foodstuffs (plants, meat, fish) and may be synthesized *in vivo* from the amino acid tryptophan. However, deficiency of other water-soluble vitamins of the B group and possibly tryptophan may also contribute to the pathogenesis of pellagra. Dietary deficiency is now rare, occurring only in areas where maize is the staple diet (southern

Africa, India). Other risk factors include prolonged isoniazid therapy without pyridoxine supplementation, Hartnup's disease, chronic alcoholism with malnutrition (in which situation an encephalopathic syndrome may occur), general malabsorption, very low protein diets, and the carcinoid syndrome.

Clinical features

Neurological features are confined to chronic disease:

- Depression, apathy, hallucinations, psychosis, irritability, insomnia, delirium, impaired consciousness (the encephalopathy of pellagra may be referred to as Jolliffe syndrome)
- +/- Extrapyramidal features, cerebellar signs, myelopathy, polyneuropathy, optic atrophy, tremor

Investigation

There are no specific investigations. Careful dietary history may be necessary, plus investigations for secondary causes (e.g., malabsorption, carcinoid syndrome) if other symptoms and signs are suggestive. Neuropathological findings reported include chromatolysis of large neurones of the motor cortex ("central neuritis" of Adolph Meyer).

Differential diagnosis

Deficiency of other water-soluble vitamins of the B group, e.g., riboflavin, pyridoxine, thiamine, and possibly also of tryptophan. Rash may resemble that seen in Hartnup's disease.

Treatment and prognosis

Treatment with niacin alone is often not effective, suggesting the possibility of other deficiencies contributing to the syndrome. Response to nicotinic acid/nicotinamide is better, but it is usual to give vitamin B complex to try to cover other deficiencies. Increasing the protein content of the diet may also be helpful. Cerebral symptoms and signs may not be completely reversible.

References

Langworthy OR. Lesions of the central nervous system characteristic of pellagra. Brain. 1931;54:291–302
Serdaru M, Hausser-Hauw C, Laplane D, et al. The clinical spectrum of alcoholic pellagra encephalopathy. Brain. 1988;111:829–842

Periodic paralysis (PP)

The periodic paralyses are autosomal dominant inherited disorders characterized by attacks of weakness, of variable frequency and duration, and with differing precipitants. These disorders were previously classified according to concurrent serum potassium ion concentrations as hyperkalemic (Gamstorp's disease, adynamia episodica hereditaria), hypokalemic or, rarely, normokalemic. With the advent of molecular genetic techniques, all these disorders have been shown to result from mutations in genes encoding ion channel proteins: hyperkalemic PP results from sodium channel (SCN4A) gene mutations, hypokalemic PP from mutations in the L-type calcium channel gene (CACNA1S), potassium channel gene (KCJN2), or even the same sodium channel gene implicated in hyperkalemic PP. Normokalemic PP also is associated with sodium channel mutations and hence is a variant of hyperkalemic PP; at the end of paralytic attacks, serum K^+ may fall, giving a false impression of the concentration during an attack. *Andersen-Tawil syndrome* is characterized by the triad of PP, ventricular arrhythmias, and specific physical features. Thyrotoxic PP, common in Asia, mostly as a sporadic disorder, is phenotypically similar to hypokalemic PP. These disorders manifest phenotype divergence or allelic heterogeneity: Mutations in the sodium channel gene SCN4A may cause hyperkalemic PP, *potassium-aggravated myotonia*, paramytonia congenita, and even hypokalemic PP.

Clinical features

- Attacks of limb muscle weakness usually begin in childhood; ocular and respiratory muscles are spared, and consciousness preserved.
- Triggers include exercise and then rest, carbohydrate load (hypokalemic PP), and prolonged fasting (hyperkalemic PP).
- Weakness lasts longer (hours to days) and is more severe in hypokalemic PP as compared to hyperkalemic PP (minutes to hours).
- There is no myotonia in hypokalemic PP, but this is seen sometimes in hyperkalemic PP.
- Females with hypokalemic PP may present with a late-onset proximal myopathy, and a persistent mild myopathy may develop later in the course of hyperkalemic PP.

Investigation

Bloods: K^+ level during an attack (sent immediately to laboratory to avoid hemolysis and false reading; often missed). Nowadays, if the diagnosis is suspected clinically, sending blood to a reference laboratory for mutation analysis is appropriate. Concurrent thyroid function tests (association with thyrotoxicosis may be known as Kitamura syndrome). Neurophysiology

(EMG) showing decrement in compound muscle action potential amplitude after a period of sustained exercise is characteristic. ECG should be routine in all PP cases to look for features suggestive of Andersen-Tawil syndrome (prominent U wave, long QT).

Differential diagnosis

PP could potentially be confused with myasthenia gravis, but usually the differentiation is straightforward, likewise with porphyria, Guillain–Barre syndrome, metabolic myopathies.

Treatment and prognosis

Avoid recognized precipitating factors. Many patients with hyperkalemic PP benefit from treatments which prevent hyperkalemia (i.e., prophylaxis for weakness): thiazide diuretics, β-adrenoreceptor agonists (e.g., salbutamol); carbonic anhydrase inhibitors (e.g., acetazolamide, dichlorphenamide) may also help. If present in hyperkalemic PP, myotonia may be treated with mexiletine. Frequency and severity of attacks diminish with age. A progressive vacuolar myopathy may develop. Andersen-Tawil syndrome may require cardiac monitoring or a pacemaker.

References

Fontaine B. Periodic paralysis. Adv Genet. 2008;63:3–23
Fontaine B, Hanna MG. Muscle ion channelopathies and related disorders. In: Karpati G, Hilton-Jones D, Bushby K, Griggs RC, eds. Disorders of Voluntary Muscle. 8th ed. Cambridge: Cambridge University Press; 2010:409–426
Platt D, Griggs R. Skeletal muscle channelopathies: new insights into the periodic paralyses and nondystrophic myotonias. Curr Opin Neurol. 2009;22:524–531

Peripheral nerve hyperexcitability (PNH)

Isaacs syndrome, Neuromyotonia

Neuromyotonia is continuous muscle activity of peripheral nerve origin, persisting after proximal nerve block or general anesthesia but abolished by depolarizing muscle relaxants and neuromuscular blocking agents. The clinical associations of neuromyotonia – paraneoplastic and autoimmune conditions – first suggested its autoimmune aetiology, subsequently confirmed by the discovery of antibodies to voltage-gated potassium channels (VGKC) in the serum of some affected patients.

Clinical features

Clinically heterogeneous:

- Muscle twitching at rest: myokymia, a wave-like rippling or a "bag of worms" below the skin
- Cramps: may be triggered by voluntary or induced muscle contraction.
- Impaired muscle relaxation: pseudomyotonia; no percussion myotonia (cf. myotonic dystrophy type 1). Muscle stiffness, muscle hypertrophy
- +/– Excessive sweating
- +/– Mild muscle weakness
- +/– Paresthesia
- +/– Absent tendon reflexes

CNS features may be present (*Morvan's syndrome*).

Neuromyotonia may occur in isolation or be a feature of other conditions such as *episodic ataxia* type I, or *hereditary motor and sensory neuropathy*. Associations include thymoma, *myasthenia gravis*, vitiligo, lymphoma, Hashimoto's thyroiditis and penicillamine treatment. An ocular variant is also described, in which spontaneous spasm in extraocular muscles may follow prolonged voluntary activation of specific muscles; this rare syndrome commonly follows irradiation for pituitary tumor but has also been reported in association with internal carotid artery aneurysm or alcohol consumption.

Investigation

Bloods: Specific test is VGKC antibody assay, found in about 35% of all PNH patients, rising to 80% in those with thymoma. Neurophysiology: EMG shows spontaneous continuous single motor unit discharges (doublet, triplet or multiplet) at high intraburst frequency (30–300 Hz). Fibrillation potentials and fasciculations are often present. Electrical stimulation of the nerve typically leads to increased spontaneous activity (after-discharges).

Investigations to search for underlying causes, especially thymoma, myasthenia gravis, lymphoma, may be undertaken.

Differential diagnosis

- Electrophysiological findings are quantitatively rather than qualitatively different from those seen in cramp- fasciculation (Denny-Brown, Foley) syndrome.
- Stiff man syndrome also results from continuous motor activity, involving spinal interneuronal networks.

Treatment and prognosis

Neuromyotonia occurring in isolation may remit spontaneously. Muscle weakness is usually mild. Anticonvulsants such as phenytoin, carbamazepine, sodium valproate, and lamotrigine may suppress neuronal repetitive firing. Immunotherapy, including plasma exchange, may be appropriate for acquired neuromyotonia. Underlying causes may influence prognosis (e.g., small-cell lung carcinoma), treatment of which may have little effect on neuromyotonia.

References

Hart IK, Maddison P, Newsom Davis J, Vincent A, Mills KR. Phenotypic variants of autoimmune peripheral nerve hyperexcitability. Brain. 2002;125:1887–1895

Isaacs H. A syndrome of continuous muscle-fibre activity. J Neurol Neurosurg Psychiatry. 1961;24:319–325

Maddison P. Neuromyotonia. Pract Neurol. 2002;2:225–229

Sathasivam S, Larner AJ. Disorders of the neuromuscular junction. In: Sinclair A, Morley JE, Vellas B, eds. Pathy's Principles and Practice of Geriatric Medicine. 5th ed. Chichester: Wiley; 2011: in press

Skeie GO, Apostolski S, Evoli A, et al. Guidelines for the treatment of autoimmune neuromuscular transmission disorders. Eur J Neurol. 2006;13:691–699

Peroneal neuropathy

Common peroneal nerve palsy

The common peroneal nerve is the lateral division of the sciatic nerve, comprising fibers from the L4-S2 spinal roots. It branches from the sciatic nerve within the popliteal fossa, giving rise to sural and lateral cutaneous sensory branches before winding around the head of the fibula where it is particularly vulnerable to compression injury. Beyond the tendinous arch formed by the peroneus longus muscle, it divides into the superficial peroneal nerve, which supplies the peroneus longus and brevis, and the deep peroneal nerve, which innervates tibialis anterior, extensor hallucis longus, and extensor digitorum longus muscles, then via its terminal portion extensor digitorum brevis.

Clinical features

- Motor: foot drop, with weak tibialis anterior, extensor hallucis longus, and extensor digitorum longus causing weak ankle dorsiflexion, ankle eversion and toe dorsiflexion; ankle inversion and foot plantar flexion are spared (cf. L5 radiculopathy); often there is no reflex loss although the ankle jerk may be reduced.
- Sensory: minimal change: may be impaired over anterolateral lower leg, dorsum of foot.

Investigation

EMG/NCS may identify site and extent of axonal injury, and distinguish peroneal neuropathy from L4-5 radiculopathy.

Differential diagnosis

Other causes of lower motor neurone (floppy) foot drop, including lumbar radiculopathy, lumbosacral plexopathy, sciatic neuropathy involving the lateral division only.

References

Katirji B. Peroneal neuropathy. Neurol Clin. 1999;17:567–591
Staal A, Van Gijn J, Spaans F. Mononeuropathies: Examination, Diagnosis and Treatment. London, UK: WB Saunders; 1999:133–141

Pick's disease

Arnold Pick originally presented (1892, 1906) reports of focal cerebral atrophy, affecting predominantly temporal and/or frontal lobes, causing linguistic or behavioral syndromes, respectively. These cases are equivalent to modern day *frontotemporal lobar degeneration* (*FTLD*). It was not until 1911 that Alois Alzheimer described the microscopic neuropathological changes in some of these cases which subsequently became known as Pick bodies and Pick cells. Latterly it became apparent that focal atrophy could also occur with other neuropathological changes. Hence, debate as to what should be included under the rubric of "Pick's disease" continues, the extreme positions being represented by those who accept only Pick body positive focal lobar atrophy (almost impossible to predict from clinical findings alone), and those who accept lobar atrophy independent of the pathological findings.

References

Graham A, Hodges J. Pick's disease: its relationship to progressive aphasia, semantic dementia and frontotemporal dementia. In: Burns A, O'Brien J, Ames D, eds. Dementia. 3rd ed. London, UK: Hodder Arnold; 2005:678–688
Kertesz A, Munoz DG eds. Pick's Disease and Pick Complex. New York, NY: Wiley; 1998

Pineal gland tumors

Numerous tumor types may arise within the pineal gland. The clinical presentation may be with neurological features (e.g., Parinaud's syndrome, hydrocephalus) or endocrine change (e.g., diabetes insipidus).

Pineal tumors may be:

- Parenchymal:
  - Pineocytoma
  - Parenchymal tumor with intermediate differentiation
  - Pineoblastoma (resembles primitive neuroectodermal tumor)
- Germ-cell tumors: germinoma, teratoma
- *Glioma*
- Metastases (e.g., lung)
- *Cysts*: simple, dermoid, epidermoid

Although tumor markers may give the diagnosis (e.g., for certain germ-cell tumors), biopsy or surgery may be necessary to identify exact tumor type.

References

De Girolami U, Fevre-Montange M, Seilhean D, Jouvet A. Pathology of tumors of the pineal region. Rev Neurol (Paris). 2008;164:882–895
Ogden AT, Bruce JN. Pineal region tumors. In: Bernstein M, Berger MS, eds. Neuro-Oncology: The Essentials. 2nd ed. New York, NY: Thieme; 2008:299–306

Piriformis syndrome

The piriformis syndrome comprises gluteal and leg pain ascribed to entrapment of the sciatic nerve by the piriformis muscle as it passes beneath it, beyond the sciatic notch. Few rigorous case reports support the existence of this entrapment neuropathy syndrome: at best, it is very unusual.

Clinical features

- Unilateral gluteal pain, +/– leg pain along back of thigh, calf
- Localized tenderness over the piriformis muscle (although this may also be found in patients with plexopathy or lumbosacral radiculopathy)
- Absent or asymmetric ipsilateral ankle jerk
- Sensory abnormalities along the lateral aspect of the foot, fifth toe

Investigation

Neurophysiology shows absent or low amplitude sural sensory nerve action potential; prolonged or dispersed tibial nerve F waves; abnormal H reflex; with normal lower limb nerve conduction velocities. Denervation potentials in gastrocnemius +/– hamstring (i.e., as in other causes of sciatic neuropathy). Neuroimaging of the lumbosacral region is normal.

Differential diagnosis

Other causes of proximal sciatic neuropathy:

- L5-S1 disc herniation
- Intrapelvic compressive lesion: carcinoma, lymphoma
- Pelvic bone lesion: sarcoma, metastasis
- Idiopathic lumbosacral plexopathy
- Intraneural neurofibroma
- Diabetic ischemic neuropathy

Treatment and prognosis

Botulinum toxin injection into the piriformis muscle has been reported. Surgical decompression may, theoretically, be appropriate.

References

Al-Memar AY, Hudson N, Thomas G, Hughes P, Wimalaratna HSK. The piriformis syndrome: a sciatic nerve entrapment. J Neurol Neurosurg Psychiatry. 1997;62:210
Stenner A, Reichel G, Hermann W. Successful treatment of pirifromis syndrome with botulinum toxin A. J Neurol. 2006;253 (suppl 2): II/110 (P434)

Pisa syndrome

The so-called Pisa syndrome, or pleurothotonus, is a rare extrapyramidal side effect caused by neuroleptic medications, or by cholinesterase inhibitors in Alzheimer's disease patients, characterized by twisting and bending of the upper thorax (hence truncal dystonia), with involuntary flexion of the neck and head, to one side. It can also be seen in extrapyramidal disorders such as Parkinson's disease and multiple system atrophy. Tilting symptoms occurring bilaterally may be labeled as "metronome Pisa syndrome."

Reference

Yokochi F. Lateral flexion in Parkinson's disease and Pisa syndrome. J Neurol. 2006;253(Suppl7):VII/17–VII/20

Pituitary disease: overview

Disease of the pituitary gland, most usually an adenoma, may produce both local effects, due to compression of adjacent neurological structures, most commonly the optic chiasm, and distant effects due to endocrinological changes. Infarction of an adenoma which has outgrown its blood supply leads to the syndrome of pituitary apoplexy, an acute medical emergency. Ischemic necrosis of the pituitary gland, occurring most often in the postpartum period (Sheehan's syndrome), can cause panhypopituitarism.

Occasionally pituitary tumors may occur in the context of familial syndromes:

- Multiple endocrine neoplasia (MEN) type 1: autosomal dominant; parathyroid, endocrine pancreas, and pituitary tumors (especially prolactinoma); linked to chromosome 11q13.
- Carney complex: familial multiple neoplasia and lentiginosis syndrome, featuring skin and cardiac myxomas, and testicular, adrenal and pituitary tumors, which has been linked to chromosome 2.
- McCune-Albright syndrome (polyostotic fibrous dysplasia): progressive fibrous dysplasia of the skull and long bones causing bone pain, fractures, and cranial nerve palsies, with brown pigmented skin patches and endocrine abnormalities such as precocious puberty may occur. Pituitary tumors may also feature.

Clinical features

- Local:
  - Chiasmal compression: bitemporal hemianopia, junctional scotoma of Traquair (pre-chiasmal compression)
  - Optic atrophy, visual failure
  - Headache: migraine, cluster headache
  - Ocular palsies (extension to cavernous sinus)
  - Seizures (extension to temporal lobe)
  - Somnolence, diabetes insipidus (hypothalamic extension)
  - CSF rhinorrhea
- Distant (endocrine):
  - Prolactinoma: secondary amenorrhea, thin skin
  - ACTH (Cushing's disease): myopathy, hypertension, osteoporosis, striae
  - GH: gigantism, acromegaly
  - LH, FSH (rare)
  - TSH (rare)
- Pituitary apoplexy:
  - Acute headache
  - Visual loss
  - Ophthalmoplegia (parasellar extension)
  - Drowsiness/coma (diagnosis may be difficult if pituitary tumor has not been previously diagnosed)

Panhypopituitarism (Simmonds syndrome): may follow tumor, apoplexy.

Investigation

Bloods: prolactin (majority of functioning tumors, 60–70%), GH, ACTH, LH, FSH, TSH. Neuroimaging: CT may show enlarged, eroded, sella turcica; MRI shows extent of tumor, its relation to optic nerves and other local structures. In apoplexy, MRI shows infarction of tumor with or without hemorrhage above the sella. Visual field mapping documents visual field defects. CSF in apoplexy shows pleocytosis +/– subarachnoid hemorrhage.

Differential diagnosis

Visual field changes may be confused with those secondary to *craniopharyngioma*. Apoplexy may be mistaken for intracerebral hemorrhage, subarachnoid hemorrhage, encephalitis or meningitis, eclampsia, idiopathic thunderclap headache.

Treatment and prognosis

Medical: prolactinoma: dopamine agonists (bromocriptine, cabergoline); acromegaly; octreotide. Surgical: excision: trans-sphenoidal approach, transcranial if suprasellar extension. Apoplexy: acute medical emergency: dexamethasone +/– surgery.

References

Chanson P, Lepeintre JF, Ducreux D. Management of pituitary apoplexy. Expert Opin Pharmacother. 2004;5:1287–1298

Kovacs K. Sheehan syndrome. Lancet. 2003;361:520–522

Kunwar S. Pituitary tumors. In: Bernstein M, Berger MS, eds. Neuro-Oncology: The Essentials. 2nd ed. New York: Thieme; 2008:334–342

Levy A. Pituitary disease: presentation, diagnosis, and management. J Neurol Neurosurg Psychiatry. 2004;75 (suppl III):iii47–iii52

Randeva HS, Schoebel J, Byrne J, Esiri M, Adams CB, Wass JA. Classical pituitary apoplexy: clinical features, management and outcome. Clin Endocrinol (Oxf). 1999;51:181–188

Stratakis CA, Carney JP, Lin JP, et al. Carney complex, a familial multiple neoplasia and lentiginosis syndrome: analysis of 11 kindreds and linkage to the short arm of chromosome 2. J Clin Investig. 1996;97:699–705

POEMS syndrome

Crow-Fukase syndrome

POEMS syndrome is a rare multisystem disorder, more common in men, characterized by osteosclerotic myeloma (plasmacytoma) with a circulating monoclonal protein, and peripheral neuropathy. Immunopathogenesis is uncertain, but the condition does improve following disappearance of the M protein. The syndrome may be a paraneoplastic phenomenon driven by plasma cell products.

Clinical features

POEMS is an acronym for the chief clinical features, although most patients do not have all five features, at least at presentation:

- P = polyneuropathy: demyelinating, predominantly motor, type, lower limbs generally more affected than upper; cranial nerves are typically spared, although papilledema may occur in up to 60%.
- O = organomegaly: hepatosplenomegaly, or lymphadenopathy.
- E = endocrinopathy: gynecomastia and impotence in males; secondary amenorrhea in females; diabetes mellitus; hypothyroidism.
- M = M protein, usually λ light chains, IgA or IgG, rarely IgM.
- S = skin changes: hyperpigmentation, hypertrichosis, skin thickening.
- +/− cardiomyopathy, pleural effusion, peripheral edema, ascites, pulmonary hypertension, renal failure, thrombotic events, congestive cardiac failure.
- Castlemann disease (angiofollicular lymphoid hyperplasia, a diffuse B-cell dyscrasia as opposed to a focal myelomatous lesion) may also be associated with a syndrome of POEMS type.

Investigation

Bloods show M protein with λ light chains on serum electrophoresis or immunofixation (latter may be required because of a low concentration of paraprotein). Endocrine bloods should be performed (TFTs, testosterone, estradiol, gonadotrophin, prolactin). CSF shows raised protein. A skeletal survey is required to identify sclerotic bone lesion(s), biopsy of which may confirm plasmacytoma. If initially negative, skeletal survey should be repeated every 6 months. Imaging of chest and abdomen is recommended. Skin biopsy and nerve biopsy may be required.

Differential diagnosis

Myeloma, *chronic inflammatory demyelinating polyradiculoneuropathy (CIDP)*, other demyelinating neuropathy such as *paraproteinemic demyelinating neuropathy (PDN)*.

Treatment and prognosis

There is no report of spontaneous remission or stabilization without treatment. Single bone lesions may be surgically excised or irradiated, although clinical improvement may not be apparent for several months thereafter. Medical treatment with a combination of prednisolone and melphalan has also been used, and autologous stem cell transplantation has been tried. Occasional reports of benefit with tamoxifen, interferon-alpha, alkylating agents and trans-retinoic acid have appeared. No evidence for benefit from plasma exchange or IVIg. Median survival is 2–3 years.

References

Caswell R, Warner T, Mehta A, Ginsberg L. POEMS syndrome. Pract Neurol 2006;6:111–116
Dispenzieri A, Kyle RA, Lacy MQ, et al. POEMS syndrome: definitions and long-term outcome. Blood. 2003;101:2496–2506

Poliomyelitis

Infection with poliovirus, a small RNA enterovirus, is usually asymptomatic or nonspecific, but occasionally paralytic disease, resulting from the neurotropic properties of the virus, may be devastating or fatal. Children are particularly vulnerable. Vaccination programmes have greatly reduced the frequency of the disease in developed countries, although occasional cases in vaccine recipients or their unvaccinated family members are still reported.

Clinical features

Incubation is between 3 and 35 days. There may be malaise, sore throat, gastrointestinal upset, headache, vomiting, fever, meningeal irritation, and low back pain.

Neurological features:

- Aseptic lymphocytic meningitis, followed by flaccid paralysis (proximal > distal, legs > arms), often asymmetric, +/– muscle pain, tenderness; areflexia (involvement of anterior horn cells), atrophy, +/– fasciculation
- Involvement of cranial nerve nuclei (10–15%), causing bulbar weakness, facial weakness less often
- Respiratory failure (bulbar involvement)
- Autonomic involvement: hyper- or hypohidrosis, systemic hypertension (less commonly hypotension), urinary retention
- Definite sensory loss very rare but documented (dorsal root ganglia involvement)
- Extraocular muscles not involved
- Rarely encephalitic illness

Investigation

Blood serology for polio virus. CSF shows increased cell count, initially poly-morphonuclear cells, later a pleocytosis; raised protein occurs late. Microbiology: stool culture for virus; pharyngeal swab for virus culture less often positive. Neurophysiology: EMG is usually normal in the acute stage, but later shows changes typical of anterior horn cell disease (fasciculations, fibrillations). Neuropathology shows degeneration of anterior horn cells of the spinal cord, motor and sensory cranial nerve nuclei, layers III and V of motor cortex, thalamus, and cerebellar vermis.

Differential diagnosis

- Acute flaccid paralysis: *Guillain–Barré syndrome*, acute intermittent *porphyria*, other viral infections (Coxsackie A and B, enterovirus EV70, 71); Japanese encephalitis and other arboviruses (e.g., West Nile virus) are reported to produce a similar acute syndrome on occasion.
- Bulbar symptoms: myasthenia gravis, diphtheria, botulism.

Treatment and prognosis

There is no specific treatment. In the acute phase, respiratory status should be monitored and supportive treatment of respiratory failure, with mechanical ventilation if need be, instituted. There is a 10% fatality rate in acute paralytic illness. In the acute phase, some muscles recover quickly, but paralysis at 1 month is permanent. Scoliosis develops in virtually all patients contracting paralytic polio before the pubertal growth spurt. A *motor neurone disease* developing 20 years or so after an attack of polio has been reported, but late deterioration, *postpolio syndrome*, may have many other causes. Prevention of poliomyelitis with oral live attenuated (Sabin) vaccine leads to excretion of virus in stools from which the nonimmune individuals can become infected.

References

Gould T. A Summer Plague – Polio and Its Survivors. New Haven, CT: Yale University Press; 1995
Howard RS. Poliomyelitis and the postpolio syndrome. BMJ. 2005; 330:1314–1318

Polyarteritis nodosa (PAN)

Systemic necrotizing vasculitis

Classical polyarteritis nodosa (cPAN) is a necrotizing *vasculitis* of small- and medium-sized arteries, especially affecting branch points and sometimes resulting in aneurysmal dilatation. Similar to *Churg–Strauss syndrome*, it may overlap with microscopic polyangiitis (mPAN). Although it may present with systemic and renal features, neurological complications may also occur.

Clinical features

Systemic features include fever, weight loss, malaise, hypertension (renal vasculitis, glomerulonephritis), skin rash, gastrointestinal features, cardiac features, but the lungs remain unaffected (cf. Churg–Strauss syndrome).

Neurological features: peripheral (ca. 60% affected) and central (ca. 20% affected) nervous system may be affected.

- Peripheral neuropathy: mononeuritis multiplex, peripheral or cranial (V, VII, VIII); distal polyneuropathy, cutaneous neuropathy, radiculopathy uncommon
- Global: headache, aseptic meningitis; dementia, psychosis, encephalopathy, depression, mania
- Focal: stroke-like syndromes causing aphasia, hemiparesis, visual field defects; rarely chorea, parkinsonism, cranial nerve involvement, cerebellar ataxia; spinal cord syndromes including infarction/necrosis, acute transverse myelopathy

Investigation

Blood hepatitis B serology may be positive; ANCA is usually negative (cf. microscopic polyangiitis); PAN has been reported on occasion as a paraneoplastic consequence of hairy cell leukemia.

Neuroimaging (CT/MRI) may show cerebral atrophy, focal/multifocal infarction, hemorrhage (all nonspecific findings); renal angiography may show presence of microaneurysms which may assist diagnosis.

CSF may show elevated pressure, protein, and cell count (lymphocytic pleocytosis in aseptic meningitis).

Neurophysiology: EMG/NCS is always abnormal with clinically apparent peripheral nervous system disease (axonal neuropathy most common) and is often abnormal in asymptomatic patients suggesting subclinical disease. EEG may show generalized slowing in encephalopathic patients. Nerve biopsy may show vasculitis of epineurial blood vessels and nerve infarction.

Differential diagnosis

Other vasculitic syndromes enter the differential, including microscopic polyangiitis.

Treatment and prognosis

CNS involvement in PAN is the second most common cause of death, following renal disease. Vigorous treatment is therefore indicated with immunosuppressive agents such as corticosteriods and cyclophosphamide.

Reference

Nadeau SE. Neurologic manifestations of systemic vasculitis. Neurol Clin. 2002; 20:123–150

Polycythemia rubra vera (PRV)

Polycythemia rubra vera (PRV) is a myeloproliferative disease characterized by increased red cell mass and blood volume, resulting in erythrocytosis (raised hematocrit) and increased blood viscosity. There may be associated neurological features, including *transient ischemic attack* and thrombotic *stroke*, less commonly cerebral hemorrhage, chorea.

Polyglucosan body disease (PGB)

Adult polyglucosan body disease (PGB) has a broad phenotype, with onset in the fifth to seventh decades. There is a positive family history in about a third of cases, sometimes associated with mutation in the gene encoding glycogen-branching enzyme. PGB is characterized by accumulation of polyglucosan bodies, composed of abnormally branched glycogen (amylopectin), in the central and peripheral nervous systems. PGB are also seen in Lafora body disease, type IV glycogenosis, and can occur incidentally with ageing (corpora amylacea).

Clinical features

Pleomorphic.

- Gait disorder, sphincter problems, sensory complaints, mixture of upper and lower motor neurone signs, cognitive decline, psychiatric features
- Peripheral (axonal) neuropathy
- Dementia (of frontal type)
- Neurogenic bladder
- Upper motor neurone signs
- +/– Amyotrophy, cerebellar signs, optic atrophy, parkinsonian syndrome, tremor

Investigation

PGB is essentially a tissue diagnosis, since all other investigations produce nonspecific findings with the exception of GBE mutations: PGB with diffuse peripheral and central involvement is allelic with Andersen disease (glycogen storage disease type IV). Neuroimaging (CT/MRI) may show extensive white matter abnormalities. Neurophysiology (EMG/NCS) may show diffuse axonal neuropathy, or denervation. Neuropsychology may show a subcortical type picture (slowness, problem-solving difficulties, impaired abstract reasoning). On nerve biopsy, PGB are large rounded intra-axonal inclusions, seen especially in myelinated fibers, up to 30 μm in diameter, metachromatic with toluidine blue staining (dark centre with lighter halo) and PAS +ve. On axillary skin biopsy, PGB may be seen in myoepithelial cells of apocrine glands. On brain biopsy, PGB seen in astrocytes.

Differential diagnosis

Very broad, in light of the variable clinical phenotype

Treatment and prognosis

No specific treatment

References

Robitaille Y, Carpenter S, Karpati G, DiMauro SD. A distinct form of polyglucosan disease with massive involvement of central and peripheral neuronal processes and astrocytes: a report of four cases and a review of the occurrence of polyglucosan bodies in other conditions such as Lafora's disease and normal ageing. Brain. 1980;103:315–336
Ziemssen F, Sindern E, Schroder JM, et al. Novel missense mutations in the glycogen-branching enzyme gene in adult polyglucosan body disease. Ann Neurol. 2000;47:536–540

Polymyalgia rheumatica (PMR)

Polymyalgia rheumatica (PMR) is a late-onset, acute illness, probably inflammatory in nature, producing muscular pain and stiffness around the shoulder girdle, usually symmetrical, but without true weakness, and which responds to adequate doses of steroids. Polymyalgia rheumatica (PMR) is strongly associated with *giant cell arteritis* (GCA).

Clinical features

- History of morning stiffness of >1 h, symmetrical shoulder and upper arm pain; illness <2 weeks in duration.
- Age usually >65 years.
- Systemic features may be present: weight loss, sweating, malaise.
- Response to steroids may be included among the diagnostic criteria.

- Examination discloses no true weakness of the shoulder girdle (cf. polymyositis) although this may be difficult to ascertain with the concurrent pain.
- Peripheral nerve problems have been reported on occasion (mononeuropathy, radiculopathy, brachial plexopathy, possibly chance concurrence, or reflection of underlying systemic vasculitis).

Investigation

Blood ESR raised (>40 mm/h), CRP, blood viscosity +/− alkaline phosphatase (transaminases usually normal). Normal creatine kinase, rheumatoid factor, autoantibodies, protein electrophoresis, and thyroid function tests may be helpful in excluding other diagnoses. Temporal artery biopsy is not considered helpful in pure PMR.

Differential diagnosis

Late-onset rheumatoid arthritis, osteoarthritis, rotator cuff disease. Myeloma. Hypothyroidism. Polymyositis, other causes of a proximal myopathy. Connective tissue disorders.

Treatment and prognosis

More than 80% of patients improve with prednisolone 15–20 mg/day. This is given for about 1 month and then weaned slowly. The majority of patients require a small maintenance dose of steroids. Prognosis is generally very good. Relapses may occur if steroids are weaned too quickly. Steroid-induced adverse effects may emerge if large doses are required to keep the disorder in check (e.g., steroid myopathy). Prophylactic bisphosphonates are indicated to prevent osteoporosis. There is a risk of subsequently developing giant cell arteritis.

Diagnostic criteria

Hunder GG, Bloch DA, Michel BA, et al. The American College of Rheumatology 1990 criteria for the classification of giant cell arteritis. Arthritis Rheumat. 1990;33:1122–1128

References

Dasgupta B, Borg FA, Hassan N, et al. BSR and BHPR guidelines for the management of polymyalgia rheumatica. Rheumatology (Oxford). 2010;49:186–190
Salvarani C, Cantini F, Hunder GG. Polymyalgia rheumatica and giant cell arteritis. Lancet. 2008;372:234–245
Weyand CM, Gorozny JJ. Giant-cell arteritis and polymyalgia rheumatica. Ann Intern Med. 2003;139:505–515

Polymyositis

Polymyositis is an idiopathic, probably autoimmune, inflammatory myopathy, most usually affecting proximal limb musculature, and occurring between the ages 30 and 60 years, although there is a smaller peak during adolescence; females predominate.

Clinical features

- Weakness of proximal limb muscles, trunk, limb girdles (may be asymmetrical), +/– neck ("dropped head syndrome"), +/– bulbar muscles (dysphonia, dysphagia), +/– respiratory muscles (rarely causes dyspnoea); extraocular muscles are not involved. Mild muscle atrophy may be seen.
- Painless myopathy in majority; pain, aching in ca. 15% of cases.
- Hyporeflexia.
- +/– Cardiac dysrhythmias.
- +/– Lung fibrosis.

There may be concurrent connective tissue or autoimmune disease, e.g., myasthenia gravis, scleroderma, Hashimoto's thyroiditis.

Investigation

Blood creatine kinase and ESR may be elevated; +/– ANA, anti-Jo1 autoantibodies; check TFTs, AchRAb, other autoantibodies for concurrent autoimmune disease, including voltage-gated calcium channel antibodies. ECG may be abnormal. EMG is myopathic, with brief low voltage action potentials, fibrillation potentials, positive sharp waves, polyphasic units. Muscle biopsy shows scattered muscle fibre necrosis and phagocytosis (macrophages); lymphocytic infiltration with predominantly CD8 T cells (cf. *dermatomyositis*); evidence of regeneration (proliferating sarcolemmal nuclei, new myofibrils, small fibers in clusters). No perifascicular atrophy (cf. dermatomyositis).

Differential diagnosis

Other inflammatory myopathies such as dermatomyositis, *inclusion body myositis*, eosinophilic myositis (may occur in context of hypereosinophilic syndrome). Metabolic myopathies such as *McArdle's disease* and mitochondrial myopathies. Myalgic disorders such as fibromyalgia, *polymyalgia rheumatica*. Muscular dystrophies such as dysferlinopathies, dystrophinopathies, and facioscapulohumeral dystrophy. Neuromuscular junction disorders such as *myasthenia gravis*, which may be present concurrently, and *Lambert–Eaton myasthenic syndrome*. Steroid myopathy may develop during treatment.

Treatment and prognosis

Treatment is initially with steroids (60–80 mg/day of prednisolone), slowly weaned as clinical and biochemical improvement progresses. Depending on duration of treatment, steroid sparing agents such as azathioprine or methotrexate may be used. Intravenous methylprednisolone may be used for quicker response if there is respiratory muscle weakness or dysphagia. Failure to respond may prompt use of mycophenolate, ciclosporin, tacrolimus, or pulsed intravenous cyclophosphamide. Rituximab and IvIg are also options for resistant cases. The majority of patients improve with steroid treatment, although there may be some residual weakness. Long-term steroid therapy mandates osteoporosis prophylaxis. Untreated patients develop muscle atrophy, fibrosis, and contracture. Most patients require treatment for 2 years, many for 5 years, and some indefinitely. Treatment of cardiac dysrhythmias as appropriate. There is only a small risk of underlying malignancy; so, polymyositis is not typically regarded as one of the *paraneoplastic syndromes* (cf. dermatomyositis).

References

Dalakas MC, Karpati G. Inflammatory myopathies. In: Karpati G, Hilton-Jones D, Bushby K, Griggs RC, eds. Disorders of Voluntary Muscle. 8th ed. Cambridge: Cambridge University Press; 2010:427–452
Mastaglia FL. When the treatment does not work: polymyositis. Pract Neurol. 2008;8:170–174

Pompe's disease [OMIM#232300]

Acid maltase deficiency, Glycogenosis type II, Late-onset glycogen storage disease type 2

Acid maltase deficiency is an autosomal recessive *glycogen storage disorder* due to deficiency of the lysosomal enzyme acid α-glucosidase, or acid maltase, in the CNS and skeletal muscle. This enzyme does not contribute to the normal control of blood glucose levels, but deficiency leads to massive accumulation of glycogen within lysosomes, with subsequent cell damage and death. The clinical phenotype is variable, with age of onset ranging from infancy to adulthood. More than 50 mutations in the acid α-glucosidase gene on chromosome 17 have been identified; gene deletions lead to more severe disease. Enzyme replacement therapy is now available.

Clinical features

- Infantile (Pompe's disease):
  - Profound weakness and hypotonia +/– muscle firmness ("woody texture"); paucity of movement; frog-leg posture, normal social interaction
  - Loss of deep tendon reflexes
  - Heart failure due to cardiomyopathy, with cardiomegaly
  - +/– Hepatosplenomegaly; macroglossia
- Late Infantile/Juvenile (Smith's disease):
  - Motor delay
  - Progressive myopathy
  - +/– Organomegaly
- Adult: (Engel's disease): two peaks, in third to fourth and sixth to seventh decades.
  - Progressive myopathy, usually of the legs.
  - Respiratory insufficiency may be presenting feature (type II respiratory failure) due to early involvement of respiratory muscles; cardiomyopathy is much less prominent than in infantile disease.
  - +/– Cranial nerve involvement (e.g., bulbar); macroglossia; distal limb involvement.

Investigation

Bloods: creatine kinase may be raised (usually only modest elevation, ~3 to 4× normal) especially in infantile and juvenile forms, but may be normal in adult onset disease. Acid α-glucosidase levels may be measured in the blood leukocytes, fibroblasts, or muscle. Normal leukocyte levels with reduced values in muscle may occur. Neurophysiology (EMG) is usually compatible with a myopathy, but variable. Myotonic discharges and neurogenic changes (fibrillations) may be found. Important to examine paraspinal muscles. Muscle biopsy characteristically shows increased glycogen within lysosomes and vacuolar change. Increased acid phosphatase may be seen especially in small fibers. Crystalloid inclusions may be seen in mitochondria. Acid α-glucosidase level may be assayed in muscle tissue. ECG may be abnormal in adult onset disease.

Differential diagnosis

Juvenile disease may be confused with *Duchenne muscular dystrophy*. Adult disease may be confused with inflammatory myopathy or *limb-girdle muscular dystrophies*.

Treatment and prognosis

In infantile (Pompe's) disease, progression is relentless with death usually by the age of 2 years. Likewise, in the juvenile form, the disease is fatal within a few months of onset of heart failure. In the adult disease, prognosis depends on the degree of respiratory involvement. Ventilatory aids such as nocturnal intermittent positive pressure ventilation may be used to support these patients. Enzyme replacement therapy with alglucosidase alpha has been reported to stabilize neuromuscular deficits over a year with mild functional improvement.

References

Müller-Felber W, Horvath R, Gempel K, et al. Late onset Pompe disease: clinical and neurophysiological spectrum of 38 patients including long-term follow-up in 18 patients. Neuromuscul Disord. 2007;17:698–706
Van der Beek NAME, Hagemans MLC, van der Ploeg AT, Reuser AJ, van Doorn PA. Pompe disease (glycogen storage disease type II): clinical features and enzyme replacement therapy. Acta Neurol Belg. 2006;106:82–86
van der Ploeg AT, Clemens PR, Corzo D, et al. A randomized study of alglucosidase alfa in late-onset Pompe's disease. N Engl J Med. 2010;362:1396–1406
Winkel LPF, Hagemans MLC, van Doorn PA, et al. The natural course of non-classic Pompe's disease: a review of 225 published cases. J Neurol. 2005;252:875–884

Porphyria

Inborn or acquired errors of porphyrin metabolism may cause visceral, dermatological, neurological, psychiatric, or mixed disorders. Those affecting the nervous system, the "neuropsychiatric porphyrias," are the autosomal dominant conditions of:

- Acute intermittent porphyria (AIP)
- Variegate porphyria (VP)
- Hereditary coproporphyria (HCP)
- Plumboporphyria

Gastrointestinal and peripheral nervous system features are thought to result from neuronal dysfunction, whereas cerebral manifestations may result from metabolic compromise, ischemia, demyelination, or oxidative stress.

Clinical features

Highly variable: systemic features include abdominal pain, cramping, +/– dermatological features such as bullae, erythema (VP, HCP).

Neurological features:

- Peripheral neuropathy: motor; proximal weakness in arms > legs (especially wrist drop); patients may become quadriparetic; flaccidity, areflexia or hyporeflexia
- Cranial nerve palsies (III, VII, X)
- Autonomic instability
- Epileptic seizures (20% in acute attacks)
- Psychosis
- Delirium

There may be a history of fasting, infection, drug exposure, or lead exposure (plumboporphyria), all these being recognized precipitating factors. Diagnosis may also need to be considered in patients with chronic refractory epilepsy, unexplained neuropathy and myopathy. The diagnosis can easily be missed and needs to be considered in patients with recurrent episodes of altered consciousness and behavior as well as in some cases labeled as Guillain–Barré syndrome.

Investigation

Liaison with a specialist laboratory familiar with diagnosis of porphyria is advisable, and essential for specialized investigations. Diagnosis requires the demonstration of porphyrin precursor accumulation (porphobilinogen, PBG, and aminolaevulinic acid, ALA) at the time of symptoms (cf. asymptomatic carriers) in either urine (AIP) or feces (HCP, VP). Light sensitivity of porphyrins mandates storage of samples in dark and prompt transmission to the laboratory for analysis. Urine PBG is a screening test, but with high frequency of false positive and false negative results; if clinical suspicion is high, the test should be repeated if initially negative. Fecal PBG can also be measured. EMG/NCS may show changes consistent with axonal neuropathy and denervation of muscles. CSF is usually normal, although there may be a nonspecific raised protein. Skin biopsy (VP, HCP) may show homogeneous PAS +ve thickening and IgG deposition in vessel walls. Underlying enzyme deficiency, e.g., δ-aminolaevulinic acid dehydratase (ALAD) in plumboporphyria requires specialist investigation.

Differential diagnosis

Guillain–Barré syndrome, other acute axonal motor neuropathies, and *poliomyelitis* in the acute phase. Weakness may lead to confusion with *critical illness myopathy*. Lead poisoning (plumbism), tyrosinemia (fumaryl acetoacetate hydrolase deficiency), hexachlorobenzene poisoning.

Treatment and prognosis

Treatment of the acute attack comprises withdrawl of precipitants, especially drugs; increasing carbohydrate intake; and treating any intercurrent infection. Symptomatic treatment of seizures may be required. Heme arginate (Normosang) given intravenously may be useful, as it compensates for heme breakdown by inhibiting ALA synthase, the rate-limiting and rate-controlling enzyme in the heme biosynthetic pathway. Acute attacks can be fatal despite supportive therapy, possibly due to cardiac arrhythmias. Prevention of attacks consists of avoidance of porphyrinogenic agents (drugs, alcohol), adequate carbohydrate intake, and the avoidance of dieting.

References

Crimlisk HL. The little imitator – porphyria: a neuropsychiatric disorder. J Neurol Neurosurg Psychiatry. 1997;62:319–328

Dyer J, Garrick DP, Ingus A, Pye IF. Plumboporphyria (ALAD deficiency) in a lead worker: a scenario for potential diagnostic confusion. Br J Ind Med. 1993;50: 1119–1121

Kauppinen R. Porphyrias. Lancet. 2005;365:241–252

Peters TJ, Mills KR. Porphyria for the neurologist: the bare essentials. Pract Neurol. 2006;6:255–258

Posterior cortical atrophy (PCA)

Visual variant of Alzheimer's disease

The syndrome of posterior cortical atrophy (PCA) is characterized by a visual disorder with visual agnosia, topographical difficulty, optic ataxia, simultanagnosia, ocular apraxia (Balint's syndrome), alexia, acalculia, and later a more generalized dementia. Visual hallucinations may sometimes occur. Functional imaging shows hypoperfusion and hypometabolism of visual cortical areas. The majority of cases have neuropathological evidence of underlying *Alzheimer's disease* (AD), although other neuropathological substrates are described. Response to cholinesterase inhibitors is exceptional.

References

Kirshner HS, Lavin PJ. Posterior cortical atrophy: a brief review. Curr Neurol Neurosci Rep. 2006;6:477–480

Mendez MF, Ghajarania M, Perryman KM. Posterior cortical atrophy: clinical characteristics and differences compared to Alzheimer's disease. Dement Geriatr Cogn Disord. 2002;14:33–40

Posterior interosseous syndrome

The posterior interosseous nerve is the purely motor terminal branch of the radial nerve in the forearm which supplies the supinator muscle, wrist, and finger extensors, hence a form of *radial neuropathy*. Posterior interosseous mononeuropathy as a consequence of entrapment, usually at the level of the supinator, is rare. It produces weakness of the wrist and finger extensors but with sparing of extensor carpi radialis (which receives a more proximal branch of the radial nerve), hence causing a wrist drop with radial deviation. There are no sensory signs, but pain in the elbow or dorsal forearm may occur. Diagnosis is by clinical history and EMG/NCS.

Reference

Staal A, Van Gijn J, Spaans F. Mononeuropathies: Examination, Diagnosis and Treatment. London: W.B. Saunders; 1999:43–46

Posterior reversible leukoencephalopathy syndrome (PRES)

Hyperperfusion encephalopathy, Reversible posterior leukoencephalopathy syndrome

Posterior reversible leukoencephalopathy syndrome (PRES) comprises rapidly evolving neurological dysfunction associated with rapidly increasing blood pressure, with marked white matter changes on brain imaging. Situations in which posterior leukoencephalopathy syndrome has been described include:

- *Eclampsia*
- Renal disease
- Hypertensive encephalopathy
- Cytotoxic/immunosuppressive drug therapy, e.g., ciclosporin, tacrolimus
- Complication of *reversible cerebral vasoconstriction syndrome*

It has also been argued that this syndrome may be a neuroradiological expression of various metabolic disorders which affect the CNS, including seizures. Pathogenesis may be autoregulatory failure with passive overdistension of cerebral arterioles causing blood-brain barrier disruption and vasogenic edema formation.

Clinical features

- Headache, nausea and vomiting, seizures, visual disturbances, altered sensorium, +/− focal neurological deficits
- Rapidly increasing blood pressure
- Rarely, spinal cord involvement

Investigation

Neuroimaging: MR brain shows edematous lesions in posterior parietal and occipital white matter, occasionally extending to basal ganglia, brain stem, cerebellum, and even cervical spinal cord; grey matter is sometimes involved. Ischemic lesions are uncommon.

Differential diagnosis

Other causes of encephalopathy; encephalitis.

Treatment and prognosis

Prompt control of blood pressure and control of precipitating factors (e.g., drugs) form the mainstay of management. With early treatment, the condition is completely reversible, but delay may be associated with permanent neurological deficits.

References

Lee VH, Wijdicks EF, Manno EM, Rabinstein AA. Clinical spectrum of reversible posterior leukoencephalopathy syndrome. Arch Neurol. 2008;65:205–210
Stott VL, Hurrell MA, Anderson TJ. Reversible posterior leukoencephalopathy syndrome: a misnomer reviewed. Intern Med J. 2005;35:83–90

Posthypoxic syndromes

Posthypoxic syndromes are a consequence of reduced oxygen supply to the brain due to reduced perfusion (ischemia), for example, following a myocardial infarction, ventricular fibrillation, hemorrhage or "shock," or a reduced amount of circulating arterial oxygen (suffocation, *carbon monoxide poisoning*, respiratory failure, anesthesia with deficient inspired oxygen). The failure of normal brain energy metabolism may have a variety of neurological consequences.

Clinical features

- Borderzone or watershed infarction (ischemic injury secondary to systemic hypotension): hippocampus, cerebellum, cerebral cortex particularly affected, brain stem relatively resistant.
- Clinical sequela: seizures, myoclonus, especially action myoclonus (*Lance-Adams syndrome*), dementia with extrapyramidal signs, Korsakoff-type amnesic state, visual agnosia, choreoathetosis, cerebellar ataxia.
- Delayed postanoxic encephalopathy.
- *Coma*, especially if hypoxia acute. Prognosis variable, but reasonable if brain stem reflexes intact. Persistent coma or a *vegetative state* may occur. Brain death is diagnosed when all brain stem reflexes are abolished, there is no natural respiration in response to hypercapnia, and the EEG is isoelectric.

Investigation

Neuroimaging (CT/MRI) may demonstrate ischemic injury, infarction. EEG may show nonspecific changes.

Differential diagnosis

Potentially broad: all other causes of coma, seizures, myoclonus, dementia, movement disorders, cerebellar ataxia, and encephalopathy, but diagnosis is usually obvious from the history.

Treatment and prognosis

Acute management involves cardiopulmonary resuscitation to try to ensure adequate oxygenation of brain tissue. Hyperbaric oxygen therapy may be appropriate in cases of carbon monoxide poisoning. Symptomatic treatment of seizures, myoclonus.

Postpolio syndrome

Late postpolio functional deterioration

Neurological deficits following paralytic *poliomyelitis* were traditionally viewed as fixed and non-progressive. In recent years, some polio survivors have re-presented with further deterioration in functional ability, pain, increased deformity, and/or muscle atrophy, on average 30 years after their acute attack. The term postpolio syndrome has been used for this late functional deterioration in polio survivors. Some authors have documented specific orthopedic, neurological, general medical, and psychiatric causes for deterioration, whereas others maintain the term postpolio syndrome for unexplained deterioration. An epidemiological survey suggests that postpolio syndrome, however defined, is rare among polio survivors.

Investigation

Multidisciplinary assessment may be required to determine the cause(s) of deterioration, including:

- Neurological opinion; creatine kinase, EMG/NCS
- Respiratory assessment, to exclude nocturnal hypoventilation or *obstructive sleep apnea-hypopnea syndrome*
- Sleep assessment (sleep study)
- Orthopedic opinion, radiology, orthotics
- +/− Psychiatric opinion

Treatment and prognosis

Dependent upon cause (orthopedic, neurological, respiratory, psychiatric), when identified.

References

Howard RS. Late post-polio functional deterioration. Pract Neurol. 2003;3:66–77
Windebank AJ, Litchy WJ, Daube JR, Iverson RA. Lack of progression of neurologic deficit in survivors of paralytic polio: a 5-year prospective population-based study. Neurology. 1996;46:80–84

Potassium-aggravated myotonia (PAM) [OMIM#608390]

Myotonia fluctuans, Myotonia permanens

This autosomal dominant disorder is one of the *myotonic syndromes*, linked to mutations in the α-subunit of the sodium channel gene SCN4A, hence is a sodium *channelopathy*, allelic with hyperkalemic *periodic paralysis* and paramyotonia congenita.

Clinical features

Variable.

- Painful cramps, stiffness without weakness; fluctuation of symptoms, cold sensitivity is usual.

- A rare form, myotonia permanens, is characterized by severe persistent myotonia.
- Myotonia fluctuans: fluctuating severity (cf. myotonia congenita); delayed onset exercise-induced myotonia (cf. myotonia congenita: reduced myotonia with exercise; paramyotonia: immediate onset exercise-induced myotonia); no effect from cooling (cf. paramyotonia); increased myotonia with K^+ load (cf. hyperkalemic periodic paralysis: weakness with K^+ load).

Investigation

Neurophysiology shows reduced CMAP amplitude with muscle cooling or exposure to K^+ ions. Neurogenetic testing reveals mutations in the SCN4A gene.

Differential diagnosis

Other causes of muscle cramp, stiffness, e.g., autosomal dominant myotonia congenita (Thomsen's disease).

Treatment and prognosis

Mexiletine is the drug of choice for myotonia; it may be required lifelong in myotonia permanens.

References

Kubota T, Kinoshita M, Sasaki R, et al. New mutation of the Na channel in the severe form of potassium-aggravated myotonia. Muscle Nerve. 2009;39:666–673
Orrell RW, Jurkat-Rott K, Lehmann-Horn F, Lane RJ. Familial cramp due to potassium-aggravated myotonia. J Neurol Neurosurg Psychiatry. 1998;65:569–572
Ricker K, Moxley RT3rd, Heine R, Lehmann-Horn F. Myotonia fluctuans. A third type of muscle sodium channel disease. Arch Neurol. 1994;51:1095–1102

Pregnancy and the nervous system: overview

Pregnancy and the puerperium may impact on a variety of chronic neurological conditions, including *epilepsy*, *migraine*, and *multiple sclerosis*. It may also increase the risk of developing *de novo* neurological illness (cerebrovascular disease), the effects of which may continue after pregnancy. *Eclampsia* is a disease encountered only during pregnancy and the puerperium which may have neurological effects.

- Neurological conditions during pregnancy
  - Cerebrovascular disease:
    - Increased incidence of stroke, probably multifactorial; increased risk of cerebral aneurysm rupture leading to intracerebral hemorrhage; increased risk of bleeding from arteriovenous malformations (especially spinal); increased risk of sinus and cortical venous thrombosis. Postpartum cardiomyopathy increases the risk of ischemic stroke.
  - Epilepsy:
    - Control of preexisting seizures may deteriorate, especially in the first trimester and in patients with poorly controlled epilepsy and/or poor compliance (altered metabolism of drugs, vomiting, impaired intake). *De novo* epilepsy may occur (estrogens may lower seizure threshold); epilepsy confined to pregnancy ("gestational epilepsy") is described but rare. Antiepileptic drug dosages may need to be increased during pregnancy to ensure optimal seizure control; monitoring of drug levels may be helpful in judging appropriate increases in dosage. Risk of teratogenicity with many antiepileptic drugs, hence need for pre-conceptual counseling and prophylactic folic acid for those planning pregnancy. Carbamazepine has been the favored drug for control of epilepsy during pregnancy, but some authors now favor lamotrigine. Risks to unborn child of uncontrolled epileptic seizures in the mother outweigh small risk of teratogenicity, so other antiepileptic medications should not be stopped once pregnancy has occurred.
  - *Idiopathic intracranial hypertension*:
    - May present in first trimester or puerperium (differential diagnosis = sinus thrombosis).
  - Migraine:
    - Tends to improve, although sometimes worsens or presents *de novo*.
  - Multiple sclerosis:
    - Decreased relapse rate during pregnancy; increased relapse rate during the puerperium.
  - *Neuropathy*:
    - *Carpal tunnel syndrome, meralgia paresthetica, Bell's palsy* are said to be more common in pregnancy; femoral, obturator, and common peroneal palsies may occur as a consequence of delivery procedures. Neuropathies associated with *porphyria* and chronic inflammatory demyelinating polyneuropathy (CIDP) may be exacerbated.
  - Neuromuscular disease:
    - *Myasthenia gravis*: no clear effect: may improve, stay stable, or deteriorate.
  - *Systemic lupus erythematosus*:
    - May be exacerbated during puerperium.

- Conditions unique to pregnancy, puerperium:
  - Eclampsia: hypertension, proteinuria, hyperreflexia, epileptic seizures.
  - Chorea gravidarum (rare).
  - Wernicke-type syndrome in patients with hyperemesis gravidarum.
  - Sheehan's syndrome (postpartum hypopituitarism, due to infarction of pituitary, usually associated with peripartum hemorrhage).

References

Confavreux C, Hutchinson M, Hours MM, Cortinovis-Tourniaire P, Moreau T. Rate of pregnancy-related relapse in multiple sclerosis. Pregnancy in Multiple Sclerosis Group. N Engl J Med. 1998;339:285–291
Donaldson JO. Neurology of Pregnancy. 2nd ed. London: W.B. Saunders; 1989
Sawle GV, Ramsay MM. The neurology of pregnancy. J Neurol Neurosurg Psychiatry. 1998;64:711–725

Primary angiitis of the central nervous system (PACNS)

Isolated angiitis of the central nervous system

Primary angiitis of the central nervous system (PACNS) is a very rare granulomatous angiitis, confined to the central nervous system (hence "isolated angiitis"), affecting small leptomeningeal, cortical, and spinal blood vessels. It may on occasion be associated with herpes zoster infection or with lymphoma.

Clinical features

- Subacute or chronic encephalopathy: headache (often insidious and progressive, not thunderclap), confusional state, cognitive decline
- Epileptic seizures
- Stroke: in <20%; ischemia > hemorrhage
- Rarely: myelopathy, radiculopathy, systemic symptoms (fever)

Investigation

Bloods are often normal although ESR may be raised. Neuroimaging (MRI) abnormal in most (>90%) cases with nonspecific cortical and subcortical infarctions and diffuse white matter hyperintensities, but may be normal. Cerebral angiography (preferable to MRA) is frequently normal but may show luminal irregularities which do not reverse. CSF is abnormal in most (>95%) cases with raised protein and/or lymphocytosis. Tissue (meningeal + cortical) biopsy is required for definitive diagnosis: Overreliance on specificity of neuroradiological appearances is the greatest diagnostic pitfall.

Differential diagnosis

Reversible cerebral vasoconstriction syndrome may be indistinguishable but usually has acute onset, often normal MRI and CSF, and angiography is always abnormal (by definition). *Neurosarcoidosis* may cause a very similar angiitis. Infections (varicella zoster. syphilis), drugs (amphetamines, cocaine), malignancy (lymphoma, angioendotheliomatosis), and systemic vasculitides (polyarteritis nodosa, Behçet's) may cause a similar clinical and radiological picture on occasion, hence the importance of biopsy. In the workup of suspected cerebral vasculitis, most patients will have a disease other than arteritis.

Treatment and prognosis

Immunosuppression (prednisolone, cyclophosphamide) is usually given, but efficacy is uncertain. Cases of spontaneous resolution have been claimed. More usually, death occurs in weeks or months. Variants, based on the size of the affected blood vessels, have been claimed: Small vessel disease, analogous to microscopic polyarteritis, has a poorer prognosis than medium vessel disease.

Diagnostic criteria

Calabrese LH, Mallek JA. Primary angiitis of the central nervous system. Report of 8 new cases, review of the literature, and proposal for diagnostic criteria. Medicine (Baltimore). 1988;67:20–39

References

McLaren K, Gillespie J, Shrestha S, Neary D, Ballardie FW. Primary angiitis of the central nervous system: emerging variants. Q J Med. 2005;98:643–654
Birnbaum J, Hellmann DB. Primary angiitis of the central nervous system. Arch Neurol. 2009;66:704–709
Chadha T, Duna GF, Calabrese LH. Primary angiitis of the CNS and its mimics. In: Kilpatrick T, Ransohoff RM, Wesselingh S, eds. Inflammatory Diseases of the Central Nervous System. Cambridge: Cambridge University Press; 2010:109–124

Primary headache associated with sexual activity (PHSA)

Coital cephalalgia, Coital headache, Sex headache

The second International Headache Society classification of headache disorders defines two clinical types of primary headache associated with sexual activity (PHSA):

- Pre-orgasmic: headache which develops gradually during the buildup of intercourse (previously type 1)
- Orgasmic: headache which occurs suddenly at orgasm (previously type 2)

The pathophysiology of PHSA is ill understood; it may be related to impaired cerebrovascular autoregulation, or release of vasoactive substances. Comorbidity with migraine is possible. Arterial hypertension is not now thought to be a risk factor.

Differential diagnosis and investigation

Symptomatic or secondary headaches associated with sexual activity also occur. The clinical similarity of orgasmic PHSA to *subarachnoid hemorrhage* (SAH), although vomiting does not usually occur, necessitates investigation with CT +/− CSF analysis if the patient presents acutely, to look for subarachnoid blood and xanthochromia, respectively. Another increasingly recognized cause of secondary headache associated with sexual activity is *reversible cerebral vasoconstriction syndrome*, often presenting with recurrent thunderclap headache, so angiography may also be indicated to exclude this condition as well as to search for an underlying aneurysm in the case of SAH. With delayed (>2 weeks) presentation, MRA is often performed but there is no evidence to indicate that this defines a pathological cause.

Treatment and prognosis

Both types of PHSA are benign with an excellent prognosis. Reassurance is usually the only treatment required. There is no evidence base beyond case series for pharmacotherapy. With recurrent type 2 headache, a course of indomethacin or ergotamine may be helpful. Some advocate the use of beta-blockers as well.

References

Frese A, Evers S. Primary headache syndromes associated with sexual activity. Pract Neurol. 2005;5:350–355

Larner AJ. Transient acute neurologic sequelae of sexual activity: headache and amnesia. J Sex Med. 2008;5:284–288
Turner IM, Harding TM. Headache and sexual activity: a review. Headache. 2008;48:1254–1256

Primary lateral sclerosis (PLS)

Progressive symmetric spinobulbar spasticity

Primary lateral sclerosis (PLS) is a rare variant of *motor neurone disease*. It is a syndrome of progressive, usually symmetrical, spinobulbar spasticity without lower motor neurone features, starting in adulthood, thought to be due to selective dysfunction or loss of the descending motor tracts, hence a motor neurone disease with exclusively upper motor neurone features.

Clinical features

- Slowly progressive spastic quadriparesis, usually symmetrical; hyperreflexia, extensor plantar responses.
- Pseudobulbar affect, spastic dysarthria.
- Mild cognitive dysfunction of frontal lobe type.
- Bladder function preserved. No clinical lower motor neurone features.

Investigation

Bloods and CSF are generally normal. Neuroimaging (MRI) excludes alternative pathology (e.g., cord compression, multiple sclerosis) and may show focal atrophy of the precentral gyrus and the corpus callosum. Functional neuroimaging (PET) may show reduced metabolism in precentral gyrus. EMG is generally normal, although may show occasional (asymptomatic) fibrillation potentials. Neuropathological reports indicate heavy loss of Betz cells from motor cortex of the precentral gyrus.

Differential diagnosis

Other causes of exclusively upper motor neurone signs, e.g., *hereditary spastic paraplegia*, and some presentations of *multiple sclerosis* (in which abdominal reflexes are said to be lost early, unlike the situation in motor neurone disease). MR imaging excludes the other likely diagnoses.

Corticobasal degeneration may be mistaken for PLS.

Treatment and prognosis

No specific treatment. Symptomatic treatment of spasticity. Disease is slowly progressive. Many cases of PLS ultimately "convert" into a more traditional ALS phenotype.

Reference

Pringle CE, Hudson AJ, Munoz DG, Kiernan JA, Brown WF, Ebers GC. Primary lateral sclerosis: clinical features, neuropathology and diagnostic criteria. Brain. 1992;115:495–520

Primary orthostatic tremor (POT)

Shaky legs syndrome, White rabbit syndrome

Primary orthostatic tremor (POT) is characterized by *tremor*, predominantly of the lower limbs, present on standing and which disappears on sitting, walking, leaning, or when the patient is lifted off the ground. The 14–18 Hz oscillation is unique, approximately twice that of *essential tremor*, and is thought to be generated by a central oscillator (peripheral loading does not alter tremor frequency).

Clinical features

- A feeling of unsteadiness, shakiness, or "legs like jelly" when standing still.
- Rapid rhythmic synchronized contractions of the leg muscles on standing, causing knee tremor.
- On auscultation with the diaphragm over lower limb muscles, a regular thumping sound, likened to helicopter rotors in the distance, may be heard.
- Arm tremor is much less frequent; a jaw tremor with features of POT has been described.

Investigation

EMG shows a pathognomonic synchronous activity in leg muscles on standing, with a frequency of 14–18 Hz, which disappears when not weight bearing.

Differential diagnosis

The clinical features of POT are very characteristic, but can be mistaken for functional illness if the clinician is not familiar with the diagnosis. Secondary causes of orthostatic tremor include *Parkinson's disease* and other parkinsonian syndromes, pontine lesions, and Graves disease, but these conditions are invariably associated with other neurological symptoms and signs.

Treatment and prognosis

A number of drugs have anecdotally been reported to be helpful in POT, including phenobarbitone, primidone, clonazepam, pramipexole, and levodopa, although the only blinded placebo-controlled study suggesting efficacy is with gabapentin. Propranolol is not helpful (cf. essential tremor). Because of impact on quality of life, there may be concurrent depression which merits treatment in its own right.

References

Heilman KM. Orthostatic tremor. Arch Neurol. 1984;41:880–881.
Ramtahal J, Larner AJ. Shaky legs? Think POT! Age Ageing. 2009;38:352–353

Primary systemic amyloidosis

Primary systemic amyloidosis is a rare, nonfamilial, multisystem disorder, usually of later life, characterized by the extracellular deposition of fibrillar proteins in a beta-pleated sheet configuration (= amyloid) composed of fragments of immunoglobulin light chains (AL = amyloid light chain). Symptoms include fatigue, renal involvement, cardiac involvement, and peripheral neuropathy (cf. *familial amyloid polyneuropathies*). Autonomic disturbance is common (orthostatic hypotension, impotence, pupillary abnormalities, impaired sweating). Investigation may reveal a monoclonal (M) band in blood or urine, but this may be subtle and missed by routine serum and urinary electrophoresis. EMG/NCS shows an axonal sensorimotor polyneuropathy. Pathological confirmation may be achieved with biopsy of abdominal fat pad or nerve. Serum amyloid P component scintigraphy (SAP scan) may show abnormal uptake of labeled SAP. Prognosis is poor due to cardiac and renal involvement.

Reference

Hu MTM, Gabriel CM, Lachmann HJ, King R, Hawkins PN, Ginsberg L. A faint in the emergency department (due to primary systemic amyloidosis neuropathy). Pract Neurol. 2004;4:104–109

Prion disease: overview

Prionoses, Transmissible spongiform encephalopathies (TSE)

Prion diseases result from accumulation of abnormal isoforms (PrP^{Sc}) of the normal cellular prion protein (PrP^C) within the brain, which have greater β-sheet and less α-helix conformation than the normal protein and hence a greater propensity to aggregate. The clinical phenotype is extremely heterogeneous, partly influenced by polymorphisms within codon 129 of the PrP gene.
  Prion diseases may be classified etiologically as:

- Sporadic: Sporadic Creutzfeldt-Jakob disease (sCJD), sporadic familial insomnia
- Inherited: Familial Creutzfeldt-Jakob disease (fCJD), Gerstmann-Sträussler-Scheinker disease (GSS), fatal familial insomnia (FFI)
- Acquired: kuru, variant Creutzfeldt-Jakob disease (vCJD; "Human BSE")
- Iatrogenic: Dura mater grafts, human pituitary–derived hormone treatments (growth hormone, gonadotrophins), corneal transplantation, intracranial electrodes

Clinical features

History generally requires an informant interview regarding disease progression and cognitive features. While the various prion diseases often have distinctive clinical phenotypes, the following features are common to many:

- Dementia
- Cerebellar syndrome (kuru, GSS, Brownell-Oppenheimer or ataxic variant of CJD)
- Myoclonus
- Encephalopathy (Nevin-Jones syndrome of CJD)
- Extrapyramidal syndrome
- Pyramidal signs
- Psychiatric disturbance: not restricted to vCJD
- Cortical blindness: Heidenhain variant of CJD
- Sensory symptoms and signs, hyperpathia: especially vCJD
- Amyotrophy (muscle wasting)
- Chorea (may be seen in vCJD)
- Akinetic mutism

Investigation

There are no specific blood abnormalities known, other than mutations in the PrP gene in inherited cases (missense mutations, deletions, insertions). Neuroimaging may show nonspecific brain atrophy. MRI may show high signal in the caudate nucleus in sCJD, and high signal in the posterior thalamus (pulvinar sign) in vCJD. CSF protein may be moderately elevated; protein markers of neuronal injury (Neuron-Specific Enolase, 14-3-3) and glial activation (S100β) may be elevated. 14-3-3 has reasonable sensitivity and specificity for CJD diagnosis. EEG may show periodic sharp wave complexes at a frequency of 2/s in a markedly abnormal background in sCJD, although they may not develop until late in the disease and hence repeated EEGs may be needed; atypical changes (focal changes, periodic lateralized epileptiform discharges) sometimes reminiscent of complex partial status epilepticus may also be seen. The EEG is typically normal in vCJD. Brain biopsy may be required, typical features including spongiform vacuolation affecting any part of the cerebral grey matter (although cases without spongiform change have been described), astrocytic proliferation, gliosis, neuronal loss, synaptic degeneration, and PrP-immunopositive amyloid plaques. Tonsil biopsy may be helpful in diagnosis of vCJD if PrP-immunopositive staining is present.

Differential diagnosis

Various disorders have been confused with prion disease including *dementia with Lewy bodies*, *Alzheimer's disease*, paraneoplastic *limbic encephalitis*, complex partial status epilepticus, cerebrovascular disease with multi-infarct dementia, lithium intoxication, and *Hashimoto's encephalopathy*.

Treatment and prognosis

There is currently no specific treatment for prion diseases which are uniformly fatal, often within weeks to months; vCJD may last more than a year; some inherited forms may continue for many years.

References

Collinge J. Molecular neurology of prion disease. J Neurol Neurosurg Psychiatry. 2005;76:906–919
Ironside JW, Ritchie DL, Head MW. Phenotypic variability in human prion diseases. Neuropathol Appl Neurobiol. 2005; 31:565–579
Telling GC ed. Prions and Prions Diseases. Current Perspectives. London: Horizon Bioscience; 2004

Progeria [OMIM#176670]

Hutchinson-Gilford syndrome

Progeria is a rare condition characterized by premature ageing. Common features, developing within the first few years of life, include short stature, alopecia, reduced subcutaneous fat (lipodystrophy), scleroderma, and joint restriction. Thinning of the bones, facial hypoplasia, and micrognathia may also be features. Premature atherosclerosis develops leading to coronary artery disease and stroke, the former being the chief cause of death, usually during the second decade. Cognition is conspicuously preserved. Classical progeria follows an autosomal dominant inheritance pattern; in nonclassical progeria, growth is less retarded and survival into adulthood is not uncommon. The cause of progeria is either mutation of the lamin A gene (hence allelic with some forms of *Emery-Dreifuss muscular dystrophy, limb-girdle muscular dystrophy* type 1B) or abnormal posttranslational processing.

Reference

Hennekam RCM. Hutchinson-Gilford Progeria syndrome: review of the phenotype. Am J Med Genet Part A. 2006;140A:2603–2624

Progressive ataxia and palatal tremor (PAPT)

The rare syndrome of progressive ataxia and palatal tremor (PAPT), a form of symptomatic palatal tremor, may be either familial or sporadic. In the latter, there is hypertrophy of inferior olivary nuclei, whereas the former shows atrophy of cervical cord and brain stem. The cause is unknown: Some sporadic cases might represent forms of *multiple system atrophy*; some familial cases might be a form of *Alexander's disease* since they are associated with a substitution in the glial fibrillary acidic protein (GFAP) gene.

Reference

Samuel M, Torun N, Tuite PJ, Sharpe JA, Lang AE. Progressive ataxia and palatal tremor (PAPT): clinical and MRI assessment with review of palatal tremors. Brain. 2004;127:1252–1268

Progressive encephalomyelitis with rigidity and myoclonus (PERM)

Progressive encephalomyelitis with rigidity and myoclonus (PERM) may be classified as a subacute polioencephalomyelitis within the spectrum of *stiff person syndrome*. It is characterized by axial muscle stiffness, rigidity, and painful muscle spasms, but in contrast to stiff man syndrome, there are often preceding or accompanying sensory symptoms or brain stem signs (ataxia, vertigo, ocular motility disorders, dysarthria). Autonomic features and myoclonus may be prominent in some cases. CSF may show a lymphocytic pleocytosis and elevated protein, sometimes with oligoclonal bands. EMG may show continuous motor unit activity. Pathology shows perivascular lymphocyte cuffing, neuronal loss in brain stem and cervical cord, especially spinal interneurones in some cases. Pathogenesis is variable, with cases reported in association with viral infection (EBV, HIV, hepatitis C), paraneoplasia, and autoantibodies to glutamate acid decarboxylase and a glycine receptor. The course is progressive but highly variable, some rapidly deteriorating to death, others being protracted. Plasmapheresis and immunosuppression have proven helpful in some cases.

Reference

Burn DJ, Ball J, Lees AJ, Behan PO, Morgan-Hughes JA. A case of progressive encephalomyelitis with rigidity and positive antiglutamic acid decarboxylase antibodies. J Neurol Neurosurg Psychiatry. 1991;54:449–451

Progressive multifocal leukoencephalopathy (PML)

Progressive multifocal leukoencephalopathy (PML) is a demyelinating disorder due to reactivated infection of oligodendroglia with the JC papovavirus, a double-stranded DNA virus, most often seen in the setting of immunocompromise, particularly AIDS (*HIV/AIDS*), but also Hodgkin's disease, lymphoma, leukemia, carcinoma, neurosarcoidosis, tuberculosis, organ transplantation, and other situations requiring therapeutic immunosuppression, including cases associated with the use of natalizumab in multiple sclerosis. Primary infection with JC virus is asymptomatic.

Clinical features

Focal or multifocal signs are related to lesion location:

- Hemiparesis; quadriparesis
- Aphasia
- Visual field defects, especially hemianopia; cortical blindness
- Ataxia
- Cranial nerve palsies
- Cognitive disturbance, dementia in later stages
- Sensory abnormalities
- Clear consciousness; headache and seizures are rare

PML occurred in about 4% of AIDS patients and in half of these was the AIDS defining illness.

Investigation

Bloods for HIV status if not already known; CD4 count is usually $<200/mm^3$. Neuroimaging (CT) shows diffuse or multiple hypodensities; on MRI,

T_2-weighted hyperintensities extend right into the gyral cores, without mass effect or enhancement. CSF for standard indices is often normal, although there may be a mild mononuclear pleocytosis and raised protein, but PCR for JC virus is positive (PCR supersedes attempts at virus culture). EEG may show nonspecific diffuse or focal slowing. Brain biopsy of affected areas shows multifocal demyelination in subcortical white matter, with foamy macrophages, loss of oligodendroglia with sparing of axons, and enlarged nuclei in remaining oligodendroglia. Immunohistochemistry, in situ hybridization, and electron microscopy may be used to show oligodendroglial inclusions composed of papovavirus particles. However, the typical clinical picture and positive CSF PCR for JC virus usually negate the requirement for brain biopsy.

Differential diagnosis

Other causes of CNS mass lesion, in the context of HIV, consider particularly lymphoma, toxoplasmosis, tuberculous or fungal abscess, focal encephalitis, metastatic Kaposi's sarcoma, and acute stroke.

Treatment and prognosis

There is no effective treatment currently known. Dismal prognosis, with large majority of patients (>80%) dead within 1 year. Survival is improved in patients receiving highly active antiretroviral therapy (HAART), a combination of nucleoside and non-nucleoside reverse transcriptase inhibitors and protease inhibitors, which reduces "virus load" (HIV RNA). Cidofovir has also been suggested to be beneficial. Occasional spontaneous remissions have also been reported.

References

Berger JR, Pall L, Lanska D, Whiteman M. Progressive multifocal leukoencephalopathy in patients with HIV infection. J Neurovirol. 1998;4:59–68
Berger JR, Cohen BA. Opportunistic infections of the nervous system in AIDS. In: Gendelman HM, Grant I, Everall IP, Lipton SA, Swindells S, eds. The Neurology of AIDS. 2nd ed. Oxford: Oxford University Press; 2005:485–529 [at 491–495]
Tan CS, Koralnik IJ. Progressive multifocal leukoencephalopathy and other disorders caused by JC virus: clinical features and pathogenesis. Lancet Neurol. 2010;9:425–437

Progressive myoclonus epilepsies (PME)

The progressive myoclonus epilepsies (PME) are a heterogeneous group of disorders of genetic origin causing a progressive clinical syndrome with myoclonus, epilepsy, and neurological deterioration with dementia and ataxia. PME is distinguished from other causes of myoclonus associated with epilepsy (e.g., idiopathic generalized epilepsies with prominent myoclonus) in consequence of the myoclonus being the predominant and initial symptom, hence also differentiating PME from progressive encephalopathies and ataxias. The myoclonus in PME is generalized, multifocal, asymmetric, erratic, and continuous for long periods of time, such that it may render the patient bed-bound and severely disabled.

Recognized causes of PME include:

- Common:
  - Unverricht-Lundborg disease (Baltic myoclonus)
  - Lafora body disease
  - Mitochondrial disorders, e.g., MERRF
  - Sialidoses
  - Neuronal ceroid lipofuscinoses: Kufs' disease
- Rare:
  - Gangliosidoses (GM1, GM2)
  - Gaucher's disease: type III
  - Neurodegeneration with brain iron accumulation
  - Dentatorubral-pallidoluysian atrophy (DRPLA)
  - Huntington's disease (childhood form)
  - Neuroaxonal dystrophy
  - Alpers disease
  - Biotin-responsive encephalopathy
  - *Action myoclonus-renal failure syndrome* (Andermann's syndrome)
  - FENIB

References

Conry JA. Progressive myoclonus epilepsies. J Child Neurol. 2002;17(Suppl 1):S80–S84

Michelucci R, Serratosa JM, Genton P, Tassinari CA. Seizures, myoclonus and cerebellar dysfunction in progressive myoclonus epilepsies. In: Guerrini R, Aicardi J, Andermann F, Hallett M, eds. Epilepsy and Movement Disorders. Cambridge: Cambridge University Press; 2002:227–249

Progressive non-fluent aphasia (PNFA)

Primary progressive aphasia (PPA)

This linguistic variant of *frontotemporal lobar degeneration* is characterized by the dissolution of language function to the point of mutism due to focal cerebral cortical degeneration involving the left perisylvian region, in the total or relative absence for two or more years of other neuropsychological deficits, e.g., of memory or visuospatial abilities. The term may also encompass a syndrome of progressive loss of speech output with dysarthria and orofacial dyspraxia. Suggested diagnostic criteria also require no disturbance of consciousness, or the presence of systemic disorders or brain disease which could account for the clinical findings. Functional imaging and pathological studies confirm the focal nature of the process. The neuropathological substrate is variable.

Clinical features

- Impaired language output: non-fluent aphasia; calculation, perception, and spatial abilities are preserved; verbal memory may be poor but non-verbal memory is preserved.
- +/− Frontal lobe signs
- +/− Orofacial dyspraxia

Investigation

Sequential neuropsychological assessment confirms the selective impairment of language function. Structural neuroimaging (CT/MRI) may show left perisylvian atrophy (low specificity and sensitivity), and functional neuroimaging (SPECT/PET) shows early defects in left temporal and perisylvian areas, extending later to left parietal and frontal lobes. EEG and CSF are usually normal.

The neuropathological substrate of PNFA is variable: nonspecific neuronal loss with gliosis and some spongiform changes ("dementia lacking distinctive histology"), AD, Pick's. Neurogenetic testing has shown that some familial cases have mutations in the tau gene (rare).

Differential diagnosis

Other dementias presenting in a focal way, e.g., *Alzheimer's disease, Creutzfeldt-Jakob disease*, but other neuropsychological deficits and/or neurological signs evolve.

Treatment and prognosis

No specific treatment. Input from a speech and language therapist may be helpful to explore other avenues for communication. Patients usually remain independent despite their deficits, and are often able to continue at work despite mutism. Gradual progression to mutism, sometimes dementia and death (median duration of illness is about 8 years).

References

Grossman M. Primary progressive aphasia: clinicopathological correlations. Nat Rev Neurol. 2010;6:88–97
Mesulam MM. Primary progressive aphasia. Ann Neurol. 2001;49:425–432

Progressive subcortical gliosis of Neumann (PSG)

Progressive subcortical glial dystrophy

Progressive subcortical gliosis of Neumann (PSG) is a rare dementing illness, sometimes familial, which may be classified with the *frontotemporal lobar degeneration* syndromes. The diagnosis is based on neuropathological findings of frontotemporal atrophy with extensive subcortical gliosis. The clinical phenotype is variable, sometimes suggesting frontotemporal dementia (Neumann originally thought it a form of Pick's disease, but later distinguished it as a separate entity) or *Alzheimer's disease*. Mutation in the gene encoding the microtubule-associated protein tau on chromosome 17 has been demonstrated in familial PSG suggesting it sometimes falls within the *frontotemporal lobar degeneration with parkinsonism linked to chromosome 17 (FTDP-17)* group.

Clinical features

- Personality change (e.g., disinhibition), psychosis, dementia, parkinsonism, aphasia.
- Late pyramidal signs.
- Supranuclear gaze palsy has been reported.

Investigation

Neuroimaging (MRI) may show frontotemporal atrophy with or without extensive subcortical white matter change, sometimes extending to basal ganglia: The changes are nonspecific. Neuropathology shows subcortical white matter gliosis/astrocytosis, including the basal ganglia and thalamus, midbrain, medulla, and sometimes the ventral horns of spinal cord. There is neuronal loss; diffuse symmetrical atrophy of cortex; neuronal tau positive inclusions but Pick bodies are absent. There are no Lewy bodies or Alzheimer type senile plaques.

Differential diagnosis

Frontotemporal dementia, Alzheimer's disease, *progressive supranuclear palsy*.

Treatment and prognosis

No specific treatment. Disease may follow a prolonged course.

References

Goedert M, Spillantini MG, Crowther RA, et al. Tau gene mutation in familial progressive subcortical gliosis. Nat Med. 1999;5:454–457
Neumann MA, Cohn R. Progressive subcortical gliosis, a rare form of presenile dementia. Brain. 1967;90:405–418

Progressive supranuclear palsy (PSP)

Steele-Richardson-Olszewski (SRO) syndrome

Progressive supranuclear palsy (PSP) is an akinetic rigid syndrome of unknown aetiology. Clinically, many cases show a characteristic phenotype with early postural instability and falls, a characteristic eye movement abnormality (supranuclear gaze palsy) and cognitive decline, for which the term "Richardson's syndrome" has been proposed, whereas others have a phenotype much more reminiscent of idiopathic *Parkinson's disease* for which the term PSP-parkinsonism has been suggested.

Clinical features

*   Extrapyramidal syndrome: bradykinesia, axial rigidity, no tremor; very occasionally PSP may present with pure akinesia
*   Postural instability leading to early falls; *en bloc* sitting, "rocket man sign," extensor rigidity (retrocollis) associated with falls backward
*   Supranuclear gaze palsy: vertical gaze failure corrected with vestibulo-ocular responses
*   Broken pursuit eye movements; saccades reduced in velocity and amplitude
*   Paucity of blinking; levator inhibition/eyelid apraxia
*   Bulbar symptoms: dysphagia, dysarthria; often prominent
*   Poor, unsustained response to anti-parkinsonian medications
*   Neuropsychological deficits, especially frontal executive functions: slow information processing, deficits in focused and divided attention, impaired initiation, memory impairment (active recall > recognition)

Investigation

No diagnostic test is available, so diagnosis remains clinical. Neuro-ophthalmology assessment of eye movements and saccade error rate may be performed. Neuropsychology shows a cognitive profile consistent with a subcortical dementia. CSF/brain tissue tau protein profile: Gel electrophoresis of tau reveals major bands of 64 and 68 kDa, and a minor band of 72 kDa (all derived from 4 C-terminal repeat tau isoforms; hence tauopathy; cf. Alzheimer's disease). Neuropathology shows neuronal loss with neurofibrillary tangles, inclusions and gliosis in basal ganglia, brain stem, cerebellar nuclei, usually sparing cortex. Some cases may be associated with mutations in the tau gene on chromosome 17, hence falling within the *frontotemporal lobar degeneration with parkinsonism linked to chromosome 17* (*FTDP-17*) group.

Differential diagnosis

* Atypical Parkinson's disease
* *Corticobasal degeneration* (overlap)
* *Multiple system atrophy*
* *Dementia with Lewy bodies*
* Vascular syndromes
* Supranuclear gaze palsy also reported in *Creutzfeldt-Jakob disease, progressive subcortical gliosis*

Treatment and prognosis

Some patients may show L-dopa responsiveness. Deep brain stimulation yet to be systematically assessed, but unlikely to be helpful in light of lack of response to levodopa.

Diagnostic criteria

Litvan I, Agid Y, Calne D, et al. Clinical research criteria for the diagnosis of progressive supranuclear palsy (Steele-Richardson-Olszewski syndrome): report of the NINDS-SPSP international workshop. Neurology. 1996;47:1–9

References

Steele JC, Richardson JC, Olszewski J. Progressive supranuclear palsy: a heterogeneous degeneration involving the brainstem, basal ganglia and cerebellum with vertical gaze and pseudobulbar palsy, nuchal dystonia and dementia. Arch Neurol. 1964;10:333–358
Williams DR, de Silva R, Paviour DC, et al. Characteristics of two distinct clinical phenotypes in pathologically proven progressive supranuclear palsy: Richardson's syndrome and PSP-parkinsonism. Brain. 2005;128:1247–1258
Williams DR, Lees AJ. Progressive supranuclear palsy: clinicopathological concepts and diagnostic challenges. Lancet Neurol. 2009; 8:270–279

Pronator teres syndrome

High median neuropathy

Pronator teres syndrome is an *entrapment neuropathy* of the median nerve, hence a *median neuropathy*, between the heads of the pronator teres muscle in the forearm.

Clinical features

- Pain along the flexor side of the proximal forearm
- Paresthesia in the median nerve distribution in the hand
- Weakness in one or more hand muscles innervated by the median nerve (abductor pollicis brevis, flexor pollicis longus, opponens pollicis, flexor digitorum profundus); pronator teres itself is not affected since branches supplying this muscle emerge proximal to where the median nerve passes under the muscle

Pressure over pronator teres may produce pain or paresthesia (Tinel sign in antecubital fossa).

It may be difficult on clinical grounds to distinguish pronator teres syndrome from anterior interosseous nerve syndrome, and indeed partial median nerve palsies located proximally (e.g., supracondylar region) may produce a picture typical of anterior interosseous neuropathy (= pseudo anterior interosseous neuropathy). EMG may confirm median nerve involvement in the forearm and hand.

Pseudomigraine

Pseudomigraine with lymphocytic pleocytosis

Migraine type headache associated with acute confusion, psychosis, focal neurological deficits (e.g., hemisensory symptoms, hemiplegia, aphasia) lasting minutes to hours, with sterile CSF lymphocytic pleocytosis, has been labeled pseudomigraine. This may occur in familial hemiplegic migraine, reversible forms of *acute disseminated encephalomyelitis (ADEM)*, and may be mistaken for epileptic seizure or stroke.

Reference

Gomez-Aranda F, Canadillas F, Marti-Masso JF, et al. Pseudomigraine with temporary neurological symptoms and lymphocytic pleocytosis. A report of 50 cases. Brain. 1997;120:1105–1113

Pseudoxanthoma elasticum (PXE)

Pseudoxanthoma elasticum is a hereditary disorder of elastic connective tissue, with both autosomal dominant and recessive types described. The principal manifestations are dermatological, but elastic tissue in coronary and cerebral arteries may also be affected, leading to cardiovascular and cerebrovascular complications. Mutations in the ABCC6 gene, an ATP-binding cassette subfamily C member 6 transporter, encoded at chromosome 16p13.1, also known as multidrug resistance–associated protein 6, underlie both autosomal dominant and recessive forms of PXE.

Clinical features

- Dermatological: flexural plaques, "chicken-skin," cutis laxa
- Ophthalmic: angioid streaks (degeneration of Bruch's membrane) leading to visual impairment, blindness
- Coronary artery disease
- Intermittent claudication
- Gastrointestinal bleeding
- Strokes: ischemia due to large or small artery disease, accelerated by hypertension (common). Co-occurrence of intracranial aneurysm, subarachnoid hemorrhage, and cervical artery dissection reported but may be fortuitous rather than causal

Investigation

Diagnosis usually obvious from skin findings; skin biopsy. Neuroimaging for cerebrovascular disease.

Treatment and prognosis

Control hypertension. Avoid platelet inhibitors, contact sports due to increased risk of bleeding.

References

Ringpfeil F, Lebwohl MG, Christiano AM, Uitto J. Pseudoxanthoma elasticum: mutations in the MRP6 gene encoding a transmembrane ATP-binding cassette (ABC) transporter. Proc Natl Acad Sci USA. 2000;97:6001–6006
van den Berg JS, Hennekam RC, Cruysberg JR, et al. Prevalence of symptomatic intracranial aneurysm and ischaemic stroke in pseudoxanthoma elasticum. Cerebrovasc Dis. 2000;10:315–319

Psittacosis

Ornithosis

Chlamydia psittaci, the causative organism of psittacosis, is transmitted from birds to humans by inhalation. Systemic symptoms include fever, myalgia, and respiratory features, especially a nonproductive cough. Neurological features are infrequent, usually an encephalitic or meningo-encephalitic illness; raised intracranial pressure has also been described. Blood serology is positive for *C. psittaci*. Differential diagnosis includes other causes of pneumonia with associated neurological features (myco-plasma, Q fever, Legionnaire's disease) and other causes of meningoen-cephalitis. Treatment is with tetracycline 0.5 mg qds, and recovery is usually complete.

Reference

Hughes P, Chidley K, Cowie J. Neurological complications in psittacosis: a case report and literature review. Respir Med. 1995; 89:637–638

Psychiatric disorders and neurological disease: overview

Disorders labeled either psychiatric or neurological in origin are likewise disorders of the nervous system, and it is therefore not surprising that there should be overlap between them, i.e., psychiatric features in neurological disease ("behavioral neurology") and a neurological origin for psychiatric symptoms (sometimes with neurological signs), often implicating the limbic system ("neuropsychiatry" or "biological psychiatry"). Close liaison between neurologists and psychiatrists may be required for the optimal management of "psychiatric" features in "neurological" disease, and to determine "neuro-logical" causes for "psychiatric" symptoms.

Many patients presenting to the neurology clinic may have primarily psy-chiatric disease, particularly those with headache, pain syndromes, complaints of poor memory, and sleep disorders. Recognition of this fact is an important first step in appropriate management.

Clinical features

- Frontal lobe pathology: impaired attention, distractibility, perseveration; personality changes: either apathy, indifference, self-neglect (abulia); or euphoria, disinhibition (may be labeled "mania" or "manic-depressive psychosis").

- Temporal lobe pathology: interictal psychosis, schizophreniform features may develop with dominant medial temporal focus. Geschwind's syndrome (hypergraphia, hyposexuality, hyperreligiosity).
- Various neurological disorders may have prominent behavioral and psychiatric features, e.g., *epilepsy, multiple sclerosis, systemic lupus erythematosus*, cerebrovascular disease, *Alzheimer's disease, dementia with Lewy bodies*, Parkinson's disease dementia, *Huntington's disease*, and *neuroacanthocytosis*.

Investigation

Neuroimaging (CT/MRI) may show focal brain lesions to account for psychiatric symptoms, e.g., frontal meningioma. EEG may show seizure activity of temporal lobe origin to account for psychiatric symptoms.

Differential diagnosis

- Abulia: psychomotor retardation of depression, catatonia, hypoactive delirium
- Disinhibition: mania, bipolar disorder, hyperactive delirium
- Psychiatric features may be seen in:
  - Neurodegenerative disease: Frontotemporal lobar degeneration (behavioral variant frotnotemporal dementia, Pick's disease), Alzheimer's disease
  - Cerebrovascular disease
  - Inflammatory disease: multiple sclerosis, systemic lupus erythematosus
  - Metabolic disease: adrenoleukodystrophy, porphyria, thyroid disease, Wilson's disease
  - Neoplasia: frontal lobe tumors

Treatment and prognosis

Of individual condition where possible. Treatments aimed at psychiatric features per se may be required, e.g., antidepressants, neuroleptics, mood stabilizers.

References

Cummings JL, Mega MS. Neuropsychiatry and Behavioral Neuroscience. Oxford: Oxford University Press; 2003

David A, Fleminger S, Kopelman M, Lovestone S, Mellers J. Lishman's Organic Psychiatry. A Textbook of Neuropsychiatry. 4th ed. Oxford: Wiley-Blackwell; 2009
Moore DP. Textbook of Clinical Neuropsychiatry. 2nd ed. London: Hodder Arnold; 2008
Trimble MR. Biological Psychiatry. 2nd ed. Chichester, UK: Wiley; 1996

Pure autonomic failure (PAF)

Bradbury-Eggleston syndrome, Idiopathic autonomic failure, Idiopathic orthostatic hypotension

Pure autonomic failure (PAF) is a rare condition characterized by an idiopathic degeneration of the postganglionic sympathetic fibers of the autonomic nervous system, with relative preservation of the parasympathetic nervous system. It is not associated with degeneration in any other neurological system (cf. *multiple system atrophy* (MSA), autonomic failure associated with *Parkinson's disease*), although some cases of MSA and *dementia with Lewy bodies* (DLB) present with isolated autonomic failure before other features develop.

Clinical features

Diagnosis is essentially clinical.
* Postural hypotension: gradual fading of consciousness when patient is standing, walking; neck ache, backache in "coathanger" distribution; symptoms worse in morning, hot weather, after meals and exercise. Recumbent/supine hypertension, reversal of diurnal blood pressure pattern (may have adverse neurological consequences)
* Visual disturbances: transient scotomata, hallucinations, tunnel vision (occipital lobe ischemia)
* Defective sweating
* Sexual dysfunction: erectile failure, followed by disturbance of ejaculation.
* Gastrointestinal: swallowing difficulty, laryngeal paresis

Investigation

Bloods: plasma noradrenaline level low in resting state, no elevation with tilting or standing. Neuropathology (postmortem) shows Lewy bodies in the sympathetic ganglia, with or without neuronal loss.

Differential diagnosis

Autonomic failure due to other neurodegenerative diseases such as MSA and DLB: other neurological and/or neuropsychological features emerge. *Dopamine β-hydroxylase deficiency* has earlier onset than PAF, and virtually absent plasma noradrenaline. Autonomic dysfunction/postural hypotension due to other conditions: diabetes mellitus, pheochromocytoma, amyloidosis, hereditary sensory and autonomic neuropathies, Guillain–Barré syndrome.

Treatment and prognosis

Management of postural hypotension: non-pharmacological interventions include increased salt intake, head-up bed tilt, and wearing a G-suit. Pharmacological treatments include fludrocortisone, ephedrine, and mido-drine. Specific management of certain symptoms, such as erectile dysfunction. The outlook is relatively good in PAF: With management of postural hypotension, life expectancy is only a little reduced.

Diagnostic criteria

Consensus statement on the definition of orthostatic hypotension, pure autonomic failure and multiple system atrophy. Clin Auton Res. 1996;6:125–126

References

Lahrmann H, Cortelli P, Hilz M, Mathias CJ, Struhal W, Tassinari M. EFNS guidelines on the diagnosis and management of orthostatic hypotension. Eur J Neurol. 2006;13:930–936
Low PA, Singer W. Management of neurogenic orthostatic hypotension: an update. Lancet Neurol. 2008;7:451–458

Q

Q fever

Q fever is a zoonotic infection caused by the obligate intracellular organism *Coxiella burnetti*, belonging to the family of *Rickettsial diseases*. A self-limiting coryzal illness is the commonest manifestation, but pneumonia and endocarditis may occur. Neurological complications are rare: meningoencephalitis is the commonest neurological feature; acute transverse myelitis has also been described. Culture-negative *endocarditis* is also a feature of *Coxiella* infection, which may result in embolic neurological sequelae. Steroid-responsive demyelinating lesions have also been reported. Diagnosis of Q fever is based on serological evidence of infection. Differential diagnosis encompasses other causes of pneumonia with associated neurological features and other causes of meningoencephalitis. Treatment is with doxycycline.

References

Maurin M, Raoult D. Q fever. Clin Microbiol Rev. 1999;12:518–553
Skiba V, Barner KC. Central nervous system manifestations of Q fever responsive to steroids. Military Med. 2009;174:857–859

Quail myopathy

Quail eater's myopathy, Quail poisoning myoglobinuria

This myopathic syndrome is characterized by muscle cramps, myalgia, *rhab-domyolysis*, and proximal weakness, often with nausea and vomiting, following consumption of quail meat. It is most common in the Mediterranean basin, for example, in Greece in the spring following the migration of quails from North Africa. The pathogenesis is unknown, but it has been suggested to reflect poisoning with hemlock or laudanum since the birds eat seeds of these plants. It is said to be the earliest myopathy to have been described, in the Bible (Numbers 11: 31–34).

Reference

Papapetropoulos T, Hadziyannis S, Ouzounellis T. On the pathogenetic mechanism of quail myopathy. JAMA. 1980;244:2263–2264

R

Rabies

The rabies virus, or related members of the genus *Lyssavirus*, family Rhabdoviridae, is transmitted to man from the saliva of affected mammals, usually dogs, through skin bites or abrasions. The virus reaches the CNS via the peripheral nerves by means of retrograde axoplasmic flow. There is a predilection for the brain stem and grey matter. The condition is almost uniformly fatal once neurological features occur. Postexposure prophylaxis is available. Person-to-person transmission is not reported other than following organ transplantation. The condition is extremely rare in the UK, where it is a notifiable disease, with fewer than 20 cases in the past 30 years, most imported from overseas.

Clinical features

- Incubation period very variable: days to months or even years
- Fever, malaise, headache, sore throat; severe pain/paresthesia at site of bite
- Anxiety, depression, agitation, insomnia
- Neurological features:
  - "Furious": hyperacusis, hydrophobia, aerophobia, pharyngeal/laryngeal spasms leading to salivary drooling, respiratory arrest, opisthotonos; episodes of hallucination, profound agitation requiring restraint, sympathetic overactivity, but fully conscious and terrified in period between attacks; seizures; coma, flaccid paralysis, death
  - "Paralytic" or "dumb": flaccid paralysis only, leading to death

History of an animal bite is not always forthcoming.

Investigation

Bloods: serology for rabies virus has been superseded by PCR of saliva and skin. CSF shows nonspecific pleocytosis. Neuroimaging (MR) may show high signal intensity lesions in the hippocampi and caudate head on T2-weighted images. Skin biopsy from the nape of the neck including hair follicles with peripheral nerve endings may show rabies virus antigen on a fluorescent antibody test. Neuropathology, rarely available antemortem, shows a primary encephalomyelitis with mononuclear cell infiltrate; characteristic Negri bodies (eosinophilic cytoplasmic inclusion body) are seen in the majority of cases.

Differential diagnosis

The "furious" syndrome is characteristic. Flaccid paralysis may be mistaken for *Guillain–Barré syndrome*, especially the acute motor axonal (AMAN) form: concurrent headache, fever, asymmetric limb weakness, bladder involvement, and cellular CSF may be clues against this diagnosis. *Encephalitis* and tetanus also enter the differential.

Treatment and prognosis

Cleansing of wound. A combination of early passive (rabies-immune serum) and active (rabies vaccine) immunization may be protective after exposure. Pre-exposure vaccination is recommended in some circumstances. Very rare reports of survival with full recovery, in context of pre- or postexposure prophylaxis, mandate full intensive care support of patients with neurological disease. The "Wisconsin protocol" (ketamine, midazolam, ribavirin, amantadine) has been reported successful in one case after a bat bite.

References

Hemachudha T, Laothamatas J, Rupprecht CE. Human rabies: a disease of complex neuropathogenetic mechanisms and diagnostic challenges. Lancet Neurol. 2002;1:101–109
Shah P, Stewart G, Fooks AR, et al. A difficult case … at least in Scotland. Pract Neurol. 2004;4:110–113
Solomon T, Marston D, Mallewa M, et al. Paralytic rabies after a two week holiday in India. BMJ. 2005;331:501–503

Radial neuropathy

The radial nerve may be compressed or damaged in the axilla, in the spiral groove of the humerus ("Saturday night palsy"), or more distally (*posterior interosseous syndrome*, superficial sensory branches). Some authors suggest the radial nerve is the most commonly injured peripheral nerve.

Clinical features

- Motor: weakness of triceps (axillary injury only), brachioradialis, supinator, wrist and finger extensors (hence wrist drop, finger drop); triceps reflex may be depressed or lost with axillary lesions.
- Sensory: loss on dorsal aspect of hand, thumb, index and middle fingers. No sensory loss with posterior interosseous lesions. Purely sensory findings occur with injury to superficial sensory branches, for example, with handcuffs (*cheiralgia paresthetica*).

Investigation

Neurophysiology (EMG/NCS) may identify reduced amplitude CMAP in radial innervated muscles and reduced or absent SNAPs. Fibrillations in triceps suggest injury at axillary level. Abnormalities beyond radial nerve territory may refute a diagnosis of mononeuropathy.

Differential diagnosis

Radiculopathy, brachial plexopathy: clinical features unlikely to be mistaken.

Reference

Staal A, Van Gijn J, Spaans F. Mononeuropathies: Examination, Diagnosis and Treatment. London: W.B. Saunders; 1999:35–48

Radiculopathies: overview

Radiculopathies are disorders of nerve roots which may cause sensory and motor features in the corresponding dermatome and myotome respectively. Radiculopathies may be single or multiple (polyradiculopathy, e.g., *cauda equina syndrome*), and may occur in conjunction with spinal cord disease (radiculomyelopathy). Causes of radiculopathy include compression, trauma (root avulsion), diabetes, neoplasia, infection/inflammation (radiculitis), and demyelination.

Clinical features

- Sensory: pain, paresthesia, sensory diminution or loss, in a radicular distribution
- Motor: lower motor neurone type weakness; hyporeflexia or areflexia

(For details on specific roots, see *Cervical cord and root disease, Lumbar cord and root disease*).

Investigation

Neurophysiology: EMG/NCS may differentiate radiculopathy from neuropathy or plexopathy: sensory nerve action potentials are normal for intrathecal root lesions, and EMG shows involvement of paraspinal muscles; neurophysiology may also be used to localize levels of radiculopathy. Neuroimaging: MRI may demonstrate compression from prolapsed intervertebral disk, metastases, spondylolisthesis; fracture; infection. Bloods: fasting glucose (to exclude diabetes); inflammatory markers; serology (if appropriate) for HIV (CMV late in the course), *neuroborreliosis*, *neurosyphilis* (tabes dorsalis), herpes zoster. CSF for protein, cell count, cytology (may need to be repeated if clinical suspicion of malignant infiltration high), oligoclonal bands.

Differential diagnosis

Plexopathies; mononeuropathies, polyneuropathies.

Treatment and prognosis

Of cause where identified, for example, surgery for compressive lesions. Symptomatic treatment with drugs for neuropathic pain may be appropriate (e.g., amitriptyline, carbamazepine, gabapentin, pregabalin).

Reference

Chad DF. Nerve root and plexus disorders. In: Bogousslavsky J, Fisher M, eds. Textbook of Neurology. Boston, MA: Butterworth-Heinemann; 1998:491–506

Radiotherapy-induced neurological disorders

Radiation therapy, most often given to inhibit or destroy neoplastic cells, is relatively nonspecific in its effects and may adversely affect normal neuronal function in brain, spinal cord, and peripheral nervous system, transiently or permanently. Neurotoxicity is more likely with high-dose therapy and in combination with chemotherapy. Some of the more common adverse effects are listed here.

Clinical features

- Cerebral injury: acute encephalopathy, early delayed encephalopathy, late encephalopathy (focal cerebral necrosis, diffuse cerebral injury: leukoencephalopathy)
- Cerebrovascular disease: occlusive disease

- Optic neuropathy, other cranial neuropathies (especially XII, X, XI)
- Myelopathy: transient, delayed progressive
- *Brachial plexopathy*: usually delayed progressive; lumbosacral plexopathy
- Intracranial tumors: meningioma, glioma, sarcoma; long latency

Investigation

Radiotherapy effects may occur after some delay (months to years) and must be differentiated from tumor recurrence or metastatic disease. Depending on the clinical presentation, imaging, EMG/NCS, and CSF analysis may be appropriate, but these seldom produce diagnostic information. One possible exception is the finding of myokymic discharges in the EMG in radiation-induced brachial plexopathy, not found in brachial plexopathy due to metastatic disease (lung, breast).

Differential diagnosis

Metastatic disease, opportunistic infection, metabolic derangement, drug toxicities.

Treatment and prognosis

Corticosteroids (e.g., dexamethasone) may reduce both the risk and the effects of radiation-induced acute encephalopathy.

References

Dropcho EJ. Neurologic complications of radiation therapy. In: Biller J, ed. Iatrogenic Neurology. Boston, MA: Butterworth-Heinemann; 1998:461–483
Keime-Guibert F, Napolitano M, Delattre JY. Neurological complications of radiotherapy and chemotherapy. J Neurol. 1998;245:695–708

Raeder's paratrigeminal syndrome

This is a rare facial pain syndrome characterized by two essential features: unilateral oculosympathetic paralysis (Horner's syndrome) and ipsilateral head, face, or retro-orbital pain related to trigeminal (V) nerve involvement. The syndrome may on occasion be due to a parasellar (middle cranial fossa) mass lesion such as tumor, aneurysm, trauma (head injury), or infection, but "idiopathic" cases are also reported, which may be due to carotid artery *dissection*, not always detected by imaging techniques. The value of this eponym has been questioned.

Clinical features

- Persistent pain in first and second divisions of the trigeminal nerve (V1 and V2): persistent, burning, throbbing, unilateral; may wake the patient at night, pain likened to that of tic douloureux
- Oculosympathetic dysfunction (Horner's syndrome): ptosis, miosis, but preserved sweating (no anhidrosis) because sudomotor fibers traveling extracranially with the external carotid artery are spared
- +/– Trigeminal sensory loss
- +/– Weakness of trigeminal innervated muscles
- +/– Other cranial nerve lesions (II, III, IV, VI)

Investigation

Neuroimaging (MRI preferable) to exclude parasellar (trigeminal ganglion) lesion, especially if signs extend beyond trigeminal involvement; MRI/MRA and/or angiography to exclude carotid artery dissection.

Differential diagnosis

As for a painful Horner's syndrome:

- Carotid artery dissection
- Cavernous sinus lesion (e.g., aneurysm)
- *Cluster headache* (lacks oculomotor or trigeminal nerve dysfunction)
- Orbital pseudotumor/"Tolosa–Hunt syndrome"
- Syringomyelia

Treatment and prognosis

Treatment of cause, if identified, plus symptomatic treatment of pain. The most important issue is to exclude other treatable causes for painful Horner's syndrome, especially carotid artery dissection.

References

Raeder JG. "Paratrigeminal" paralysis of oculo-pupillary sympathetic. Brain. 1924;47:149–158
Solomon S. Raeder syndrome. Arch Neurol. 2001;58:661–662

Ramsay Hunt syndromes

James Ramsay Hunt (1874–1937) described a variety of neurological syndromes, including:

- Dyssynergia cerebellaris myoclonica: a syndrome probably encompassing *progressive myoclonus epilepsies* such as *Unverricht–Lundborg disease, Lafora body disease*
- Herpes zoster oticus: herpetic inflammation of the Gasserian (geniculate) ganglion causing zoster of the outer ear or oropharynx with acute facial (VII) nerve palsy, with or without acoustic nerve involvement (tinnitus, vertigo, deafness)
- Juvenile paralysis agitans with progressive globus pallidus atrophy
- Palsy of the deep palmar branch of the ulnar nerve (pure motor ulnar neuropathy), a form of *entrapment neuropathy*

References

Pearce JMS. Some syndromes of James Ramsay Hunt. Pract. Neurol. 2007;7:182–185
Sweeney CJ, Gilden DH. Ramsay Hunt syndrome. J Neurol Neurosurg Psychiatry. 2001;71:149–154

Rasmussen's encephalitis (RE), Rasmussen's syndrome

Chronic encephalitis and epilepsy, Kojewnikoff's syndrome, Kozhevnikov syndrome

Rasmussen and colleagues originally described a syndrome of chronic partial *epilepsy* with progressive focal neurological deficits and cognitive decline, associated with neuropathological features of a focal chronic *encephalitis*. Onset of Rasmussen's encephalitis (RE) is usually in childhood, although adult onset cases are described, with a relentlessly progressive course for several years until the disease process may appear to "burn out." Partial forms with pathology confined to the temporal lobes and presenting as intractable temporal lobe epilepsy have also been reported, sometimes with focal movement disorders. The condition may be related to viral infection, particularly with cytomegalovirus which has been identified in brain tissue in some cases, but etiology in most cases remains obscure.

Clinical features

- Seizures: focal, secondary generalized, epilepsia partialis continua; often poorly controlled despite multiple antiepileptic drugs
- Focal signs: hemiparesis/hemiplegia, hemianopia, hemisensory loss
- Cognitive decline

Investigation

No specific blood tests; autoantibodies to the glutamate receptor 3 (GluR3) do not discriminate RE from other causes of epilepsy, and their assay is not recommended. Neuroimaging (CT/MRI) shows focal, usually hemispheric, brain atrophy. EEG shows epileptiform and nonepileptiform lateralized abnormalities, with multiple independent interictal epileptiform abnormalities. CSF shows no specific abnormalities, but pleocytosis, oligoclonal bands may be present in some. Neuropsychology may show cognitive deficits appropriate to affected hemisphere. Brain biopsy may be required for diagnosis: classical features are inflammation with microglial nodules, neuronophagia, perivascular lymphocyte cuffing, and glial scarring. However, findings may be nonspecific later in the disease when the inflammatory process may have "burned out."

Differential diagnosis

Space-occupying lesions, slow-growing neoplasms. Neuronal migration disorders, cortical dysplasia. There may be an association with *Parry–Romberg syndrome* in some cases.

Treatment and prognosis

Seizures are usually only partially responsive to standard antiepileptic medications; polytherapy is common. Epilepsy surgery may be considered: hemispherectomy will stop the seizures but is only recommended when the patient is already hemiplegic. Immunotherapy (high-dose steroids, intravenous immunoglobulins, plasma exchange, tacrolimus) is probably beneficial, especially early in the course. Antivirals (ganciclovir; zidovudine) have also been reported of benefit in individual cases.

References

Andermann F, ed. Chronic Encephalitis and Epilepsy: Rasmussen's Syndrome. Boston, MA: Butterworth-Heinemann; 1991
Bien CG, Granata T, Antozzi C, et al. Pathogenesis, diagnosis and treatment of Rasmussen encephalitis: a European consensus statement. Brain. 2005;128:454–471

Rapid-onset dystonia parkinsonism [OMIM#128235]

DYT12

Rapid-onset dystonia parkinsonism is an autosomal dominant disorder characterized by abrupt onset of *dystonia* with features of parkinsonisim, a rostrocaudal gradient and prominent bulbar findings, resulting from mutations in the ATP1A3 gene. There is often a lack of response to dopaminergic agents.

Reference

Brashear A, Dobyns WB, de Carvalho Aquiar P, et al. The phenotypic spectrum of rapid-onset dystonia-parkinsonism (RDP) and mutations in the ATP1A3 gene. Brain. 2007;130:828–835

Reflex epilepsies

Reflex, or evoked, epilepsies are those forms of *epilepsy* in which seizures are precipitated in response to discrete or specific stimuli. Examples include:

- In response to simple stimuli:
  - Photosensitive epilepsy (most common), for example, television, possibly computer/video games; idiopathic photosensitive occipital lobe epilepsy; Jeavons syndrome (eyelid myoclonia with absences)
  - Hot water/hot bath epilepsy
  - Startle epilepsy
  - Eating epilepsy
- In response to complex stimuli:
  - Reading epilepsy
  - Musicogenic epilepsy
  - Performing mathematical calculations

Reference

Panayiotopoulos CP. A Clinical Guide to Epileptic Syndromes and Their Treatment. Based on the ILAE Classifications and Practice Parameter Guidelines. 2nd ed. London: Springer; 2007:437–471

Refsum's disease

Hereditary motor and sensory neuropathy (HMSN) type IV,
Heredopathia atactica polyneuritiformis,
Phytanic acid storage disease

Refsum's disease is an autosomal recessive disorder of peroxisome function, with deficiency of phytanoyl-CoA 2-hydroxylase (PAHX), leading to the accumulation of phytanic acid, a branched chain fatty acid, in the nervous system and elsewhere. Mutant forms of PAHX have been shown to be responsible for some, but not all, cases of Refsum's disease. The majority of cases present in the first or second decade of life with the classic triad of ataxia, retinitis pigmentosa, and polyneuropathy.

Clinical features

- Night blindness (nyctalopia) due to retinal pigmentary degeneration (retinitis pigmentosa); early concentric field defect
- Hypertrophic polyneuropathy, affecting the legs first; pes cavus, wasting, weakness, areflexia, distal sensory disturbance (especially proprioception) leading to gait disturbance
- +/– Cerebellar ataxia (slurred speech, intention tremor)
- Sensorineural hearing loss
- Anosmia
- Cognition normal
- Systemic features: short fourth metatarsals leading to overriding toes, ichythyosis (especially of shins), cardiac conduction abnormalities, cataracts, growth retardation, hepatomegaly

Investigation

Raised phytanic acid in blood and urine. Nonspecific elevation in CSF protein. EMG/NCS shows reduced motor conduction velocities, reduced or absent sensory nerve action potentials. Electroretinogram may be absent. ECG may show cardiac conduction abnormalities. Neuroimaging (MRI) may show thickening of affected nerves.

Differential diagnosis

- Nerve thickening: Charcot–Marie–Tooth type of *hereditary motor and sensory neuropathy* (HMSN), Déjerine–Sottas (HMSN type III)
- Relapsing–remitting course: Inflammatory polyneuropathies
- Hereditary pigmentary retinal degenerations: Alstrom's syndrome, Cockayne syndrome, Usher's syndrome
- Raised phytanic acid levels: mitochondrial disease can cause potentially misleading increase, as can some other rare peroxisomal disorders

Treatment and prognosis

All phytanic acid is of dietary origin; hence, dietary restriction reduces blood levels. Plasma exchange has been tried. Exacerbations and remissions of the neuropathy are recognized. Survival may be for decades, but sudden unexpected death, perhaps related to cardiac conduction defects, is reported.

References

Refsum S. Heredopathia atactica polyneuritiformis: a familial syndrome not hitherto described. A contribution to the clinical study of the hereditary diseases of the nervous system. Acta Psychiatr Scand Suppl. 1946;38:1–303

Wierzbicki AS, Lloyd MD, Schofiled CJ, Feher MD, Gibberd FB. Refsum's disease: a peroxisomal disorder affecting phytanic acid alpha-oxidation. J Neurochem. 2002;80:727–735

Relapsing polychondritis

Relapsing polychondritis is a very rare condition characterized by recurrent inflammatory episodes affecting the cartilage of the ear, nose, trachea, and larynx. It may be complicated by systemic and cerebral vasculitis, which may manifest as neurological features in 5% of patients, as aseptic meningitis, encephalopathy, epileptic seizures, stroke or transient ischemic attacks, ischemic optic neuropathy, cranial nerve palsies (VIII, VII, VI, II), and limbic encephalitis. Symptoms usually respond well to steroids with or without other immunosuppression such as cyclophosphamide.

Diagnostic criteria

McAdam LP, O'Hanlan MA, Bluestone R, et al. Relapsing polychondritis: prospective study of 23 patients and a review of the literature. Medicine. 1976;55:193–215

Reference

Irani SR, Soni A, Beynon H, Athwal BS. Relapsing "encephalo" polychondritis. Pract Neurol. 2006;6:372–375

REM sleep behavior disorder (REMBD)

REM sleep behavior disorder (REMBD) is a syndrome of stereotypic behaviors occurring during REM sleep in which the usual muscular atonia, originally described by Jouvet, is lost. Bizarre behaviors may represent the acting out of dreams, of which the patient may have a relatively clear recollection when woken or on the following day (cf. pavor nocturnus or night terrors). Investigation with polysomnography may be required. In older individuals, there is a link with parkinsonian syndromes such as *Parkinson's disease*, *dementia with Lewy bodies*, and *multiple system atrophy*, and occasional reports of pathologically confirmed Alzheimer's disease with REMBD have been reported. Monitoring for the emergence of these conditions may be appropriate in older individuals. Structural lesions in the brain stem may also cause

REMBD, implicating the dorsal midbrain and pons. Generally, clonazepam is of clinical benefit in REMBD.

Reference

Boeve BF, Silber MH, Saper CB, et al. Pathophysiology of REM sleep behaviour disorder and relevance to neurodegenerative disease. Brain. 2007;130:2770–2788

Renal disease and the nervous system: overview

A number of multisystem conditions may affect both the renal and nervous systems. Uremia, dialysis, and renal transplantation may all be associated with neurological syndromes.

Clinical features

- Conditions affecting both the kidneys and the nervous system:
  - Vasculitides:
    - Primary: *polyarteritis nodosa, Churg–Strauss syndrome, Wegener's granulomatosis*
    - Secondary: infection (hepatitis B), toxins, neoplasia (lymphoid malignancy)
  - Connective tissue diseases: *rheumatoid arthritis, systemic lupus erythematosus, Sjögren's syndrome*
  - Plasma cell dyscrasias: myeloma, *POEMS syndrome*, MGUS, Waldenström's macroglobulinemia
  - Genetically determined disease: *Von Hippel–Lindau disease*, polycystic kidney disease, *Wilson's disease, Fabry's disease*, Alport's syndrome
  - Renal disease leading to vitamin D (1,25-dihydroxycholecalciferol) deficiency; may lead to apparent limb weakness from osteomalacia
- Conditions affecting both renal system and muscle:
  - *Rhabdomyolysis*
- Uremia and the nervous system:
  - CNS:
    - Encephalopathy with myoclonus and asterixis; probably multifactorial etiology
    - Aseptic meningitis
  - PNS:
    - Distal sensorimotor axonal neuropathy, affecting especially large myelinated axons, with secondary demyelination
    - Isolated mononeuropathies (e.g., *carpal tunnel syndrome*)
    - Vestibulocochlear (VIII) nerve: (exclude drug toxicity, hereditary conditions causing hearing loss and nephropathy)
    - Myopathy: proximal wasting and weakness (exclude primary hyperparathyroidism and osteomalacia)

- Dialysis:
  - Dialysis dysequilibrium syndrome: restlessness, nausea, headache, cramps, progressing to delirium, myoclonus, epileptic seizures, raised intracranial pressure, cardiac arrhythmias; now very rare, and a diagnosis of exclusion
  - Wernicke's syndrome: may be atypical, without ophthalmoplegia
  - *Subdural hematoma*
  - Dialysis dementia
- Complications of renal transplantation:
  - Intraoperative: compression of femoral nerve, lateral cutaneous nerve of thigh; conus medullaris syndrome (spinal cord ischemia from iliac artery manipulation)
  - Postoperative:
    - Side effects of immunosuppressive drugs:
    - Steroids: hypertension
    - Ciclosporin A: tremor, seizures, *posterior reversible leukoencephalopathy syndrome*
    - FK506: posterior reversible leukoencephalopathy syndrome
  - Opportunistic infection, for example:
    - Viral: CMV, EBV, JC virus causing *progressive multifocal leukoencephalopathy*
    - Fungal: aspergillus, Cryptococcus
    - Bacterial: Nocardia, Listeria
  - Lymphoproliferative disease: primary CNS *lymphoma*, possibly related to EBV infection of B lymphocytes
  - Rejection encephalopathy

Investigation

- Monitor renal function: Blood: urea, creatinine, creatinine clearance; markers of inflammation, autoantibodies, serology for infection (e.g., hepatitis B) Urine: examine urine for cells, casts.
- Neuroimaging: CT/MRI to look for evidence of inflammation, infarction; subdural hematoma; MRA or catheter angiography in patients with polycystic kidney disease and family history of subarachnoid (and/or intracerebral) hemorrhage.
- Neurophysiology: EEG shows slowing, especially frontally, with excess delta and theta in uremic encephalopathy. EMG/NCS shows slowing of proximal nerve conduction as the earliest finding in uremic neuropathy, followed by reduced conduction velocity and action potential amplitudes.
- CSF: raised protein, lymphocyte count in uremic aseptic meningitis; organisms in immunosuppression related opportunistic infection; Indian ink stain for fungi, PCR for viruses, culture.

Differential diagnosis

As the aforegoing lists show, differential diagnosis is broad and requires a high index of clinical suspicion. In uremic encephalopathy, encephalopathy secondary to the underlying cause of the renal failure (e.g., hypertension, diabetes mellitus, SLE, thrombotic thrombocytopenic purpura), must be distinguished from encephalopathy secondary to the treatment of renal failure (e.g., dialysis syndromes).

Treatment and prognosis

Many of the features associated with uremia improve with dialysis and may resolve entirely following successful renal transplantation.

Reference

Burn DJ, Bates D. Neurology and the kidney. J Neurol Neurosurg Psychiatry. 1998; 65:810–821

Respiratory failure: overview

Neurogenic respiratory failure

Respiratory failure may result from a variety of neurological disorders as well as primary respiratory disease. Recognized neurological causes include:

- Myopathy: acid maltase deficiency (AMD); nemaline, centronuclear myopathies; *limb girdle muscular dystrophies*, types 1B, 2C-F, 2I
- Neuromuscular disease: *myasthenia gravis*
- Neuropathy: *Guillain–Barré syndrome*
- Neuronopathy: *motor neurone disease*; *poliomyelitis*
- Myelopathy: high cervical cord lesions (involving C3–C5): structural, inflammatory (e.g., multiple sclerosis)
- Primary central hypoventilation: *Wolfram syndrome*

Clinical features

- Respiratory symptoms and signs may be minimal prior to the development of respiratory failure.
- Paradoxical diaphragm movement may be seen.

- Metabolic encephalopathy, +/– asterixis, papilledema.
- Respiratory arrest.

Investigation

See individual entries for the investigation of specific neurological disorders.

In patients with conditions which might lead to respiratory failure, monitoring of respiratory parameters and intervention before the development of respiratory failure is required, by means of:

- Forced vital capacity: may be difficult if weak facial muscles preclude good lip seal around vitalograph/spirometer
- Arterial blood gases
- Chest radiograph; X-ray screening of diaphragm movement

Differential diagnosis

- Other causes of encephalopathy.
- In those already ventilated who prove difficult to wean, critical illness polyneuropathy may contribute.

Treatment and prognosis

- Prevention if possible.
- Recumbent position may further compromise respiration with diaphragm weakness.
- Avoid respiratory depressant drugs.
- If required, ventilation.
- In some chronic stable disorders, patients may compensate for respiratory failure, but also may require intermittent positive pressure ventilation, now most easily delivered by means of nocturnal CPAP or NIPPY.

References

Howard RS, Davidson C. Long term ventilation in neurogenic respiratory failure. J Neurol Neurosurg Psychiatry. 2003;74(Suppl III):iii24–iii30

Howard RS, El Kabir D, Williams AJ. Neurogenic respiratory failure. In: RJ Greenwood, MP Barnes, TM McMillan, CD Ward, eds. Handbook of Neurological Rehabilitation. 2nd ed. Hove, UK: Psychology Press; 2003:313–325

Hutchinson D, Whyte K. Neuromuscular disease and respiratory failure. Pract Neurol. 2008;8:229–237

Restless legs syndrome (RLS)

Anxietas tibiarum, Ekbom's syndrome

Restless legs syndrome (RLS) is characterized by intense discomfort within the legs associated with a desire to move them; movement temporarily relieves the discomfort. It is frequently associated with periodic limb movement disorder (PLMD, or periodic limb movements of sleep, PLMS). The pathogenesis is not understood but may relate to a central imbalance of serotoninergic and dopaminergic pathways, possibly at the level of the basal ganglia, linked in some way with disordered brain iron metabolism. A number of linked genetic loci have been defined in familial RLS.

Clinical features

- History of urge or compulsion to move legs due to deep discomfort; often worse at rest or during the evening or night; sensory symptoms eased or relieved by activity, hot baths. Restless arms may be an extension, or even the presentation, of RLS.
- History of leg movements during sleep (periodic movements of sleep, "nocturnal myoclonus"): brief slow periodic movements varying from dorsiflexion of big toe to triple flexion; bed partner may report being kicked at night.
- Secondary insomnia, excessive daytime somnolence, depression, subjective memory complaints.
- Normal neurological examination, unless accompanied by concurrent neurological disease, e.g., essential tremor.

RLS may be:

- Primary or idiopathic: in up to one third of cases the condition is hereditary with evidence for autosomal dominant transmission with variable penetrance.
- Secondary or symptomatic: need to exclude concurrent peripheral neuropathy, uremia, and iron deficiency.

Investigation

Diagnosis of RLS is essentially clinical. Blood biochemistry and iron status may be examined to look for secondary causes. Sleep studies may record PLMS.

Differential diagnosis

Akathisia associated with neuroleptic drug use. *Painful legs and moving toes (PLMT)*. PLMD may be confused with hypnic jerks, *REM sleep behavior disorder*, nocturnal epilepsy, or abnormal movements secondary to associated *obstructive sleep apnea-hypopnea syndrome* (OSAHS).

Treatment and prognosis

Good sleep hygiene and avoidance of aggravating factors may help, including drugs such as tricyclic antidepressants (amitriptyline), nifedipine, antiemetics, phenytoin, but generally pharmacotherapy is required for RLS:

- Dopamine agonists: non-ergot (ropinirole, pramipexole, rotigotine; ergot: cabergoline).
- Levodopa preparations: dyskinesias do not develop with long-term levodopa use for RLS (cf. *Parkinson's disease*).
- Antiepileptics: gabapentin, carbamazepine.
- Benzodiazepines: clonazepam.
- Opioids: oxycodone, dextropropoxyphene.
- Adrenergic drugs: clonidine, propranolol.
- Iron therapy.

Symptoms of RLS generally persist.

Diagnostic criteria

Allen RP, Picchietti D, Hening WA, Trenkwalder C, Walters AS, Montplaisir J. Restless legs syndrome: diagnostic criteria, special considerations, and epidemiology. A report from the restless legs syndrome diagnosis and epidemiology workshop at the National Institutes of Health. Sleep Med. 2003;4:101–119

References

Chaudhuri KR, Ferini-Strambi L, Rye D, eds. Restless Legs Syndrome. Oxford: Oxford University Press; 2009
Ekbom KA. Restless legs syndrome. Neurology. 1960;10:868–873
Freedom T, Merchut MP. Arm restlessness as the initial symptom in restless legs syndrome. Arch Neurol. 2003;60:1013–1015
Hening WA, Allen RP, Chokroverty S, Earley CJ, eds. Restless Legs Syndrome. Philadelphia, PA : Saunders Elsevier; 2009

Reversible cerebral vasoconstriction syndromes (RCVS)

Conditions that have been associated with reversible cerebral vasoconstriction include migraine, thunderclap headache, effort-induced headaches including *primary headache associated with sexual activity*, pre-eclampsia and eclampsia, the postpartum state, and the use of sympathomimetic drugs, and have attracted a wide variety of names (Call–Fleming syndrome, postpartum cerebral angiopathy, reversible cerebral segmental vasoconstriction syndrome). These cases are usually monophasic and benign and need to be distinguished from vasculitides which require immunosuppression. Cases are more common in women than men (M:F = 4:1).

Clinical features

- Hyperacute onset: "worst" headache in less than 1 min, + nausea, vomiting, photophobia; may be precipitated by exercise or sexual activity
- Focal neurological signs (hemiparesis, visual field defects) due to transient ischemic attack or stroke
- Seizures may develop secondary to ischemia
- +/– Hypertension

Investigation

Bloods generally normal, likewise CSF (moderately elevated protein in some cases). Neuroimaging (CT/MRI) may show single or multiple ischemic or hemorrhagic infarcts, frequently in watershed or border zone regions. Cerebral angiography shows diffuse multifocal areas of stenosis and ectasia, and long areas of smooth symmetric narrowing in multiple vascular beds, although these changes are not specific.

Differential diagnosis

Subarachnoid hemorrhage, CNS vasculitis including *primary angiitis of the central nervous system, posterior reversible leukoencephalopathy syndrome.* Differential diagnosis of angiographic changes includes CNS vasculitis, atherosclerosis, infectious arteritis.

Treatment and prognosis

No controlled studies, but calcium channel blocker such as verapamil may be given for headache, plus prednisolone if there is no prompt response or if there is additional TIA or stroke. Treatment of hypertension as appropriate. Response may be monitored not only by cessation of clinical symptomatology but also by repeat cerebral angiography after 6–12 weeks to demonstrate reversion of angiographic findings, without which the diagnosis of RCVS cannot be sustained. The long-term prognosis is very good if the acute complications are appropriately managed.

Diagnostic criteria

Calabrese LH, Dodick DW, Schwedt TJ, et al. Narrative review: reversible cerebral vasoconstriction syndromes. Ann Intern Med. 2007;146:34–44

References

Ducros A, Boukobza M, Porcher R, et al. The clinical and radiological spectrum of reversible cerebral vasoconstriction syndrome. A prospective series of 67 patients. Brain. 2007;130:3091–3101
Ducros A, Bousser M-G. Reversible cerebral vasoconstriction syndrome. Pract Neurol. 2009;9:256–267

Rhabdomyolysis

Crush syndrome, Necrotizing polymyopathy

Rhabdomyolysis is a syndrome of necrotizing myopathy causing muscle pain, tenderness, weakness, and areflexia, which develops over about 24–48 h. Muscle swelling may cause secondary ischemic injury due to the development of a compartment syndrome. Release of intracellular contents may lead to myoglobinuria, acute renal failure, and death.

There are many recognized causes of rhabdomyolysis, including:

- Crush injury (e.g., earthquake survivors)
- Alcohol intoxication, drug use and prolonged drug-induced coma
- Electrolyte disturbances (hypernatremia, hyperglycemia, hypokalemia, hypophosphatemia, hyperosmolality)
- Certain infections
- Metabolic myopathies

Some cases remain idiopathic, and may recur (Meyer–Betz disease).

Clinical features

- Muscle pain, tenderness, weakness, and areflexia
- Oliguria, dark urine
- History of trauma, alcohol intoxication, drug use

Investigation

Blood shows raised creatine kinase, usually >1,000 U/L, sometimes >100,000 U/L. Urine shows myoglobinuria (dipstick +ve for hemoglobin but no hematuria or hemoglobinuria on examination of urine). EMG may show a severe myopathic picture.

Differential diagnosis

Other acute and/or painful myopathies, such as *polymyositis*.

Treatment and prognosis

Removal of the cause of muscle necrosis if identified. Full supportive care with particularly careful monitoring of electrolytes and renal function, with dialysis if required. The ultimate prognosis is very good if the acute complications are appropriately managed.

References

Bywaters EGL, Beall D. Crush injuries with impairment of renal function. BMJ. 1941;i:427–432
Khan FY. Rhabdomyolysis: a review of the literature. Neth J Med. 2009;67:272–283

Rheumatoid arthritis

Rheumatoid arthritis is a multisystem chronic inflammatory disorder classified with the connective tissue disorders, characterized by a symmetrical polyarthritis; lung and heart may also be affected. Neurological features may be due to direct involvement by rheumatoid nodules, vasculitis, or a consequence of bone disease.

Clinical features

- Neurological:
    - CNS: Rheumatoid nodules: meningeal: often asymptomatic; parenchymal (very rare) may cause seizures
    - Vasculitis (very rare, in context of multisystem rheumatoid vasculitis): seizures, hemiparesis, cranial nerve palsy, dementia
    - Spinal cord compression: most commonly due to atlanto–axial joint subluxation (may also rarely cause vertebral artery compression); occasionally due to rheumatoid nodules
    - PNS: Entrapment/compression neuropathies (e.g., carpal tunnel syndrome, ulnar nerve) due to inflamed synovial joints

- Distal sensorimotor polyneuropathy (segmental demyelination + lesser axonal changes, ?vasculitic): mild, vibration sense particularly affected
- Mononeuritis multiplex (axonal sensorimotor; vasculitic)
- Autonomic neuropathy is reported
- Rheumatological: oligoarticular arthritis, usually symmetrical; rheumatoid nodules
- Pulmonary: pleurisy, pneumonitis, interstitial fibrosis (Caplan's syndrome)
- Eyes: sicca syndrome; Sjögren's syndrome may coexist
- Hematology: anemia; iron deficiency; splenomegaly, hypersplenism (Felty's syndrome)
- Cardiac: pericarditis (causing a rub), pericardial effusion
- Kidney: amyloidosis

Investigation

Blood shows positive serology for rheumatoid factor (false positives occur, e.g., systemic lupus erythematosus). Imaging: plain radiology shows typical articular changes. MRI cervical spine indicated in cases of myelopathy. CSF may show nonspecific raised protein. Neurophysiology (EMG/NCS) to elucidate peripheral nervous system involvement: for example, *entrapment neuropathy*, mononeuropathy multiplex, symmetrical polyneuropathy.

Differential diagnosis

Other, seronegative, arthritides. Neurological features may overlap with other connective tissue diseases such as *systemic lupus erythematosus*, *Sjögren's syndrome*, *systemic sclerosis*; and cerebral *vasculitis*.

Treatment and prognosis

Vasculitis: immunosuppression, as for any vasculitis. Cervical subluxation: conservative: analgesia, protection from trauma (e.g., at intubation); majority remain stable or improve; deterioration may necessitate surgical stabilization. Neuropathy: if mild, conservative treatment reasonable; if severe and/or progressive, immunosuppression as for systemic vasculitis may be tried.

References

Keersmaeker A, Truyen L, Ramon F, Cras P, De Clerck L, Martin JJ. Cervical myelopathy due to rheumatoid arthritis: case report and review of the literature. Acta Neurol Belg. 1998;98:284–288
Nadeau S. Neurologic manifestations of connective tissue disease. Neurol Clin. 2002;20:151–178

Rickettsial disease

Rickettsia are obligate intracellular parasites (Gram-negative coccobacilli) which have a life cycle involving an animal reservoir, an insect vector (lice, fleas, ticks, mites), and man. Diseases falling into this category, their causative agents, and insect vectors, include:

- Epidemic *typhus* (*Rickettsia prowazekii*; human body louse)
- Endemic (or murine) typhus (*Rickettsia typhi*, *R. mooseri*; fleas)
- Scrub typhus or tsutsugamushi fever (*Rickettsia orientalis* recently renamed as a new genus with only one species, *Orientia tsutsugamushi*; trombiculid mites, chiggers)
- *Q fever* (*Coxiella burnetii*; no necessary insect vector)
- Rocky Mountain spotted fever (*Rickettsia rickettsiii*; various ticks)

Exposure to wildlife or livestock may be an important clue to diagnosis. Although uncommon in the developed world, about one third of cases are said to develop neurological features. Severity of disease is variable.

Clinical features

- Bacteremic illness: fever, headache, prostration
- Deliruim, stupor, coma, +/– focal neurological signs
- Meningitis, encephalitis, myelitis
- Macular rash (not in Q fever): necrotic ulcer and eschar in scrub typhus
- Lymphadenopathy: local, general
- +/– Disseminated intravascular coagulation
- Q fever: atypical pneumonia, culture negative endocarditis

Investigation

Bloods: Weil–Felix test for the presence of heterophile antibodies to strains of *Proteus mirabilis*, may be negative in up to 50% of cases. Serology: species-specific ELISA, immunofluorescent antibody tests (IFAT), PCR. CSF may be normal, or show a modest lymphocytic pleocytosis.

Differential diagnosis

Other causes of acute infective or inflammatory CNS disease, for example, viral meningitis.

Treatment and prognosis

Antibiotics (tetracycline, chloramphenicol) +/– supportive care as appropriate. Early appropriate treatment is associated with good prognosis; neurological sequelae are rare.

Reference

Cowan G. Rickettsial diseases: the typhus group of fevers – a review. Postgrad Med J. 2000;76:269–272

Rigid spine syndrome [OMIM#602771]

Rigid spine muscular dystrophy

The rigid spine syndrome is a *congenital muscular dystrophy*, presenting with motor delay and axial rigidity, predominantly of the spine causing limitation of neck and trunk flexion. There may also be scoliosis, proximal myopathy, respiratory disturbance, and cardiac changes. Blood creatine kinase may be elevated, EMG is myopathic, and muscle biopsy shows a nonspecific merosin-positive dystrophy; there may be overlap with *multi-minicore disease*. The differential diagnosis encompasses Duchenne, Becker, and Emery–Dreifuss dystrophies, and *ankylosing spondylitis*. The condition is linked to chromosome 1p and deficiency in the protein selenoprotein N1 results from mutations in this gene. Botulinum toxin injections may help the axial rigidity.

Reference

Moghadaszadeh B, Petit N, Jaillard C, et al. Mutations in SEPN1 cause congenital muscular dystrophy with spinal rigidity and restrictive respiratory syndrome. Nat Genet. 2001;29:17–18

Riley–Day syndrome [OMIM#223900]

Familial dysautonomia, Hereditary sensory and autonomic neuropathy (HSAN) III

An autosomal recessive neuropathy, now classified as *hereditary sensory and autonomic neuropathy (HSAN)* type III, occurring principally in Ashkenazi Jewish kindreds. It affects peripheral autonomic, sensory, and motor neurones and causes predominantly autonomic symptoms. Linked to chromosome 9q31-q33, mutations have been identified in the inhibitor of kappa light polypeptide (IKBKAP) gene. Clinical features include:

- Neurological: decreased pain and temperature sensation, but relatively preserved tactile sense; reduced vibration sensation from teenage years. Progressive sensory ataxia (adult years). Decreased tendon reflexes. Below average IQ in ca. one third; otherwise normal intelligence
- Vasomotor: orthostatic hypotension, hyperhidrosis, blotchy skin
- Ocular: lack of overflow tears, corneal analgesia

- Orthopedic: kyphoscoliosis
- Gastrointestinal: swallowing difficulties, esophageal dilatation, reduced gastric motility. Absence of fungiform papillae on the tongue
- Respiratory: apneic episodes; risk of pneumonia

Family history of similar disorder

Investigation

Neurophysiology (EMG/NCS) shows reduced conduction velocities and CMAP amplitude; raised thermal thresholds. Bloods may show normal or elevated supine plasma noradrenaline levels, but no increase on standing. Neurogenetic testing for mutation in the IKBKAP gene (over 90% of patients have the same splice site mutation). Nerve biopsy shows reduction in unmyelinated fibers and small myelinated fibers. Neuropathology shows hypoplastic sympathetic ganglia; loss of neurones in dorsal roots, Lissauer's tracts, and intermediolateral grey column of spinal cord.

Differential diagnosis

Other causes of orthostatic hypotension (autonomic neuropathies, *pure autonomic failure*), and of hereditary sensory neuropathy.

Treatment and prognosis

No specific treatment. Symptomatic therapy for orthostatic hypotension, gastrointestinal symptoms; careful attention to posture when swallowing to avoid aspiration. Perhaps only 20% of patients survive to adulthood; pneumonia is the commonest cause of death.

Reference

Anderson SL, Coli R, Daly IW, et al. Familial dysautonomia is caused by mutations of the IKAP gene. Am J Hum Genet. 2001;68:753–758

Rippling muscle disease (RMD) [OMIM#606072]

Rippling muscle disease (RMD) is a benign *myopathy* with symptoms and signs of muscular hyperexcitability, which is usually inherited as an autosomal dominant condition, but may also be autosomal recessive or sporadic. It is associated with mutations in the gene encoding the protein caveolin 3

(CAV3) and hence is allelic with *limb-girdle muscular dystrophy* type 1c, and some cases of *idiopathic hyperCKemia*, hypertrophic cardiomyopathy, and congenital *long QT syndrome*. It is not a channelopathy.

Clinical features include:

- Complaints of muscle stiffness and exercise-induced myalgia
- Cramp-like sensations
- Self-propagating rippling of muscles, visible from the surface, induced by stretch or percussion
- Myoedema, or muscle mounding, representing electrically silent muscle contractions provoked by mechanical stimuli or stretch

References

Betz RC, Schoser BGH, Kasper D, et al. Mutations in CAV3 cause mechanical hyper-irritability of skeletal muscle in rippling muscle disease. Nat Genet. 2001;28:218–219
Torbergsen T. Rippling muscle disease: a review. Muscle Nerve. 2002; Suppl 11: S103–S107

Rosai–Dorfman disease

Sinus histiocytosis with massive lymphadenopathy

Rosai–Dorfman disease is an idiopathic histioproliferative disease usually affecting systemic lymph nodes, although extranodal and, very rarely, CNS involvement is also described. CNS lesions are often mistaken for *meningioma*. The condition is more common in Afro-Caribbeans.

Clinical features

- Bilateral painless lymphadenopathy, especially cervical
- Fever, weight loss
- Focal neurological signs, seizures if intracranial involvement

Investigation

Blood may show a polyclonal hypergammaglobulinemia. In cases with CNS involvement, neuroimaging (CT/MRI) may show multiple well-circumscribed mass lesions with dural attachment and homogeneous enhancement with contrast, resembling meningioma. Biopsy shows proliferation of histiocytes, infiltration with plasma cells; lymphophagocytosis (emperipolesis) is characteristic. S100 protein staining of cytoplasm may be seen.

Differential diagnosis

Clinically and radiologically it may be impossible to distinguish Rosai–Dorfman disease from multiple meningioma. Multifocal CNS lymphoma may present a similar picture. Multiple metastases and neurosarcoidosis must also be considered.

Treatment and prognosis

The condition usually resolves spontaneously, hence the importance of making a pathological diagnosis and avoiding inappropriate and potentially toxic therapies.

References

Petzold A, Thom M, Powell M, Plant GT. Relapsing intracranial Rosai-Dorfman disease. J Neurol Neurosurg Psychiatry. 2001;71:538–541
Wang Y, Gao X, Tang W, Jiang C. Rosai-Dorfman disease isolated to the central nervous system: a report of six cases. Neuropathology. 2010;30:154–158

Ross syndrome

Ross syndrome consists of a combination of

- Progressive segmental hyperhidrosis with widespread hypohidrosis or anhidrosis
- Tonic (Holmes–Adie) pupil
- Hyporeflexia or areflexia

Clinical heterogeneity is reported (i.e., not all these features may be present). There is phenotypic overlap between Ross syndrome and *Holmes–Adie syndrome* and Harlequin syndrome (isolated progressive segmental hypohidrosis).

Evidence from clinical studies and skin biopsies of reduced cholinergic sweat gland innervation supports the concept of a selective degenerative process affecting predominantly postganglionic skin sympathetic fibers, especially cholinergic sudomotor neurones, in Ross syndrome.

References

Nolano M, Provitera V, Estraneo A, et al. Ross syndrome: a rare or a misknown disorder of thermoregulation? A skin innervation study on 12 subjects. Brain. 2006;129:2119–2131
Ross AT. Progressive selective sudomotor denervation. Neurology. 1958;8:809–817

Roussy–Lévy syndrome [OMIM#180800]

Hereditary areflexic dystasia

Roussy–Lévy syndrome is a hereditary sensory ataxia with onset in infancy. Its nosological position was for many years controversial due to its similarities to *Friedreich's ataxia* and Charcot–Marie–Tooth (CMT) syndrome: some authorities included it in the peroneal muscular atrophy/*hereditary motor and sensory neuropathy* (*HMSN*) group as a variant of CMT1; others regarded it as an entirely separate entity. Tissue from the original family was shown to have a novel missense mutation in the P_0 gene, indicating that the original Roussy–Lévy syndrome was a subtype of CMT-1B. Other families with mutations in the PMP22 gene, hence CMT-1A, have also been described.

Clinical features

- Pes cavus, areflexia, atrophy (legs > hands)
- Sensory impairment: vibration, position sense causing sensory ataxia
- Kyphoscoliosis
- +/− Extensor plantar response(s)
- +/− Action tremor
- No cerebellar ataxia, autonomic dysfunction, or nerve thickening

Investigation

Neurophysiology (EMG/NCS) shows sensorimotor demyelinating polyneuropathy; sensory responses may be absent and motor conduction velocities slowed. There may be denervation changes. Neurogenetic testing (PMP22, P_0) may be undertaken.

Differential diagnosis

- Friedreich's ataxia
- Hereditary motor and sensory neuropathy (HMSN)

Treatment and prognosis

Follow-up of four of the original seven cases of Roussy and Lévy after 30 years found little change in the condition.

References

Planté-Bordeneuve V, Guiochon-Mantel A, Lacroix C, Lapresle J, Said G. The Roussy-Lévy family: from the original description to the gene. Ann Neurol. 1999;46:770–773
Zubair S, Holland NR, Beson B, Parke JT, Prodan CI. A novel point mutation in the PMP22 gene in a family with Roussy-Levy syndrome. J Neurol. 2008;255:1417–1418

Rubella

Infection with the rubella virus, an RNA virus of the Togaviridae family, may have various consequences for the nervous system. Of these, congenital rubella syndrome is the most common, despite the availability of vaccination, and the only one associated with direct viral invasion and replication within brain. A postinfectious *encephalitis* following acute infection with rubella virus is described, as is progressive rubella panencephalitis, an extremely rare condition thought to represent either reactivation of latent viral infection causing a subacute or chronic viral illness, or an autoimmune reaction. Patients with progressive rubella panencephalitis may have features of congenital rubella syndrome, but then develop decline of intellect and behavior with seizures, ataxia, and progressive dementia. Oligoclonal bands and raised rubella-specific antibody titers are found in the CSF. Neuropathologically there is white matter destruction but no inclusion bodies are seen. There is no specific treatment and death occurs within a few years, although spontaneous remissions have been reported.

Reference

Frey TK. Neurological aspects of rubella virus infection. Intervirology. 1997;40:167–175

"Rucksack paralysis"

Carrying a heavy backpack may be followed by a *brachial plexopathy* (akin to *Erb's palsy, Erb–Duchenne palsy*) or an isolated *long thoracic nerve palsy*. This may be due to direct nerve trauma or, in the case of *neuralgic amyotrophy*, to exercise-induced inflammatory disease.

S

Sandhoff's disease [OMIM#268800]

β-Hexosaminidase A and B deficiency, GM2 gangliosidosis

Although this rare form of gangliosidosis, clinically almost indistinguishable from *Tay-Sachs disease*, usually has late-infantile onset, occasional adult-onset cases are reported presenting with spinocerebellar degeneration. Enzyme activity (total; HexA, HexB) can be measured in plasma, leukocytes, or fibroblasts, and neuroimaging (CT/MRI) may show typical bright thalami and cerebellar atrophy. Neurogenetic testing may show mutations in the hexosaminidase A and B genes.

Reference

Hara A, Uyama E, Uchino M, et al. Adult Sandhoff's disease: R505Q and I207V substitutions in the HEXB gene of the first Japanese case. J Neurol Sci. 1998;155:86–91

Saphenous neuropathy

The saphenous nerve is a cutaneous branch of the femoral nerve which emerges from the parent trunk distal to Hunter's canal and medial and superior to the knee. It accompanies the saphenous vein in the medial part of the leg to the medial aspect of the foot supplying sensory innervation to these areas. Saphenous neuropathy, resulting in sensory loss to these areas, most commonly follows surgical injury to the nerve (e.g., saphenous vein removal, knee surgery).

Sarcoglycanopathy

Sarcoglycans are a group of five distinct, dystrophin-associated, transmembrane proteins. Deficiency of four of these proteins results in autosomal recessive *limb-girdle muscular dystrophy*, often the severe childhood variants previously known as SCARMD (*severe childhood autosomal recessive muscular dystrophy*):

- α-Sarcoglycan (adhalin): LGMD type 2D, linkage to chromosome 17q
- β-Sarcoglycan: LGMD type 2E, linkage to chromosome 4q
- γ-Sarcoglycan: LGMD type 2C, linkage to chromosome 13q
- δ-Sarcoglycan: LGMD type 2F, linkage to chromosome 5q

The hip abduction sign, abduction of the thighs when rising from the ground due to the relative weakness of hip adductors with relatively preserved strength in hip abductors, seems to be a sensitive and specific sign in sarcoglycanopathies. Since sarcoglycans are expressed in cardiac as well as skeletal muscle, concurrent cardiomyopathy may also occur. These conditions may be confused clinically with *Duchenne muscular dystrophy* but are genetically distinct.

Abnormalities of ε-sarcoglycan, linked to chromosome 7q21, have been associated with the *myoclonus-dystonia syndrome (MDS)*, or DYT11.

Satoyoshi syndrome

Komuragaeri disease, Myospasm gravis

Satayoshi syndrome is a progressive syndrome of painful intermittent generalized muscle spasms, alopecia, diarrhea, with secondary skeletal abnormalities and endocrinopathy with amenorrhea. It is believed to be an autoimmune condition because of the frequent presence of autoantibodies directed against acetylcholine receptors (in the absence of myasthenia gravis or thymoma) and the response to steroids, intravenous immunoglobulin, and tacrolimus. Carbamazepine may be helpful for painful muscle spasms.

References

Heger S, Kuester RM, Volk R, Stephani U, Sippell WG. Satoyoshi syndrome: a rare multisystemic disorder requiring systemic and symptomatic treatment. Brain Dev. 2006;28:300–304
Satoyoshi E. A syndrome of progressive muscle spasm, alopecia, and diarrhea. Neurology. 1978;28:458–471

Scapuloperoneal syndrome

Scapuloperoneal syndrome, as its name implies, describes periscapular wasting and weakness with associated scapular winging, and wasting and weakness of tibialis anterior causing weak ankle dorsiflexion or *foot drop*. This phenotype may be:

- Myogenic:
  - *Facioscapulohumeral (FSH) dystrophy*: "forme fruste" without the facial weakness in some cases
  - *Emery–Dreifuss syndrome* (consider this if cardiomyopathy, contractures present)
- Neurogenic:
  - Scapuloperoneal *spinal muscular atrophy* (rare; genetically heterogeneous).
  - *Dawidenkow syndrome* (may be additional sensory findings)

Despite electrophysiological studies and muscle biopsy, it may be difficult to differentiate myogenic and neurogenic syndromes.

References

Tawil R, Myers GJ, Weiffenbach B, et al. Scapuloperoneal syndromes: absence of linkage to the 4q35 FSHD locus. Arch Neurol. 1995;52:1069–1072
Milanov I, Ishpekova B. Differential diagnosis of scapuloperoneal syndrome. Electromyogr Clin Neurophysiol. 1997;37:73–78

Scheuermann's disease

Juvenile kyphosis

Scheuermann's disease refers to thoracic or thoracolumbar kyphosis in adolescents causing *low back pain* with exercise. The syndrome is usually benign, but occasionally spinal cord compression from thoracic disk herniation or severe kyphosis may occur and necessitate surgical intervention.

Schilder's disease

Diffuse sclerosis, Encephalitis periaxalis diffusa, Myelinoclastic diffuse sclerosis

Schilder's disease is a rare, non-familial, acute, or subacute demyelinating disorder of children or young adults, of unknown cause, classified with the *leukodystrophies*. It may be a devastating monophasic illness, or a relapsing-remitting disorder without full recovery. Schilder's disease may be a variant of *multiple sclerosis* (some authors regard it as a "transitional" form); clinical manifestations are similar although cortical features (dementia, hemiplegia, cortical blindness, and deafness) are more prominent. One of the original cases reported resembled *adrenoleukodystrophy*.

Clinical features

- Hemiplegia
- Visual field defects; cortical blindness
- Pseudobulbar palsy
- Deafness
- Dementia
- Intracranial hypertension
- Psychiatric features

Investigation

There is no diagnostic test, but diagnostic criteria (pre-MRI era) have been suggested:

- Subacute or chronic demyelinating disorder with one or two symmetric bilateral lesions involving the centrum semiovale (at least 3×2 cm).
- No other lesions demonstrable clinically or by imaging.
- No involvement of adrenal glands, peripheral nervous system.
- Histological findings identical to multiple sclerosis, but large sharply demarcated foci, may involve whole lobe.

Investigations aiming to exclude other disorders include:

- Bloods: lactate, amino acids, arylsulfatase A, C26/C22 very long chain fatty acid ratio: all normal.
- CSF: lactate normal; oligoclonal bands usually negative; myelin basic protein elevated.
- MRI: confluent or multifocal areas of high signal on T_2-weighted images, confined to white matter; may show mass effect during acute deteriorations. May be mistaken for brain tumor.
- Brain biopsy: inflammatory perivascular infiltrate with demyelination; cystic lesions in severe cases; axonal damage.

Differential diagnosis

- Multiple sclerosis
- Other leukodystrophy, e.g., X-ALD, MLD

- Encephalomyelitides, e.g., ADEM
- Diffuse cerebral neoplasm
- *Mitochondrial disease*
- *Primary CNS angiitis*

Treatment and prognosis

Corticosteroids may improve the outcome of single episodes, but their effect, if any, on the course of the disease is unknown.

References

Bacigaluppi S, Polonara G, Zavanone ML, et al. Schilder's disease: non-invasive diagnosis? A case report and review. Neurol Sci. 2009;30:421–430
Schilder P. Zur Kenntnis der sogenannten diffusen Sklerose. Z Gesamte Neurol Psychiatr. 1912;10:1–60

Schistosomiasis

Bilharziasis

Trematode *Schistosoma* parasites gain access to the human body via larvae (cercariae) shed by the intermediate snail host in water. They may affect spinal cord and brain.

Clinical features

- Cerebral (*S. japonicum*):
  - Acute: meningoencephalitis
    - Focal signs (hemiplegia, spasticity, cranial nerve palsy)
    - Epileptic seizures (part of Katayama fever)
  - Chronic: raised intracranial pressure
    - Epileptic seizures
    - Mass lesion
    - Cerebral *vasculitis*
- Spinal (*S. mansoni* in South America, *S. haematobium* in Africa):
  - cauda equina and conus medullaris syndromes
  - paraplegia: transverse myelitis, cord infarct, granulomatous cord compression

Investigation

Blood: eosinophilia; serology for Schistosoma. Stool: ova (often not helpful). CSF: eosinophilic pleocytosis. Neuroimaging: brain (CT/MRI) dense multi-nodular lesions with enhancement, edema (nonspecific); spinal cord MRI: swelling, arachnoiditis, granuloma. Tissue: biopsy or rectum, liver, bladder.

Differential diagnosis

Other causes of meningoencephalitis, epileptic seizures, paraplegia, conus medullaris, and cauda equina syndrome. Travel history may be key to focusing differential diagnosis.

Treatment and prognosis

Antischistosomal treatment: praziquantel, metrifonate, oxamniquine, +/– corticosteroids. Surgical decompression.

Reference

Bill P. Schistosomiasis and the nervous system. Pract Neurol. 2003;3:12–21

Schnitzler's syndrome

Schnitzler's syndrome of chronic urticaria has occasionally been reported with neurological features, of an inflammatory small vessel CNS disease and peripheral neuropathy.

Reference

Gossrau G, Pfeiffer C, Meurer M, Reichmann H, Lampe JB. Schnitzler's syndrome with neurological findings. J Neurol. 2003;250:1248–1250

Schwartz–Jampel syndrome [OMIM#255800]

Chondrodystrophic myotonia

Schwartz–Jampel syndrome is a rare autosomal recessive condition characterized by neurological and morphological features, the former characterized clinically by myotonia and continuous EMG activity which originates at the level of the muscle membrane. It results from mutations in the HSPG2 gene which encodes perlecan, a major component of basement membranes.

Clinical features

- Neurological:
  - Muscle stiffness, myotonia (action and percussion); blepharospasm, blepharophimosis; high-pitched voice
- Morphological:
  - Short stature, oculofacial abnormalities, bone and joint deformities

Investigation

Neurophysiology: NCS are normal, including repetitive nerve stimulation and neuromuscular junction transmission; EMG shows persistent spontaneous activity and myotonic discharges.

Differential diagnosis

Other *myotonic syndromes*, but morphological features render confusion unlikely.

Treatment and prognosis

No specific treatment.

References

Schwartz O, Jampel RS. Congenital blepharophimosis associated with a unique generalized myopathy. Arch Ophthalmol. 1962;68:52–57
Stum M, Davoine CS, Vicart S, et al. Spectrum of HSPG2 (Perlecan) mutations in patients with Schwartz-Jampel syndrome. Hum Mutat. 2006;27:1082–1091

Sciatic neuropathy

Containing fibers from the L4-S3 roots, the sciatic nerve exits the pelvis via the sciatic notch, runs under the piriformis muscle, descends into the posterior thigh, and divides above the knee into peroneal and tibial branches. This division is reflected more proximally by two trunks, lateral and medial, and lateral sciatic nerve trunk injury may produce a picture identical to that with isolated peroneal nerve involvement. Most cases of sciatic neuropathy relate to trauma: pelvic injury, hip injury, compression by tumor, hematoma, and, possibly, the piriformis muscle (*piriformis syndrome*).

Clinical features

- Motor:
  - Complete lesions cause weakness of all muscles below the knee as well as hamstrings (biceps femoris, semitendinosus, semimembranosus) with loss or depression of ankle and hamstring reflexes. However, lateral trunk injury is more common, producing foot drop as in a *peroneal neuropathy* (weak tibialis anterior, extensor hallucis longus, and extensor digitorum longus).
- Sensory:
  - Loss in the distribution of the peroneal and tibial nerves, hence whole foot, lateral calf.

Pelvic examination for mass lesions may be indicated.

Investigation

Neurophysiology (EMG/NCS) helps to distinguish sciatic mononeuropathy from common peroneal nerve palsy, radiculopathy, lumbosacral plexopathy.

Differential diagnosis

- Lumbar radiculopathy, especially L5-S1
- *Lumbosacral plexopathies*
- Peroneal neuropathy, *tibial neuropathy*

Reference

Staal A, Van Gijn J, Spaans F. Mononeuropathies: Examination, Diagnosis and Treatment. London: W.B. Saunders; 1999:117–123

Sciatica

Sciatica (literally "hip pain") is a clinical syndrome of nerve root/radicular pain or referred pain involving the spinal roots L4, L5, or S1, from which the sciatic nerve takes its origin. Patients may also use the term to refer to more chronic back, buttock, and leg pain which is consequent on an acute event or due to other pathologies, including musculoskeletal problems. A rare catamenial variant is described, due to implantation of endometriosis in the sciatic nerve.

Clinical features

- Pain: radiating from lower back to buttock, posterior thigh, posterolateral or anterolateral foot. If due to intervertebral disk prolapse, pain may develop acutely when bending or lifting a heavy object. Pain is exacerbated by maneuvers which raise intracranial pressure (coughing, sneezing, straining, jugular vein compression), and by local stretching (straight leg raising, Lasègue's sign).
- Motor signs: loss of ankle jerk (L5, S1); weakness, atrophy, +/- fasciculation if anterior roots involved.

Investigation

Neurophysiology (EMG/NCS) to look for evidence of radiculopathy. Neuroimaging (MRI) to look for root compression (e.g., disk). CSF may be required if no compressive lesion found on imaging, especially if malignant infiltration is suspected.

Differential diagnosis

History not likely to be mistaken for plexopathy, neuropathy.

Treatment and prognosis

Pain usually settles with rest and adequate analgesia. If not, or if neurological signs develop (wasting, weakness), investigation should be pursued. Surgical decompression may be required. Surgery (microdiskectomy) leads to quicker resolution of symptoms compared to conservative management, but the long-term outcome was the same in both groups.

References

Fairbank JCT. Sciatica: an archaic term. BMJ. 2007;335:112
Kellgren J. Sciatica. Lancet. 1941;i:561–564
Koes BW, van Tulder MW, Peul WC. Diagnosis and treatment of sciatica. BMJ. 2007;334:1313–1317
Peul WCF, van Houwellingen HC, van den Hout WB, et al. Surgery versus prolonged conservative treatment for sciatica. N Engl J Med. 2007;356:2245–2256

Scoliosis: overview

Kyphoscoliosis

Scoliosis is abnormal curvature of the spine in the lateral plane; kyphosis is abnormal curvature anteroposteriorly; kyphoscoliosis is a combination of both.

Although perhaps 70% of childhood scoliosis is idiopathic, particularly in girls (F:M = 8:1), scoliosis may reflect an underlying neurological or muscular disorder; it was a common sequela of paralytic *poliomyelitis*. Certainly neurological investigation is appropriate if in addition to scoliosis there are neurological signs such as back pain, bowel and/or bladder problems, leg or foot weakness, or a midline patch of hair, pigmentation, or a mass over the spinal column. If so, in addition to plain radiographs of the spine, other neurological investigations such as MR imaging may be indicated. Kyphoscoliosis may contribute to respiratory compromise. The differential diagnosis of scoliosis includes:

- Upper motor neurone disorders:
  - Cerebral palsy (spastic, quadriparetic, athetoid, dystonia)
  - Primary *dystonia* syndromes
  - *Spinocerebellar ataxia; Friedreich's ataxia*
  - Spinal cord tumor
  - *Syringomyelia*
  - *Neurofibromatosis*
- Lower motor neurone disorders:
  - Neuropathies, e.g., *Charcot–Marie–Tooth disease* (peroneal muscular atrophy)
- Myopathies, e.g., *nemaline myopathy*
- Abnormalities of bone:
  - Congenital: Hemivertebra
  - *Diastematomyelia*
  - Acquired: Pott's disease of the spine (*tuberculosis*)
- Idiopathic scoliosis

Semantic dementia (SD)

Progressive fluent aphasia, Semantic aphasia with associative agnosia

Semantic dementia (SD) is one of the variants of *frontotemporal lobar degeneration (FTLD)* of the brain, characterized by a loss of word meaning. Atrophy of the left anterior medial and inferior temporal gyri may be of particular importance as the neuroanatomical substrate of semantic memory, either alone or as part of a functional network. Right-sided lesions seem less common, although this may be an artifact consequent upon the more obvious effects upon language, as opposed to visual semantic function (e.g., prosopagnosia) of left-sided pathology.

Clinical features

- Left-sided lesions more common (ca. 3:1): Progressive fluent aphasia with preserved syntax; impaired naming (anomia), loss of word meaning; with or without surface dyslexia and dysgraphia. Calculation spared.
- Right-sided lesions: job loss, loss of insight, social awkwardness, difficulty with person identification.
- Semantic memory impairment with relative preservation of episodic memory (cf. episodic memory disturbance in *Alzheimer's disease*); new learning (recognition memory) preserved early in disease.
- Associative agnosia: impairment of object identity on both visual and tactile presentation.

Investigation

Neuropsychological profile: semantic index of the Addenbroooke's Cognitive Examination may be helpful. Neuroimaging: volumetric MR brain imaging shows asymmetric atrophy (usually L > R) affecting all anterior temporal lobe structures (especially entorhinal cortex, amygdala, anterior medial and inferior temporal gyri, and anterior fusiform gyrus) with an anteroposterior gradient of atrophy (cf. Alzheimer's disease: symmetrical atrophy, especially medial temporal lobe structures including hippocampus; with no anteroposterior gradient).

Neuropathological substrate is variable as in other FTLD syndromes, but ubiquitin-positive tau-negative neuronal inclusions are most common in SD.

Differential diagnosis

- Alzheimer's disease
- *Primary nonfluent aphasia*

Treatment and prognosis

No specific treatment; no response to cholinesterase inhibitors.

References

Hodges JR, Patterson K. Semantic dementia: a unique clinicopathological syndrome. Lancet Neurol. 2007;6:1004–1014
Thompson SA, Patterson K, Hodges JR. Left/right asymmetry of atrophy in semantic dementia: behavioural-cognitive implications. Neurology. 2003;61:1196–1203

Sengers syndrome

First described in 1975, this is a very rare syndrome, possibly inherited as an autosomal recessive condition, comprising congenital cataracts, hypertrophic cardiomyopathy, mitochondrial myopathy, and lactic acidosis. Pathologically, muscle biopsy shows abnormal arrangement and loss of mitochondrial cristae, crystals within the mitochondrial matrix, and lipid and glycogen deposits. Despite this clinical and histopathological evidence suggesting a *mitochondrial disease*, there is no evidence from biochemical studies for abnormal function of the mitochondrial respiratory chain. Evidence for deficiency of adenine nucleotide translocator 1 (ANT1), a transmembrane transport protein, in muscle tissue from Sengers syndrome patients has been presented, but there is no genetic mutation suggesting the deficiency results from transcriptional, translational, or posttranslational events.

Reference

Jordens EZ, Palmieri L, Huizing M, et al. Adenine nucleotide translocator 1 deficiency associated with Sengers syndrome. Ann Neurol. 2002;52:95–99

Septo-optic dysplasia

De Morsier's syndrome

Septo-optic dysplasia, or De Morsier's syndrome, is a developmental disorder of the nervous system characterized by bilateral optic nerve and chiasmal hypoplasia with reduced visual acuity, small optic disks, and an absent septum pellucidum. Hypothalamic-pituitary axis disturbances also occur, ranging from isolated growth hormone deficiency to panhypopituitarism.

Serotonin syndrome

Serotonin syndrome refers to symptoms associated with a state of increasing central intrasynaptic serotonin release. The clinical features include:

- Mental status change, agitation, irritability, confusion, headache
- Myoclonus, shivering, tremor, incoordination, hyperreflexia
- Diaphoresis, fever, hyperpyrexia, diarrhea

Clinically it resembles the *neuroleptic malignant syndrome*, and some authors classify it as a form of "malignant catatonia."

Serotonin syndrome was initially reported in the context of an interaction between monoamine oxidase inhibitors and selective serotinin reuptake inhibitors (SSRIs), but may also occur with combinations of selegiline and SSRIs or tricyclic antidepressants.

The syndrome is usually brief, but may persist despite drug withdrawal, mandating full supportive care.

References

Mann SC, Caroff SN, Keck PE, Lazarus A. Neuroleptic Malignant Syndrome and Related Conditions. 2nd ed. Washington, DC: American Psychiatric Association; 2003:75–92

Sternbach H. The serotonin syndrome. Am J Psychiatry. 1991;148:705–713

Shapiro syndrome

Shapiro syndrome is the rare concurrence of agenesis of the corpus callosum with a hypothalamic disturbance of thermoregulation producing a syndrome akin to *spontaneous periodic hypothermia*, with episodic hyperhidrosis and hypothermia. Early speculations that these phenomena might be epileptiform, so-called diencephalic epilepsy, have not been confirmed: antiepileptic medications are helpful in only a minority of cases. Clonidine has been reported to be beneficial.

References

Shapiro WR, Williams GH, Plum F. Spontaneous recurrent hypothermia accompanying agenesis of the corpus callosum. Brain. 1969;92:423–436

Shenoy C. Shapiro syndrome. Q J Med. 2008;101:61–62

Walker BR, Anderson JAM, Edwards CRW. Clonidine therapy for Shapiro's syndrome. Q J Med. 1992;82:235–245

Shoulder–hand syndrome

Pain in the shoulder and arm with secondary vasomotor changes in the hand may occur in an immobile arm following a stroke or myocardial infarction, with osteoporosis and atrophy of cutaneous and subcutaneous tissues (of Sudeck type). This condition probably falls within the rubric of *complex regional pain syndromes*.

Sialidosis

α-Neuraminidase deficiency, Mucolipidosis type I (ML type I)

Sialidosis is related to deficiency in lysosomal acid α-neuraminidase (or N-acetyl neuraminidase, sialidase) and mutations in the sialidase gene on chromosome 6p, with resulting excretion of large quantities of sialyl oligosaccharides. The clinical syndromes are heterogeneous, encompassing cortical myoclonus, visual loss, and cognitive features.

Clinical features

- Type I (Cherry red spot-myoclonus syndrome):
  - Autosomal recessive disorder due to isolated α-neuraminidase deficiency
  - Onset in late childhood, adolescence
  - Progressive visual loss, polymyoclonus, seizures (tonic-clonic), macular cherry red spot, optic atrophy, intellectual deterioration, +/– cerebellar ataxia, painful peripheral neuropathy. No dysmorphism
- Type II:
  - Congenital, infantile, and juvenile forms recognized
  - Autosomal recessive congenital form; often stillborn
  - Early infantile hepatosplenomegaly
  - Dysmorphism: depressed nasal bridge
  - Macular cherry red spot
  - Severe psychomotor retardation
  - Myoclonus, seizures with longer survival
  - +/– Nephrosialidosis (secondary renal dysfunction, proteinuria)
  - Angiokeratoma corporis diffusum may be prominent

Investigation

- Types I and II:
  - Urine: thin layer chromatography shows increased sialic acid containing oligosaccharides
  - α-Neuraminidase enzyme assay in fibroblasts, leukocytes
  - Bone marrow: foamy histiocytes
- Type I:
  - Imaging: cerebral/cerebellar atrophy
  - Blood film: vacuolated lymphocytes

Differential diagnosis

- Type I:
  - Myoclonic epilepsy with ragged red fibers (MERRF)
  - Unverricht–Lundborg syndrome
  - Lafora body disease
  - Lipofuscinosis (neuronal ceroid lipofuscinosis type II)
  - Late onset GM2 gangliosidosis
  - Dentatorubral-pallidoluysian atrophy (DRPLA)
  - Benign essential familial myoclonus
  - Andermann syndrome: action-myoclonus-renal failure syndrome

- Type II:
  - GM1 gangliosidosis
  - Hurler syndrome: similar dysmorphism, but no corneal clouding
  - Angiokeratoma corporis diffusum: Fabry's disease, fucosidosis

Treatment and prognosis

No specific treatment available; prenatal diagnosis possible. Symptomatic treatment for myoclonus, epileptic seizures. Early infantile form usually leads to death in the second year.

Reference

Rapin I, Goldfischer S, Katzman R, et al. The cherry-red spot-myoclonus syndrome. Ann Neurol. 1978;3:234–242

Sickle-cell disease

Stroke syndromes and epileptic seizures may complicate this hemoglobinopathy which may lead to occlusion of small intracerebral vessels.

Reference

Prengler M, Pavlakis SG, Prohovnik I, et al. Sickle cell disease: the neurological complications. Ann Neurol. 2002;51:543–552

Silver syndrome [OMIM#270685]

Spastic paraplegia 17

An autosomal dominant form of complicated *hereditary spastic paraplegia* associated with amyotrophy of hand muscles, now designated SPG17. Linked to chromosome 11q12-q14, it is caused by mutations in the BSCL2 gene, and is allelic with distal spinal muscular atrophy type 5.

Sjögren's syndrome

Sjögren's syndrome is an autoimmune disorder of exocrine glands, occurring either as a primary disorder or secondary to another connective tissue disorder (e.g., *rheumatoid arthritis*); it more often affects women than men.

Neurological complications may affect both the peripheral and the central nervous systems. Their pathogenesis is uncertain; small vessel *vasculitis* may be relevant in some cases.

Clinical features

- Neurological:
  - Peripheral (10–30%):
    - Distal symmetrical sensory neuropathy
    - Sensorimotor neuropathy
    - Polyradiculopathy
    - Mononeuropathy multiplex
    - *Trigeminal sensory neuropathy*
    - Sensory ataxic neuronopathy or ganglionopathy (rare, but virtually pathognomonic)
  - Central:
    - *Aseptic meningitis*, meningoencephalitis, encephalopathy
    - *Stroke, transient ischemic attack (TIA)*; focal neurological deficits (hemisphere, brainstem)
    - Epileptic seizures
    - Acute *transverse myelitis*/chronic myelopathy
    - Psychiatric disturbance
    - Dementia (rare)
    - Parkinsonism (rare)
    - Dystonia (rare)
    - Multiple sclerosis-like syndrome: optic neuropathy, cerebellar ataxia, internuclear ophthalmoplegia (significance debated)
- Non-neurological:
  - Sicca syndrome: salivary glands (xerostomia), lacrimal glands (xerophthalmia): 50%
  - Features of connective tissue disease (e.g., rheumatoid arthritis)
  - Vasculitic skin rash
  - Interstitial nephritis
  - Lymphadenopathy
  - Interstitial pneumonitis (rare)

Investigation

Bloods: +ve ANA (speckled), anti-Ro (SSA), anti-La (SSB) (75–80%). Schirmer's test of tear production: (<5 mm wetness in 5 min). Tissue: salivary gland (lip) biopsy shows destruction/fibrosis of glandular tissue with lymphocytic infiltrate. With neurological features, the following investigations may be indicated: EMG/NCS if peripheral nerve disease; neuroimaging (MRI) may show multifocal white matter lesions, mostly subcortical; CSF may show raised protein, white cell count, pressure, and oligoclonal bands in encephalopathy.

Differential diagnosis

Broad: other causes of peripheral neuropathy, stroke; MS. Sensory ataxic neuronopathy or ganglionopathy may be seen in anti-Hu (paraneoplastic) syndrome.

Treatment and prognosis

Immunosuppression: prednisolone +/− cyclophosphamide. No controlled trials.

Diagnostic criteria

Vitali C. Classification criteria for Sjögren's syndrome. Ann Rheum Dis. 2003;62:94–95

References

Delalande S, de Seze J, Fauchais AL, et al. Neurologic manifestations in primary Sjögren syndrome: a study of 82 patients. Medicine (Baltimore). 2004;83:280–291
Fox RI. Sjögren's syndrome. Lancet. 2005;366:321–331
Lafitte C, Amoura Z, Cacoub P, et al. Neurological complications of primary Sjögren's syndrome. J Neurol. 2001;248:577–584

Sleep apnea syndromes: overview

Sleep apnea refers to a temporary cessation or absence of breathing during sleep. Sleep apnea syndromes may be broadly divided into three categories: obstructive, central, and mixed:

- Obstructive: cessation of airflow through nose and mouth with persistence of respiratory effort, diaphragmatic and intercostal muscle activity. Upper airway resistance may lead to paradoxical breathing, with thorax and abdomen moving in opposite directions. The obstructive pattern may

be seen in *obstructive sleep apnea-hypopnea syndrome (OSAHS)* and in upper airway resistance syndrome (UARS). Partial obstruction of nocturnal breathing, with or without snoring, may also occur as a consequence of obesity or neuromuscular disorder affecting pharyngeal muscles.
- Central: cessation of airflow through nose and mouth with no respiratory effort, in the absence of diaphragmatic and intercostal muscle activity. Central sleep apnea (CSA) may occur with lower brainstem lesions (infarction, poliomyelitis, syringobulbia) with loss of automatic breathing, especially during sleep (primary hypoventilation, Ondine's curse), or may be idiopathic. Cheyne–Stokes breathing, a waxing and waning depth of respiration, is a special type of central apnea, characterized by a crescendo–decrescendo sequence separated by central apneas; it may be seen with neurological disorders and congestive heart failure.
- Mixed: initial cessation of airflow with no respiratory effort (i.e., central apnea) is followed by a period of upper airway obstructive sleep apnea.

Sleep disorders: overview

Sleep disorders are classified in the International Classification of Sleep Disorders (ICSD-2) into eight broad categories (with several subcategories), viz:

- Insomnias
- Sleep-related breathing disorders, such as *sleep apnea syndromes*
- Hypersominas of central origin, such as *narcolepsy*
- Circadian rhythm sleep disorders
- *Parasomnias*
- Sleep-related movement disorders, such as *restless legs syndrome*
- Isolated symptoms, apparently normal variants, and unresolved issues
- Other sleep disorders

Two appendices in ICSD-2 list:

- Sleep disorders associated with conditions classifiable elsewhere, such as *fatal familial insomnia*
- Other psychiatric and behavioral disorders frequently encountered in the differential diagnosis of sleep disorders, such as *somatoform disorders*

Reference

Chokroverty S. Sleep and its disorders. In: Bradley WG, Daroff RB, Fenichel GM, Jankovic J, eds. Neurology in Clinical Practice. 5th ed. Philadelphia, PA: Butterworth-Heinemann Elsevier; 2008:1947–2009

Sneddon's syndrome

A noninflammatory thrombo-occlusive arteriolar vasculopathy, affecting skin and brain and often (but not always) associated with antiphospholipid antibodies. The disorder occurs primarily in young patients, with a female preponderance.

Clinical features

- Livedo reticularis
- Recurrent strokes in the absence of obvious risk factors
- Focal neurological signs
- Epileptic seizures: more common in antibody positive patients
- Cognitive decline
- Thrombocytopenia
- Mitral regurgitation

Investigation

Bloods: antiphospholipid antibodies, thrombocytopenia. Neuroimaging: brain CT/MRI for ischemic infarcts in middle cerebral artery territory.

Differential diagnosis

Skin lesions usually make the diagnosis obvious. Other vasculopathies and vasculitides must be considered, e.g., collagen vascular diseases (*systemic lupus erythematosus*, *Sjögren's syndrome*), cerebral *vasculitis*, *primary angiitis of the CNS*, *Susac's syndrome*, *fibromuscular dysplasia*.

Treatment and prognosis

Anticoagulation is recommended if antiphospholipid antibodies are present. Aspirin and immunosuppressive therapy have been tried but their place remains to be defined; they may be of more use in antibody negative patients. Existing cognitive impairment does not reverse; the aim is to prevent further decline.

References

Sneddon IB. Cerebrovascular lesions and livedo reticularis. Br J Dermatol. 1965;77:180–185

Frances C, Papo T, Wechsler B, Laporte JL, Biousse V, Piette JC. Sneddon syndrome with or without antiphospholipid antibodies: a comparative study in 46 patients. Medicine (Baltimore). 1999;78:209–219

Solvent exposure

Exposure to organic solvents, either accidentally or recreationally (e.g., glue sniffing), may occasionally be associated with neurological problems, especially if exposure is acute and occurs in poorly ventilated locations:

- Acute cerebellar ataxia, e.g., with toluene, carbon tetrachloride.
- Psychosis, cognitive impairment, pyramidal signs: toluene ("glue sniffers' encephalopathy").
- Encephalopathy + behavioral disturbances with acute inhalation of carbon disulfide; chronic exposure may lead to extrapyramidal signs, retinopathy, peripheral neuropathy.
- Neuropathy, predominantly motor +/– dysautonomia with acute use of/ exposure to hexacarbon solvents; with long-term exposure, a chronic demyelinating sensorimotor neuropathy may develop.

Whether low level chronic exposure to solvents over prolonged periods leads to adverse effects, such as "painter's encephalopathy," is less certain. A review of 40 studies found no reliable conclusions as to brain atrophy and deficits in neurophysiological studies.

References

Ogden JA. Fractured Minds. A Case-Study Approach to Clinical Neuropsychology. 2nd ed. Oxford: Oxford University Press; 2005:222–236

Ridgway P, Nixon TE, Leach JP. Occupational exposure to organic solvents and long-term nervous system damage detectable by brain imaging, neurophysiology or histopathology. Food Chem Toxicol. 2003;41:153–187

Somatoform disorders

Classifications of mental disorders recognize a number of somatoform disorders which may often be seen in neurological clinics. Many of these patients would in the past have been given a label of hysteria (or conversion hysteria) but this is now seldom helpful, at least in part because of the pejorative overtones of this term.

The somatoform disorders include:

- Somatization disorder, Briquet's syndrome:
  - Polysymptomatic disorder, onset before age 30, usually in females. Multiple physical complaints may include:
    - Neurological (or pseudoneurological): amnesia, dysphagia, aphonia, deafness, double vision, blurred vision, blindness, loss of consciousness/fainting, seizure or convulsion, difficulty walking, paralysis, muscle weakness, urinary retention, difficulty urinating

- ○ Gastrointestinal: nausea, vomiting, bloating, pain, diarrhea, food intolerance
- ○ Cardiopulmonary: dyspnoea, palpitations, chest pain, dizziness.
- ○ Pain: back, joints, extremities, during urination; headache
- ○ Sexual/reproductive: dyspareunia, sexual indifference, impotence, menstrual pain, menstrual irregularity
- Conversion disorder:
  - One or more symptoms affecting motor or sensory function, not fully explicable by a medical condition, e.g., monosymptomatic pseudoparalysis
- Hypochondriasis:
  - Preoccupation with, or fear of, having a serious disease in spite of previous (negative) investigations and reassurance
- Body dysmorphic disorder:
  - Preoccupation with an imagined defect in appearance (may also be classified amongst the obsessive-compulsive disorders)
- Pain disorder:
  - Pain is predominant symptom, and psychological factors are judged to have an important role in pathogenesis and maintenance.

Diagnosis is often difficult (no diagnostic tests, but lots of negatives). Many patients have been repeatedly investigated under the auspices of various specialties and remain unreassured despite normal findings. Clues to the diagnosis include discrepancy between extent of symptoms and paucity or absence of findings on neurological examination, hemianesthesia (more often on the left) with clear demarcation at the midline, patches of anesthesia. Identification of present or past psychopathology, including personality disorder and previous episodes of conversion, may also assist in diagnosis. Management is often very difficult: avoidance of invasive procedures or investigations, and of addictive medications, is desirable. Previous reports of a high rate of organic diagnoses emerging in patients previously labeled "hysterical," dating from the time of Slater in the 1960s, have not been borne out by more recent studies; psychiatric comorbidity, either psychiatric disease or personality disorder, was, however, high.

References

Crimlisk HL, Bhatia K, Cope H, David A, Marsden CD, Ron MA. Slater revisited: 6 year follow up study of patients with medically unexplained motor symptoms. BMJ. 1998;316:582–586

Lamberty GJ. Understanding Somatisation in the Practice of Clinical Neuropsychology. Oxford: Oxford University Press; 2007

Trimble M. Somatoform Disorders. A Medicolegal Guide. Cambridge: Cambridge University Press; 2004

Sparganosis

Infection with the larval tapeworm of the genus *Spirometra*, from drinking contaminated water or eating infected fish or snakes, is the cause of sparganosis, a disease most often seen in the east of Asia and Africa. The mobile worm causes subcutaneous swellings on chest and legs, and may penetrate the CNS to cause epileptic seizures or focal signs (*cysts*, infarcts). Serial brain imaging may reveal parasite mobility. Investigations reveal eosinophilia and serological evidence of infection, but histology is required for definitive diagnosis. Treatment is by excision; antihelminthic medications are not effective. Tuberculoma enters the differential diagnosis.

Reference

Rengarajan S, Nanjegowda N, Bhat D, et al. Cerebral sparganosis: a diagnostic challenge. Br J Neurosurg. 2008;22:784–786

Spasmodic dysphonia

Spasmodic dysphonia is a *dystonia* of the vocal cords, of which two types are described:

- Adductor-type: causing speech to sound strangled, strained, or fading away to nothing, accompanied by a complaint of tightness in the throat.
- Abductor-type: if the cords are abducted, a breathy whispering speech results, sometimes likened to that of Marilyn Monroe.

There may often be a superimposed tremulous component. Men and women are equally affected, usually in the 30–50 years age range. An early-onset generalized dystonia with prominent spasmodic dysphonia (DYT6) results from mutations in the THAP1 gene. Spasmodic dysphonia may be treated with botulinum toxin injections into the vocal cords under direct visualization, by a practitioner experienced with these injections.

Spinal and bulbar muscular atrophy (SBMA) [OMIM#313200]

Kennedy's syndrome, X-linked bulbospinal neuronopathy (XLBSN)

A pure lower motor neurone, X-linked recessive, syndrome with onset in the third to fifth decades, it was the first neurological condition demonstrated to be a *trinucleotide repeat disease*, with a CAG expansion in the androgen receptor gene.

Clinical features

- Hand and pelvic muscles may be affected first, with bulbar features thereafter, possibly after a long latent period; alternatively dysarthria and dysphagia may predate limb weakness by years. Tendon reflexes are lost. No upper motor neurone signs.
- Fasciculations: limb, tongue, facial muscles.
- Postural tremor of the arms may be seen.
- Gynecomastia (60–90%); hypogonadism, testicular atrophy, infertility.
- Diabetes mellitus (10–20%).
- Respiratory muscle weakness rare.

Investigation

Bloods show elevated creatine kinase, up to ten times normal; no consistent changes in sex hormone levels. Neurophysiology (EMG/NCS): motor studies show chronic lower motor neurone change; + absent or diminished sensory nerve action potentials. Sensory evoked potentials may be abnormal, despite the absence of sensory signs. Central motor conduction times are normal. Neurogenetic testing shows a CAG expansion in exon 1 of androgen receptor gene.

Differential diagnosis

Often misdiagnosed as *motor neurone disease*; prolonged survival may lead to revision of this misdiagnosis. Other differentials include:

- Adult-onset spinal muscular atrophy
- Hereditary motor and sensory neuropathy
- Limb girdle dystrophy
- Facioscapulohumeral (FSH) dystrophy

Treatment and prognosis

No specific treatment. Usually only slowly progressive, with survival to seventh or eighth decade. Rapid onset of disability may occur.

References

La Spada AR, Wilson EM, Lubahn DB, et al. Androgen receptor gene mutations in X-linked spinal and bulbar muscular atrophy. Nature. 1991;352:77–79

Rhodes LE, Freeman BK, Auh S, et al. Clinical features of spinal and bulbar muscular atrophy. Brain. 2009;132:3242–3251

Thomas PS Jr, La Spada AR. Spinal and bulbar muscular atrophy (Kennedy's disease): a sex-limited, polyglutamine repeat expansion disorder. In: Beal MF, Lang AE, Ludolph A, eds. Neurodegenerative Diseases. Neurobiology, Pathogenesis and Therapeutics. Cambridge: Cambridge University Press; 2005:803–816

Spina bifida

Spinal dysraphism

Incomplete closure of the caudal neural tube during development may produce various deformities, ranging from the mild and entirely incidental spina bifida occulta, to the severe, with exposure of neural tissue to the surface (rachischisis). These defects may be associated with abnormal neurological function of the lower limbs, with or without sphincter involvement. Associated *tethered cord syndrome* may lead to development of neurological problems in later life. Spina bifida may be a teratogenic consequence of drug therapy (e.g., certain antiepileptic drugs).

Clinical features

- Open spinal dysraphism (OSD):
  - Rachischisis: exposure of neural tissue to surface; evident at birth; severe disability
  - Meningomyelocoele: most common variant; sac of dura, arachnoid and neural tissue, evident at birth; severe disability likely
  - Meningocoele: protruding sac of dura and arachnoid only; seldom neurological consequences

All OSD are associated with *Chiari malformation* type II.

- Closed spinal dysraphism (CSD) = skin-covered:
  - With spinal mass: lipoma, dural defect, meningocele.
  - Without spinal mass:
    - Simple: tight filum terminale, intradural lipoma.
    - Spina bifida occulta: incomplete closure of the vertebral laminae; may be evident only as dimpling of the skin or a hairy patch over the lumbar spine, or only seen radiologically. May be asymptomatic or may present with progressive lower limb sensorimotor and sphincter dysfunction in later life due to cord tethering.
    - Complex: split cord malformation (diastematomyelia); caudal regression.

Investigation

Neuroimaging to assess extent of deformity may help in planning surgery.

Differential diagnosis

Severe degrees of dysraphism are unlikely to be mistaken, but the progressive paraparesis of cord tethering has a broad differential, including structural and inflammatory *spinal cord disease*.

Treatment and prognosis

Surgical intervention for more severe deficits; cord tethering seldom amenable to surgery. Symptomatic treatment for deficits.

Reference

Tortori-Donati P, Rossi A, Cama A. Spinal dysraphism: a review of neuroradiological features with embryological correlations and proposal for a new classification. Neuroradiology. 2000;42:471–491

Spinal cord disease: overview

Spinal cord diseases may produce:

- *Myelopathy*, which may be intramedullary or extramedullary; the latter may be intradural or extradural in origin. Although clinical features may give pointers to these subtypes, neuroimaging is more certain in defining the locus of pathology. Certain pathologies have a predilection for certain parts of the cord, which may help in defining the cause of a myelopathy, along with the temporal pattern of disease.
- +/− Segmental radiculopathy: especially with extradural lesions.

Common causes of spinal cord disease and dysfunction include:

- Structural anomalies: Spina bifida, *syringomyelia*, dural arteriovenous fistula, AVM
- Trauma
- Compression: Spondylotic myelopathy, extradural tumors, *atlanto–axial dislocation* or subluxation in *rheumatoid arthritis*
- Inflammation: demyelination (*multiple sclerosis*), myelitis, *arachnoiditis*
- Neoplasia: intramedullary *tumors* (primary, metastatic); extramedullary tumors
- *Spinal cord vascular diseases*: anterior spinal artery syndrome, spinal arteriovenous malformation, angioma
- Metabolic: *subacute combined degeneration of the cord* (vitamin B_{12} deficiency), X-linked *adrenoleukodystrophy* (adrenomyeloneuropathy)
- Infection: *neurosyphilis*, HIV-related vacuolar myelopathy, HTLV-1 myelopathy

- Radiation myelopathy
- Neurodegeneration: *spinocerebellar ataxia, hereditary spastic paraplegia*

Investigation

Imaging of the cord, preferably with MRI, is the most reliable way of local-izing spinal cord disease and may give clues to diagnosis (tumor, inflamma-tion, compression). CSF examination may also be indicated, especially for inflammatory disorders.

Differential diagnosis

Very occasionally, compressive spinal cord disease may be mimicked by Guillain–Barré syndrome.

Reference

Larner AJ. Diseases of the spinal cord. In: Cox TM, et al. eds. Oxford Textbook of Medicine. 5th ed. Oxford: Oxford University Press; 2010:5039–5045

Spinal cord vascular diseases

Vascular damage to the spinal cord most commonly results from:

- Infarction, secondary to anterior spinal artery occlusion (this may be iat-rogenic, e.g., during thoraco-abdominal aneurysm repair). Both posterior spinal artery syndrome and venous infarction are uncommon.
- Hemorrhage within the cord (hematomyelia) and/or venous hypertension due to spinal angiomas: Broadly these may be divided into *dural arterio-venous fistulas* (AVF), usually acquired, and *arteriovenous malformations* (AVMs), usually developmental.

Clinical features

- *Anterior spinal artery syndrome (ASAS):*
  - Anterior 2/3 of the cord may be infarcted with loss of descending motor and ascending sensory pathway integrity; posterior column function is preserved.
- Posterior spinal artery syndrome:
  - Posterior 1/3 of the cord damaged, causing global sensory loss at level of lesion, loss of proprioception/vibration below the level, normal tem-perature/pain sensation, motor function preserved, reflexes lost below lesion; much less common than ASAS.

- Spinal dural arteriovenous fistula (DAVF):
  - Present in middle age and beyond, most commonly in men, with a progressive painful myelopathy; venous hypertension causes hypoxia of the cord, which may progress to irreversible necrosis (Foix–Alajouanine syndrome; subacute necrotizing myelopathy). Stepwise progression may occur.
- Spinal arteriovenous malformations (AVM):
  - Tend to present earlier than DAVF, on average in the third decade but sometimes in childhood; may be at any level, on the surface of the cord, within the parenchyma, or both. High flow lesions which may have arterial aneurysms on the supplying vessels. Spinal hemorrhage is predominant manifestation, presenting with acute painful paraplegia, back pain, sciatica, with or without meningism and disturbance of consciousness; blood may track intracranially, simulating *subarachnoid hemorrhage*. Progressive neurological dysfunction less consistent than with DAVF. The presence of a spinal bruit (ca. 10%) and/or segmentally related cutaneous malformations may give a clue to the presence of an intradural AVM.
- Metameric vascular malformations:
  - Spinal angioma in association with AVM of other organs or cutaneous angiomas: neurofibromatosis, hemangioblastomas, cerebral aneurysms; Cobb syndrome, Klippel–Trénaunay–Weber syndrome.
- *Cavernoma, cavernous hemagioma.*

Investigation

Neuroimaging: MR of cord preferred; however, AVF/AVMs may not be seen in some cases, and if index of suspicion is high, then myelography may be undertaken; spinal MRA is available in some centers. Catheter angiography to define feeding vessels may be helpful in planning treatment. CSF blood staining and/or xanthochromia may confirm spinal SAH.

Differential diagnosis

- ASAS: unlikely to be mistaken for other causes of myelopathy
- DAVF: other causes of progressive myelopathy
- AVM hemorrhage: intracerebral subarachnoid hemorrhage (intracranial angiography negative)

Treatment and prognosis

ASAS: supportive care and rehabilitation. Some authorities recommend a trial of steroids on the basis of their apparent utility in spinal trauma.

Anticoagulation or antiplatelet therapy may be considered if there is an embolic cause. Spinal AVF/AVM: Some are amenable to surgical resection, others to embolization by interventional radiology.

References

Aminoff MJ. Spinal Angiomas. Oxford: Blackwell Scientific; 1976
Lamin S, Bhattacharya JJ. Vascular anatomy of the spinal cord and cord ischaemia. Pract Neurol. 2003;3:92–95
Spetzler RF, Detwiler PW, Rijna HA, Porter RW. Modified classification of spinal cord vascular lesions. J Neurosurg. 2002;96(2 Suppl):145–156

Spinal muscular atrophy (SMA)

Hereditary motor neuropathy (HMN)

The spinal muscular atrophies (SMA) are a heterogeneous group of inherited disorders affecting motor neurones (hence "hereditary motor neuropathies"), principally the anterior horn cells (α-motor neurones) of the spinal cord but also those of the bulbar motor nuclei, resulting in neurogenic muscle atrophy and weakness. Current clinical classification of these conditions, based on age of onset, pattern of weakness, and mode of inheritance, reflects ignorance of the basic biochemical defect(s):

* Childhood onset, proximal weakness:
  - Type I (SMA1): Werdnig–Hoffmann (infantile) disease: autosomal recessive [OMIM#253300]
  - Type II (SMA2): Intermediate: autosomal recessive [OMIM#253550]
  - Type III (SMA3): Kugelberg–Welander (juvenile): autosomal recessive [OMIM#253400]
  - Chronic proximal dominant SMA: autosomal dominant
* Childhood onset, others:
  - Distal SMA (DSMA1): autosomal recessive/autosomal dominant [OMIM#604320]
  - Bulbar SMA: Fazio–Londe disease: autosomal recessive/autosomal dominant
  - Bulbar SMA + deafness: Brown Vialetto Van Laere syndrome
  - SMA + external ophthalmoplegia: autosomal recessive
* Adult onset:
  - Proximal SMA: autosomal recessive [Type IV, SMA4, OMIM#271150] or autosomal dominant [OMIM#182980]
  - *Spinal and bulbar muscular atrophy* (SBMA, Kennedy's syndrome): X-linked

- Distal SMA (*O'Sullivan-McLeod syndrome*): autosomal recessive/autosomal dominant
- Chronic asymmetric SMA (CASMA, Hirayama disease, monomelic SMA): ?not genetic

At the genetic level, childhood onset proximal SMA types I, II, and III have all been linked to chromosome 5q, and two unrelated genes in this region have been identified as responsible for SMA: survival motor neuron (SMN) and neuronal apoptosis inhibitory protein (NAIP).

Clinical features

- Muscle wasting, weakness, fasciculation of limb +/– bulbar muscles; +/– ophthalmoplegia; no sensory findings.

Investigation

Bloods: creatine kinase normal in SMA type I, but elevated in SMA type III. EMG shows active and chronic denervation, fasciculations; polyphasic motor unit potentials indicative of reinnervation in SMA type III. Neurogenetic testing to look for deletions in SMN and NAIP genes on chromosome 5.

Differential diagnosis

Motor neurone disease in adults

Treatment and prognosis

No specific treatment, supportive treatment. Prognosis varies with syndrome, e.g., death by age 2 years in Werdnig–Hoffmann disease; normal life expectancy in some of the other conditions.

References

Lefebvre S, Burglen S, Reboullet S, et al. Identification and characterization of a spinal muscular atrophy-determining gene. Cell. 1995;80:155–165
Lunn MR, Wang CH. Spinal muscular atrophy. Lancet. 2008;371: 2120–2133

Spinal stenosis

Lumbar canal stenosis, Neurogenic claudication, Pseudoclaudication

Spinal stenosis is a syndrome of exertional back and leg pain, usually asymmetric, due to narrowing of the spinal canal. Pain is thought to be a consequence of the failure to meet or respond to the exercise-induced increase in metabolic rate of nervous tissue (cauda equina) within a stenosed lumbar canal. It is most common in the third to fifth decades of life. Spinal stenosis must be differentiated from arterial insufficiency of the legs (claudication).

Clinical features

The history is the most important part of evaluation:

- Leg pain induced by walking or standing, relieved by rest within minutes (cf. seconds for vascular claudication); sitting with flexed posture may ease pain (cf. standing in vascular claudication). Bicycling typically does not induce pain.
- Ambulatory distance before onset of pain may be variable (cf. fixed distance in vascular claudication).
- Numbness, paraesthesia, weakness, heaviness in legs may also be evident.
- Spinal movements may be limited; back pain is common.
- Neurological examination may be unremarkable at rest; mild nerve root dysfunction (e.g., L5) may be found.
- Peripheral pulses should be intact.

Investigation

Neuroimaging: lumbar region CT/MRI may show canal stenosis, most often at L4/5 and L3/4, as a consequence of hypertrophic facet joints, bulging of intervertebral disks, posterior osteophytes, hypertrophic ligamentum flavum, vertebral subluxations, or any combination thereof. In addition, there may be "redundancy," buckling, or kinking, of nerve roots of the cauda equina above the canal stenosis. All these changes are, however, nonspecific, and may be seen in the absence of any history of exercise-induced pain; hence, it is the conjunction of history, examination and radiological changes which establishes the diagnosis. Neurophysiology (EMG/NCS) may show mild root dysfunction.

Differential diagnosis

- Arterial insufficiency (claudication)
- Spinal cord disease, e.g., multiple sclerosis
- Degenerative hip disease
- Metabolic muscle disease, e.g., myophosphorylase deficiency, phospho-fructokinase deficiency, carnitine palmitoyl transferase deficiency (often associated with cramps)

Treatment and prognosis

A randomized trial suggested that patients who undergo surgery show more improvement than those managed conservatively.

References

Weinstein JN, Tosteson TD, Lurie JD, et al. Surgical versus nonsurgical therapy for lumbar spinal stenosis. N Engl J Med. 2008;358:794–810

Yates DA. Spinal stenosis. J R Soc Med. 1981;74:334–342

Spinocerebellar ataxia (SCA)

The classification of autosomal dominant cerebellar ataxias (ADCA), which are usually of late-onset (>25 years), is to some extent becoming clearer as the genes for these conditions are discovered. Many of these conditions are *trinucleotide repeat diseases*, with the number of repeats correlating with the severity of the disease; the greater the number, the younger the onset and the greater disease severity. In addition, these disorders show anticipation, with increasing severity of the condition in succeeding generations due to the increased expansion of the triplet repeat. The disorders are characterized by a progressive cerebellar syndrome often in conjunction with signs of other CNS dysfunction, such as parkinsonism, dystonia, peripheral neuropathy, ophthalmoplegia, pigmentary retinopathy, optic atrophy and dementia. Although genetically distinct, many of the diseases are phenotypically similar; hence, a place remains for the phenotypic classification of autosomal dominant cerebellar ataxias.

Autosomal recessive and X-linked spinocerebellar atrophies have also been described.

Gene	Locus	Mutation	Clinical classification	Protein/gene
SCA1	6p23–24	CAG	ADCA type I (ca. 13–35%)	Ataxin-1 [OMIM#164400]
SCA2	12q23–24	CAG	ADCA type I (ca. 21–40%)	Ataxin-2 [OMIM#183090]
SCA3	14q32	CAG	ADCA type I (ca. 17–40%), including *Machado–Joseph disease* + ADCA type III	Ataxin-3 [OMIM#109150]
SCA4	16q22.1	Probably not a CAG repeat disorder	Ataxia with sensory neuropathy (Biemond's ataxia)	
SCA5	11q13	Deletions, missense mutations	ADCA type III	Beta-III spectrin [OMIM#600224]
SCA6	19p13	CAG	ADCA type III; allelic with episodic ataxia type 2 and familial hemiplegic migraine	CACNA1A [OMIM#183086]
SCA7	3p12	CAG	ADCA type II	Ataxin-7 [OMIM#164500]
SCA8	13q21	CTA/CTG	ADCA type I	Ataxin-8 [OMIM#608768]
SCA9	Reserved			
SCA10	22q13	ATTCT expansion	ADCA type III	ATXN10 [OMIM#603516]
SCA11	15q14–21		ADCA type III	Tau tubulin kinase-2 (TTBK2) [OMIM#604432]
SCA12	5q32	CAG	ADCA type I	PPP2R2B [OMIM#604326]
SCA13	19q13	Point mutations	ADCA type I	KCNC3 [OMIM#605259]
SCA14	19q13	Point mutations	ADCA type III	Protein kinase C gamma gene (PRKCG) [OMIM#605361]

SCA15	3p24	Deletion, point mutations	ADCA type III	Type 1 inositol 1,4,5-triphosphate receptor (ITPR1) [OMIM#606658]
SCA16	= SCA15			
SCA17	6q27	CAG	Huntington's disease-like phenotype (HDL4)	TATA-binding protein (TBP) gene [OMIM#607136]
SCA18	7q22-q32		+ Sensory features	
SCA19	1p21-q21		ADCA type III	
SCA20	11			
SCA21	7p21			
SCA22	1p21-q21		?? = SCA 19 ADCA type III	
SCA23	20p13-p12.3			
SCA24	Now SCAR4			
SCA25	2p21-p13		Saccadic intrusions + Severe sensory neuropathy	
SCA26	19p13.3			
SCA27	13q34	Point mutation	ADCA type III	Fibroblast growth factor 14 (FGF14) [OMIM#609307]
SCA28	18p11	Missense mutations		Mitochondrial protease gene AFG3L2
SCA29	3p26			
SCA30				
SCA31	16q21-q22	Intronic insertion with TGGAA repeats	ADCA type III	BEAN gene [OMIM#117210]

Differential diagnosis

A spinocerebellar syndrome may also occur in:

- Multiple sclerosis
- Vitamin E deficiency
- GM2 gangliosidoses
- Mitochondrial disease

References

Giunti P, Wood NW. The inherited ataxias. Adv Clin Neurosci Rehabil. 2007;7(5):18–21
Margolis RL. Dominant spinocerebellar ataxias: a molecular approach to classification, diagnosis, pathogenesis and the future. Expert Rev Mol Diagn. 2003;3:715–732

Spontaneous intracranial hypotension (SIH)

Essential aliquorrheoa, Low-pressure headache, Schaltenbrand's syndrome

Spontaneous intracranial hypotension is a rare syndrome characterized by postural headache and low CSF opening pressure. Leakage of cerebrospinal fluid is thought to be the cause: Most often this is idiopathic, but it may follow rupture of a spinal arachnoid cyst (e.g., in *Marfan's syndrome*). Low-pressure headache is, of course, more commonly iatrogenic, as a consequence of a lumbar puncture or neurosurgery; head trauma is also a cause. Acute *subdural hematoma* has been reported as a complication of spontaneous intracranial hypotension.

Clinical features

- Low-pressure headache: worse with erect posture (cf. raised intracranial pressure), usually within 15 min of sitting or standing.
- +/– Nausea, vomiting, and vertigo.
- +/– Tinnitus.
- +/– Abducens nerve palsy (unilateral, bilateral).
- If increasing headache, focal signs, and impaired level of consciousness, consider subdural hematoma.
- Hyperacute onset may occur (secondary *thunderclap headache*).

Investigation

Neuroimaging (MRI) may show thin subdural effusions (hygroma) without mass effect. Meningeal enhancement with contrast is the earliest and most frequent feature. Venous sinus dilatation +/- subdural hematoma may be seen. Radioisotope studies may demonstrate the leak. CSF shows low opening pressure.

Differential diagnosis

Meningeal infiltration

Treatment and prognosis

It may be impossible to identify the site of CSF leakage. Headache may take months to resolve spontaneously. An epidural blood patch may help (also used for iatrogenic low-pressure headache). Epidural saline has also been reported to help.

References

Nour EM, Charles TJ, White RP. Spontaneous intracranial hypotension. Br J Hosp Med. 2006;67:44-45
Wetherby S, Imam I. Spontaneous intracranial hypotension – diagnosis and management. Adv Clin Neurosci Rehabil. 2006;6(1):32-34

Spontaneous periodic hypothermia

A rare syndrome characterized by episodes, lasting minutes to hours, of hypothermia (rectal temperature <30°C), bradycardia, salivation, nausea, vomiting, vasodilatation, sweating and lacrimation, suggesting autonomic dysfunction. Epileptic seizures may occur (so-called diencephalic seizures). Between attacks there are no abnormal neurological signs. The syndrome has been described in association with cholesteatoma of the third ventricle, but is often idiopathic. A posterior hypothalamic lesion is suspected.

Reference

Kloos RT. Spontaneous periodic hypothermia. Medicine (Baltimore). 1995;74:268-280

Startle syndromes: overview

The physiological startle reflex is a rapid, generalized motor response to a sudden, unexpected, surprise stimulus (usually auditory, but also tactile and visual) which may be followed by behavioral phenomena such as laughter.

The reflex habituates markedly and is heightened by fear. Exaggerated startle responses, in which the motor response is too violent, and/or the triggering stimuli would not affect a normal individual, or there are atypical behavioral phenomena, occur in a variety of circumstances:

- Hyperekplexia: hereditary, symptomatic
- Startle epilepsy
- A syndrome variously known in different parts of the world as latah, myriachit, Jumping Frenchmen of Maine, Ragin' Cajuns of Louisiana
- Often seen in stiff man syndrome

Clinical features

- Exaggerated startle: shock-like movement, with eye blink, grimace, abduction of arms, flexion of neck, trunk, elbows, hips, knees; patient may fall; there may be urinary incontinence.
- Behavioral features: echolalia, coprolalia, echopraxia, striking posture, automatic obedience (response to commands such as "jump," "throw").

Investigation

Diagnosis is essentially clinical, from history and observation of the response. Laboratory testing of such phenomena has not proven easy. EEG may be undertaken to look for evidence of epilepsy.

Differential diagnosis

The excessive features usually make differentiation from physiological startle responses easy.

Treatment and prognosis

Symptomatic treatment with clonazepam or diazepam may be tried. Condition does not remit.

References

Brown P. Neurophysiology of the startle syndrome and hyperekplexia. Adv Neurol. 2002;89:153–159
Manford MR, Fish DR, Shorvon SD. Startle provoked epileptic seizures: features in 19 patients. J Neurol Neurosurg Psychiatry. 1996;61:151–156

Status epilepticus

Status epilepticus has been described as the maximum expression of *epilepsy*, and may be defined as a condition in which epileptic activity persists for 30 min or more, without full recovery of consciousness between seizures. Status epilepticus may manifest as a wide range of clinical symptoms, with highly variable pathophysiological, anatomical, and etiological basis. The most common forms are:

- Generalized convulsive status epilepticus
- Nonconvulsive status epilepticus (NCSE): includes absence status and complex partial status
- Simple partial status epilepticus: repeated focal motor seizures, focal impairment of function (e.g., aphasia), epilepsia partialis continua (EPC)
- Pseudostatus epilepticus

Clinical features

- A previous history of seizure disorder (although status may emerge *de novo*); recent change in antiepileptic drug therapy.
- Acute cerebral insult: *meningitis, encephalitis,* head trauma, hypoxia, hypoglycemia, drug intoxication.
- Encephalopathy, +/– convulsive motor seizures.
- Nonconvulsive status may manifest as a behavioral change.

Investigation

EEG may be helpful in diagnosing nonconvulsive status, and differentiating epileptic from non-epileptic (pseudo) status. Search for a precipitating event which mandates treatment in its own right, although treatment of generalized convulsive status epilepticus takes precedence over investigation. Bloods for metabolic derangements: hypoxia, hypoglycemia; toxicology screen; leukocytosis, raised ESR, CRP (signs of infection). Urine for infection. Neuroimaging (CT, MRI) for acute cerebral event. CSF to look for evidence of meningitis.

Differential diagnosis

- Convulsive status: pseudostatus epilepticus
- Nonconvulsive status: other encephalopathies

Treatment and prognosis

Generalized convulsive status epilepticus is an acute medical emergency, with a substantial mortality and neurological morbidity; prognosis is better if there is a previous history of epilepsy or there is a benign reversible cause. Inadequate seizure control can lead to multiple organ failure (e.g., *rhabdomyolysis*, acute tubular necrosis, disseminated intravascular coagulation). Once diagnosed, the following standardized treatment plan is recommended:

- Maintain airway, adequate oxygenation.
- Maintain blood pressure.
- Establish intravenous access (preferably two lines): one for normal saline.
- Give:
  - Intravenous benzodiazepine: lorazepam preferred to diazepam.
  - Intravenous phenytoin (or fos-phenytoin) infusion, monitoring blood pressure, ECG.
  - Intravenous phenolbarbitone or, less often, chlormethiazole may also be used.
- If seizures continue for 60–90 min despite these interventions, the next step is anesthesia, endotracheal intubation and ventilation; intravenous thiopentone or propofol are the most commonly used agents. Full ITU monitoring, including EEG monitoring, and supportive care are required.

Increasingly frequent seizures may precede the development of generalized convulsive status epilepticus: lorazepam at this stage may abort deterioration into full-blown status. With nonconvulsive status and simple partial status, the urgency is less, since neurones are not thought to be dying as a consequence of seizure activity. Complex partial status may be controlled with intravenous benzodiazepines and phenytoin. Absence status may be terminated with intravenous benzodiazepines. Simple partial status may be controlled with intravenous phenytoin.

References

Kelso ARC, Cock HR. Status epilepticus. Pract Neurol. 2005;5:322–333
Scholtes FB, Renier WO, Meinardi H. Non-convulsive status epilepticus: causes, treatment, and outcome in 65 patients. J Neurol Neurosurg Psychiatry. 1996;61:93–95
Shorvon S. Status Epilepticus: Its Clinical Features and Treatment in Children and Adults. Cambridge: Cambridge University Press; 1994
Shorvon S, Baulac M, Cross H, et al. The drug treatment of status epilepticus in Europe: consensus document from a workshop at the first London Colloquium on Status Epilepticus. Epilepsia. 2008;49:1277–1285
Walker MC. Treatment of nonconvulsive status epilepticus. Int Rev Neurobiol. 2007;81:287–297

Stiffness: overview

Stiff man syndrome was first described by Moersch and Woltman in 1956. This condition is presumed to be an autoimmune disorder associated with increased motor unit activity in the lower limbs and paraspinal/abdominal muscles. It presents with slowly increasing stiffness of the legs with jerking and falls, usually in the fourth to fifth decades, with equal sex incidence. It is associated with other autoimmune disorders and many patients have anti-bodies to glutamic acid decarboxylase (GAD) and concurrent insulin-dependent *diabetes mellitus* (IDDM). The pathophysiology is unknown: It is thought that anti-GAD antibodies may interfere with spinal inhibitory interneurones ("spinal interneuronitis"), and since GAD is also found in islet cells, they may be important in development of IDDM. Stiffness is also a feature of a syndrome of *progressive encephalomyelitis with rigidity and myoclonus (PERM)*, which is probably related. The therapeutic role of immunosuppressive therapy is debated; symptomatic treatment with baclofen and benzodiazepines may be used.

Clinical features

- Complaint of tightness and/or stiffness of axial and lower limb musculature; on examination, there is increased stiffness of the lower limbs, often made worse by sensory stimuli; hyperlordosis of the lumbar spine with increased tone in the paraspinal muscles.
- Often there are associated intermittent painful spasms precipitated by voluntary movement, fright, sounds. Such stimulus-sensitive jerks ("jerking stiff man syndrome") are believed to be of brainstem origin.
- May be associated with excessive startle response, which coupled to the above features leads to falls.
- No sphincter abnormalities; upper limb involvement rare.
- No sensory abnormalities.
- Reflexes may be brisk, plantars flexor.
- Associated disorders:
  - IDDM (30–60%)
  - Epilepsy (10–15%)
  - Autoimmune thyroid disease, vitiligo, and pernicious anemia.

Investigation

Bloods may show diabetes mellitus. Sixty percent of patients have positive anti-GAD antibodies; there may be other associated autoantibodies including pancreatic islet cell, gastric parietal cell and thyroid microsomal antibodies. Neuroimaging shows normal brain and spinal cord; plain radiology may confirm lumbar hyperlordosis. Neurophysiology shows normal NCS, but EMG shows continuous motor unit activity in paraspinal and lower limb muscles. CSF is often difficult to obtain because of hyperlordosis. Oligoclonal bands are found in about 50% of patients, with normal protein, no cells.

Differential diagnosis

- Progressive encephalomyelitis with rigidity (+/– myoclonus; PERM)
- *Peripheral nerve hyperexcitability* (neuromyotonia, Isaacs syndrome)
- Stiff limb syndrome
- *Schwartz–Jampel syndrome*
- Non-organic

Treatment and prognosis

- Symptomatic:
  - Benzodiazepines: usually diazepam, high doses (>30 mg/day).
  - Baclofen: usually at high dose (~90 mg/day).
  - Other medications with anecdotal evidence of benefit include clonazepam, sodium valproate, tizanidine, and vigabatrin.
  - Baclofen pumps have been tried with variable success.
- Immunotherapy:
  - Prednisolone, azathioprine, and plasma exchange have all been tried with variable success.
  - IVIg (0.4 g/kg/day) has been shown to be useful in this condition.

Prognosis is relatively benign, most patients remain ambulant. Major cause of death is from complications of IDDM.

References

Barker R, Revesz T, Thom M, Marsden CD, Brown P. Review of 23 patients affected by the stiff man syndrome: clinical subdivision into stiff trunk (man) syndrome, stiff limb syndrome, and progressive encephalomyelitis with rigidity. J Neurol Neurosurg Psychiatr. 1998;65:633–640
Meinck H-M, Thompson PD. Stiff man syndrome and related conditions. Mov Disord. 2002;17:853–866

Stroke: overview

Cerebrovascular disease is one of the most common causes of morbidity and mortality in the adult population. *Spinal cord vascular diseases* are by contrast quite uncommon. The diagnosis of stroke is suggested on the basis of a clinical history of sudden onset, focal neurological deficit, without alternative explanation (although the differential diagnosis is broad); moreover, cerebrovascular disease may sometimes have a subacute or stuttering onset. Most usually "stroke" reflects atheromatous and/or thrombotic disease of cerebral vasculature (arterial or venous), less often embolism (including arterial dissection) or hemodynamic compromise. A wide variety of vasculopathies, both inflammatory (vasculitides) and noninflammatory, may also result in cerebro-vascular disease. Once the diagnosis of acute arterial cerebrovascular disease is made, a number of other considerations, relevant to pathophysiology and management, need to be addressed:

- Thromboembolic or hemorrhagic? The majority of strokes (85%) are isch-emic in origin, due to thromboembolic disease, with some due to arterial *dissection*, other vasculopathies, *vasculitis*, and *migraine*. A smaller per-centage (ca. 10%) result from hemorrhage, the remainder being accounted for by *subarachnoid hemorrhage*. These various possibilities cannot be reli-ably differentiated on clinical grounds alone; imaging is required.
- Cardioembolic or vascular? For ischemic strokes of embolic origin, either from heart or major vessels, anticoagulation may be indicated. A search for an embolic source may sometimes be necessary.
- Anterior or posterior circulation? Events in carotid artery territory may be distinguished from those in vertebrobasilar artery territory, the latter affecting brainstem (*brainstem vascular syndromes*), cerebellum and occipital lobes. In up to 20% of people, a single anterior cerebral artery supplies both anterior territories, which may lead to bilateral signs follow-ing an infarct.

Clinical features

A number of clinical syndromes have been defined on the basis of the pri-mary site of the vascular lesion and the resulting neurological signs:

- Total Anterior Circulation Infarct/Syndrome (TACI/TACS):
  - e.g., Due to carotid occlusion: hemiparesis, hemianopia, +/– cortical dysfunction (aphasia, agnosia, apraxia, visuospatial dysfunction); gener-ally has a poor prognosis.
- Partial Anterior Circulation Infarct/Syndrome (PACI/PACS):
  - Two out of three of hemiparesis, hemianopia, and cortical dysfunction; better prognosis than TACI.
- Posterior Circulation Infarct/Syndrome (POCI/POCS):
  - Brainstem strokes and/or occipital infarction with homonymous hemiano-pia with macular sparing, e.g., *top of the basilar syndrome*. Variable prog-nosis. There are many eponymous brainstem stroke syndromes (some of which are interpreted differently by different authors) including:
  - Midbrain:
    - Benedikt's syndrome
    - Claude's syndrome
    - Nothnagel's syndrome
    - Weber's syndrome
  - Pons:
    - Foville syndrome
    - Locked-in syndrome

  ○ Marie–Foix syndrome
  ○ Millard-Gubler syndrome
  ○ Raymond syndrome
  ○ Raymond–Céstan syndrome
 – Medulla:
  ○ Avellis syndrome
  ○ Babinski–Nageotte syndrome
  ○ Céstan syndrome
  ○ Lateral medullary syndrome (Wallenberg's syndrome)
  ○ Medial medullary syndrome (Déjerine's anterior bulbar syndrome)
  ○ Opalski's syndrome
• *Lacunar syndromes* (LACS):
 – Thrombosis of perforating cerebral arteries supplying the basal ganglia, pons, and internal capsule. Miller Fisher defined a number of lacunar syndromes including:
  ○ Pure motor hemiparesis.
  ○ Dysarthria-clumsy hand syndrome.
  ○ Pure sensory stroke.
  ○ Ataxic hemiparesis (especially crural paresis).
 – Multiple subcortical infarcts can lead to a syndrome of gait and cognitive disturbance, sometimes referred to as *Binswanger's disease* or encephalopathy.
 – Lacunar syndromes are generally not associated with a proximal embolic cause.
• *Transient Ischemic Attack (TIA)*:
 – Focal neurological deficits of less than 24 h duration (usually less than 30 min), with complete recovery, affecting either the eye (ocular TIA, amaurosis fugax), one hemisphere, or both homolateral eye and hemisphere (high risk situation). Reversible neurological deficits of greater than 24 h duration may be labeled minor stroke or reversible ischemic neurological deficit (RIND). For patients seen within 24 h of onset of focal neurological deficit, one cannot know whether the diagnosis is stroke or TIA, and hence the name "brain attack" has been suggested, emphasizing the need for prompt assessment and, possibly, treatment.
• Borderzone/Watershed Infarcts: resulting from low cerebral perfusion pressure, e.g., in cardiac arrest.
• *Intracerebral Hemorrhage* (ICH).

A system for categorization of ischemic stroke subtypes based on etiology has been developed (TOAST):

• Large artery atherosclerosis.
• Cardioembolism.
• Small vessel occlusion.
• Stroke of other determined etiology.
• Stroke of undetermined etiology.

Investigation

Bloods: glucose (hyperglycemia associated with worse prognosis); ESR, FBC, clotting, electrolytes; autoantibodies if vasculitis suspected; VDRL; lactate/pyruvate if mitochondrial disorder suspected; thrombophilia screen sometimes indicated. ECG to look for arrhythmia, particularly for atrial fibrillation. Imaging: CXR for enlarged heart, unfolded aorta. Neuroimaging (CT/MRI) may confirm vascular cause for neurological events, and is the only reliable way to differentiate hemorrhage from infarction; also helps to localize pathology. Newer diffusion weighted and perfusion weighted imaging may also help to identify stroke. MRI/MRA may assist in the diagnosis of dissection. Echocardiogram (transthoracic and/or transesophageal) may be required if it is appropriate to search for cardiac embolic source. Carotid Doppler ultrasonography may be required to search for carotid stenosis if anterior circulation infarct, transient ischemic attack (some centers, depending upon local expertise, prefer MRA or catheter angiography).

Differential diagnosis

Broad:

- Decompensation of previous stroke
- *Venous sinus thrombosis*, other forms of venous stroke
- Migraine (especially hemiplegic migraine)
- Epileptic seizure (e.g., Todd's paresis post-ictally)
- *Traumatic brain injury*
- *Subdural hematoma*
- Cerebral *abscess*
- *Tumors* (especially meningioma)
- Demyelination (*multiple sclerosis*)
- Some *mitochondrial diseases* (encephalomyopathies)

Treatment and prognosis

Acute: nursing in a dedicated stroke unit, rather than a general medical ward, is associated with a better outcome. This may be related to improved access to medical, nursing, and ancillary care (physiotherapy, speech therapy, occupational therapy).

Aspirin reduces mortality and stroke recurrence following thromboembolic stroke but is contraindicated in hemorrhagic stroke (it causes a small increase in hemorrhagic events in ischemic stroke). Thrombolysis may have a role in certain situations if given early (probably within three to 6 h of stroke onset) but carries a risk of intracranial bleeding. For patients in atrial fibrillation, anticoagulation is the treatment of choice, probably beginning around 2 weeks after stroke to avoid risk of hemorrhagic transformation of an ischemic stroke. For patients with symptomatic carotid stenosis >70–80% surgery (endarterectomy) is advised; <70% antiplatelet agents (aspirin, aspirin + dipyridamole, clopidogrel).

For secondary prevention, control of risk factors is key: hypertension (probably should not be reduced acutely, because of loss or impairment of cerebral autoregulation associated with acute stroke); atrial fibrillation (anti-coagulation); control of cholesterol levels (statin); smoking cessation; optimal control of diabetes.

Neuropsychiatric sequelae of stroke are well-recognized, particularly depression, which mandate specific treatment in their own right.

Grading of neurological and behavioral deficits of stroke at presentation (for example with the National Institute of Health Stroke Scale [NIHSS]) may be predictive of recovery or progression.

Reference

Warlow C, Van Gijn J, Sandercock P, Hankey G, Dennis M, Bamford J, Wardlaw J, Sudlow C, Rinkel G, Rothwell P. Stroke. Practical Management. 3rd ed. Oxford: Blackwell Publishing; 2008

Strongyloidiasis

Infection with the nematode *Strongyloides stercoralis*, a parasite endemic to many tropical and subtropical regions, is the cause of strongyloidiasis. Infectious filariform larvae may develop many decades after initial infection, most often in the context of chronic illness or immunosuppression, leading to overwhelming autoinfection ("hyperinfection"). There is a risk of concurrent bacterial superinfection.

Clinical features

- Initial infection may be entirely asymptomatic.
- Disseminated strongyloidiasis may cause:
  - Abdominal pain, jaundice
  - Asthma-like symptoms
  - Acute pyogenic meningitis, progressing to coma; or subacute meningoencephalitis

Investigation

Bloods may show eosinophilia. Stool examination for larvae. CSF may show eosinophilic pleocytosis.

Differential diagnosis

Meningitis, vasculitis

Treatment and prognosis

Supportive therapy, treatment of bacterial superinfection. Anti-helminthics: thiabendazole, mebendazole; efficacy may be improved if immunosuppression can be suspended or reduced. Steroids are contraindicated because they facilitate autoinfection.

Reference

Gill GV, Welch E, Bailey JW, Bell DR, Beeching NJ. Chronic Strongyloides stercoralis infection in former British Far East prisoners of war. Q J Med. 2004;97:789–795

Strychnine poisoning

Strychnine is a potent alkaloid from the seeds of the *Strychnos nux-vomica* plant, which antagonizes the action of the inhibitory neurotransmitter glycine at its receptors in the spinal cord interneurones and Renshaw cells, so facilitating synaptic transmission. Cases of strychnine poisoning now only result from exposure to the drug when used as a rodenticide: less than 100 mg may prove fatal in an adult (less in a child).

Clinical features

- Stiffness and spasms of limb, face (causing risus sardonicus), neck muscles, reflex excitability
- Heightened awareness (hyperalert), visual hallucinations
- Tetanic convulsions with opisthotonos, lasting 30 s to 2 min
- No clouding of consciousness
- During convulsions: respiratory arrest, rhabdomyolysis, myoglobinuria, lactic acidosis; death

Differential diagnosis

Tetanus (including risus sardonicus). Other causes of *stiffness*, e.g., stiff man/ stiff person syndrome, stiff limb syndrome, progressive encephalomyelitis with rigidity, neuromyotonia, Schwartz–Jampel syndrome.

Treatment and prognosis

Nursing in darkened room, minimize external stimuli.

Diazepam or phenobarbital (GABA agonists) for convulsions; neuromuscular blockade (e.g., pancuronium) + ventilation may be required. Empty stomach (gastric lavage) + charcoal instillation.

Monitor for renal failure and hepatic necrosis; appropriate fluid support. The drug is rapidly metabolized, so support may only be required for a short period of time.

Reference

Scully RE, Mark EJ, McNeely WF, et al. Case records of the Massachusetts General Hospital (Case 12–2001). N Engl J Med. 2001;344:1232–1239

Sturge–Weber syndrome

Encephalotrigeminal angiomatosis, Krabbe–Weber–Dimitri disease, Meningofacial angiomatosis

Sturge–Weber syndrome describes angiomatous malformations of the face and parieto-occipital cortex; the latter may lead to *epilepsy*, progressive ischemia of the cortex, and focal signs. The ultimate cause of this syndrome is unknown. Venous dysplasia with resulting venous hypertension has been suggested. Although classified with the *neurocutaneous syndromes*, there is no evidence of a genetic basis and no predisposition to neoplasia.

Clinical features

- Neurological:
  - Angioma of meninges, brain, especially parieto-occipital cortex
  - Focal epilepsy
  - Focal signs: hemiparesis, hemianopia, hemiatrophy, hemisensory deficits
  - Learning disability
  - Onset of ipsilateral limb neurological symptoms and signs after trauma has been labeled Fegeler syndrome
- Dermatological:
  - Vascular nevus (nevus flammeus, port-wine nevus) covering large part of face and cranium (ophthalmic division of V most often affected) and sometimes trunk; present at birth; unilateral more often than bilateral

- Ocular:
  - Hemangioma of choroid, episclera, iris, ciliary body
  - Glaucoma, buphthalmos, blindness

Investigation

- Imaging:
  - Skull X-ray: tramline calcification outlining parieto-occipital cortical convolutions from second year
  - Brain imaging (MRI): abnormalities of cortex; atrophy
  - Angiography: abnormal meningeal vessels usually not well seen (cf. *arteriovenous malformations*)

Differential diagnosis

Other hemangiomatous conditions with neurological features, e.g., *von Hippel–Lindau disease*, *ataxia telangiectasia* (Louis–Bar syndrome), *Fabry's disease*, and *hereditary hemorrhagic telangiectasia* (Osler–Weber–Rendu syndrome), are unlikely to be confused with Sturge–Weber syndrome.

Treatment and prognosis

No specific treatment. Symptomatic treatment of epilepsy, spasticity. Early onset seizures are associated with a poor cognitive prognosis.

References

Jung A, Raman A, Rowland Hill C. Acute hemiparesis in Sturge-Weber syndrome. Pract Neurol. 2009;9:169–171
Parsa CF. Sturge-Weber syndrome: a unified pathophysiologic mechanism. Curr Treat Options Neurol. 2008;10:47–54

Subacute combined degeneration of the spinal cord (SACDOC)

Subacute combined degeneration of the spinal cord (SACDOC) is one of the neurological consequences of *vitamin B₁₂ deficiency*. The dorsal and lateral parts of the spinal cord (i.e., dorsal columns, spinocerebellar and pyramidal tracts) are principally affected, especially in the cervical region although changes may extend to the thoracic and even lumbar regions. This produces a syndrome of sensory ataxia (especially if there is superadded peripheral neuropathy as a consequence of vitamin B_{12} deficiency): Loss of vibration or joint position sense in the legs is the most consistent abnormality. In addition, there may be mild spasticity, with or without Lhermitte's sign, and sphincter involvement; reflexes may be brisk, or there may be a combination of brisk knee jerks, absent ankle jerks, and upgoing plantars. MR scanning of the cervical cord may show increased signal on T_2-weighted images in the dorsal cord extending over several or many segments ("longitudinal myelitis"). EMG/NCS may show a peripheral neuropathy, usually of axonal type.

Common variable immunodeficiency (CVID) may be associated with SACDOC secondary to chronic gastritis or pernicious anemia.

Overuse of nitrous oxide analgesia may produce a very similar clinical and neuroradiological syndrome. A similar clinical picture of myeloneuropathy has been reported in *copper deficiency–associated myeloneuropathy*.

The clinical and radiological changes of SACDOC may resolve with repletion vitamin B_{12} therapy, but there is an inverse correlation between delay to diagnosis and treatment and extent of recovery.

References

Hemmer B, Glocker FX, Schumacher M, Deuschl G, Lücking CH. Subacute combined degeneration: clinical, electrophysiological, and magnetic resonance imaging findings. J Neurol Neurosurg Psychiatry. 1998;65:822–827

Larner AJ, Zeman AZJ, Antoun NM, Allen CMC. MRI appearances in subacute combined degeneration of the spinal cord due to vitamin B_{12} deficiency. J Neurol Neurosurg Psychiatry. 1997;62:99–100

Subacute motor neuronopathy

Subacute, progressive, painless, asymmetrical lower motor neurone type weakness, affecting arms more than legs, may be seen in the context of an underlying *lymphoma*, and known as subacute motor neuronopathy. There may be associated monoclonal gammopathy, raised CSF protein and oligoclonal bands. The disease may simulate *motor neurone disease*. The course of the neurological syndrome may not reflect that of the underlying lymphoma, and is often benign with spontaneous remission. Association with thymoma and myasthenia-like features have also been reported.

Reference

Schold SC, Cho ES, Somasundaram M, Posner JB. Subacute motor neuronopathy: a remote effect of lymphoma. Ann Neurol. 1979;5:271–287

Subacute myelo-optic neuropathy (SMON)

This syndrome was seen in Japan in the 1960s and was thought to be a complication, direct or indirect, of consumption of the anti-diarrheal agent clioquinol (iodochlorhydroxyquinoline). More recently, it has been suggested that these cases may have represented examples of *copper deficiency–associated myeloneuropathy*.

References

Konagaya M, Matsumoto A, Takase S, et al. Clinical analysis of longstanding subacute myelo-optico-neuropathy: sequelae of clioquinol at 32 years after its ban. J Neurol Sci. 2004;218:85–90

Meade TW. Subacute myelo-optic neuropathy and clioquinol. An epidemiological case-history for diagnosis. Br J Prev Soc Med. 1975;29:157–169

Schaumburg H, Herskovitz S. Copper deficiency myeloneuropathy: a clue to clioquinol-induced subacute myelo-optic neuropathy? Neurology. 2008;71:622–623

Subacute sclerosing panencephalitis (SSPE)

Dawson's encephalitis

Subacute sclerosing panencephalitis (SSPE) is a chronic reactivation of latent measles virus infection causing progressive inflammation and gliosis of the brain. Defective maturation of virus in neural cells follows primary infection, usually in the first 2 years of life. Symptoms then emerge from around age 14 years, although occasional adult cases are reported. In some children and adults, another form of subacute measles encephalitis has been described that develops months (not years) after the primary infection and which leads to death within days or weeks. The illness is characterized by focal neurological signs, intractable focal seizures, stupor, and coma. It is thought to occur in immunocompromised people, unlike SSPE, but has histological features similar to SSPE.

Clinical features

- Change in behavior; decline in intellect, personality
- Myoclonus
- Epileptic seizures
- Progressive dementia
- Ataxia
- Progressive rigidity
- Autonomic dysfunction
- Late stages: pyramidal signs, stupor, decorticate posture, coma

Investigation

Neuroimaging (CT/MRI) may show involvement of periventricular and subcortical white matter. EEG shows characteristic (pathognomonic) periodic complexes, bursts of 2–3 per second high voltage waves, with background slowing (i.e., burst suppression). CSF shows no cells, normal glucose, high protein with oligoclonal bands (CSF only); detection of measles virus–specific antibodies is diagnostic. Neuropathology shows nerve cell destruction in all sites except cerebellum; lymphocytic and mononuclear infiltrates; eosinophilic inclusions in cytoplasm and nuclei of both neurones and glial cells.

Differential diagnosis

Prion disease, especially *variant Creutzfeldt–Jakob disease (vCJD)*. Metabolic disorders.

Treatment and prognosis

Course is slowly progressive with death usually occurring in 1–3 years. No specific treatment is available, although a variety of antiviral and immunomodulatory drugs have been used (e.g., isoprinosine, amantadine, corticosteroids, IVIg, and intrathecal alpha-interferon) without conclusive evidence to support their use.

References

Connolly JH, Allen IV, Hurwitz LJ, Millar JH. Measles-virus antibody and antigen in subacute sclerosing panencephalitis. Lancet. 1967;1:542–544
Heath CA, Smith C, Davenport R, Donnan GA. Progressive cognitive decline and myoclonus in a young woman: clinicopathological conference at the Edinburgh Advanced Neurology Course, 2007. Pract Neurol. 2008;8:296–302

Subarachnoid hemorrhage (SAH)

Bleeding into the subarachnoid space usually originates from a ruptured *aneurysm* or *arteriovenous malformation* (intracranial, spinal). Both lesions are usually clinically silent prior to rupture although some patients give a (usually retrospective) history of events suggestive of "sentinel" or "warning" bleeds (= "missed SAH").

Recognized risk factors for SAH include:

- Smoking
- Hypertension

- +ve family history of SAH, especially if associated with polycystic kidney disease, *neurofibromatosis* (NF-1), *Marfan's syndrome, Ehlers–Danlos syndrome* type IV, *fibromuscular dysplasia*

Clinical features

- Sudden (instantaneous) onset of severe pain, especially occipital in location ("hit on the back of the head"), often during stress or exercise, with nausea, vomiting, sometimes brief loss of consciousness.
- Nuchal rigidity, secondary to chemical meningitis.
- Subhyaloid (venous) hemorrhage in around 25%.
- +/– Vitreal hemorrhage: Terson's syndrome is the name given to preretinal hemorrhages which break into the vitreous cavity, as occurs in perhaps half of cases.
- Focal signs, e.g., oculomotor nerve palsy, may occur secondary to raised intracranial pressure and mass effect; may be a consequence of arterial vasospasm, occurring in up to 25% of patients 4–12 days following the original bleed, or due to embolism from intra-aneurysmal thrombus.

Clinical grading scales for the classification of SAH have been devised, such as that of Hunt and Hess:

- I: Asymptomatic, or mild headache, slight nuchal rigidity
- II: Moderate to severe headache, nuchal rigidity, no neurological deficit other than cranial nerve palsy
- III: Mild focal neurological deficit, drowsiness or confusion
- IV: Stupor, moderate to severe hemiparesis, possible early decerebrate rigidity
- V: Deep coma, decerebrate rigidity, moribund appearance

Though widely used, this system is neither reliable nor valid. Another classification, based around the Glasgow Coma Scale, itself highly reliable and valid, is the World Federation of Neurological Surgeons scale:

- I GCS 15, focal deficit absent
- II GCS 14–13, focal deficit absent
- III GCS 14–13, focal deficit present
- IV GCS 12–7, focal deficit present or absent
- V GCS 6–3, focal deficit present or absent

Investigation

Neuroimaging: CT is modality of choice for imaging subarachnoid blood in the acute phase; scans may be normal in a small percentage of patients with SAH, particularly if scanned very early (<12 h) after onset. If imaging is negative but clinical suspicion is high, lumbar puncture for CSF is mandatory to look for blood staining and xanthochromia, ideally using spectrophotometry rather than the naked eye; these changes are present for up to 10–14 days following an acute bleed, but may not be found if LP is performed within 12 h of onset. If SAH is confirmed, angiography to look for an aneurysmal bleeding source is indicated: Catheter angiography remains the investigation of choice currently, rather than magnetic resonance angiography (MRA). Perimesencephalic bleeds (i.e., blood confined to the cisterns around the midbrain, ventral to the pons; = 10% of SAH, two thirds of angiogram negative SAH) may not require angiography, because of the lack of association with an underlying aneurysm. In patients presenting >2 weeks after event, appropriate investigation is uncertain; MRA is often deployed.

Differential diagnosis

Broad (cf. *intracerebral hemorrhage*):

- Headache:
  - *Migraine*
  - Tension type headache
  - *Primary headache associated with sexual activity*
  - Idiopathic *thunderclap headache*
- Meningitis:
  - Bacterial, viral
- Injury:
  - Head, cervical spine
- Intoxication:
  - Drug, alcohol
- Hypertension:
  - Hypertensive encephalopathy, eclampsia
- Cervial disk herniation
- Pituitary apoplexy

Treatment and prognosis

Acute medical management includes monitoring of neurological status, fluid balance (central line recommended); there is some evidence to support the use of nimodipine to reduce the risk of vasospasm. Surgical clipping of an aneurysm (if one is found) reduces the risk of rebleeding, which carries a significant mortality. This has been the standard treatment, but in recent years, endovascular coiling techniques with detachable platinum coils have been increasingly used, initially in patients with high surgical risk and with aneurysms of the posterior cerebral circulation, particularly those arising from the basilar artery. Recent evidence suggests that coiling is better than surgery for the majority of patients. Prognosis correlates with the clinical grading on admission. Up to 30% of survivors have persisting sensorimotor and/or neuropsychological deficits, and as SAH affects younger people, there is a considerable impact on long-term mortality. By contrast, perimesencephalic bleeds have an excellent prognosis and no risk of rebleeding. *Superficial siderosis of the central nervous system* may be a consequence of subarachnoid hemorrhage. Screening of asymptomatic family members has been suggested in the past, but is of doubtful value unless there is a history of polycystic kidney disease. Small aneurysms (<10 mm diameter) have a very low rupture rate, less than the risk associated with surgery, suggesting they should be managed conservatively.

References

Dorhout Mees SM, Rinkel GJ, Feigin VL, et al. Calcium antagonists for aneurysmal subarachnoid haemorrhage. Cochrane Database Syst Rev. 2007 July;18(3):CD000277

Hütter BO. Neuropsychological Sequelae of Subarachnoid Hemorrhage and Its Treatment. Berlin: Springer; 2000

Molyneux AJ, Kerr RS, Birks J, et al. Risk of recurrent subarachnoid haemorrhage, death, or dependence and standardised mortality ratios after clipping or coiling of an intracranial aneurysm in the International Subarachnoid Aneurysm Trial (ISAT): long-term follow-up. Lancet Neurol. 2009;8:427–433

Rinkel GJ, Klijn CJ. Prevention and treatment of medical and neurological complications in patients with aneurysmal subarachnoid haemorrhage. Pract Neurol. 2009;9:195–209

Subclavian steal syndrome

A hemodynamically significant stenosis of the subclavian artery located proximal to the origin of the vertebral artery may lead to reversal of blood flow in the vertebral artery, toward the axillary artery, sometimes provoked by ipsilateral arm exercise. This may cause neurological signs (vertebrobasilar *transient ischemic attack*), accompanied by typical signs (asymmetric blood pressure in the arms, supraclavicular bruit). However, asymptomatic steal, demonstrated at ultrasonography or angiographically, is much more common than symptomatic, perhaps because of collateral brainstem blood flow. Symptomatic subclavian steal may be treated surgically (endarterectomy, angioplasty).

Reference

Hennerici M, Klemm C, Rautenberg W. The subclavian steal phenomenon: a common vascular disorder with rare neurological deficits. Neurology. 1988;38:669–673

Subdural empyema

Subdural empyema is purulent bacterial infection between the dura and pia mater which may spread over the hemispheres to lie in the parafalcine region (cf. cerebral *abscess*). Raised intracranial pressure and epileptic seizures may result. It occurs most commonly after trauma (including neurosurgery), although nontraumatic cases are well recognized, for example, in association with severe middle ear and paranasal sinus disease. Other infective processes, such as meningitis (10%), cerebral abscess (20–25%), and cerebral venous thrombosis (20–40%), may also be present. It typically affects men between the ages of 10 and 30 years, and may be clinically occult in the early stages.

Clinical features

- Headache: frontal, generalized
- Fever, malaise, meningism
- Drowsiness (rapid decline)
- Focal neurological deficits: hemiparesis, aphasia, cranial nerve lesions
- +/– Papilledema, raised intracranial pressure
- +/– Seizures: focal, generalized (especially postoperative)

A past history of sinus disease is common

Investigation

Neuroimaging: CT may be normal initially, needing to be repeated if clinical suspicion is high or there is no access to MRI. Subdural collection, hemisphere swelling may be evident. The patient may require sedation if restless to ensure adequate scan quality. Skull/sinus X-rays may show sinus opacification (frontal > ethmoid > maxillary). CSF shows a mild to moderate pleocytosis, raised protein, normal glucose; Gram stain may be normal.

Differential diagnosis

- Cerebral abscess
- Bacterial *meningitis* (partially treated)

Treatment and prognosis

Surgery: formal exploration is preferred to burr holes to aspirate pus and give appropriate antibiotic therapy. Microbiology: Common organisms are

Streptococcus milleri, Staphylococcus aureus, and *Escherichia coli*; appropriate antibiotics include penicillin, metronidazole. Control of seizures may be difficult; prophylaxis may be indicated. Complete recovery may occur, but residual disability and seizures are possible. There remains an appreciable mortality rate.

References

De Bonis P, Anile C, Pompucci A, Labonia M, Lucantoni C, Mangiola A. Cranial and spinal subdural empyema. Br J Neurosurg. 2009;23:335–340
Kubik CS, Adams RD. Subdural empyema. Brain. 1943;66:18–42

Subdural hematoma (SDH)

Collections of blood in the subdural space are more often cranial than spinal. Cranial subdural hematoma may be acute (occurring within 72 h of head injury), subacute, or chronic. The latter condition presents a particular diagnostic challenge as no history of head trauma may be forthcoming. Furthermore, subdural hematoma may mimic other neurological syndromes; the presenting features may be non-localizing, and imaging apparently normal. A high index of clinical suspicion is therefore necessary, particularly in elderly patients with altered behavior. Besides head trauma (often in the context of alcohol overindulgence), other recognized risk factors for subdural hematoma include anticoagulation, chronic renal failure/hemodialysis, and, although rare, *spontaneous intracranial hypotension*.

Clinical features

- Cranial:
  - Headache
  - Cognitive impairment; fluctuating state of arousal
  - Neurological signs may be absent, but sometimes there is accompanying papilledema, pyramidal signs, brainstem compression, aphasia
- Spinal:
  - Acute spinal cord compression

Investigation

Bloods: clotting studies, especially INR in a patient receiving therapeutic anticoagulation with warfarin. Neuroimaging: CT may show subdural collection, effacement of cortical sulci, midline shift. However, isodense collections may be missed; bilateral lesions may not be accompanied by midline shift. MRI is more sensitive in such cases; it is the imaging modality of choice for spinal hematoma.

Differential diagnosis

- Cranial:
  - Acute confusional states, *delirium*
  - Evolving mass lesions, e.g., *tumor*, cerebral *abscess*
  - *Dementia*
- Spinal:
  - Spinal epidural or intramedullary hemorrhage, abscess; tumor; acute inflammatory myelopathy

Treatment and prognosis

Evacuation of clot; through burr holes for cranial SDH, especially if acute (if patient is anticoagulated, this will need to be reversed before surgery). In chronic cases, conservative management may be preferable. Reaccumulation of cranial subdural collections may occur.

References

McKissock W, Richardson A, Bloom WH. Subdural haematoma – a review of 389 cases. Lancet. 1960;1:1365–1369
Plaha P, Malhotra D, Heuer D, Whitfield P. Management of chronic subdural haematoma. Adv Clin Neurosci Rehabil. 2008;8(5):12,14–15

Subependymal giant-cell astrocytoma (SEGA)

Subependymal giant-cell astrocytoma (SEGA) is classified as a noninvasive (WHO Grade I) astrocytic tumor. Lesions typically occur near the interventricular foramen of Monro, obstruction of which may cause hydrocephalus and raised intracranial pressure. Damage to the fornix may cause an anterograde amnesic syndrome. Although the tumor is benign, local invasion may occur. SEGA is reported to develop in 6–14% of patients with the *neurocutaneous syndrome* of *tuberous sclerosis (TS)*, and some authors state that SEGA only occurs in TS. Solitary SEGA is rare, and has been suggested to represent a *forme fruste* of TS.

References

Ibrahim I, Young CA, Larner AJ. Fornix damage from solitary subependymal giant cell astrocytoma causing postoperative amnesic syndrome. Br J Hosp Med. 2009;70:478–479
Kawahara I, Tsutsumi K, Hirose M, Matsuo Y, Yokoyama H. Solitary subependymal giant cell astrocytoma: a forme fruste of tuberous sclerosis complex? [in Japanese]. No To Shinkei. 2004;56:585–591

Sudden unexplained death in epilepsy (SUDEP)

The increased mortality in patients with *epilepsy* may be in part attributable to both the underlying disease and to epileptic seizures. At least part of this excess mortality is ascribed to SUDEP, which may be defined as sudden unexpected nontraumatic and non-drowning death in an individual with epilepsy with or without evidence for a seizure, and excluding documented *status epilepticus*, where postmortem does not reveal a cause for death. It is believed likely that SUDEP is a seizure-related phenomenon, mainly in the context of a generalized tonic-clonic seizure, whose prevention rests on optimization of seizure control.

References

Surges R, Thijs RD, Tan HL, Sander JW. Sudden unexpected death in epilepsy: risk factors and potential pathomechanisms. Nat Rev Neurol. 2009;5:492–504
Tomson T, Nashef L, Ryvlin P. Sudden unexpected death in epilepsy: current knowledge and future directions. Lancet Neurol. 2008;7:1021–1031

SUNCT syndrome, SUNA syndrome

*S*hort-lasting *u*nilateral *n*euralgiform headache with *c*onjunctival injection and *t*earing (SUNCT) syndrome, and *s*hort-lasting *u*nilateral *n*euralgiform headache with cranial *a*utonomic features (SUNA) are paroxysmal disorders falling within the *trigeminal autonomic cephalalgias* group of the *headache* classification, characterized by attacks of unilateral facial pain lasting seconds to minutes (rarely up to 2 h) and occurring five to six times per hour, sometimes precipitated by neck movement. Men are more commonly affected than women. The duration of attacks distinguishes SUNCT from *cluster headache* and *paroxysmal hemicrania*, although underlying pathophysiological mechanisms may be similar.

Clinical features

* Characteristic history of unilateral paroxysms of pain, in an orbital, supraorbital, or temporal distribution, without a refractory period (cf. trigeminal neuralgia)
* Conjunctival injection, tearing
* Other autonomic phenomena: sweating on the forehead, rhinorrhea

Condition is occasionally secondary/symptomatic, so there may be symptoms and signs related to the underlying pathology such as *pituitary disease*. SUNCT has been associated with the use of dopaminergic agents to treat pituitary prolactinoma.

Investigation

Diagnosis is by history. Imaging to look for secondary causes (e.g., pituitary tumor, cerebellopontine angle AVM) is recommended.

Differential diagnosis

- Cluster headache
- Paroxysmal (episodic) hemicranias
- *Trigeminal neuralgia*
- Other causes of *facial pain*

Treatment and prognosis

Treatments include gabapentin, lamotrigine, verapamil. Indomethacin does not help (cf. paroxysmal hemicrania).

References

Cohen AS, Matharu MS, Goadsby PJ. Short-lasting unilateral neuralgiform headache attacks with conjunctival injection and tearing (SUNCT) or cranial autonomic features (SUNA) – a prospective clinical study of SUNCT and SUNA. Brain. 2006;129:2746–2760
Larner AJ. Headache induced by dopamine agonists prescribed for prolactinoma: think SUNCT! Int J Clin Pract. 2006;60:360–361
Williams MH, Broadley SA. SUNCT and SUNA: clinical features and medical treatment. J Clin Neurosci. 2008;15:526–534

Superficial siderosis of the central nervous system

Siderosis is deposition of hemosiderin in the superficial layers of the CNS close to CSF (i.e., subpial, subependymal deposition) as a consequence of chronic *subarachnoid hemorrhage*, with associated gliosis, neuronal loss, and demyelination.

Clinical features

- Sensorineural deafness
- Cerebellar ataxia
- Pyramidal signs; anterior horn cell dysfunction
- Dementia
- Bladder disturbance
- Anosmia

Investigation

Pure tone audiometry to confirm sensorineural hearing loss; speech audiogram is much worse than expected on the basis of pure tone audiometry. Neuroimaging with MRI shows signal void around affected areas of brain corresponding to hemosiderin on T_2-weighted scans. Angiography may identify a bleeding source. CSF shows elevated protein and ferritin.

Differential diagnosis

- Meningeal infiltration (inflammation, infection, tumor)
- Intrinsic brain stem lesion
- Can mimic multiple sclerosis, motor neurone disease

Treatment and prognosis

Treatment of bleeding source if found (ideally by surgical ablation). Cochlear implants may help speech appreciation. Value of iron-chelating agents (e.g., trientine) has not been proved. If no bleeding point is identified, there is usually relentless progression of neurological signs with a grave prognosis.

Reference

Fearnley JM, Stevens JM, Rudge P. Superficial siderosis of the central nervous system. Brain. 1995;118:1051–1066

Superior oblique myokymia

Superior oblique myokymia is a syndrome of intermittent uniocular oscillopsia and diplopia due to involuntary eye movements, usually following a superior oblique (trochlear nerve) palsy. It has been suggested that some cases result from neurovascular compression of the trochlear nerve. Episodic involuntary eye movements (vertical, torsional, or oblique) may be precipitated by tiredness, reading. Slit-lamp examination may be the best way to observe eye movements. Treatment with carbamazepine or gabapentin may help. In the event of failure, surgical interventions may be tried.

Reference

Kattah JC, FitzGibbon EJ. Superior oblique myokymia. Curr Neurol Neurosci Rep. 2003;3:395–400

Susac syndrome

Retinocochleocerebral vasculopathy

Susac's syndrome is a rare, idiopathic, noninflammatory vasculopathy affecting principally young women, usually following a monophasic but fluctuating course, and causing small infarcts in the cochlea, retina, and brain.

Clinical features

- Sensorineural deafness
- Branch retinal arteriolar occlusions
- Encephalopathy +/– acute psychiatric features (easy to overlook hearing loss in this situation)
- Upper motor neurone limb signs: spasticity, hyperreflexia, Babinski sign
- Cranial nerve palsies (III, VI, VII)
- Cognitive dysfunction (impaired short-term memory)
- Epileptic seizures

Investigation

Neuroimaging: MRI shows multifocal high-intensity lesions on T_2-weighted scans, affecting white and (to a lesser extent) grey matter; lesions (infarcts) show enhancement with gadolinium during attacks. EEG may show diffuse slowing +/– seizure activity. CSF shows raised protein, lymphocytic pleocytosis. Pure tone audiometry shows bilateral sensorineural hearing loss, especially at low frequencies. Muscle biopsy (not routine) may show a microangiopathy affecting the endothelium, similar to *dermatomyositis*.

Differential diagnosis

- *Multiple sclerosis*
- Systemic vasculitides/vasculopathies
- *Mitochondrial disease*
- *Adrenoleukodystrophy*

Treatment and prognosis

Treatment effects are difficult to assess because of rarity of condition and monophasic and variable natural history. Immunosuppression with high-dose corticosteroids (prednisolone) +/– IVIg, cyclophosphamide, mycophenylate, methotrexate, rituximab, plasmapheresis have all been tried. Antiplatelet treatment with aspirin and anticoagulation with warfarin have also been used, although a procoagulant state has not been demonstrated.

References

Rennebohm RM, Susac JO. Treatment of Susac's syndrome. J Neurol Sci. 2007;257:215–220
Susac JO, Egan RA, Rennebohm RM, Lubow M. Susac's syndrome: 1975–2005. Microangiopathy/autoimmune endotheliopathy. J Neurol Sci. 2007;257:270–272
Susac JO, Hardman JM, Selhorst JB. Microangiopathy of the brain and retina. Neurology. 1979;29:313–316

Sweet's syndrome

Acute febrile neutrophilic dermatosis

This multisystem inflammatory disorder consists of acute multiple asymmetric erythematous edematous mucocutaneous plaques with dense neutrophil infiltration, with or without blood neutrophilia and aseptic neutrophilic infiltration of various organs, including the nervous system. "Neuro-Sweet disease" may manifest as *meningitis* or as a relapsing-remitting *encephalitis*. CSF lymphocytosis may be found in these cases. The clinical picture overlaps with that of *Behçet's disease*, diagnostic criteria for which may be fulfilled. However, unlike Behçet's, there is a strong association with certain HLA types (B54, Cw1). Drug-induced Sweet's syndrome has been reported. Sweet's syndrome is an exquisitely steroid-sensitive disease.

References

Hisanaga K, Iwasaki Y, Itoyama Y, Neuro-Sweet Disease Study Group. Neuro-sweet disease: clinical manifestations and criteria for diagnosis. Neurology. 2005;64:1756–1761
Nobeyama Y, Kamide R. Sweet's syndrome with neurologic manifestation: case report and literature review. Int J Dermatol. 2003;42:438–443

Sydenham's chorea

Rheumatic chorea, St Vitus' dance

Sydenham's chorea is a choreiform movement disorder related to group A streptococcal infection. The condition usually occurs in childhood and early adult life, and is more common in females. It is usually self-limiting but more persistent neurobehavioral features sometimes occur. An association with rheumatic heart disease was noted more than a century ago. Chorea may occur several months after infection. There may be an analogy with pediatric autoimmune neuropsychiatric disorders associated with streptococcal infection (PANDAS). Sydenham's chorea is now uncommon in developed countries.

Clinical features

- Chorea: generalized > hemichorea; insidious onset, progressive course, gradual spontaneous resolution
- +/– Psychiatric symptoms, e.g., obsessive-compulsive behavior, attention deficit hyperactivity disorder
- No cognitive deterioration (cf. *Huntington's disease*)

Investigation

No diagnostic test; many investigations seek to rule out other causes of chorea. Bloods: ASO titers, anti-basal ganglia antibodies; ANA, anticardiolipin antibodies; glucose, osmolality, thyroid function tests, hematocrit, hemoglobin. Neuroimaging: CT is usually normal, but MRI may show diffuse enlargement of basal ganglia (caudate, putamen, globus pallidus); PET scan may show striatal hypermetabolism.

Differential diagnosis

Other causes of chorea: Huntington's disease, *neuroacanthocytosis*, *thyroid diseases*, *systemic lupus erythematosus*, hyperosmolar non-ketotic syndrome (HONKS), *polycythemia rubra vera*, drug-induced (oral contraceptive pill, phenytoin).

Treatment and prognosis

May or may not require treatment: valproate, dopamine antagonists (e.g., risperidone, haloperidol) have been used. In severe cases, IVIg, plasmapheresis, and immunosuppression (intravenous methylprednisolone) have been tried. Condition generally resolves spontaneously, but may recur within 2 years.

References

Cardoso F. Sydenham's chorea. Curr Treat Options Neurol. 2008;10:230–235
Gordon N. Sydenham's chorea, and its complications affecting the nervous system. Brain Dev. 2009;31:11–14

Syncope

Syncope is a sudden, transient (<30 min) loss of consciousness and postural tone, leading to collapse, as a consequence of reduced cerebral blood flow. Syncope may be classified as:

- Neurally mediated:
  - Peripheral vascular reflex (vasovagal) syncope
  - Carotid sinus syncope
  - Situational syncope:
    - Cough/post-tusive
    - Micturition
    - Swallow/deglutition
- Orthostatic (postural) syncope (as in *autonomic failure*)
- Cardiac:
  - Arrhythmia: bradycardia, tachyarrhythmia
  - Valvular disease: aortic stenosis, hypertrophic subaortic stenosis
- Metabolic: Hypoglycemia
- Idiopathic ("syncope of unknown origin"); Psychogenic

Syncopal attacks may provoke secondary (anoxic) epileptic seizures which may confuse the diagnosis.

Clinical features

- Peripheral vascular reflex mechanisms (vasovagal syncope; common): premonitory symptoms (presyncope) include light-headedness (often described as "dizziness"), weakness, feeling of distance, blacking of vision, nausea and sweating (useful to exclude epileptic seizure); gradual slump to ground; pallor; there may be some twitching movements at the periphery, or even marked and repeated myoclonic jerks, but not tonic-clonic movements (unless there is a secondary anoxic seizure); nonetheless, an untrained observer may mistake these for a "convulsion" or "seizure"; urinary incontinence may occur even in the absence of epileptic seizure (some studies do not find incontinence a useful discriminator between seizure and syncope). A slow pulse may be detected. Rapid recovery, no prolonged post-ictal confusion; prolonged disorientation (> few minutes) after a blackout increases the likelihood that it was an epileptic seizure (as does increasing age).
- Provoking features: cough syncope, micturition syncope: valsalva maneuver associated with these activities may trigger an attack. In swallow syncope, associated with metastatic disease of the glossopharyngeal or vagus nerves, or *glossopharyngeal neuralgia*, swallowing stimulates baroreceptor nerves causing profound bradycardia.
- Orthostatic (postural) syncope: events similar to above associated with change in posture from lying or sitting to standing.

- Cardiac: may be triggered by exercise. There may be signs of aortic stenosis, sick sinus syndrome, *long QT syndromes* (e.g., Romano–Ward syndrome, Jervell–Lange-Nielsen syndrome), cardiac dysrhythmia.

Investigation

Neural: diagnosis is largely by history alone; eyewitness account may be helpful (but see caveat above concerning twitching/convulsive movements).

Standing/lying blood pressure: if orthostatic syncope suspected (of no value in vasovagal syncope); may need to wait a few minutes after standing before drop occurs.

Bloods to exclude anemia and hyponatremia may be appropriate.

ECG: to exclude short PR interval, long QT interval; +/− echocardiogram to exclude aortic stenosis, hypertrophic obstructive cardiomyopathy.

Tilt table testing: to exclude orthostatic syncope.

Neurophysiology: EEG: may be indicated if seizure seems more likely than syncope as cause of loss of consciousness

Differential diagnosis

- Epileptic seizure (atonic)
- *Drop attacks*
- *Transient ischemic attack* (rarely associated with loss of consciousness)

Treatment and prognosis

Reassurance is often all that is required for vasovagal attacks. Syncope of unknown origin is a useful diagnosis since it has an excellent prognosis. Drugs such as fludrocortisone, β-blockers, and serotonin reuptake inhibitors are sometimes used. For cardiogenic syncope, specific treatment (from cardiologists!) may be available, e.g., for arrhythmias.

References

European Heart Rhythm Association (EHRA). Guidelines for the diagnosis and management of syncope (version 2009): the Task Force for the Diagnosis and Management of Syncope of the European Society of Cardiology (ESC). Eur Heart J. 2009;30:2631–2171

Fox RH, Williams L, Gowers WR. Vagal attacks. Lancet. 1907;169:1804–1805

Larner AJ. Syncope. In: Cox TM, et al. eds. Oxford Textbook of Medicine. 5th ed. Oxford: Oxford University Press; 2010: 4838–4841

Soteriades ES, Evans JC, Larson MG, et al. Incidence and prognosis of syncope. N Engl J Med. 2002;347:878–885

Syndrome of inappropriate ADH secretion (SIADH)

Inappropriate (autonomous) production of antidiuretic hormone (ADH) leads to "water intoxication" with hyponatremia and inappropriate antidiuresis; thirst is also abnormal. The resulting hyponatremia may have neurological consequences, but only if severe (plasma sodium concentration < 120 mmol/L). Treatment should be aimed at the underlying cause where possible, rather than to the electrolyte disturbance itself.

Various causes of sIADH are described including:

- Ectopic ADH production, most commonly by oat cell carcinoma of the lung
- Drug-induced, e.g., carbamazepine, vincristine, *cis*-platinum
- Nonspecific effect of intracranial tumor
- Following *subarachnoid hemorrhage*, especially anterior communicating artery aneurysm rupture (although low sodium may be due to *cerebral salt wasting* in some SAH patients)
- Following bacterial meningitis, viral encephalitis, tuberculous meningitis
- Head injury
- Diabetic ketoacidosis
- *Porphyria* (acute attacks)

Clinical features

- Confusional state, lethargy, disorientation (encephalopathy)
- Muscle weakness, ataxia, tremulousness
- Epileptic seizures
- Focal signs
- Coma

Investigation

Normal renal and adrenal functions are *sine qua non* for the diagnosis of SIADH.

Concurrent studies of blood and urine show:

- Hyponatremia (Na^+ < 128 mmol/L) and reduced plasma osmolality
- Increased urinary sodium excretion, urine osmolality > 300 mosmol/L
- Normal renal, hepatic, adrenal, thyroid function
- No volume depletion/dehydration
- No diuretic usage

Cause may be obvious (e.g., SAH, meningitis, head injury); if not, chest radiography/CT/MRI to look for lung tumor; review all drug therapy.

Differential diagnosis

Other causes of encephalopathy, coma; hyponatremia (e.g., cerebral salt wasting syndrome).

Treatment and prognosis

Identify and treat primary cause where possible.
  Specific treatment of SIADH:

- Restrict fluid intake to 0.5–1.5 L/day (dependent on the severity of hyponatremia); in some circumstances, care is needed as restriction itself may be hazardous, e.g., bacterial meningitis, SAH, increasing the risk of cerebral infarction.
- Agents to induce nephrogenic diabetes insipidus have occasionally been used, e.g., demeclocycline (demethylchlortetracycline), lithium, phenytoin.
- Occasionally, sodium replacement may be indicated (2N NaCl); however, rapid correction is best avoided since it increases the risk of "osmotic demyelination syndrome" or *central pontine and extrapontine myelinolysis*.

Reference

Robertson GL. Syndrome of inappropriate antidiuresis. N Engl J Med. 1989;321: 538–539

Synucleinopathy

Lewy bodies are eosinophilic neuronal inclusions, found in various neurological disorders, classically idiopathic *Parkinson's disease*, within the cell bodies of surviving substantia nigra neurones. These inclusions are also immunopositive for the protein α-synuclein. A large kindred of autosomal dominant Parkinson's disease, the Contursi kindred, was linked to a substitution mutation in the gene encoding α-synuclein, labeled PD1, in 1997. The mutation occurs in a position which may disrupt protein α-helical structure in favor of β-sheet; it is possible that self-aggregation of the mutant protein might be the result. α-Synuclein immunohistochemistry has shown this protein to be the major filamentous component of Lewy bodies in both PD and *dementia with Lewy bodies (DLB)*, hence the use of "synucleinopathy" as a generic term. α-Synuclein is also present in *Alzheimer's disease* (a *tauopathy*) cases with Lewy bodies. The glial cytoplasmic inclusions of *multiple system atrophy* also contain α-synuclein, although Lewy bodies are not seen. *REM behavior disorder* is common to several of these synuclein disorders, and may precede more obvious motor features.

References

Polymeropoulos MH, Lavedan C, Leroy E, et al. Mutation in the α-synuclein gene identified in families with Parkinson's disease. Science. 1997;276:2045–2047

Spillantini MG, Crowther RA, Jakes R, Hasegawa M, Goedert M. α-synuclein in filamentous inclusions of Lewy bodies from Parkinson's disease and dementia with Lewy bodies. Proc Natl Acad Sci USA. 1998;95:6469–6473

Syringomyelia and syringobulbia

Cystic myelopathy

Syringomyelia, or syringohydromyelia, is an expanding fluid-filled cavity within the spinal cord, which gradually impinges on nervous tissue, initially the crossing spinothalamic fibers of the ventral funiculus of the cord producing a suspended (vest-like, "cuirasse") and dissociated sensory loss (pain and temperature affected, other modalities spared), but eventually involving descending motor pathways causing a paraparesis, and anterior horn cells causing localized lower motor neurone signs. The cavity may extend into the brainstem, where it is known as syringobulbia, causing cranial nerve signs. The cause of such cavities is uncertain but may relate to disordered CSF hydrodynamics. Syringomyelia is often associated with structural anomalies of the foramen magnum (*Chiari malformations*) and *hydrocephalus*, but there are other recognized causes and associations. A simple classification is as follows:

- Developmental
- Acquired:
  - Sequel to:
    - Spinal cord trauma ("cystic myelopathy")
    - Spinal cord tumors
    - Arachnoiditis
    - Intrinsic spinal cord inflammation (rare)
- Idiopathic

Clinical features

- Early: dissociated sensory loss (spinothalamic) in suspended pattern; may be asymmetrical; painless trauma to fingers and hands may occur
- Late: upper limb radicular features; Charcot joints in upper limb; lower limb upper motor neurone features
- Very late: dorsal column loss
- +/– autonomic features

Investigation

Neuroimaging (MRI) shows cavity within cord; views of the foramen magnum for Chiari malformations, and the brain for hydrocephalus, should be included. Neurophysiology (EMG/NCS) may show denervation changes with fibrillation potentials, causing confusion with *motor neurone disease* if sensory signs are minimal.

Differential diagnosis

Other intrinsic spinal cord pathologies, such as tumor, trauma, inflammation. A selective loss of pain and temperature modalities with relative preservation of vibration and position sense (pseudosyringomyelia) may also be seen in amyloid polyneuropathy and *Tangier disease* (small fiber sensory neuropathy). Predominance of motor signs may lead to suspicion of MND.

Treatment and prognosis

Where possible, treatment is of the cause, e.g., foramen magnum decompression, tumor resection, treatment of inflammatory disorders. In idiopathic cases, the judgment as to whether some form of surgical intervention will be beneficial is difficult. Some cavities are slowly but relentlessly progressive and lead to significant disability.

References

Brodbelt AR, Stoodley MA. Post-traumatic syringomyelia: a review. J Clin Neurosci. 2003;10:401–408
Larner AJ, Muqit MMK, Glickman S. Concurrent syrinx and inflammatory CNS disease detected by magnetic resonance imaging: an illustrative case and review of the literature. Medicine (Baltimore). 2002;81:41–50
Levine DN. The pathogenesis of syringomyelia associated with lesions at the foramen magnum: a critical review of existing theories and proposal of a new hypothesis. J Neurol Sci. 2004;220:3–21

Systemic lupus erythematosus (SLE)

Systemic lupus erythematosus (SLE) is a multisystem autoimmune disorder of the *collagen vascular disorder* group; very rarely there may be a true vasculitis. It is more common in women and Afro-Caribbeans. Diagnostic criteria are available, as is a disease activity index.

Clinical features

- Neurological: occur in 25–75% of patients affected in different series, but uncommon as a presenting sign of SLE.
  - CNS:
    - Headache: migraine, venous sinus thrombosis, idiopathic intracranial hypertension, aseptic meningitis
    - Psychiatric: hallucinations, delusions, schizophreniform psychosis, depression
    - *Delirium*: "lupus encephalopathy"
    - Arterial strokes, repeated TIAs: associated with anticardiolipin antibodies (secondary *antiphospholipid syndrome*); cerebral embolism secondary to *endocarditis*; venous sinus thrombosis; may cause focal signs, hemiparesis, aphasia
    - Cognitive impairment, dementia: may be reversible (not if due to multiple infarcts)
    - Chorea, choreoathetosis, ballism, parkinsonism, tremor (rare)
    - Myelopathy: acute or subacute (rare)
    - Cranial nerve palsy (III, IV, V, VI) (rare)
    - Optic neuropathy (rare)
    - Cerebellar ataxia (rare)
  - PNS:
    - Peripheral neuropathy:
    - Acute or subacute symmetrical demyelinating polyneuropathy
    - Guillain–Barré syndrome-like illness
    - Mononeuropathy, single or multiple
    - + Iatrogenic neurological problems, e.g., opportunistic infection in immunosuppressed patient
- Non-neurological:
  - Systemic: fever, malaise
  - Rheumatological: symmetrical non-erosive arthritis of large and small joints
  - Dermatological: malar (butterfly) rash, maculopapular rash, livedo reticularis, photosensitivity
  - Renal: glomerulonephritis
  - Pulmonary: pleurisy, pneumonitis
  - Cardiac: pericarditis, Libman–Sacks endocarditis
  - Hematological: anemia, thrombocytopenia, lupus anticoagulant (predisposing to arterial and venous thromboses)

Investigation

Bloods: anemia, leucopenia, thrombocytopenia; lupus anticoagulant (prolonged activated partial thromboplastin time and Russell Viper Venom time). Serology: positive ANA (usually > 1/160), anti-ds DNA (50%), anti-Ro (30%), anti-La (15%), anti-Sm (75%), anti-RNP (30%), anticardiolipin (IgG, IgM,

IgA antiphospholipid); false-positive VDRL. Neuroimaging (CT/MRI) brain infarcts, hemorrhage; multiple subcortical lesions more prevalent than periventricular lesions; MRI cord to exclude compression in cases of myelopathy. CSF may show raised protein, pleocytosis; positive oligoclonal bands in around 50%; low glucose may be found in association with myelopathy. Hunt for secondary/iatrogenic problems, e.g., complications of immunosuppression.

Differential diagnosis

Other multisystem disorders: Behçet's disease, vasculitic syndromes; multiple sclerosis.

Treatment and prognosis

No randomized controlled trial data available. Inflammation: steroids +/– azathioprine, cyclophosphamide (oral, IV pulsed); plasma exchange for acute fulminant cases; IVIg. Stroke with anticardiolipin antibodies (NB positive in 25% of normal population): warfarin (aim for INR > 3). Symptomatic treatment of epilepsy, psychosis, chorea. Treatment of opportunistic infection.

Prognosis is reasonable, but neurological involvement is second only to renal disease as a cause of death.

Diagnostic criteria

Tan EM, Cohen AS, Fries JF, et al. The 1982 revised criteria for the classification of systemic lupus erythematosus. Arthritis Rheum. 1982;25:1271–1277

References

Bombardier C, Gladman DD, Urowitz MB, Caron D, Chang CH. Derivation of the SLEDAI. A disease activity index for lupus patients. The Committee on Prognosis Studies in SLE. Arthritis Rheum. 1992;35:630–640
Joseph FG, Scolding NJ. Neurolupus. Pract Neurol. 2010;10:4–15

Systemic sclerosis

Progressive systemic sclerosis, Scleroderma

Systemic sclerosis is a disorder of excess collagen deposition in blood vessels (hence a *collagen vascular disorder*) affecting particularly the skin but also other organs. Nervous system involvement is rare.

Clinical features

- Neurological:
  - PNS:
    - ○ Trigeminal sensory neuropathy +/– pain
    - ○ Peripheral neuropathy (sensorimotor axonopathy)
    - ○ Myopathy, *dermatomyositis* (overlap syndrome, sclerodermatomyositis)
  - CNS:
    - ○ Cerebral angiopathy
    - ○ Focal hemisphere/brainstem signs, extrapyramidal signs
    - ○ Myelopathy
    - ○ Cognitive decline, dementia (rare, but potentially reversible)
- Non-neurological:
  - Dermatological: scleroderma: calcinosis, Raynaud's phenomenon, telangiectasia (= CREST syndrome when combined with esophageal strictures); limited forms of cutaneous scleroderma occur (morphea, some cases of *Parry–Romberg syndrome, coup de sabre*)
  - Pleura, pericardia, kidney (glomerulonephritis), and eye may be involved.

Investigation

Serology: anti-centromere antibodies (85%); anti-SCL70 (50%); raised creatine kinase with muscle involvement. CSF may show: raised protein.

Differential diagnosis

Other collagen vascular disorders; eosinophilic fasciitis may mimic skin lesions.

Treatment and prognosis

Very difficult: no disease-modifying drugs known; symptomatic treatment of trigeminal sensory neuropathy (e.g., carbamazepine, gabapentin). Prognosis reasonable, renal and cardiac involvement being the principal causes of death.

Reference

Scolding N. Neurological complications of rheumatological and connective tissue disorders. In: Scolding NJ, ed. Immunological and Inflammatory Disorders of the Central Nervous System. Oxford: Butterworth Heinemann; 1999:147–180

T

Takayasu's arteritis

Aortic arch/branch disease, Pulseless disease

Takayasu's disease is a form of *vasculitis* affecting large blood vessels, especially the aorta and the proximal portions of its major branches, occurring particularly in young women.

Clinical features

- Neurological:
  - Syncope, especially related to exercise
  - Headache
  - TIA (carotid territory)
  - Completed stroke (hemiparesis)
  - +/– Epileptic seizures
  - +/– Myelopathy
- Absence of peripheral pulses, different blood pressure in two arms, bruits
- Acute limb ischemia
- Hypertension, angina, heart murmurs (valvular incompetence)
- Visceral infarctions

Investigation

Bloods: anemia, raised ESR, hypergammaglobulinemia. Neuroimaging: angiography (MRA, catheter) is first-line investigation if diagnosis is suspected. Pathology is similar to *giant cell arteritis*; vasa vasorum are involved. Cellular infiltrate is in the adventitia and outer media (cf. elastic lamina in giant cell arteritis).

Differential diagnosis

Other vasculitides affecting large vessels (e.g., giant cell arteritis), although these tend not to affect the aorta and its major branches. Occlusive atheromatous vascular disease.

714

Treatment and prognosis

Steroids, +/– methotrexate, cyclophosphamide. Surgery for some stenoses.

References

Numano F, Okawara M, Inomata H, Kobayashi Y. Takayasu's arteritis. Lancet. 2000;356:1023–1025
Salvarani C, Cantini F, Boiardi L, Hunder GG. Laboratory investigations useful in giant cell arteritis and Takayasu's arteritis. Clin Exp Rheumatol. 2003;21(Suppl 32):S23–S28

Tangier disease [OMIM#205400]

Analphalipoproteinemia, Familial high-density lipoprotein deficiency

Tangier disease is a very rare autosomal recessive disorder affecting the reticuloendothelial system and peripheral nerves, with onset in childhood, resulting from severe deficiency of plasma high-density lipoproteins (HDL) leading to cholesterol ester deposition in many tissues. The condition was originally described in individuals originating from Tangier Island, Virginia. Mutations in a gene on chromosome 9q31 encoding the ATP binding cassette transporter 1 (ABCA1) protein are responsible.

Clinical features

Two neuropathic variants are described:

- Progressive symmetrical neuropathy: faciobrachial muscle wasting and weakness with dissociated pain and temperature loss.
- Relapsing multifocal mononeuropathies (cranial, trunk, limb nerves).

Other features include:

- Enlarged yellow-orange tonsils (cholesterol-laden).
- Early atherosclerosis.

Investigation

Bloods show low (virtually zero) HDL and serum cholesterol, with raised or normal triglycerides; the lipid profile is diagnostic. Neurophysiology (EMG/NCS) shows reduced motor conduction velocities and reduced amplitude sensory nerve action potentials. Nerve biopsy in the multifocal mononeuropathy variant shows segmental demyelination/remyelination; in the symmetrical variant, there is loss of small myelinated and unmyelinated fibers and lipid vacuoles in Schwann cells. Bone marrow examination shows fat-laden macrophages. Neurogenetic testing shows mutation (insertion, deletion) of the ABCA1 gene.

Differential diagnosis

Progressive symmetrical neuropathy may be mistaken for *syringomyelia*; multifocal mononeuropathy variant may be confused with vasculitic neuropathies and *hereditary neuropathy with liability to pressure palsies*.

Treatment and prognosis

No specific treatment known.

References

Brousseau ME, Schaefer EJ, Dupuis J, et al. Novel mutations in the gene encoding ATP-binding cassette 1 in four Tangier disease kindreds. J Lipid Res. 2000;41:433–441
Frederickson DS, Altrocchi PH, Avioli LV, Goodman DS, Goodman HL. Tangier disease. Ann Intern Med. 1961;55:1016–1031
Pollock M, Nukada H, Frith RW, Simcock JP, Allpress S. Peripheral neuropathy in Tangier disease. Brain. 1983;106:911–928

Tarlov cyst

Perineural cyst, Sacral nerve root cyst

Cysts of the sacral nerve roots are sufficiently common to be regarded as normal variants. Often asymmetrical, with imaging density as for CSF, they may enlarge the nerve root/sheath complex and cause benign expansion of the sacral nerve root canal. They may sometimes be associated with sciatica-like pain. They are well-visualized by MR imaging. There may be electro-physiological abnormalities, specifically abnormal sural sensory nerve action potentials (SNAPs) but motor nerve conduction studies are normal.

References

Cattaneo L, Pavesi G, Mancia D. Sural nerve abnormalities in sacral perineural (Tarlov) cysts. J Neurol. 2001;248:623–624
Tarlov IM. Sacral Nerve Root Cysts. Another Cause of the Sciatic or Cauda Equina Syndrome. Springfield, CT: Charles C Thomas; 1953

Tauopathy

Tauopathy is the generic name for conditions resulting from abnormal processing of the microtubule-associated protein tau, which is an important component of the neuronal cytoskeleton. These conditions may result from mutations within the gene encoding tau on chromosome 17. Various phenotypes have been described, including:

- *Frontotemporal dementia with parkinsonism linked to chromosome 17 (FTDP-17).*
- Disinhibition-dementia-parkinsonism-amyotrophy-complex (DDPAC).
- Pallido-ponto-nigral degeneration (PPND).
- Familial *progressive subcortical gliosis* of Neumann (PSG).

A number of other neurodegenerative conditions may be described as tauopathies, even though they are not linked to tau gene mutations, since there is abnormal tau protein processing, manifested as intraneuronal neurofibrillary tangles and neuropil threads, or abnormal tau protein isoform profiles. Some are associated with tau gene polymorphisms, which seem to be risk factors for disease development:

- Alzheimer's disease (AD)
- Argyrophilic grain disease (AGD)
- Corticobasal degeneration (CBD)
- Pick's disease (FTLD-tau)
- Progressive supranuclear palsy (PSP)

Reference

Lee VM, Goedert M, Trojanowski JQ. Neurodegenerative tauopathies. Annu Rev Neurosci. 2001;24:1121–1159

Tay–Sachs disease [OMIM#272800]

β-hexosaminidase A deficiency, GM2 gangliosidosis

Tay–Sachs disease is the most common form of the severe late-infantile variant of GM2 gangliosidosis. Formerly common among Ashkenazi Jews, the incidence has dropped as a result of carrier screening and prenatal diagnosis. Unlike GM1 gangliosidosis, visceromegaly and bone involvement are not features of GM2 gangliosidosis, with the exception of *Sandhoff disease.*

Clinical features

- Type 1: Infantile: Tay–Sachs disease, Familial amaurotic idiocy
  - Total hexosaminadase A deficiency: mutations in α-subunit, chromosome 15q23
  - Onset in first 3–6 months of life
  - Developmental delay and then regression
  - Progressive irritability with exaggerated startle response (auditory myoclonus)
  - Macrocephaly
  - Hypotonia, which then develops into spasticity
  - Myoclonic seizures: difficult to control
  - Visual failure: macular cherry-red spot (Tay sign)
  - Deafness
- Type 2: Juvenile:
  - Reduced hexosaminidase A activity
  - Onset from 2–6 years of age
  - Gait difficulty with ataxia initially
  - Spastic paraplegia and decerebrate rigidity
  - Intellectual decline, dementia
  - Polymyoclonus
  - Epileptic seizures
  - Dystonia
  - Visual loss is a late feature
- Type 3: Adult:
  - Partial hexosaminidase A deficiency
  - Onset over 15 years of age
  - Variable phenotype: either slowly progressive muscular atrophy, spinocerebellar syndrome, or speech loss, dysarthria, spastic paraparesis, cerebellar ataxia, dystonia, choreoathetosis

Investigation

Bloods: vacuolated leukocytes may be seen; enzyme deficiency may be measured in plasma, leukocytes, or fibroblasts. Neuroimaging (CT/MRI) may show typical bright thalami. Neurophysiology: abnormal EEG, abnormal ERG/VEP. Neurogenetic testing for mutations in hexosaminidase α-subunit (chromosome 15q23), β-subunit (chromosome 5), or GM2 glycoprotein activator gene (chromosome 5q32–33).

Differential diagnosis

Sandhoff disease.

Treatment and prognosis

No specific treatment. Type 1 patients typically die before the age of 3 years; type 2 patients typically die in second decade of life; type 3 patients may survive to middle adulthood.

Reference

Shapiro BE, Logigian EL, Kolodny EH, Pastores GM. Late-onset Tay-Sachs disease: the spectrum of peripheral neuropathy in 30 affected patients. Muscle Nerve. 2008;38:1012–1015

Teratoma

A *germ-cell tumor*, an example of a *pineal gland tumor* in which it often occurs as a radiologically and histologically heterogeneous lesion with multiloculated cysts. There may be raised serum and CSF levels of α-fetoprotein.

Tetanus

Infection with the Gram-negative anaerobic bacillus *Clostridium tetani*, particularly in necrotic wounds or septic abortion, may result in tetanus due to release of the bacterial exotoxin. Tetanus is now very rare in industrialized countries due to the widespread availability of immunization with tetanus toxoid.

Clinical features

- Stiffness, pain, rigidity in voluntary muscles, leading to involuntary spasms, e.g., in the jaw (trismus), and dystonic movements in the face (risus sardonicus), back (opisthotonos), abdomen, neck, pharynx, and larynx causing dysphagia and respiratory failure.
- Minimal fever.
- Ophthalmoplegia, facial weakness rare.
- History and/or signs of responsible wound, trauma, intravenous drug use.

Investigation

Diagnosis is usually clinically obvious, although the wound site may not always be obvious. CSF is normal (cf. *Rabies*) but EMG may show continuous muscle unit activity.

Differential diagnosis

- Drug-induced *dystonia*
- Rabies
- *Strychnine poisoning*
- *Progressive encephalomyelitis with rigidity and myoclonus* (PERM)

Treatment and prognosis

Debridement of the wound, clearing all necrotic tissue. Intravenous antibiotics (benzylpenicillin); antitetanus immunoglobulin. Supportive nursing including sedation, paralysis/intubation/ventilation if respiration is threatened. Recovery occurs over several months; 10% case fatality. Prevention is with tetanus toxoid immunization.

References

Farrar JJ, Yen LM, Cook T, et al. Tetanus. J Neurol Neurosurg Psychiatry. 2000;69: 292–301
Thwaites CL. Tetanus. Pract. Neurol. 2002;2:130–137

Tethered cord syndrome

Low conus syndrome

Malascent of the conus medullaris of the spinal cord during development may have various causes: intradural fibrous adhesions, intradural lipomas, *diastematomyelia*, tight filum terminale. These result in a syndrome characterized by lower limb sensorimotor dysfunction and pain, which may present at any time between birth and the second or third decade of life.

Clinical features

- Progressive lower limb sensorimotor segmental deficits
- Intense pain in perineo-gluteal region
- Non-dermatomal leg pain

- Cutaneous stigmata of spinal dysraphism, e.g., subcutaneous lipoma, midline hypertrichosis, sacral naevus
- Bladder or bowel dysfunction
- Mild lower limb upper motor neurone signs, ascribed to longitudinal stresses transmitted within the spinal cord

Investigation

Plain spinal radiography: spina bifida in >95%. MRI may show tethering and cause thereof

Differential diagnosis

- Multiple lumbosacral radiculopathy
- *Cauda equina syndrome*

Treatment and prognosis

Some causes of tethered cord syndrome may be amenable to surgical correction.

Reference

Pang D, Wilberger JE. Tethered cord syndrome in adults. J Neurosurg. 1982;57:32–47

Thalamic syndromes: overview

A variety of clinical syndromes may result from damage to the thalamus. The *DéjerineRoussy syndrome*, first described in 1906, is characterized by contralateral hemisensory loss; there may be associated hemiparesis if the internal capsule is also involved (capsular-thalamic lesion). Delayed onset pain syndrome, various movement disorders (dystonia, chorea, tremor, myoclonus), and dementia have also been described with thalamic pathology. Stroke (hemorrhage or infarct) and tumor are the most common causes of thalamic syndromes.

Clinical features

- Acute:
  - Hemisensory loss: dissociated pain and temperature or light touch and vibration; proprioceptive loss is usual, often with astereognosis; *cheiro–oral syndrome*.

- Hemiparesis, often transient.
- Hemiataxia–hypesthesia (lateral thalamic syndrome).
- Delayed:
    - Pain (thalamic pain): spontaneous or evoked by stimulation; unpleasant, persistent.
    - Complex involuntary movements: dystonia, athetosis, chorea associated with proprioceptive sensory loss ("pseudochoreoathetosis"), with or without intention/action tremor and jerky myoclonus associated with cerebellar ataxia.

Investigation

Neuroimaging: MRI is modality of choice.

Differential diagnosis

A similar clinical picture can sometimes be produced by lesions of the parietal lobe (pseudothalamic syndromes; *Verger–Déjerine syndrome, Déjerine–Mouzon syndrome*), medial lemniscus, or dorsolateral medulla.

Treatment and prognosis

Pain may be resistant to many analgesics and electrical stimulation.

References

Kim JS. Delayed onset mixed involuntary movements after thalamic stroke. Clinical, radiological and pathophysiological findings. Brain. 2001;124:299–309
Melo TP, Bogousslavsky J. Hemiataxia-hypesthesia: a thalamic stroke. J Neurol Neurosurg Psychiatry. 1992;55:581–584
Schmahmann JD. Vascular syndromes of the thalamus. Stroke. 2003;34:2264–2278

Thoracic outlet syndromes (TOS)

Cervical rib syndrome, Cervicobrachial neurovascular compression syndrome, Naffziger's syndrome, Neurogenic outlet syndrome, Scalenus syndrome

Angulation of the fibers from C8 and T1 roots entering the brachial plexus over an abnormal cervical rib or, more commonly, a fibrous band extending from C7 to the first rib, can cause wasting and weakness in the hand and medial forearm with paresthesia (neurogenic thoracic outlet syndrome). Angulation of the sub-clavian artery may cause Raynaud's phenomenon, aneurysmal dilatation, and emboli (vascular thoracic outlet syndrome). The neurogenic and vascular syn-dromes seldom occur concurrently. Division of the band or rib may improve symptoms, but careful case selection is required, since these abnormal structures may be incidental to sensory hand and arm symptoms. Unambiguous cases of thoracic outlet syndrome are rare. Most cervical ribs or bands are asymptomatic.

Clinical features

- Motor:
  - Wasting, weakness of intrinsic hand muscles, medial forearm, wrist, and finger flexors (i.e., muscles innervated by both the median, after medial forearm and ulnar nerves).
- Sensory:
  - Numbness, paresthesiae, medial border of forearm, hand +/− pain.
  - +/− Horner's syndrome.

Investigation

Imaging: Cervical spine plain films may identify a cervical rib, or elongated C7 transverse process. MRI of the thoracic outlet has been reported useful in some centers for identifying angulation of the lower cords of the brachial plexus. Neurophysiology (EMG/NCS) is required to exclude radiculopathy and neuropathy. Typically, there is reduced amplitude of ulnar sensory poten-tials with normal median sensory potential, +/− reduced amplitude of median and ulnar compound motor action potentials; fibrillation potentials in muscles innervated by the lower trunk of the brachial plexus may be seen. SSEPs have been found helpful by some investigators.

Differential diagnosis

- C8, T1 radiculopathies
- *Carpal tunnel syndrome* (thenar wasting)
- *Ulnar neuropathy, median neuropathy*

Treatment and prognosis

In carefully selected cases, removal of the rib or band leads to improvement, sensory symptoms showing greater benefit than motor. In the absence of gen-erally agreed diagnostic criteria for TOS, treatment is difficult to evaluate systematically.

References

Gilliatt RW, Willison RG, Dietz V, Williams IR. Peripheral nerve conduction in patients with a cervical rib and band. Ann Neurol. 1978;4:124–129

Povlsen B, Belzberg A, Hansson T, Dorsi M. Treatment for thoracic outlet syndrome. Cochrane Database Syst Rev. 2010;(1):CD007218.

Wilbourn AJ. The thoracic outlet syndrome is overdiagnosed. Arch Neurol. 1990;47:328–330

Thunderclap headache

Severe explosive *headache*, sudden and unexpected like a clap of thunder, mandates urgent investigation to exclude *subarachnoid hemorrhage*. However, many such headaches are idiopathic, benign, and recurrent, presumably a variant of migraine. Other symptomatic causes may also be identified. Whether thunderclap headache is a marker for unruptured intracranial aneurysm, as originally claimed, is now thought doubtful, and extensive investigation to exclude aneurysm is not recommended.

Clinical features

- Instantaneous or hyperacute onset of head pain (<30 s).
- Very severe pain intensity.
- Headache may occur spontaneously or be precipitated by Valsalva maneuver, sexual activity, or exercise.
- Duration usually 1 h to 10 days; may be up to 4 weeks.
- Headache may recur over a 7-day period but not regularly over subsequent weeks and months.

Investigation

Investigation is always required to rule out secondary causes. Neuroimaging: CT to exclude subarachnoid hemorrhage; if negative, proceed to CSF examination to look for blood, xanthochromia; opening pressure. If CT, CSF are normal, then additional investigations to look for an unruptured intracranial aneurysm are unwarranted. Other secondary causes may be disclosed with MRI. MR angiography: may show segmental vasoconstriction, reversible.

Differential diagnosis

- *Primary headache associated with sexual activity.*
- *Reversible cerebral vasoconstriction syndrome.*

- Secondary causes of thunderclap headache include:
  - Subarachnoid hemorrhage
  - Cerebral venous sinus thrombosis
  - Intracranial hematoma
  - Cervical artery *dissection*
  - Pituitary apoplexy
  - Spontaneous intracranial hypotension
  - Acute hypertensive crisis
  - Colloid cyst of the third ventricle

Treatment and prognosis

Prognosis of idiopathic thunderclap headache is excellent, although headaches may be recurrent.

Reference

Matharu MS, Schwedt TJ, Dodick DW. Thunderclap headache: an approach to a neurologic emergency. Curr Neurol Neurosci Rep. 2007;7:101–109

Thyroid disease and the nervous system: overview

A broad spectrum of neurological disorders may be associated with thyroid gland dysfunction, both over- and underactivity. Since thyroid dysfunction is often treatable, thyroid disease should be frequently considered in the differential diagnosis of neurological syndromes.

Clinical features

- Hyperthyroidism: Thyrotoxicosis
  - Neuromuscular symptoms (67%): myopathy, polyneuropathy (distal sensorimotor)
  - Tremor (= enhanced physiological tremor)
  - Cognitive and mental changes: insomnia, poor concentration, reduced attention span; delirium (rare)
  - Epileptic seizures (rare); exacerbation of underlying seizure disorder; *Hashimoto's encephalopathy*
  - Headache: migraine or tension-type
  - Thyroid ophthalmopathy, dysthyroid eye disease, Graves' disease: eyelid retraction, exophthalmos, restrictive ophthalmopathy due to edema of intraorbital tissues, +/– optic neuropathy (rare)

- Chorea (rare)
- Parkinsonism: may be chance concurrence of two common conditions
- Acute neuropathy (Basedow's paraplegia; rare)
- Association with other neurological disorders, e.g., *myasthenia gravis*, thyrotoxic *periodic paralysis* (Kitamura syndrome)
- Hypothyroidism:
  - Neuromuscular symptoms (75%): myopathy, mononeuropathy, sensorimotor axonal polyneuropathy, carpal tunnel syndrome, slow-relaxing ("hung-up") tendon reflexes (pseudomyotonia; Woltman's sign)
  - Epileptic seizures; Hashimoto's encephalopathy
  - Cognitive slowing; dementia, coma
  - Neuropsychiatric syndromes: psychosis ("myxedema madness"), delirium
  - Cerebellar ataxia (controversial: one case reported as such was later shown to have pathology of multiple system atrophy)
  - Hearing loss, vestibular dysfunction (congenital): Pendred's syndrome

Investigation

Bloods: measurement of thyroid function tests, namely, thyroid stimulating hormone (TSH), thyroxine (T4) +/− tri-iodothyronine (T3). Thyroid autoantibodies (thyroglobulin, microsomal): may be present in high titer despite normal thyroid function tests in Hashimoto's encephalopathy. CSF may show raised protein in Hashimoto's encephalopathy. Neurophysiology (EMG/NCS) required to investigate neuromuscular disorder. Neuroimaging, EEG may be needed to exclude other disorders.

Differential diagnosis

Of individual features.

Treatment and prognosis

Many features resolve with adequate treatment of the thyroid disorder.

References

Duyff RF, van den Bosch J, Laman DM, Potter van Loon B-J, Linssen WHJP. Neuromuscular findings in thyroid dysfunction: a prospective clinical and electrodiagnostic study. J Neurol Neurosurg Psychiatry. 2000;68:750–755

Mistry N, Wass J, Turner MR. When to consider thyroid dysfunction in the neurology clinic. Pract Neurol. 2009;9:145–156

Swanson JW, Kelly JJ, McConahey WM. Neurologic aspects of thyroid dysfunction. Mayo Clin Proc. 1981;56:504–512

Tibial muscular dystrophy [OMIM#600334]

Udd myopathy

Common in Finland, this *distal myopathy* is characterized by weakness in ankle dorsiflexion beginning in the fourth decade, with visible atrophy in the anterior compartment of lower leg muscles. Progression is slow and often asymmetrical, with development of foot drop and sometimes proximal lower limb weakness. Serum creatine kinase may be mildly elevated. Fatty degeneration of anterior tibial muscles is seen on MRI. The condition results from mutations in the titin gene and hence is allelic with *limb girdle muscular dystrophy* type 2J.

Reference

Hackman P, Marchand S, Sarparanta J, et al. Truncating mutations in C terminal titin may cause more severe tibial muscular dystrophy (TMD). Neuromuscul Disord. 2008;18:922–928

Tibial neuropathy

The tibial nerve emerges from the medial trunk of the sciatic nerve, carrying fibers from L5-S2 roots, to supply gastrocnemius, soleus, tibialis posterior, flexor digitorum, hallucis longus, and all intrinsic foot flexor muscles. At the ankle, the nerve runs posterior to the medial malleolus under the flexor retinaculum, which forms the tarsal tunnel, wherein the tibial nerve may be compressed (an *entrapment neuropathy* analogous to the *carpal tunnel syndrome* in the wrist, but a very much rarer entity). Tibial neuropathy is much less frequent than *peroneal neuropathy*.

Clinical features

- Motor:
  - Weak ankle plantar flexion and inversion may be evident; more distal lesions may cause weakness of intrinsic toe flexors only; no reflex loss.
- Sensory:
  - Loss of sensation on sole of foot.

Tarsal tunnel syndrome: perimalleolar pain, pain +/– paresthesia in the foot, wasting of intrinsic foot muscles.

Investigation

EMG/NCS may confirm or refute diagnosis, distinguishing isolated tibial neuropathy from radiculopathy or sciatic neuropathy. Slowing of distal tibial motor conduction may be observed in tarsal tunnel syndrome.

Differential diagnosis

- Lumbar radiculopathy
- *Lumbosacral plexopathies*
- *Sciatic neuropathy*

References

McNamara B. The tibial nerve and tarsal tunnel syndrome. Adva Clin Neurosci Rehab. 2003;3(4):18
Staal A, Van Gijn J, Spaans F. Mononeuropathies: Examination, Diagnosis and Treatment. London: W.B. Saunders; 1999:125–132

Tolosa–Hunt syndrome

Orbital pseudotumor

Originally described in the 1950s, this is a clinical syndrome occurring most often in the fourth to sixth decades, comprising severe periorbital pain with any combination of ophthalmoplegia, diplopia, and facial sensory symptoms reflecting multiple cranial nerve palsies (II, IV, VI, V), and usually responsive to treatment with systemic corticosteroids. It is now known to reflect granulomatous inflammation in the cavernous sinus and/or superior orbital fissure, and may be known as orbital pseudotumor, for which reason some authorities prefer to abandon completely the term "Tolosa–Hunt syndrome." Wegener's granulomatosis, sarcoidosis, and lymphoma enter the differential diagnosis. *Ophthalmoplegic migraine* enters the differential diagnosis, as do other causes of *cavernous sinus disease* or the superior orbital fissure syndrome. Imaging of this area, preferably with MRI, is therefore mandatory in any patient presenting with these clinical features. Should corticosteroids fail or be contraindicated, other immunosuppressive agents or radiotherapy may be used.

References

La Mantia L, Curone M, Rapoport AM, et al. Tolosa-Hunt syndrome: critical literature review based on IHS 2004 criteria. Cephalalgia. 2006;26:772–781

Tolosa E. Periarteritic lesions of the carotid siphon with the clinical features of a carotid infraclinoidal aneurysm. J Neurol Neurosurg Psychiatry. 1954;17:300–302

Top of the basilar syndrome

Rostral basilar artery syndrome

"Top of the basilar" syndrome is the result of infarction of midbrain, thalamus, and portions of the occipital and temporal lobes due to occlusion of the rostral basilar artery, usually due to an embolus, resulting in severe visual, oculomotor, and behavioral features without prominent motor or sensory features. It may be classified with the *brainstem vascular syndromes*.

Clinical features

- Behavioral features: acute confusional state invariable, +/– drowsiness, coma
  - Posterior hemisphere:
    - Visual agnosia
    - Anosognosia
    - *Klüver–Bucy syndrome*
    - Color anomia, amnesia
    - Topographic disorientation
    - Anton's syndrome
    - Balint's syndrome
    - Charcot–Wilbrand syndrome
  - Brainstem/diencephalon:
    - Peduncular hallucinosis
    - Change in sleep/wake cycle
    - Pathological crying
- Ophthalmic/visual features
  - Posterior hemisphere:
    - Homonymous hemianopia
    - Visual hallucinations
    - Visual illusory phenomena (allesthesia, palinopsia)
  - Brainstem/diencephalon:
    - Internuclear ophthalmoplegia
    - Vertical gaze paresis
    - *Parinaud's syndrome*
    - Weber syndrome
    - Benedikt syndrome
    - Nothnagel syndrome
- Motor features.
    - Cerebellar ataxia

Investigation

Bloods to look for evidence of vasculitis. Neuroimaging (MRI) to show extent of infarction, and any abnormalities in the basilar artery (occlusion). Echocardiography may be required to look for embolic source.

Differential diagnosis

Other causes of *delirium* (acute confusional state).

Treatment and prognosis

The outlook is poor if there is a previous history of hypertension and vertebrobasilar ischemic episodes; in the absence of these features, the syndrome may be reversible with a good prognosis. Secondary prevention measures and appropriate treatment of any embolic source are indicated.

References

Caplan LR. "Top of the basilar" syndrome. Neurology. 1980;30:72–79
Mehler MF. The rostral basilar artery syndrome: diagnosis, etiology, prognosis. Neurology. 1989;39:9–16

Tourette syndrome (TS)

Gilles de la Tourette syndrome

Tourette syndrome is a condition of multiple vocal and motor tics of variable severity, more common in males (M:F = 4:1), sometimes occurring in conjunction with an obsessive-compulsive disorder. The condition typically develops in adolescence. Twin studies show greater concordance in monozygotic as compared to dizygotic twins, suggesting a genetic component. The pathoanatomical substrate was thought to be in the basal ganglia, since drugs that interfere with dopaminergic neurotransmission have been tried with some success, but more recently functional imaging studies have implicated the cingulate and orbitofrontal cortex. Other neurotransmitters, such as serotonin and opioids, may also be involved. The condition persists despite therapy in the majority of cases, although periods of long remission are not uncommon. Although the name derives from the French neurologist who described the condition in 1885, previous accounts may be detected in earlier medical and nonmedical literature: Dr Samuel Johnson (1709–1784) was a noted sufferer.

Clinical features

- Motor tics: multiple and multifocal; present for >12 months.
- Vocal tics: including animal noises and, in some cases, coprolalia; palilalia (repeating one's own words), echolalia, and echopraxia may occur.
- Obsessive-compulsive disorder (OCD) is relatively common; less frequently, attention deficit hyperactivity is seen.
- Often the tics wax and wane in time and change in their nature and location.
- Self-injurious compulsions may occur.
- Tourette syndrome has been reported in 6–8% of subjects with autism.

Investigation

Structural neuroimaging (CT, MRI) is normal; functional imaging (SPECT, PET) may show increased activity in cingulate and orbitofrontal cortex. CSF is normal. Neurophysiology is usually noncontributory although nonspecific EEG abnormalities are not uncommon; no *bereitschaftpotential*, unlike the same movements mimicked by the patient. Neuropsychological assessment may reveal deficits, especially in attentional domains.

Differential diagnosis

- Simple tics
- Startle syndromes

Treatment and prognosis

The course of the illness is unpredictable, but the majority of patients have lifelong disease. However, the condition often varies with time and often improves after puberty, which means that drug therapy should be initiated and monitored with care. A number of agents have been tried, including:

- Haloperidol (e.g., 0.25 mg/day increasing to 2–10 mg a day)
- Sulpiride (e.g., 100–400 mg/day)
- Topiramate

Pimozide, clonidine, tetrabenazine, risperidone, quetiapine, and aripiprazole have all been tried.

Concurrent OCD should be treated with serotonin reuptake inhibitors (clomipramine, SSRIs).

References

Jankovic J. Tourette's syndrome. N Engl J Med. 2001;345:1184–1192
Kushner HI. A Cursing Brain? The Histories of Tourette Syndrome. Cambridge, MA: Harvard University Press; 1999

Leckman JF. Tourette's syndrome. Lancet. 2002;360:1577–1586

Rampello L, Alvano A, Battaglia G, Bruno V, Raffaele R, Nicoletti F. Tic disorders: from pathophysiology to treatment. J Neurol. 2006;253:1–15

The Tourette Syndrome Classification Study group. Definitions and classification of tic disorders. Arch Neuro. 1993;50:1013–1016

Toxocariasis

Visceral larva migrans

Nematode larvae of the dog and cat ascarids, *Toxoplasma canis* and *Toxoplasma cati*, may infect children playing with infected animals or in contact with contaminated soil. A pulmonary syndrome with hepatomegaly and eosinophilia is the commonest clinical manifestation. Neurological features, though rare, include focal deficits (hemiparesis), encephalopathy, epileptic seizures, and a retinal inflammatory mass (ocular larva migrans). Diagnosis may be confirmed by ELISA. Treatment is with antihelminthic drugs such as thiabendazole or mebendazole, supplemented with steroids to reduce inflammatory complications of infection.

Toxoplasmosis

Toxoplasma gondii, an obligate intracellular protozoan parasite, causes congenital or acquired infection, the latter most usually due to contact with cat feces. Most of these infections are asymptomatic but may become manifest (opportunistic infection) in the context of immunosuppression, particularly *HIV/AIDS*-related, in which toxoplasmosis is top of the differential diagnosis for multiple enhancing brain lesions.

Clinical features

* Rash, lymphadenopathy
* Meningoencephalitis
* Inflammatory myopathy
* Focal cerebral mass lesions

Investigation

Bloods: raised creatine kinase; serology (may be –ve in AIDS). Neuroimaging (CT/MRI): multiple (> single) nodular brain lesions. CSF shows lymphocytic pleocytosis, increased protein; organisms in sediment. Investigation for underlying immunodeficiency required (e.g., HIV test, CD4 count).

Differential diagnosis

* In immunocompetent: other causes of brain *abscess*.
* In context of HIV/AIDS, immunocompromise: other causes of brain abscess; cerebral *lymphoma, tuberculosis*, cryptococcal meningitis, *progressive multifocal leukoencephalopathy (PML)*.

Treatment and prognosis

Sulphadiazine, pyrimethamine: 4 weeks in immunocompetent patients, lifelong in immunodeficient. Regression of lesions is typical in HIV; cerebral biopsy may be considered if no improvement occurs, but since treatment for the treatable alternatives (TB, cryptococcal meningitis) is likely to have been instituted, and the other conditions (cerebral lymphoma, PML) are essentially untreatable, not all would proceed to biopsy.

Reference

Porter SB, Sande MA. Toxoplasmosis of the central nervous system. N Engl J Med. 1992;327:1643–1648

Transient epileptic amnesia (TEA)

An *epilepsy* syndrome characterized by recurrent episodes of transient amnesia.

Clinical features

* Recurrent, witnessed episodes of transient amnesia, often manifested by recurrent questioning; attacks are usually brief (1 h or less); attacks often occur on waking.
* Co-occurrence of other seizure types (not in all patients).
* Persistent interictal defects in autobiographical memory have been observed in some patients.

Investigation

Neurophysiology: EEG may show epileptiform abnormalities of temporal lobe origin, more evident on sleep EEG. Neuroimaging is usually normal. Neuropsychology assessment may show persistent interictal defects in autobiographical memory.

Differential diagnosis

Transient global amnesia.

Treatment and prognosis

Generally responds favorably to standard antiepileptic medications (carbamazepine).

References

Butler CR, Graham KS, Hodges JR, Kapur N, Wardlaw JM, Zeman AZ. The syndrome of transient epileptic amnesia. Ann Neurol. 2007;61:587–598
Kapur N. Transient epileptic amnesia: a clinical update and a reformulation. J Neurol Neurosurg Psychiatry. 1993;56:1184–1190

Transient global amnesia (TGA)

A syndrome consisting of an abrupt attack of impaired anterograde memory, of brief duation (<24 h) without clouding of consciousness or focal neurological signs. The etiology of this temporary deactivation of mesial temporal and thalamic structures is unknown, but may be triggered by physical or emotional stressors (e.g., sea bathing, pain, sexual intercourse). A previous history of migraine may be found. A reported association between transient global amnesia and patent foramen ovale remains to be confirmed. Drug-induced cases (e.g., clioquinol) are also reported.

Clinical features

- Abrupt onset of repeated questioning; implicit memory functions are usually intact (e.g., driving).
- Absence of other neurological symptoms and signs.
- Resolution within 24 h with no recollection of amnesic period.
- Informant interview may be helpful, particularly if the patient is seen after resolution of the episode (as is usual).

Investigation

Neuropsychology assessment:

- During attack:
  - Dense, severe, anterograde amnesia
  - Variably severe retrograde amnesia
  - Working memory intact

- Semantic memory intact usually
- Non-declarative/procedural/implicit memory intact
- After attack:
  - Often entirely normal
  - May be subtle impairment of anterograde verbal memory

Neuroimaging: structural imaging usually normal; functional imaging (e.g., SPECT scan) during attack may show hypoperfusion of medial temporal lobe +/− thalamus. Jugular vein valve incompetence said to be more common in cases than controls. Neurophysiology: EEG is normal.

Differential diagnosis

- *Transient epileptic amnesia*
- *Migraine*
- Head injury
- Vertebrobasilar circulation *transient ischemic attack* (usually accompanied by other neurological symptoms and signs)
- Drug toxicity
- Psychogenic amnesia

Treatment and prognosis

No specific treatment. Majority of attacks occur in isolation and quoted recurrence rate is low (3% per year).

Diagnostic criteria

Hodges JR, Warlow CP. Syndromes of transient amnesia: towards a classification: a study of 153 cases. J Neurol Neurosurg Psychiatry. 1990;53:834–843

References

Bartsch T, Deuschl G. Transient global amnesia: functional anatomy and clinical implications. Lancet Neurology. 2010;9:205–214
Fisher CM, Adams RD. Transient global amnesia. Acta Neurol. Scand. 1964;40 (Suppl 9):1–81
Larner AJ. Transient global amnesia in the district general hospital. Int J Clin Pract. 2007;61:255–258

Transient ischemic attack (TIA)

Transient ischemic attacks (TIAs) are temporary focal neurological deficits, presumed to be due to ischemia of nervous tissue; most last less than 30 min, although by definition they may last up to 24 h (longer reversible events may be labeled "reversible ischemic neurological deficits" [RIND]). A distinction may be drawn between embolic TIAs, usually reflecting a source from ipsilateral *carotid artery disease* or heart disease (e.g., atrial fibrillation, *endocarditis*), and hemodynamic TIAs, where inadequate perfusion pressure is causal. Embolic events are the more common.

Clinical features

- Embolic TIAs:
  - Anterior/Carotid circulation TIA:
    - Ocular TIA/amaurosis fugax/transient monocular blindness: brief episode unilateral visual loss.
  - Hemisphere TIA/transient hemispheral attacks:
    - Contralateral motor or sensory dysfunction, aphasia, homonymous hemianopia or combination thereof.
  - Vertebrobasilar circulation TIA:
    - Bilateral or shifting motor/sensory dysfunction, complete or partial loss of vision in homonymous fields, combination thereof; *subclavian steal syndrome*.

Previous TIA is a risk factor for stroke: predictive scoring systems (e.g., ABCD, ABCD2) have been developed. Increasing frequency of TIA ("crescendo TIA"), particularly hemisphere TIA or combination of hemisphere and ocular TIA, is thought particularly ominous. On examination, there may be an ipsilateral carotid artery bruit, reflecting turbulent blood flow; but carotid bruits may be asymptomatic, in which case probably best left alone; moreover, some critically stenosed carotid arteries may not have a bruit. Evidence of concurrent coronary artery disease should be sought, since this may influence decisions regarding surgery for symptomatic carotid artery stenosis. Look for hypertension, stigmata of hypercholesterolemia (modifiable risk factors for TIA), and smoking history.

- Hamodynamic TIAs:
  - Carotid territory: "*Limb shaking*": recurrent, involuntary, irregular movements described as shaking, trembling, twitching, flapping; associated with severely stenosed or occluded carotid, exhausted cerebral vasomotor reactivity.

Investigation

Imaging of the carotid artery for stenotic change: options include Doppler ultrasonography in skilled hands, MRA, and digital subtraction angiography. Degree of stenosis is important for deciding on most appropriate management (medical or surgical). Neuroimaging (CT/MRI) for ischemic damage ipsilateral to a stenotic artery (suggestive of symptomatic effect). Imaging of the heart: echocardiography (transthoracic, transesophageal) to look for embolic source if carotids clear; this may extend to a bubble echocardiogram if a right to left shunt is being looked for. Blood cholesterol, glucose may be checked.

Differential diagnosis

TIA and minor stroke are overdiagnosed: 27% of those referred with this diagnosis were "undone" in a neurovascular clinic, the revised diagnoses for transient neurological symptoms including:

- *Migraine*
- *Epilepsy*
- Hyperventilation
- Multiple sclerosis
- Unclassified (the largest group)

Treatment and prognosis

Treat the modifiable risk factors: hypertension, hypercholesterolemia (statin). Smoking cessation, reduce alcohol intake, adopt a healthy diet. Manage diabetes mellitus.

- Medical: antiplatelet agents (aspirin, clopidogrel) reduce risk of ischemic stroke; probably ticlopidine, dipyridamole, also. Warfarin is indicated for TIA in context of atrial fibrillation, and may be indicated for mild carotid stenosis which continues to be symptomatic despite antiplatelet therapy and is not suitable for surgery.
- Surgery: symptomatic stenosis of >70% is best managed with surgery (carotid endarterectomy) or stenting, greater restenosis rate with stenting.

References

Giles MF, Rothwell PM. Systematic review and pooled analysis of published and unpublished validations of the ABCD and ABCD2 transient ischemic attack risk scores. Stroke. 2010;41:667–673

Martin PJ, Young G, Enevoldson TP, Humphrey PRD. Overdiagnosis of TIA and minor stroke: experience at a regional neurovascular clinic. QJM. 1997;90:759–763

Sudlow C. Preventing further vascular events after a stroke or transient ischaemic attack: an update on medical management. Pract Neurol. 2008;8:141–157

Swain S, Turner C, Tyrrell P, Rudd A, Guideline Development Group. Diagnosis and initial management of acute stroke and transient ischaemic attack: summary of NICE guidance. BMJ. 2008;337:a786

Transient unresponsiveness of the elderly

Idiopathic recurrent stupor, Psychogenic unresponsiveness

This ill understood condition of the elderly is characterized by recurrent self-limited episodes of unresponsiveness with no obvious structural, toxic, meta-bolic, convulsive or psychiatric disorder, and no specific neuroimaging or EEG signature. Flumazenil may reverse some of these episodes. It is self-evidently a diagnosis of exclusion (if not desperation).

Transient episodes of unresponsiveness without loss of muscle tone may represent one extreme of fluctuating attention and cognition in *dementia with Lewy bodies*.

References

Haimovic JC, Beresford HR. Transient unresponsiveness in the elderly. Arch Neurol. 1992;49:35–37
Tinuper P, Montagna P, Plazzi G, et al. Idiopathic recurring stupor. Neurology. 1994;44:621–625

Transverse myelitis

Transverse myelopathy

Transverse myelitis is an acute or subacute spinal cord syndrome, sometimes par-tial and sometimes complete. The condition is etiologically heterogeneous; pri-mary or idiopathic cases occur, but most are secondary, with an inflammatory or immunopathogenic basis, with a wide variety of underlying diagnoses, including:

* Post-infectious (varicella, EBV, mycoplasma, herpes zoster): may be a localized form of post-infectious encephalomyelitis or *acute disseminated encephalomyelitis (ADEM)*.
* Post-vaccination (e.g., influenza).
* *Multiple sclerosis* (MS).
* *Neuromyelitis optica* (Devic's syndrome).
* *Neurosarcoidosis*.
* Collagen vascular disease: *systemic lupus erythematosus (SLE), Sjögren's syndrome, antiphospholipid syndrome, giant cell arteritis*.
* Idiopathic; clincally isolated syndrome.

Clinical features

Variable:

- Lower limb weakness (paraparesis, paraplegia), paresthesia
- Urinary retention, incontinence
- +/– Pain in the spine

Symptoms usually evolve rapidly, may extend cranially.

Usually a monophasic illness, involving a complete spinal cord segment. Recurrent cases are described.

Phenotype differs in idiopathic vs. MS transverse myelitis: latter is usually partial, whereas idiopathic is usually complete.

Investigation

Neuroimaging: spinal cord MRI may show swelling of and signal change within the spinal cord; this may involve part of or the whole anteroposterior diameter of the cord, and single, multiple, or several contiguous cord segments ("longitudinal myelitis"). There may be patchy enhancement with gadolinium in the acute stage. Longitudinal myelitis is not typical of multiple sclerosis, which tends to affect single segments; inflammatory lesions on brain MRI may support a diagnosis of multiple sclerosis. CSF may show a moderate pleocytosis, raised protein; +/– oligoclonal bands. Blood tests may include autoantibodies for certain collagen vascular diseases and serology for infective agents. Neurophysiology: central motor conduction time (CMCT) to tibialis anterior abnormal in 90% in one series, CMCT to abductor digiti minimi in 30%; tibial somatosensory evoked potential (SEP) abnormal in 77%, median SEP in 15%; EMG evidence of denervation in 51%; suggests pronounced involvement of dorsal region of spinal cord.

Differential diagnosis

Spinal cord vascular disease: infarction, subarachnoid hemorrhage.

Treatment and prognosis

Of cause where established: intravenous steroids for MS, post-infectious, post-vaccination; immunosuppression for SLE; anticoagulation for antiphospholipid antibody syndrome. Partial syndromes are more likely to improve; complete syndromes less so. Isolated transverse myelitis, particularly if partial, may be the harbinger of more widespread inflammation, i.e., a clinically isolated syndrome heralding MS.

Reference

Transverse Myelitis Consortium Working Group. Proposed diagnostic criteria and nosology of acute transverse myelitis. Neurology. 2002;59:499–505

Traumatic brain injury (TBI)

Traumatic brain injury (TBI) may be classified as

- Primary: related to the impact, the severity of injury per se.
- Secondary: evolving after the primary impact, for anything up to 1 week.

Although preventive (epidemiological) measures may reduce the severity and frequency of primary brain injury, secondary injury is potentially amenable to medical intervention. Timely (i.e., early) transfer to a trauma center with neurosurgical facilities is probably the optimum management, in order to monitor and treat brain swelling, raised intracranial pressure, falling cerebral perfusion pressure, hypotension and hypoxemia, recognized causes of secondary injury due to brain ischemia.

Clinical features

TBI may be graded according to Glasgow Coma Scale (GCS) score at presentation:

- Severe: GCS 3–8; loss of consciousness >24 h; may be accompanying *subdural hematoma*, brain contusion.
- Moderate: GCS 9–13; patient lethargic, stuporous; loss of consciousness or amnesia 30 min to 24 h; may be accompanying skull fracture.
- Mild (MTBI): GCS 13–15; often no more than concussion; loss of consciousness or amnesia <30 min.

Concussion may be defined as an immediate and transient impairment of consciousness following head injury; there need not be loss of consciousness although this usually occurs briefly. There is usually amnesia for the events surrounding the injury (retrograde and anterograde). Modern classification of head injury has tended to abandon the term concussion in favor of description of the severity of head injury (as measured by the Glasgow Coma Scale).

Investigation

Neuroimaging may be needed to define the extent of cerebral injury (e.g., contusion) and complications that may be amenable to neurosurgical intervention, e.g., subdural/extradural hematoma, parenchymal hematoma (temporal, frontal), and subarachnoid hemorrhage.

Differential diagnosis

Usually TBI is obvious, but occasionally there may be difficulty, e.g., someone suffering a subarachnoid hemorrhage when driving leading to an accident or falling downstairs. MTBI may be confused with other causes of amnesia, e.g., *transient epileptic amnesia* and psychogenic amnesia.

Treatment and prognosis

Treatment at the scene of any accident may be crucial, because of the time factor in preventing secondary injury. Intubation and hand ventilation may be required to prevent hypoxemia, as well as intravenous access for fluids to prevent hypotension (both recognized to increase the risk of secondary injury). Once the patient is stabilized, transfer to a trauma center is recommended; some would advocate helicopter transfer if the distances involved are large. Following neuroimaging, if immediate neurosurgical intervention is not required, arrangements for ICP monitoring should be made (ventricular catheter preferred to a bolt); normal ICP = 0–10 mmHg; intervention probably appropriate if ICP > 15–20 mmHg, by means of:

- Ventricular drainage of CSF.
- Hyperventilation (but may risk hypocapnic vasoconstriction and brain ischemia).
- Diuretics (but may risk hypovolemia and brain ischemia).
- Mannitol (but may only be given intermittently).

Repeat imaging may be appropriate to define cause of rising ICP.

Monitoring of central venous pressure may assist in decisions regarding hypotension and fluid balance.

The place of prophylactic steroids and antiepileptic medications in TBI remains uncertain; clearly, any epileptic seizures should be treated as they may be associated with worsening of brain ischemia.

Prognosis is dependent on severity of TBI:

- Moderate, Severe: linear correlation between GCS score 3–9 and outcome of death, *vegetative state*, and severe neurological disability.
- Mild: full recovery usual, may be residual concentration or short-term memory problems. A post-concussion syndrome of headaches, dizziness, difficulty concentrating, irritability, loss of confidence, anxiety, and depression is common. This syndrome is of variable severity and is not related to the severity of the original injury; psychological factors, perhaps related to legal claims ("accident neurosis," "compensation neurosis") may contribute in some, but not all, circumstances. Epidemiological studies suggest that head injuries severe enough to produce concussion are a risk factor for the later development of *Alzheimer's disease*.

Posttraumatic epileptic seizures may be described as:

- Early: within 7 days of TBI.
- Late: more than 7 days after TBI.

Mild and moderate TBI is associated with a small increased risk of *epilepsy*; severe TBI with a substantial increase in risk. There is currently no strong evidence that prophylactic antiepileptic medication alters these risks, i.e., they relate to primary rather than secondary brain injury.

References

Anderson T, Heitger M, Macleod AD. Concussion and mild head injury. Pract Neurol. 2006;6:342–357

Chadwick D. Seizures and epilepsy after traumatic brain injury. Lancet. 2000;355:334–336

Ghajar J. Traumatic brain injury. Lancet. 2000;356:923–929

McCrea MA. Mild Traumatic Brain Injury and Postconcussion Syndrome. The New Evidence Base for Diagnosis and Treatment. Oxford: Oxford University Press; 2008

McCrory PR, Berkovic SF. Concussion. Neurology. 2001;57:2283–2289

Quality Standards Committee of the American Academy of Neurology. The management of concussions in sports. Neurology. 1997;48:581–585

Tremor: overview

Tremor is an involuntary movement, roughly rhythmic and sinusoidal, although some tremors (e.g., dystonic) are irregular in amplitude and periodicity. Many types of tremor are recognized.

Clinical features

- Physiological tremor: normal; exacerbated by anxiety states, hyperthyroidism, drugs (especially β2 agonists).
- Rest tremor: present when limb supported against gravity and no voluntary muscle activation, e.g., 4–6 Hz "pill-rolling" hand tremor of *Parkinson's disease* (PD); Holmes's/midbrain/rubral tremor due to lesions interrupting cerebellothalamic and/or cerebello-olivary projections (most commonly seen in *multiple sclerosis*).
- Action tremor: present during any voluntary muscle contraction; various subdivisions:
  - Postural tremor: present during voluntary maintenance of posture opposed by gravity, e.g., arm tremor of *essential tremor (ET)*; 6 Hz postural tremor sometimes seen in PD, may predate emergence of akinesia/

rigidity/rest tremor; modest postural tremor of cerebellar disease; some drug-induced tremors; tremor of IgM *paraproteinemic demyelinating neuropathy (PDN)*.

- Kinetic tremor: present with movement, often with an exacerbation at the end of a goal-directed movement (intention tremor), e.g., cerebellar/midbrain tremor (3–5 Hz).
- Task-specific tremor: evident during the performance of a highly skilled activity, e.g., primary writing tremor.
- Isometric tremor: present when voluntary muscle contraction is opposed by a stationary object, e.g., *primary orthostatic tremor (POT)* (14–16 Hz).
- Dystonic tremor: in which there is jerking of a limb or body part (e.g., head and neck) with a degree of rhythmicity but underpinned by an abnormal posturing of the affected body part.
- Psychogenic tremors: difficult to classify, with changing characteristics; the frequency with which such tremors are observed varies greatly between different clinics.

Diagnosis is usually clinical, based on the appearance of the tremor and the circumstances in which it occurs. Other neurological features may also help, e.g., bradykinesia and rigidity in PD, ataxia in cerebellar disease, and peripheral sensory deficits in neuropathy. Family history may help (ET). Drug history is also crucial, along with response to alcohol.

Investigation

Bloods: thyroid function tests to exclude hyperthyroidism; immunoglobulins and electrophoretic strip. Neurophysiology: EMG may be useful for determining tremor frequency, and diagnostic in POT.

Differential diagnosis

Tremor is unlikely to be mistaken for dystonia or myoclonus.

Treatment and prognosis

See individual entries; in brief:

- ET: propranolol, topiramate, alcohol, primidone, alprazolam, flunarizine, nicardipine; deep brain stimulation.
- PD: levodopa, anticholinergics (e.g., benzhexol); deep brain stimulation.

- POT: clonazepam, gabapentin, primidone, and levodopa.
- Cerebellar: isoniazid, ondansetron, carbamazepine, clonazepam, primidone, propranolol (but most pharmacotherapy ineffectual); limb weights, deep brain stimulation surgery.

Reference

Deuschl G, Bain P, Brin M, an Ad Hoc Scientific Committee. Consensus statement of the Movement Disorder Society on tremor. Mov Disord. 1998;13(Suppl 3): 2–23

Trichinosis

Trichinosis is infection with the nematode worm *Trichinella spiralis*, due to ingestion of undercooked pork containing encysted *T. spiralis* larvae (hence Ambrose Bierce's definition of trichinosis as "the pig's reply to proponents of porcophagy"). Gastric juices free the larvae that then develop in the duodenum and jejunum to form new larvae that spread via the lymphatics and the blood stream to all tissues. They survive only in muscle to encyst and calcify.

Clinical features

- Acute (1–2 days): mild gastroenteritis.
- Subacute (1–6 weeks): fever, painful tender muscles, edematous eyelids, +/− headache, stiff neck, confusional state.
- Chronic (months):
  - Myalgia of inflammatory myopathy, affecting extraocular muscles, tongue, proximal limb muscles, diaphragm, myocardium (emboli may lead to brain infarction).
  - CNS disease (from larval invasion): meningoencephalitis, cranial vessel thrombosis.

Investigation

Bloods show eosinophilia, mild increase in creatine kinase; serology (ELISA) is +ve by third week. Neuroimaging (CT/MRI) may show multiple infarcts or hemorrhagic lesions. CSF may show lymphocytosis, + (rarely) parasites. Neurophysiology (EMG) shows fibrillation potentials (disconnection of muscle fibers from end plates). Muscle biopsy shows an inflammatory myopathy; segmental necrosis of muscle fibers with eosinophil infiltrate (cf. *eosinophilic syndromes*); observation of *Trichinella* larvae is diagnostic.

Differential diagnosis

Other causes of inflammatory myopathy (*polymyositis*).

Treatment and prognosis

Often asymptomatic. Thiabendazole or albendazole (anti-helminthics), +/– prednisolone (anti-inflammatory). The value of steroids is not definitively established, and may theoretically enhance larval dissemination. Recovery is usual.

References

Bundy DAP, Michael E. Trichinosis. In: Cox FEG, ed. The Wellcome Trust Illustrated History of Tropical Diseases. London: Wellcome Trust; 1996:310–317

Kramer MD, Aita JF. Trichinosis with central nervous system involvement. A case report and review of the literature. Neurology. 1972;22:485–491

Trigeminal autonomic cephalalagias (TACS): overview

The trigeminal autonomic cephalalagias (TACs) are a group of primary *headache* disorders that include:

- *Cluster headache*
- *Paroxysmal hemicrania*
- *SUNCT syndrome, SUNA syndrome*

Hemicrania continua may also fall within this category.

All these disorders are characterized by unilateral attacks of pain within the distribution of the trigeminal nerve with autonomic features. Functional imaging indicates a hypothalamic activation during attacks, and hypothalamic deep brain stimulation is a successful treatment. Hence, the hypothalamus seems to be crucial to the pathophysiology of these disorders.

References

Leone M, Bussone G. Pathophysiology of trigeminal autonomic cephalalgias. Lancet Neurol. 2009;8:755–764

Larner AJ. Trigeminal autonomic cephalalgias: frequency in a general neurology clinic setting. J Headache Pain. 2008;9:325–326

Trigeminal neuralgia (TN)

Fothergill's disease, Tic douloureux

A syndrome of neuropathic pain in the distribution of the sensory branches of the trigeminal nerve, especially mandibular and maxillary divisions (rarely ophthalmic), occurring in middle to late life and slightly more common in women. Although most cases are idiopathic/primary, symptomatic/secondary causes are recognized, especially *multiple sclerosis*. This may be one of the *neurovascular compression syndromes*.

Clinical features

History is usually typical and diagnostic:

- Brief, severe, paroxysmal, lancinating, unilateral, facial pain, causing patient to wince or even cry (bilateral symptoms suggest secondary cause). In some cases, pain can be so severe that it stops people eating or talking.
- Frequently recurrent.
- May be initiated by stimulation of specific facial "trigger zones," e.g., by washing, shaving, chewing, wind on the face (hence may be a form of allodynia).
- There is usually a refractory period following a paroxysm during which a further attack cannot be triggered; said not to occur in cases secondary to structural pathology such as MS or aneurysms.
- Sensory/motor cranial nerve deficit usually absent (may not be so in symptomatic group).

"Pretrigeminal neuralgia" was first described by Sir Charles Symonds in 1949 as an atypical early manifestation of TN, characterized by dull continuous pain in the upper or lower jaw, which changed with time to classic TN, and may respond to TN therapies.

Investigation

Neuroimaging (MRI) is undertaken to exclude secondary/symptomatic causes, e.g., multiple sclerosis, basilar artery aneurysm, acoustic/trigeminal neuroma, tortuous blood vessel(s) (usually posterior cerebellar artery) impinging on trigeminal nerve. Normal in idiopathic cases.

Differential diagnosis

- Postherpetic neuralgia
- Cluster headache
- Chronic paroxysmal (episodic) hemicrania (CPH)
- SUNCT syndrome
- Atypical facial pain

Treatment and prognosis

Medical: Carbamazepine (commence with low doses, increase slowly to avoid toxicity, up to doses of 600–1,200 mg/day) and oxcarbazepine (better tolerability) are first-line treatments. If these fail or cannot be tolerated, then phenytoin, baclofen, gabapentin, or lamotrigine may be tried.

Surgical: (Percutaneous) Radiofrequency thermocoagulation; gamma knife or microvascular decompression (latter requires posterior fossa craniotomy), especially if there is radiological evidence of a vascular loop contacting the dorsal root entry zone of the symptomatic trigeminal nerve. May be followed by anesthesia dolorosa.

References

Cruccu G, Gronseth G, Alksne J, et al. AAN-EFNS guidelines on trigeminal neuralgia management. Eur J Neurol. 2008;15:1013–1028

Evans RW, Graff-Radford SB, Bassiur JP. Pretrigeminal neuralgia. Headache. 2005;45:242–244

Fothergill J. On a painful affliction of the face. Med Observ Enquir. 1773;5:129–142

Jorns TP, Zakrzewska JM. Evidence-based approach to the medical management of trigeminal neuralgia. Br J Neurosurg. 2007;21:253–261

Sarsam Z, Garcia-Finana M, Nurmikko TJ, Varma TR, Elderidge P. The long-term outcome of microvascular decompression for trigeminal neuralgia. Br J Neurosurg. 2010;24:18–25

Zakrzewska JM. Insights: Facts and Stories Behind Trigeminal Neuralgia. Gainesville, FL: Trigeminal Neuralgia Association; 2007

Trigeminal sensory neuropathy (TSN)

Trigeminal sensory neuropathy is usually a slowly evolving, unilateral or bilateral, facial numbness, with or without pain, paresthesia, and disturbed taste sensation. Electrophysiological testing of the blink reflex may show a modest prolongation of latency suggesting an afferent defect, consistent with a lesion in the trigeminal ganglion or proximal part of the main trigeminal divisions. *Systemic sclerosis* (scleroderma), *Sjögren's syndrome*, and mixed connective tissue disease are frequent causes, but infiltrating skull base tumors and other inflammatory disorders enter the differential diagnosis; some cases remain idiopathic.

Reference

Lecky BR, Hughes RA, Murray NM. Trigeminal sensory neuropathy. A study of 22 cases. Brain. 1987;110:1463–1485

Trinucleotide repeat diseases: overview

Polyglutamine disease, PolyQ disease, Triplet repeat disease

A number of inherited neurodegenerative conditions have been linked to expansions of a trinucleotide repeat sequence in a gene cosegregating with the disease. Since these repeats are potentially unstable during meiosis, increasing in size with successive generations, this may explain the clinical observation of anticipation in many of these conditions (i.e., presents earlier in subsequent generations). The biochemical mechanism(s) by which expansions cause disease is uncertain, but many of the repeats encode polyglutamine, proteins containing which may aggregate into insoluble fibrils, which may manifest as pathological inclusions ("aggregopathies"); this would represent a toxic gain of function rather than a loss of function. However, not all trinucleotide repeats are in coding sequences so this cannot be the only mechanism. Moreover, genotype/phenotype correlation is not perfect, some disease-free individuals harboring pathological repeats, some affected individuals having "normal" numbers of repeats.

Disorders shown to be trinucleotide repeat diseases are as follows:

- Spinal and bulbar muscular atrophy (SBMA), Kennedy's syndrome
- Huntington's disease (HD)
- Dentatorubral-pallidoluysian atrophy (DRPLA)
- Spinocerebellar ataxia (SCA), types 1, 2, 3 (Machado–Joseph disease), 6, 7, 17 (SCA10 = quintuplet expansion ATTCT; SCA31 = intronic TGGAA expansion)
- Friedreich's ataxia (FA)
- Myotonic dystrophy type 1 (MD type 2 = quadruplet expansion CCTG)
- Fragile X syndromes (FRAX, FRAXE)
- Oculopharyngeal muscular dystrophy (OPMD)

Disease	Gene	Triplet	Location	Protein	Normal	Abnormal
SBMA	Androgen receptor	CAG	Exon	Polyglutamine	9–34	38–75
HD	Huntingtin	CAG	Exon	Polyglutamine	9–34	36–125
SCA1	ATXN1	CAG	Exon	Polyglutamine	6–36	39–81
SCA2	ATXN2	CAG	Exon	Polyglutamine	15–34	34–64
SCA3 (MJD)	ATXN3	CAG	Exon	Polyglutamine	12–40	60–84
SCA6	CACNA1A	CAG	Exon	Polyglutamine	4–16	21–27
SCA7	ATXN7	CAG	Exon	Polyglutamine	6–17	34–130
SCA8	ATXN8	CTA/CTG				
SCA10	ATXN10	ATTCT				
SCA12	PPP2R2B	CAG		Polyglutamine		
SCA17	TATA-binding protein (TBP)	CAG		Polyglutamine		
SCA31	BEAN	TGGAA	Intron			
DRPLA		CAG	Exon	Polyglutamine	3–36	49–88
FRAX	FMR1	CGG??	5′	Untranslated	7–50	50–1,500
FRAXE	FMR2	GCC??	??			
MD type 1	DMPK	CTG	3′	Untranslated	5–40	40–3,000
MD type 2	ZFN9	CCTG				
FA	Frataxin	GAA	Intron	Untranslated	6–30	90–1,700
OPMD	PAB2	GCG	Exon	Polyalanine	6–7	8–13

Investigation

Trinucleotide repeats form the basis for rapid diagnostic tests for the associated diseases using PCR technology, but care is needed in interpreting results because of the imperfect genotype/phenotype correlations. Genetic counseling is required before diagnostic and predictive gene testing.

Treatment and prognosis

Most of these conditions are progressive and lack specific treatment. However, if they have a shared pathogenesis related to the intraneuronal accumulation of pathological proteins, generic therapy to block protein aggregation might theoretically be applicable to many of the diseases in this category.

References

Paulson HL, Fishbeck KH. Trinucleotide repeats in neurogenetic disorders. Ann Rev Neurosci. 1996;19:79–107
Perutz MF. Glutamine repeats and neurodegenerative diseases: molecular aspects. Trends Biochem Sci. 1999;24:58–63
Rosenberg RN. DNA-triplet repeats and neurologic disease. N Engl J Med. 1996;335:1222–1224

Troyer syndrome

Troyer syndrome is an autosomal recessive, complicated *hereditary spastic paraplegia*, seen in high frequency among the Old Order Amish community. In addition to lower limb spasticity, the additional features are short stature, mental retardation, dysarthria (pseudobulbar palsy), and marked atrophy of small hand muscles. The condition maps to chromosome 13q12.3 and has been associated with frameshift mutations in the SPG20 gene, encoding the protein spartin.

References

Patel H, Cross H, Proukakis C, et al. SPG20 is mutated in Troyer syndrome, an hereditary spastic paraplegia. Nat Genet. 2002;31:347–348
Proukakis C, Cross H, Patel H, Patton MA, Valentine A, Crosby AH. Troyer syndrome revisited. A clinical and radiological study of a complicated hereditary spastic paraplegia. J Neurol. 2004;251:1105–1110

Trypanosomiasis

African sleeping sickness

African trypanosomiasis results from infection with the protozoan *Trypanosoma brucei gambiense* in West Africa or *Trypanosoma brucei rhodesiense* in East Africa, transmitted to humans by tsetse flies (*Glossina* species). These produce either a chronic illness (Gambian, West African), which may not become clinically apparent for up to 1 year after infection, or a more acute progressive illness (Rhodesian, East African). Both are characterized by daytime hypersomnia with nocturnal insomnia (African sleeping sickness). South American trypanosomiasis (Chagas' disease) results from infection with *Trypanosoma cruzi*, transmitted to humans by the bite of reduviid bugs. As with the African disease, the sequence of local lymphadenopathy, hematogenous spread and chronic meningoencephalitis is seen.

Clinical features

- African:
  - Local: chancre (trypanoma) at site of bite: hard, painful.
  - Dissemination: headache, fever, tachycardia.
  - Systemic: recurrent episodes lasting several days with asymptomatic periods of weeks in between.
    - Gambian:
      Lymphadenopathy, nontender, especially posterior cervical location with consistency likened to ripe plums (Winterbottom's sign). Subtle neurological changes: indifference, reversal of sleep–wake cycle, tremor.
      Somnolence and insomnia, tremor, incoordination, thermoregulatory dysfunction, hyperreflexia.
      Stupor, coma, death.
    - East African: onset within days of bite.
      Lymphadenopathy unusual.
      Other symptoms similar to Gambian but more acute; early CNS invasion, death rapid (cardiac failure).
- South American:
  - Acute flu-like illness; inoculation chagoma may be seen; Romana's sign (unilateral conjunctivitis and edema from ocular contamination by bug feces).
  - Asymptomatic phase.
  - Chronic phase: destruction of cardiac and gastrointestinal autonomic nerves: postural hypotension, arrhythmias; esophageal achalasia. Chronic meningoencephalitis; a predominantly sensory peripheral neuropathy may occur.

Investigation

Bloods: anemia, monocytosis, raised IgM (nonspecific); indirect fluorescent antibody test for trypanosomes. Tissue: blood smears, CSF examination, bone marrow aspirate, to look for trypanosomes, the diagnostic test if present. CSF: raised protein, pleocytosis (with morular cells), raised IgM.

Differential diagnosis

Disturbance of sleep–wake cycle with systemic illness following time in Africa unlikely to be mistaken for anything else. Other causes of autonomic neuropathy should be considered with Chagas' disease.

Treatment and prognosis

Suramin (East African): may cause albuminuria, +/– shock, febrile reactions, rash.
    Pentamidine (West African): may cause hypotension, fever, rash.
    Organic arsenicals for CSF penetration: melarsopol, may cause optic atrophy, rash, encephalopathy.
    Despite these, deaths still occur.

Reference

Kennedy P. The Fatal Sleep. Edinburgh, UK: Luath Press; 2007

Tuberculosis (TB) and the nervous system: overview

Infection with *Mycobacterium* species (most usually *M. tuberculosis*) may produce a number of neurological syndromes, ranging from meningitis, *tuberculous meningitis (TBM)*, to a cerebral mass lesion, tuberculoma. Disease of bone, tuberculous infection of vertebra(e) (osteitis) may cause vertebral collapse and spinal deformity, with or without spinal cord compression (Pott's disease or paraplegia). Tracking of pus into the epidural space may also cause spinal cord compression. Tuberculous infections increased in relation to concurrent *HIV/AIDS*. Most patients have evidence of active tuberculosis elsewhere, but on occasion the infection is confined to the nervous system.

Clinical features

- Tuberculoma:
  - May occur concurrently with TBM; may be asymptomatic, depending on precise location.
  - Focal signs.
  - Epileptic seizures.
- Spinal cord syndrome (Pott's disease):
  - Arachnoiditis, paraplegia, with or without involvement of the vertebral column.
  - Kyphosis of spine due to collapsed infected vertebra(e).

Investigation

- Tuberculoma:
  - Brain imaging for mass lesion(s).
  - CSF: because of proximity of mass lesion to meninges, CSF may contain raised protein, lymphocytes.
  - +/− Stereotactic biopsy.
- Spinal cord syndrome (Pott's disease):
  - Imaging of spine and spinal cord: plain radiology and MRI.

Look for evidence of tuberculous disease elsewhere, e.g., chest X-ray, sputum, bronchial washings: early morning urine samples; bone marrow aspirate; look for acid-fast bacilli (Ziehl–Neelsen stain).

Consider checking HIV status.

Differential diagnosis

- Tuberculoma:
  - Other mass lesions: bacterial abscess, tumor.
- Spinal cord syndrome (Pott's disease):
  - Other causes of cord compression; hydatid disease of the spine.

Treatment and prognosis

Antituberculous chemotherapy: intravenous triple therapy probably required:

- Isoniazid (+ prophylactic pyridoxine to prevent neuropathy).
- Pyrizinamide.
- Rifampicin.
- +/− Ethambutol, streptomycin (these drugs cross inflamed meninges, so worth using in first 3 months).

Monitor liver function tests, abnormality may necessitate cessation of isoniazid; monitor visual acuity and color vision; deterioration may require ethambutol to be stopped. Resistance to drugs is evident in some cases. No need for intrathecal therapy. Duration of treatment uncertain; may need to switch to oral therapy for up to 1 year. If risk of noncompliance, directly observed therapy (DOT) regimens may be used. If tuberculoma is unresponsive to antituberculous therapy, surgical excision may be attempted. In Pott's disease, in addition to antituberculous therapy, surgical exploration and excision of infective focus may be undertaken if possible; intervertebral grafting may be required.

References

Garg RK, Sharma R, Kar AM, et al. Neurological complications of military tuberculosis. Clin Neurol Neurosurg. 2010;112:188–192
Leonard JM, Des Prez RM. Tuberculosis and the central nervous system. In: Aminoff MJ, ed. Neurology and General Medicine: The Neurological Aspects of Medical Disorders. 2nd ed. New York: Churchill Livingstone, 1995:703–716
Shaw BA. Pott's disease with paraparesis. N Engl J Med. 1996;334:958–959

Tuberculous meningitis (TBM)

In tuberculous meningitis (TBM), the basal meninges are particularly affected, sometimes with hydrocephalus as a complication. The pathological process, tubercles with central caseation surrounded by epithelioid cells, may invade the underlying brain to produce a meningoencephalitis.

Clinical features

- Fever, headache, irritability, lethargy, vomiting.
- Meningeal irritation (nuchal rigidity: Kernig's sign, Brudzinski's sign).
- Epileptic seizures: may be due to meningitis per se, hydrocephalus, hyponatremia.
- Altered level of consciousness: may be staged as I (fully responsive), II (drowsy, often with cranial nerve palsies), III (unconscious).
- Focal signs: cranial nerve palsies (inflammatory exudates in subarachnoid space): III, IV, VI > VII > VIII; hemiparesis (inflammation of arteries leading to infarction); gaze palsies, internuclear ophthalmoplegia.
- Ischemia: cortex, brainstem.
- Hydrocephalus, raised intracranial pressure, papilledema.
- Stupor, coma, death (if untreated).

Clinical grading of TBM, based on modified British Medical Research Council clinical criteria:

- I: Alert and orientated without focal neurological deficit.
- II: Glasgow Coma Score (GCS) 14–10 with or without focal neurological deficit or GCS 15 with focal neurological deficit.
- III: GCS < 10 with or without focal neurological deficit.

Investigation

Bloods are usually unremarkable but may show low sodium if there is associated *syndrome of inappropriate ADH secretion*. Neuroimaging in cases of raised intracranial pressure, focal signs: MRI shows enhancement of basal meninges; hydrocephalus; infarction. Chest radiograph may give evidence of TB elsewhere. CSF typically shows raised pressure, protein, cell count (increasing proportion of lymphocytes with increasing duration of illness); low glucose *vs.* serum (hypoglycorrhacia); PCR may be used to demonstrate *M. tuberculosis* but its sensitivity is not as high as was hoped; therefore, traditional culture methods are still required although slow (weeks). In many cases of suspected TB of the nervous system, the diagnosis is not proven, yet the patient improves with anti-TB therapy.

Differential diagnosis

Other meningitides:

- Bacterial: *Listeria*, partially treated bacterial meningitis, focal parameningeal infection (*subdural empyema*), *neurosyphilis*.
- Fungal: cryptococcosis; coccidioidomycosis, histoplasmosis, candidiasis.
- Viral: HSV, HIV, Japanese encephalitis.
- Others: toxoplasmosis, neurosarcoidosis, neoplastic meningitis, venous sinus thrombosis.
- Focal features of acute onset may prompt consideration of cerebrovascular disease.
- In context of HIV, also need to consider toxoplasmosis, cerebral lymphoma, PML.

Treatment and prognosis

Steroids are often recommended in conjunction with antituberculous therapy to prevent subarachnoid blockage. Shunting may be undertaken if CSF pathways are blocked, but revision for shunt blockage is often necessary. Complete recovery is possible if the diagnosis is made early and appropriate therapy instituted.

Poor prognostic features are increasing age (>60 years), prolonged duration of illness before diagnosis (>2 months), and impaired consciousness at presentation. Delayed diagnosis is associated with a high mortality rate, especially among infants, HIV-positive patients, although the treatment and prognosis of TBM is similar in HIV +ve and –ve patients. Neurological sequelae are common (25–40%): epileptic seizures, cranial nerve palsies, hemiplegia, and paraplegia.

References

British Medical Research Council. Streptomycin treatment of tuberculous meningitis. BMJ. 1948;i:582–597
Parsons M. Tuberculous Meningitis. A Handbook for Clinicians. Oxford: Oxford University Press; 1979
Thwaites G, Chau TTH, Mai NTH, Drobniewski F, McAdam K, Farrar J. Tuberculous meningitis. J Neurol Neurosurg Psychiatry. 2000;68:289–299

Tuberous sclerosis [OMIM#191100, #613254]

Bourneville disease, Epiloia, Pringle disease, Tuberose sclerosis

Tuberous sclerosis is an autosomal dominant condition characterized by multiple hamartomas of ectodermal structures, hence a *neurocutaneous syndrome*. New mutations account for 70% of cases. The condition is clinically and genetically heterogeneous; chromosomal linkage to two loci has been established, at 9q34 (TSC1) encoding "hamartin," and at 16p13 (TSC2) encoding "tuberin." These may be tumor suppressor genes.

Clinical features

- Neurological:
  - Epilepsy (75%): often early onset
  - Mental retardation (50%)
  - Astrocytomas (5–10%)
  - Raised intracranial pressure (rare)
- Dermatological:
  - Hypopigmented "ash leaf" patches (80–90%)
  - Adenoma sebaceum (facial angiofibromas) (40–90%)
  - Shagreen patches (= subepidermal fibrosis) (20–40%)
  - Forehead fibrous plaque (25%)
  - Ungual fibromas (15–50%)
- Ocular:
  - Optic nerve/retina hamartoma (= phakoma) (50%)

- Renal:
  - Angiomyolipoma (60%)
  - Renal cysts (20%)
  - Renal cell carcinoma
- Cardiac rhabdomyoma
- Rectal polyps
- Lung fibrosis

Investigation

Neuroimaging: CT/MRI for intracranial mass lesions; CT better for detecting calcification. Renal imaging (ultrasound/CT) for cysts, tumors. Echocardiography for rhabdomyoma. Woods (UV) lamp examination of the skin. Neurogenetic testing.

Differential diagnosis

Other early onset epilepsy syndromes unlikely to be mistaken if typical dermatological features are looked for.

Treatment and prognosis

Morbidity most usually due to CNS complications, e.g., *status epilepticus*; occasionally renal (e.g., bleed from angiomyolipoma, development of renal cell carcinoma).

Symptomatic treatment of epilepsy, raised intracranial pressure (shunting); resection of brain/renal tumors sometimes possible. Progressive course. Genetic counseling for family may be appropriate.

References

Curatolo P. Tuberous Sclerosis Complex. From Basic Science to Clinical Phenotypes. Cambridge: MacKeith Press; 2003
Orlova KA, Crino PB. The tuberous sclerosis complex. Ann NY Acad Sci. 2010;1184:87–105

Tumors: overview

Tumors affecting the nervous system may arise from:

- Glia: glioma, oligodendroglioma, ependymoma, schwannoma (e.g., VIII nerve: *vestibular schwannoma*/acoustic neuroma; spinal roots: neurofibroma)
- Meninges: *meningioma*

- Extraneous sites:
  - Proximate, e.g., nasopharyngeal carcinoma, choroid plexus papilloma
  - Distant: metastases from bronchus, breast, melanoma
- Lymphoid cells: lymphoma; angioendotheliomatosis
- Pituitary gland: pituitary adenoma
- Primitive germ cells: teratoma, germinoma, epidermoid/dermoid
- Neural elements (rare in adults): primitive neuroectodermal tumors (PNET, e.g., medulloblastoma); central neurocytoma; ganglioglioma
- Developmental residua: (e.g., notochordal elements: chordoma; Rathke's pouch: craniopharyngioma)
- Vascular endothelia: hemangioblastoma
- Hamartoma: tuberous sclerosis

Of these, the most common in adults are glioma, meningioma, and distant metastases. Tumors in children have a different frequency and distribution (more infratentorial lesions in children).

Tumors can also have distant, non-metastatic effects on the nervous system (*paraneoplastic syndromes*)

Clinical features

- Consequences of raised intracranial pressure:
  - Headache, with postural features (worse on lying, bending, straining); may cause nocturnal waking.
  - Transient visual obscurations, papilledema.
  - "False localizing signs," especially VIth nerve palsy, sometimes IIIrd nerve palsy with transtentorial temporal lobe herniation; Kernohan's (notch) syndrome.
  - Cushing reflex, Cushing response: hypertension, bradycardia.
- Focal effects (legion): these signs are usually gradually progressive, but spontaneous "remissions" may occur, erroneously suggesting an inflammatory etiology:
  - Hemiparesis/monoparesis/paraparesis.
  - Visual field defects: homonymous hemianopia, bitemporal hemianopia.
  - Epileptic seizures: focal, secondary generalized.
  - Personality change, cognitive decline (e.g., focal meningioma, subfrontal lesions; primary CNS lymphoma).
  - Stroke-like episodes (especially meningioma; bleed into a tumor).
  - Anosmia (olfactory groove meningioma).
  - Tumors of the spinal cord can be primary or secondary and present with local +/−radicular pain with a compressive spinal cord syndrome.
- Endocrine effects (functioning pituitary tumors)

- Somnolence, galactorrhea, reduced facial hair growth and need for shaving: prolactinoma.
- Cushingoid appearance.
- Acromegaly.
• Certain tumors have a predilection for certain sites:
  - Meningioma: olfactory groove, petrous apex, falx.
  - Chordoma: skull base, spinal column.

Investigation

Neuroimaging (CT/MRI +/– contrast medium) may be diagnostic or highly suggestive of diagnosis: mass lesion (meningioma, glioma, lymphoma, pituitary lesion) +/– mass effect, midline shift, vasogenic edema. Stereotactic biopsy may be indicated for diagnosis, or open biopsy for diagnosis, debulking, and resection (if possible).

Differential diagnosis

Very broad:

• Other mass lesions: cyst, hematoma, abscess; occasionally an inflammatory mass (*multiple sclerosis, neurosarcoidosis*)
• Cord compression: degenerative bone disease, *Paget's disease*
• Stroke-like episodes: cerebrovascular disease, mitochondrial disease (MELAS)
• Cognitive/personality changes: neurodegenerative disease, depression/affective disorder, *leukodystrophies*

Treatment and prognosis

Some tumor types are amenable to complete surgical resection (certain meningiomas). Radiotherapy, either external or internal from implanted rods or seeds, is required for radiosensitive tumors (glioma, lymphoma). Symptomatic treatment includes steroids (dexamethasone) to reduce cerebral edema, analgesia for headache, other pain syndromes from nerve compression. Prognosis is very variable dependent on tumor type and location, ranging from a life expectancy of only weeks (glioblastoma multiforme) to complete recovery.

References

Behin A, Hoang-Xuan K, Carpentier AF, Delattre J-Y. Primary brain tumours in adults. Lancet. 2003;361:323–331

Bernstein M, Berger MS, eds. Neuro-oncology. The Essentials. 2nd ed. New York: Thieme; 2008

De Angelis LM. Brain tumors. N Engl J Med. 2001;344:114–123

Grant R. Overview: brain tumour diagnosis and management/Royal College of Physicians guidelines. J Neurol Neurosurg Psychiatry. 2004;75(Suppl II):ii18–ii23

Typhus

A number of different types of typhus, a *rickettsial disease*, are described, caused by various *Rickettsia*, Gram-negative coccobacilli, which have a life cycle involving an animal reservoir, an insect vector (lice, fleas, ticks, mites), and man:

- Epidemic or louse-borne typhus (*Rickettsia prowazekii*; human body louse): jail fever, ship fever, camp fever, famine fever.
- Endemic (or murine) typhus (*Rickettsia typhi*, *R. mooseri*; fleas).
- Scrub typhus or tsutsugamushi fever (*Rickettsia orientalis* recently renamed as a new genus with only one species, *Orientia tsutsugamushi*; trombiculid mites, chiggers).

Exposure to wildlife or livestock may be an important clue to diagnosis. Although uncommon in the developed world, about one third of cases are said to develop neurological features. Severity of disease is variable.

Clinical features

- Bacteremic illness: fever, headache, prostration
- *Delirium*, stupor, coma
- +/– Focal neurological signs
- Meningitis, encephalitis, myelitis
- Macular rash: necrotic ulcer and eschar in scrub typhus
- Lymphadenopathy: local, general
- +/– Disseminated intravascular coagulation

Investigation

Bloods: Weil–Felix test for the presence of heterophile antibodies to strains of *Proteus mirabilis*; may be negative in up to 50% of cases. Serology: species specific ELISA, immunofluorescent antibody tests (IFAT), PCR. CSF may show a modest lymphocytic pleocytosis

Differential diagnosis

Other causes of acute infective or inflammatory CNS disease, e.g., viral *meningitis*.

Treatment and prognosis

Although a cause of catastrophic epidemics in the past, associated with conditions of filth and poverty, and which may have influenced the course of history, early treatment with antibiotics (tetracycline, chloramphenicol) +/− supportive care as appropriate means the condition is now associated with good prognosis; neurological sequelae are rare. Untreated, the condition may be fatal.

Reference

Cowan G. Rickettsial diseases: the typhus group of fevers – a review. Postgrad Med J. 2000;76:269–272

U

Ullrich's congenital muscular dystrophy [OMIM#254090]

Ullrich's disease is a congenital muscular dystrophy, first described in 1930, and also known as hypotonic-sclerotic *muscular dystrophy*. It is characterized by generalized muscle weakness and wasting, contractures of proximal joints, hyperflexibility of distal joints, and a progressive course. Intellect and sensory function are normal. Creatine kinase is normal but muscle biopsy shows dystrophic features. Deficiency of collagen VI may result from mutations within three different genes encoding subunits of collagen VI: COL6A1, COL6A2, COL6A3; hence, this disorder is allelic with *Bethlem myopathy*. Early and prominent contractures also occur in *Emery–Dreifuss muscular dystrophy*.

Reference

Higuchi I, Shiraishi T, Hashiguchi T, et al. Frameshift mutation in the collagen VI gene causes Ullrich's disease. Ann Neurol. 2001;50:261–265

Ulnar neuropathy

The ulnar nerve carries fibers from spinal roots C7, C8, and T1. It supplies most of the small muscles of the hand (with the exception of those supplied by the median nerve), the long flexors of the ring and little finger, and the flexor of the ulnar side of the wrist (flexor carpi ulnaris). In perhaps 2% of individuals, all small hand muscles are supplied by the ulnar nerve ("all ulnar hand"). Lesions of the ulnar nerve may occur at the elbow, wrist, and in the hand, each producing a slightly different pattern of deficits which may be of localizing value. The common causes of ulnar neuropathy are trauma, fracture/dislocation of surrounding bones, and compression (e.g., in the cubital tunnel, Guyon's canal).

Clinical features

- Motor: wasting of the small hand muscles supplied by the ulnar nerve, especially evident in the first dorsal interosseous muscle (DIO), abductor digiti minimi (ADM), but eventually evident in all interossei and medial lumbricals producing dorsal guttering. With ulnar nerve lesions above the elbow an abnormal posture of the hand, claw hand or *main en griffe*, is seen, with hyperextension at the metacarpophalangeal joints (fifth, fourth, and, to a lesser extent, third finger) and flexion at the interphalangeal joints caused by the unopposed action of long finger extensors and flexors. Froment's prehensile thumb sign may be observed. In distal lesions there may be only motor findings ("Pure motor ulnar neuropathy").
- Sensory: pain along inner forearm; paresthesia/sensory impairment in little finger and medial half of ring finger, ulnar side of palm.

More restricted weakness and sensory loss in more distal lesions, that is, in wrist or palm (see *Ramsay Hunt syndrome*).

There may be a prior history of elbow trauma (with or without fracture), sometimes years before, hence "tardy ulnar palsy."

Sites of ulnar nerve *entrapment neuropathy* are:

- *Cubital tunnel syndrome*
- Wrist, Guyon's canal: deep or superficial terminal branches

Investigation

EMG/NCS: reduced amplitude and delay of ulnar sensory nerve action potential from little finger; reduced motor nerve conduction velocity across lesion (e.g., at medial epicondyle); reduced compound muscle action potential; increased distal motor latency to ADM, DIO.

Differential diagnosis

- Radiculopathy: C8/T1 root lesions; no splitting of sensory loss in ring finger
- Plexopathy: lower part of brachial plexus (*Klumpke's palsy*); no splitting of ring finger sensory loss
- Non-neurogenic causes of clawing: Dupuytren's contracture, *camptodactyly*

Treatment and prognosis

For lesions at the elbow, avoid pressure, repetitive flexion/extension; surgical decompression and/or transposition is an option. For lesions in the wrist or hand, removal of a compressing lesion may be possible.

References

Capitani D, Beer S. Handlebar palsy – a compression syndrome of the deep terminal (motor) branch of the ulnar nerve in biking. J Neurol. 2002;249:1441–1445

Larner AJ. Pitfalls in the diagnosis of ulnar neuropathy: remember the deep palmar branch. Br J Hosp Med. 2010;71:654–655

Staal A, Van Gijn J, Spaans F. Mononeuropathies: Examination, Diagnosis and Treatment. London: W.B. Saunders; 1999:69–84

Stewart J. Ulnar neuropathies: where, why, and what to do? Pract Neurol. 2006;6:218–229

Unverricht–Lundborg disease [OMIM#254800]

Baltic myoclonus (epilepsy), Dyssynergia cerebellaris myoclonica

Unverricht–Lundborg disease is an autosomal recessive condition with onset between age 6–15 years, equal sex incidence, but variable geographical distribution. It presents with myoclonus which is progressively more difficult to control. Ataxia and tremor develop; tonic–clonic seizures may occur but are not usually a serious problem. There is slow intellectual decline. Unverricht–Lundborg disease is the most common cause of *progressive myoclonus epilepsy* (PME).

Clinical features

- Polymyoclonus of cortical origin: spontaneous, action-induced, stimulus-sensitive, progressive
- Tonic–clonic epileptic seizures
- Cerebellar ataxia
- Tremor
- Dementia (mild, slowly progressive)

Investigation

Bloods: no diagnostic biochemical or pathological abnormality yet demonstrated.

Neuroimaging (CT/MRI): atrophy may occur, not specific. Neurophysiology: EEG shows potentials time-locked to myoclonus; generalized spike and slow wave discharges, slow background activity, +/− photosensitivity; SSEPs may show giant cortical potentials (not specific). Neurogenetic testing shows: mutations in EPM1 gene encoding cystatin B on chromosome 21q22.3.

Differential diagnosis

Differential diagnosis of progressive myoclonus epilepsy (PME):

- *Lafora body disease*
- Sialidosis (types I and II)
- *Myoclonic epilepsy with ragged red fibers (MERRF)*
- *Neuronal ceroid lipofuscinosis (NCL)*
- *Gaucher's disease*
- Neuroaxonal dystrophy
- *Dentatorubral-pallidoluysian atrophy (DRPLA)*
- Biotin-responsive encephalopathy

Treatment and prognosis

Symptomatic therapy: for myoclonus and epilepsy: sodium valproate, levetiracetam; for myoclonus: benzodiazepines (e.g., clonazepam), piracetam. Phenytoin may aggravate neurological symptoms and hasten cerebellar degeneration. Carbamazepine, oxcarbazepine, tiagabine, vigabatrin, gabapentin, pregabalin may aggravate myoclonus and myoclonic seizures.

Reference

Kalviainen R, Khyuppenen J, Koskenkorva P, et al. Clinical picture of EPM1-Unverricht-Lundborg disease. Epilepsia. 2008;49:549–556

Urbach–Wiethe disease [OMIM#247100]

Lipoid proteinosis

An extremely rare autosomal recessive disease associated with bilateral calcification of the amygdalae but sparing the hippocampus, causing deficits in emotional processing and judgment and in memory. It results from mutations in the extracellular matrix protein 1 (ECM1) gene.

Reference

Siebert M, Markowitsch HJ, Bartel P. Amygdala, affect and cognition: evidence from 10 patients with Urbach-Wiethe disease. Brain. 2003;126:2627–2637

Urea cycle enzyme defects (UCED): overview

Deficiencies of any of the six enzymes which comprise the urea (Krebs–Henseleit) cycle which converts ammonia to urea can result in a hyperammonemic syndrome, leading to coma and death, usually in the neonatal period. Partial defects may have a delayed onset until adolescence or even adulthood. In addition to hyperammonemia, there may be concurrent respiratory alkalosis, citrullinemia, and increases in urinary orotic acid. *Ornithine transcarbamoylase (OTC) deficiency*, probably the most common of the urea cycle disorders, is X-linked; carrier mothers may show signs of mild neurological dysfunction.

The urea cycle pathway involves the following reactions:

- Carbamoylphosphate synthase I (CPS-I) catalyzes the condensation of ammonium with bicarbonate to form carbamoylphosphate; *N*-acetylglutamate (NAG) is an obligatory effector (not substrate) for this reaction, itself produced by *N*-acetylglutamate synthetase (NAGS).
- Ornithine transcarbamoylase (OTC) condenses carbamoylphosphate with ornithine to produce citrulline.
- Argininosuccinic acid (ASA) synthase catalyzes condensation of citrulline with aspartate to form argininosuccinic acid.
- Argininosuccinic acid (ASA) lyase cleaves ASA to produce arginine and fumarate.
- Arginase cleaves arginine to urea and ornithine.
- A transport system returns ornithine to the intramitochondrial compartment.

The following UCED are recognized:

- Carbamoylphosphate synthase I (CPS-I) deficiency: low or undetectable plasma citrulline levels; absence of urinary orotic acid
- *N*-acetylglutamate synthetase (NAGS) deficiency: low or undetectable plasma citrulline levels; absence of urinary orotic acid
- Ornithine transcarbamoylase (OTC) deficiency: low or undetectable plasma citrulline levels, normal plasma ornithine; raised urinary orotic acid
- Argininosuccinic acid (ASA) synthase deficiency: markedly elevated citrulline levels ($>1,000$ µmol/L) = citrullinemia
- Argininosuccinic acid (ASA) lyase deficiency: normal or modestly elevated plasma citrulline; argininosuccinic aciduria; arginine deficiency, secondary deficiency of ornithine within mitochondria

- Arginase deficiency: normal or modestly elevated plasma citrulline, raised plasma arginine; argininosuccinic aciduria

Clinical features

- Neonatal failure to thrive; poor feeding, vomiting.
- Rigidity, opisthotonos; severe hypertonia.
- Seizures: usually myoclonic.
- Hyperpnoea.
- Hepatomegaly.
- Coma, atonia, death.
- No dysmorphism.
- Arginase deficiency presents in later infancy and early childhood with "cerebral palsy."

Investigation

Bloods: hyperammonemia (ca. 1,000 μM, NR 15–45); respiratory alkalosis; no ketoacidosis. Urea may be normal or reduced; normal glucose. Liver-related blood tests are normal or near normal (cf. hepatic failure as a cause of hyperammonemia), with the exception of OTC deficiency. Citrulline, ornithine may be raised in plasma in some defects.

Urine: orotic acid elevated in OTC deficiency.

CSF: raised ammonia.

Imaging: MRI brain may show diffuse, partly reversible, high signal change.

Neurogenetics: DNA analysis for specific genes in some cases.

Other: specific enzyme assays on liver biopsy.

The key parameters in interpretation of UCED are:

Plasma citrulline: elevated in ASA synthase deficiency.

Urinary orotic acid: elevated in OTC deficiency; absent in CPS-I deficiency, NAGS deficiency.

Differential diagnosis

- Severe hepatocellular dysfunction: viral infection, intoxication, inborn errors of metabolism
- Organic acidemias, for example, methylmalonic acidemia, proprionic acidemia
- Reye's syndrome
- *Mitochondrial diseases*

Treatment and prognosis

Reduce blood ammonia concentration: hemodialysis, intravenous sodium benzoate, intravenous sodium phenylacetate. High-calorie, low-protein diet (increased protein intake may precipitate exacerbations).

Argininosuccinic acid (ASA) lyase deficiency causing arginine deficiency: therapeutic response to arginine (4 mmol/kg intravenously) is dramatic.

Liver transplantation corrects enzyme deficiency.

If appropriate treatment is not instituted early, then death results. Survivors may also have neurological sequelae. Intermittent episodes of hyperammonemia with clinical deterioration may be provoked by excess protein intake or infection.

Valproate should be avoided as it may cause liver failure.

References

Batshaw ML. Inborn errors of urea synthesis. Ann Neurol. 1994;35:133–141
Steiner RD, Cederbaum SD. Laboratory evaluation of urea cycle disorders. J Pediatr. 2001;138(suppl 1):S21–S29
Testai FD, Gorelick PB. Inherited metabolic disorders and stroke part 2: homocystinuria, organic acidurias, and urea cycle disorders. Arch Neurol. 2010;67:148–153

Usher's syndromes

Usher's syndrome is a clinically and genetically heterogeneous autosomal recessive disorder characterized by hereditary hearing loss and slowly progressive *retinitis pigmentosa*. Various subtypes have been defined, for example, Type I (severe hearing loss, abnormal vestibular function) accounting for 50–70% of cases, and Type II (moderate hearing loss, normal vestibular function) accounting for most of the rest. Clinical features include sensorineural hearing loss, probably of cochlear origin; mutism; retinitis pigmentosa presenting with nyctalopia in late childhood or adolescence. Vestibular hypofunction occurs in some patients. Nystagmus is rare. There is no obesity, diabetes mellitus, peripheral neuropathy, skin or skeletal involvement. *Mitochondrial disease* enters the differential diagnosis.

References

Hallgren B. Retinitis pigmentosa combined with congenital deafness; with vestibulo-cerebellar ataxia and mental abnormality in a proportion of cases. A clinical and genetico-statistical study. Acta Psychiatr Neurol Scand. 1959;34(suppl 138):1–101
Smith RJH, Berlin CI, Hejtmancik JF, et al. Clinical diagnosis of the Usher syndrome. Am J Hum Genet. 1994;50:32–38

V

Van Buchem's syndrome

Hyperostosis cranialis generalisata, Sclerosteosis

This autosomal recessive syndrome of osteosclerosis affects the ribs, clavicles, long bones, and pelvis as well as the skull (cf. hyperostosis cranialis interna), causing a prominent jaw and hypertelorism. About half of cases develop involvement of the facial (VII) and vestibulocochlear (VIII) nerve, but optic nerve involvement and raised intracranial pressure are rare.

Reference

Van Buchem FS. Hyperostosis cranialis generalisata: eight new cases. Acta Med Scand 1971;189:257–267

Vanishing white matter disease (VWMD) [OMIM#603896]

Childhood ataxia with central nervous system hypomyelination, Cree leukoencephalopathy, Fatal infantile leukodystrophy, Myelinolysis centralis diffusa, Ovarioleukodystrophy

Vanishing white matter disease (VWMD) encompasses a group of disorders due to mutations in the gene encoding eukaryotic initiation factor 2B (eIF2B), previously known by a variety of different names but all characterized by an inherited leucoencephalopathy or orthochromatic *leukodystrophy* with striking cavitary lesions in cerebral white matter. Most often of childhood onset, cases may present up to the third decade. The classical clinical phenotype is dominated by cerebellar ataxia but there may also be progressive mental deterioration, spasticity, and epilepsy. Ovarian pathology and glaucoma have also been noted as associations. There is evident sensitivity to minor head trauma, febrile illness, and acute fright, all of which may trigger rapid neurological deterioration and unexplained coma. MR imaging of brain is usually diagnostic, showing diffuse symmetrical white matter change and cerebellar vermian atrophy, with cavitary lesions. Pathologically, oligodendrocytes and astrocytes are predominantly affected. Prognosis is generally poor, with death usual a few years after onset.

Reference

Van der Knaap MS, Pronk JC, Scheper GC. Vanishing white matter disease. Lancet Neurol. 2006;5:413–423

Variant Creutzfeldt–Jakob disease (vCJD)

"Human BSE"

Although only around 200 cases of variant Creutzfeldt–Jakob disease (vCJD) have been described, almost all in the UK, the condition has attracted huge attention and research effort since it is believed to be an iatrogenic *prion disease*, caused by the transmission of the prion agent which causes bovine spongiform encephalopathy (BSE) into the human food chain and across the species barrier.

Clinical features

- Psychiatric features predominate in the early stages, including dysphoria, withdrawal, anxiety, insomnia, and loss of interest.
- Neurological features precede (15%) or coincide with (22%) psychiatric features; these include poor memory, pain (hyperpathia), sensory symptoms, unsteadiness of gait, and dysarthria. Chorea is also described.

Investigation

Bloods: no specific abnormalities. Neuroimaging (MR) may show high signal change in the posterior thalamus (pulvinar sign). CSF may show elevated protein markers of neuronal injury (Neuron-Specific Enolase, 14-3-3) and glial activation (S100β) but this finding is nonspecific. EEG is typically normal in vCJD (cf. sporadic *Creutzfeldt–Jakob disease (CJD)*, in which periodic complexes may be seen). Tonsil biopsy may be helpful if PrP-immunopositive staining is present. Brain biopsy features are as for sporadic CJD but *kuru*-type PrP-immunopositive amyloid plaques are abundant. Neurogenetic testing shows no mutations in PrP gene; almost all cases of vCJD described thus far have had the MM genotype at codon 129 of the PrP gene, whether there will be a surge of VV and MV cases in the future is uncertain.

Differential diagnosis

- Sporadic, iatrogenic, or inherited CJD
- *Wilson's disease*
- *Limbic encephalitis*
- Cerebral vasculitis
- *Hashimoto's encephalopathy*

Diagnosis may be very difficult in the early stages if psychiatric features occur in isolation.

Treatment and prognosis

No specific treatment. Intraventricular pentosan polyphosphate has been given in some cases and in an observational study was found to be associated with longer mean survival than reported values for the natural history of vCJD.

References

Bone I, Belton L, Walker AS, Darbyshire J. Intraventricular pentosan polyphosphate in human prion diseases: an observational study in the UK. Eur J Neurol. 2008;15:458–464

Collinge J. Variant Creutzfeldt-Jakob disease. Lancet. 1999;354:317–323

Spencer MS, Knight RSG, Will RG. First hundred cases of variant Creutzfeldt-Jakob disease: retrospective case note review of early psychiatric and neurological features. BMJ. 2002;324:1479–1482

Varicella zoster virus (VZV) and the nervous system

Varicella zoster virus (VZV) may be associated with various neurological syndromes:

- Peripheral nervous system:
  - Herpes zoster (shingles) and herpes zoster oticus (*Ramsay Hunt syndrome*)
  - Radiculoneuropathy
  - Ganglionitis
  - Postherpetic neuralgia
- Central nervous system:
  - Myelitis, *encephalitis*, encephalomyelitis
  - Arteritis (large or small vessel)
  - Ventriculitis, meningitis

VZV has also been implicated in some cases of Reye's syndrome, *Guillain–Barré syndrome*, and progressive outer retinal necrosis (PORN) syndrome.

References

Gardner-Thorpe C, Foster JB, Barwick DD. Unusual manifestations of herpes zoster. A clinical and electrophysiological study. J Neurol Sci. 1976;28:427–447
Gilden DH, Kleinschmidt-DeMasters BK, LaGuardia JJ, Mahalingam R, Cohrs RJ. Neurologic complications of the reactivation of varicella-zoster virus. N Engl J Med. 2000;342:635–645

Vascular dementia (VaD), vascular cognitive impairment (VCI)

Cerebrovascular disease may cause cognitive impairment, as well as sensory and motor dysfunction. Vascular dementia (VaD) and lesser degrees of cognitive dysfunction, known as vascular cognitive impairment (VCI), are often proposed as the cause of cognitive decline, particularly in elderly patients. VCI may follow any cerebrovascular disorder (small or large vessel ischemia due to thrombosis or embolism, inflammatory vascular disorders such as vasculitis, vasculopathies, or hematological disorders).

Recognized varieties of vascular cognitive impairment include:

- Multi-infarct dementia (MID): multiple large vessel infarcts involving cortical and subcortical areas, usually from large vessel occlusions
- Strategic infarct dementia: single or multiple infarcts affecting structures crucial for cognitive function, for example, bilateral hippocampal infarcts, bilateral thalamic infarctions, paramedian-mesencephalic-diencephalic infarcts
- Subcortical vascular cognitive impairment: white matter disease due to small vessel ischemia, for example, *Binswanger's disease*, multiple lacunar infarcts
- Familial vascular encephalopathies, for example, *CADASIL*

Because of the emphasis on memory decline as a key feature in *Alzheimer's disease (AD)*, cases of VCI and VaD may be overlooked if assessment with cognitive instruments designed for identification of AD are used. Although VaD is sometimes said to be the second most common cause of cognitive decline after AD, cases of pure vascular dementia are rare. Cerebrovascular change may often coexist with AD (there are shared risk factors), prompting a more integrative approach to classification with a continuum running from pure AD to pure VaD through entities such as "AD with vascular lesions" and "VaD with AD changes."

Clinical features

- Focal signs are more likely than in other dementia syndromes, for example, hemiparesis, aphasia, *marche à petit pas*.
- Cognitive syndrome: executive, subcortical and frontal lobe dysfunction said to predominate over disorders of memory and language (cf. AD); behavioral features may also be prominent (e.g., emotional lability).
- The classical teaching that vascular dementia has a sudden onset and/or stepwise progression does not always hold true; a considerable proportion has a gradual onset and progression.
- History of hypertension, other cardiovascular risk factors is common.

Investigation

Neuroimaging: the finding of vascular changes on CT/MRI may, or may not, correlate with cognitive/behavioral syndrome. The tightest correlation is in (rare) examples of strategic infarct dementia. Functional imaging (SPECT) may show multifocal, patchy deficits. Blood tests should check cholesterol; homocysteine may be a risk factor for cerebrovascular disease but what, if any, response may be made to an elevated level is currently unknown. CSF shows no specific findings.

Differential diagnosis

- Alzheimer's disease (may be concurrent with cerebrovascular disease)
- Dementia with Lewy bodies
- Frontotemporal lobar degeneration

Treatment and prognosis

There is no licensed treatment for vascular dementia currently. Trials of cholinesterase inhibitors have suggested symptomatic benefit greater than placebo, but less than seen in Alzheimer's disease. Control of risk factors for cerebrovascular disease (hypertension, hypercholesterolemia) is appropriate.

References

Bowler JV, Hachinski V, eds. Vascular Cognitive Impairment: Preventable Dementia. Oxford: Oxford University Press; 2003
Moorhouse P, Rockwood K. Vascular cognitive impairment: current concepts and clinical developments. Lancet Neurol. 2008;7:246–255

O'Brien J, Ames D, Gustafson L, Folstein M, Chiu E eds. Cerebrovascular Disease, Cognitive Impairment and Dementia. London: Martin Dunitz; 2004

Román GC, Tatemichi TK, Erkinjuntti T, et al. Vascular dementia: diagnostic criteria for research studies. Report of the NINDS-AIREN international workshop. Neurology. 1993;43:250–260

Wahlund LO, Erkinjuntti T, Gauthier S, eds. Vascular Cognitive Impairment in Clinical Practice. Cambridge: Cambridge University Press; 2009

Vascular malformations: overview

A wide terminology has been applied to vascular malformations, and not always in a standardized way. A recent classification draws a clear distinction between: "malformations" in which there is normal endothelial cell turnover, and growth, if it occurs at all, is by hypertrophy; and hemangiomas, in which endothelial hyperplasia occurs. In *arteriovenous malformations* (*AVM*) there is a tangled anastomosis of vessels, whereas in an arteriovenous fistula (AVF) there is a direct high flow connection between artery and vein. Malformations and fisutlae may be in the brain parenchyma or in the dura.

- Benign proliferating vascular anomalies:
  - Hemangioma
- Nonproliferating vascular anomalies:
  - Capillary malformation: telangiectasis
  - Venous malformation: developmental venous anomaly
  - Cavernous malformation: *cavernoma*
  - Arterial malformation: angiodysplasia, aneurysm
  - Arteriovenous shunting: brain AVM, brain AVF, dural AVF, vein of Galen AVF
  - Mixed malformations

References

Chaloupka JC, Huddle DC. Classification of vascular malformations of the central nervous system. Neuroimaging Clin North Am. 1998;8:295–321

Vasculitis

The vasculitides are inflammatory disorders of blood vessels which may produce neurological symptoms and signs if intracerebral vessels or the vasa nervorum of the peripheral nervous system are involved. The inflammation may be autoimmune in origin, for example, associated with markers for lupus or with anti-neutrophil cytoplasmic antibodies (ANCA). This may occur in the context of a variety of disorders, typically affecting vessels of differing caliber:

- Large arteries: Giant cell arteritis, Kawasaki disease, classical Polyarteritis nodosa, Takayasu's arteritis
- Medium arteries: Churg–Strauss syndrome, Microscopic polyangiitis, Wegener's granulomatosis
- Small vessels: Cryoglobulinemia

Vasculits may also occur on occasion in a variety of other conditions, such as rheumatoid arthritis, Sjögren's syndrome, systemic lupus erythematosus, sarcoidosis, syphilis, other infections (hepatitis B, C), and following use of certain recreational drugs (e.g., amphetamines, cocaine).

Clinical features

Very diverse.

- Central nervous system:
  - Acute/subacute encephalopathy
  - Multiple sclerosis-like presentation: relapsing–remitting disorder + features atypical of MS, such as epileptic seizures
  - Rapidly progressive space-occupying lesion
- Peripheral nervous system:
  - Mononeuritis multiplex
  - Mononeuropathies

Investigation

Bloods may show raised ESR, CRP; autoantibody profile may show positive ANA, anti-ds DNA, ANCA, cryoglobulins; check hepatitis serology; drug screen. Neuroimaging (MRI) may show periventricular white matter abnormalities akin to those of MS, or frank infarctions. SPECT may show patchy focal ischemic deficits. Cerebral angiography, although once used as the criterion for the diagnosis of vasculitis, is not specific, nor is it sensitive; its main use is to exclude atheromatous disease as a cause of the neurological syndrome. CSF may show oligoclonal bands. Ophthalmological slit-lamp examination of the anterior segment may show inflammatory changes in CNS vasculitis; fluorescein angiogram may corroborate this. Biopsy for histopathology is the gold standard investigation for the diagnosis of vasculitis, but the procedure is not without risk and the false-negative rate must also be taken into consideration; biopsy may be helpful in ruling out other diagnoses.

Differential diagnosis

Other causes of encephalopathy:

- Inflammatory CNS/PNS disease, for example, multiple sclerosis, neurosarcoidosis, SLE
- Tumor
- Mitochondrial disease, for example, MELAS
- Other vasculopathies, for example, fibromuscular dysplasia, moyamoya disease, amyloid angiopathy, CADASIL, Marfan's syndrome, pseudoxanthoma elasticum, Fabry's disease, homocystinuria, Ehlers–Danlos syndrome
- Infection
- Cholesterol embolization syndrome
- Vasculitic neuropathy:
  - Polyarteritis nodosa
  - Nonsystemic vasculitic neuropathy
  - Rheumatoid arthritis
  - Other connective tissue disease
  - HIV
  - Wegener's granulomatosis

Treatment and prognosis

Steroids may be adequate for localized disease, but for systemic or CNS disease, steroids in combination with cyclophosphamide are generally required. This treatment may need to be lifelong.

References

Salvarani C, Brown RD Jr, Calamia KT, et al. Primary central nervous system vasculitis: analysis of 101 patients. Ann Neurol. 2007;62:442–451
Scolding NJ, Wilson H, Hohlfeld R, et al. The recognition, diagnosis and management of cerebral vasculitis: a European survey. Eur J Neurol. 2002;9:343–347

Vegetative states

Apallic syndrome, Coma vigil, Minimally conscious state, Neocortical death

Following head injury or extensive ischemic-hypoxic brain injury, for example, following resuscitation after prolonged cardiac arrest, cognitive brain function may be lost due to neocortical damage (*brain death*) whilst vegetative functions are preserved due to intact brain stem centers. A persistent vegetative state (PVS) may be diagnosed if this persists for more than 12 months following trauma (UK; 6 months in USA) or for more than 6 months following anoxia (UK; 3 months in USA). Functional imaging studies have led some authorities to suggest that a subset of patients retain islands of preserved cognitive function.

Clinical features

- No awareness of self or environment, for example, to noxious visual stimuli (visual threat), auditory or tactile stimuli.
- Preserved autonomic, respiratory function.
- Primitive postural and reflex limb movements may be observed.
- Brain stem reflexes may be preserved.
- No reasonable prospect of improvement.
- Repeated and prolonged observations may be necessary to ensure the absence of awareness; other sources of information (nursing observations, relatives) should also be consulted.

Investigation

Clinical observation over time is the key investigation.

Differential diagnosis

- *Coma*
- Abulia/akinetic mutism
- *Locked-in syndrome*
- Catatonia

Treatment and prognosis

In persistent vegetative state the prognosis is poor; however, very occasional well-substantiated reports of very late recovery have appeared. Withdrawal of medical treatment requires the approval of the High Court, which decides whether continued treatment is in the patient's best interests, though serious ethical questions remain. Death usually occurs within 14 days of withdrawal of treatment.

References

Coleman MR, ed. The Assessment and Rehabilitation of Vegetative and Minimally Conscious Patients. Hove: Psychology Press; 2005

Coleman MR, Rodd JM, Davis MH, et al. Do vegetative patients retain aspects of language comprehension? Evidence from fMRI. Brain. 2007;130:2494–2507

Jennett B. The Vegetative State. Medical Facts, Ethical and Legal Dilemmas. Cambridge: Cambridge University Press; 2002

McLean SAM. Permanent vegetative state and the law. J Neurol, Neurosurg Psychiatry. 2001;71(Suppl 1):i26–i27

Wade DT, Johnston C. The permanent vegetative state: practical guidelines on diagnosis and management. Br Med J. 1999;319:841–844

Zeman A. The persistent vegetative state: conscious of nothing? Pract Neurol. 2002;2:214–217

Venous sinus thrombosis (VST)

Cerebral venous thrombosis, Cortical venous thrombosis (CVT), Sagittal sinus thrombosis (SST)

Thrombosis of the venous sinuses (sagittal, lateral) or cortical veins (venous stroke) may have an acute or subacute onset and produce a variety of clinical features. Although many cases are idiopathic, recognized risk factors, some of which are amenable to modification, include use of the oral contraceptive pill, other drugs (tetracyclines), localized intracranial infection (e.g., middle ear, +/– *cholesteatoma*, leading to lateral sinus thrombosis), thrombophilia, malignancy, vasculopathic inflammatory disease (*systemic lupus erythematosus, Behçet's disease, polyarteritis nodosa*), the puerperium, and possibly *neurosarcoidosis*.

Clinical features

Very variable:

- *Headache*: nonspecific, sometimes "thunderclap headache" +/– papilledema (especially sagittal sinus thrombosis)
- Epileptic seizures
- Focal signs: motor, sensory, visual deficits (often bilateral), aphasia (especially with cortical venous thrombosis causing infarction)

Investigation

Neuroimaging: infarction not confined to a single arterial territory is suggestive of venous thrombosis, +/- edema, hemorrhage (may even be subarachnoid blood). Delta sign may be evident on contrast-enhanced CT in sagittal sinus thrombosis, but not reliably so. MRI with attention to the veins (MRV) may confirm absence of flow voids; catheter angiography with attention to the venous phase may be required on occasion. Other investigations attempt to define cause, especially studies of the clotting system (anti-thrombin III, protein C, protein S). CSF may show increased protein, pleocytosis.

Differential diagnosis

Broad:

- Headache: from acute onset severe (e.g., subarachnoid hemorrhage) to chronic mild (tension-type headache)
- Epileptic seizures: encephalitis, meningitis
- Focal signs: arterial *stroke, intracerebral hemorrhage*; cerebral *abscess*; *subdural hematoma*
- CSF: *aseptic meningitis*

Treatment and prognosis

Anticoagulation with heparin/warfarin, even in the presence of cerebral hemorrhage, is the treatment of choice, although robust evidence (systematic reviews, randomized controlled trials) is not available. It should probably be maintained for 3–12 months. Thrombolysis is unproven. Symptomatic treatment of epileptic seizures; prophylactic anticonvulsants are sometimes recommended, with withdrawal at 6–12 months if the patient remains seizure free. Symptomatic treatment of raised intracranial pressure (deteriorating consciousness, visual failure). If established, the underlying cause may mandate specific treatment. The mortality of the acute condition is up to 30%. Although some patients make a full recovery, neurological sequelae may occur.

References

De Bruijn SFTM, Stam J, for the Cerebral Venous Sinus Thrombosis Group. Randomized, placebo-controlled trial of anticoagulant treatment with low-molecular-weight heparin for cerebral sinus thrombosis. Stroke. 1999;30:484–488
Stam J. Thrombosis of the cerebral veins and sinuses. N Engl J Med. 2005;352: 1791–1798

Verger–Déjerine syndrome

The Verger–Déjerine syndrome is an anterior parietal lobe syndrome characterized by contralateral impairment of discriminative sensory function (position sense, localization of touch and pain, two-point discrimination) but with relative sparing of primary or elementary sensory modalities (cf. *Déjerine–Mouzon syndrome*).

Vernant's disease

Recurrent optic neuromyelitis with endocrinopathies

Vernant and colleagues described eight Antillean women with a syndrome of recurrent optic and spinal cord inflammation, with dissociated sensory loss and sometimes with syrinx formation, associated with various endocrine disturbances. Whether this is a unique disease, or simply a variant of *neuromyelitis optica* (Devic's disease), which it resembles in its neurological features, has yet to be determined.

References

Román G. Tropical myeloneuropathies revisited. Curr Opin Neurol. 1998;11:539–544
Vernant J-C, Cabre P, Smadja D, et al. Recurrent optic neuromyelitis with endocrinopathies: a new syndrome. Neurology. 1997;48:58–64

Vestibular neuritis

Vestibular neuronitis

Vestibular neuritis, often known as labyrinthitis, reflects the acute loss of vestibular function unilaterally.

Clinical features

- Vertigo, nausea, vomiting for several hours, blurred vision, disequilibrium; patient often prostrated by the symptoms
- No hearing loss, tinnitus, fullness in the ears (cf. Ménière's disease)
- May be prior history of viral infection
- Horizontal-torsional nystagmus; increased in intensity with loss of fixation; abnormal head thrust test. Positive Unterberger's test

Investigation

Diagnosis is essentially clinical. Additional investigations are seldom required if the history and examination are consistent with the diagnosis. In centers with specialist interest, videonystagmography may be undertaken, showing spontaneous vestibular nystagmus that increases with loss of fixation; caloric testing shows absence of responses unilaterally. "Vestibular function tests" generally address only one-fifth of the vestibular system, so their normality does not exclude a peripheral vestibular disorder. Neuroimaging is normal. Audiometry is normal in vestibular neuritis; it may show high-frequency hearing loss with a more generalized labyrinthitis (cf. low-tone sensorineural hearing loss with Ménière's disease).

Differential diagnosis

Other causes of an acute vestibular syndrome:

- Vestibular migraine
- Endolymphatic hydrops: "vestibular-only" Ménière's disease
- Demyelinating disorder: unlikely in absence of other neurological signs
- Infarction of labyrinth, brain stem

Treatment and prognosis

Symptoms gradually settle spontaneously by a process of vestibular compensation in most patients. A course of steroids may decrease the duration of symptoms. Vestibular suppressants and antiemetic medications may be given as needed.

Reference

Strupp M, Zingler VC, Arbusow V et al. Methylprednisolone, valacyclovir, or the combination for vestibular neuritis. N Engl J Med. 2004;351:354–361

Vestibular paroxysmia

Vestibular paroxysmia is a cause of recurrent short spells of vertigo, believed to be one of the *neurovascular compression syndromes* involving the vestibular nerve, demonstrable on MRI. Hyperventilation-induced nystagmus may be present in 70% of cases. Carbamazepine and oxcarbazepine reduce attack frequency, duration, and severity.

References

Brandt T, Dieterich M. Vestibular paroxysmia: vascular compression of the eighth nerve? Lancet. 1994;343:798–799
Hüfner K, Barresi D, Glaser M et al. Vestibular paroxysmia: diagnostic features and medical treatment. Neurology. 2008;71:1006–1014

Vestibular schwannoma

Acoustic neurinoma, Acoustic neuroma

Vestibular schwannomas, also known as acoustic neuromas or neurinomas, are benign tumors arising from the Schwann cells of the vestibular component of the vestibulocochlear (VIII) cranial nerve in the region of the internal auditory meatus, first described pathologically by Leyden in 1776. Their rate of division is slow which means that they present insidiously and can grow to considerable size before the diagnosis is made, although occasionally intratumoral hemorrhage causes acute presentation. The typical presentation is with progressive sensorineural hearing loss with local involvement of the fifth and seventh cranial nerves and ipsilateral cerebellar signs. There may be associated brain stem compression with long tract signs and hydrocephalus. Classification may be based on extent of tumor growth and its relation to the brain stem (T1-T4B). Vestibular schwannomas are a feature of *neurofibromatosis* (*NF*), particularly NF2 in which bilateral tumors may occur: increased division of Schwann cells may be due to loss of a tumor suppressor gene. Vestibular schwannomas are treated surgically, but because of the late presentation there is often a significant morbidity associated. Vestibular schwannomas account for 2–8% of all primary intracranial neoplasms, with an incidence of 1:100,000, female preponderance, and usual presentation around 40–50 years of age. In contrast, NF2 nearly always presents before the age of 21 years.

Pathology usually shows an encapsulated oval tumor, 2–3.5 cm in diameter. Histologically the tumor may be classified as either:

- Antoni A: whorls of elongated spindle cells
- Antoni B: disorganized myxoid tissue with abundant ground substance and scattered stellate cells

Occasionally tumors are cystic or hemorrhagic; it is rare to find evidence of many mitoses.

Clinical features

- Sensorineural hearing loss: usually the earliest symptom; may be associated with tinnitus and vertigo. However the slow compression of the vestibular nerve allows for compensation and acute attacks of vertigo are rare.
- Local cranial nerve involvement:
  - Trigeminal (V) nerve: loss of sensation beginning with V1; loss of the corneal reflex may be the earliest sign, followed by facial dysaesthesia
  - Facial (VII) nerve: lower motor neurone facial weakness
  - Abducens (VI) nerve: diplopia, rare
  - Glossopharyngeal (IX), vagal (X) nerves: occasionally dysphagia

- Local pressure effects:
  - Cerebellar ataxia: ipsilateral to the lesion due to compression of cerebellum, although the patient may complain of unsteadiness before ataxia is clinically apparent
  - Headache: due to hydrocephalus from compression of fourth ventricle with raised intracranial pressure and papilledema: late features
  - Long tract signs: from compression of brain stem
  - Ipsilateral horizontal gaze paresis: occasionally occurs from local brain stem compression

Investigation

Neuroimaging: MRI with special views of the internal auditory meatus. Neurophysiology: BSAEP always abnormal, even in the absence of hearing loss (audiogram).

Differential diagnosis

- Other causes of the *cerebellopontine angle syndrome*, for example, meningioma, dermoid cyst, cholesteatoma.
- Ménière's disease.
- Posterior fossa demyelination.
- Posterior fossa stroke.
- Occasionally, a meningitic process (granulomatous or syphilitic) can mimic an acoustic neuroma.

Treatment and prognosis

Surgical removal involves either a posterior fossa craniotomy or a translabyrinthine approach, in which case no attempt is made to save hearing. In such circumstances there is usually a combined approach involving both neurosurgical and ENT teams. If the tumor is small (<2 cm in diameter) then there is a 50% chance of preserving hearing, but the likelihood falls with larger tumors. Furthermore, with large tumors, preservation of Vth to XIIth cranial nerves may prove difficult, and a significant morbidity from dysphagia may ensue.

Reference

Samii M, Gerganov VM. Vestibular schwannomas. In: Bernstein M, Berger MS, eds. Neuro-Oncology. The Essentials. 2nd ed. New York: Thieme; 2008:353–358

Visual loss: overview

Causes of visual loss may be classified according to their time course (transient, sudden nonprogressive, progressive) and laterality (unilateral, bilateral).

- Transient visual loss:
  - Monocular:
    - Vascular:
      - Ocular transient ischemic attack (amaurosis fugax)
      - Migraine
      - Hypoperfusion: hypotension, hyperviscosity (more usually bilateral)
      - Partial retinal vein occlusion
      - Vasculitis (e.g., giant cell arteritis)
    - Ocular: angle closure glaucoma
    - Inflammation: Uhthoff's phenomenon
    - Psychogenic
  - Binocular:
    - Transient visual obscurations, papilledema
    - Vascular:
      - Migraine
      - Hypoperfusion: hypotension, hyperviscosity
    - Epilepsy
    - Psychogenic
- Sudden, nonprogressive visual loss:
  - Monocular:
    - Central or branch retinal artery/vein occlusion
    - Anterior *ischemic optic neuropathy*
    - Retinal detachment
    - Vitreous hemorrhage
    - Psychogenic
  - Bilateral:
    - Occipital lobe infarctions
    - Pituitary apoplexy
    - *Leber's hereditary optic neuropathy* (*LHON*)
    - Psychogenic
- Progressive visual loss:
  - Hereditary optic neuropathy
  - Anterior visual pathway compression: tumor, aneurysm, dysthyroid eye disease
  - Anterior visual pathway inflammation: *optic neuritis*, sarcoidosis, meningitis
  - Toxic and nutritional optic neuropathies
  - Drug-induced optic neuropathy
  - Paraneoplastic retinal degeneration
  - Low-tension glaucoma

Vitamin B$_{12}$ deficiency

Cobalamin deficiency

Vitamin B$_{12}$ or cobalamin is involved in DNA synthesis throughout the body as well as myelination in the nervous system. A deficiency of this vitamin may cause a megaloblastic anemia, glossitis, and hypospermia (all due to impaired peripheral DNA synthesis) and a variety of neurological disorders:

- Peripheral neuropathy, usually of axonal type
- *Subacute combined degeneration of the cord*, affecting principally the dorsal and lateral columns
- Optic neuropathy: typically with centrocaecal scotoma
- Cognitive decline
- Leukoencephalopathy (rare)
- *Imerslund–Gräsbeck syndrome* (rare)

It is well attested that the neurological manifestations of vitamin B$_{12}$ deficiency can occur in the absence of a megaloblastic anemia.

The most common cause of vitamin B$_{12}$ deficiency is pernicious anemia, the autoimmune destruction of gastric parietal cells that produce the intrinsic factor (IF) which is essential for absorption of vitamin B$_{12}$ in the terminal ileum. Correction of the vitamin deficiency in the early stages by parenteral vitamin B$_{12}$ injections can reverse the neurological deficits, but there is a well-recognized inverse relationship between duration of deficiency and extent of neurological recovery following repletion. Hence, early recognition is important; cases are still missed. The incidence of vitamin B$_{12}$ deficiency is 1–3% in individuals over the age of 65 years in European populations and may be higher in populations from the Indian subcontinent.

Total body stores of vitamin B$_{12}$ amount to 2–5 mg, of which 50% is stored in liver. The average Western diet contains 20 µg/day, but required daily intake is only 6 µg/day. It usually takes 2–5 years to develop deficiency by depleting body stores.

Recognized causes of vitamin B$_{12}$ deficiency include:

- Nutritional deficiency
- Pernicious anemia (usually ~60 years old, F:M = 1–2:1)
- Gastric or ileal resection
- Gastrointestinal disease: tropical sprue, Crohn's disease, *diphyllobothriasis*
- Antibody deficiency: *common variable immunodeficiency* syndrome (CVID)
- Functional vitamin B$_{12}$ deficiency may follow overuse of nitrous oxide

Cobalamin is a cofactor to two enzymes: methionine synthase and methylmalonyl-CoA mutase; the former seems most significant for the consequences of vitamin B$_{12}$ deficiency, since it catalyzes the transfer of a methyl group from methyltetrahydrofolate to homocysteine to form methionine; if this reaction is impaired it eventually leads to impaired DNA synthesis.

Clinical features

- History:
  - Dietary: vegan, vegetarian
  - Previous surgery to gastrointestinal tract, or disease thereof
  - Family history
- Systemic features:
  - Megaloblastic anemia
  - Glossitis, *burning mouth syndrome*
  - Hypospermia/azoospermia
  - Features of GI disease and/or other autoimmune disorders (e.g., grey hair, lemon tinge to skin in pernicious anemia)
- Neurological features:
  - Peripheral neuropathy: usually starts with symmetric paresthesiae involving the feet and fingers with loss of joint position sense and vibration perception. It is usually an axonal neuropathy although demyelinating features are sometimes found; there is occasional involvement of the autonomic nervous system.
  - Subacute combined degeneration of the spinal cord (SACDOC): affects dorsal and lateral parts of the spinal cord (i.e., dorsal columns, spinocerebellar and pyramidal tracts). It presents with sensory ataxia (especially with superadded peripheral neuropathy) and mild spasticity +/− Lhermitte's sign and sphincter involvement. Sensory level not seen.
  - Optic neuropathy: typically with centrocaecal scotoma.
  - Cognitive decline; although often stated to be a cause of reversible dementia, this is in fact extremely rare.
  - Leukoencephalopathy.
  - Other nonspecific complaints are common, including anosmia, reduced manual dexterity.

Investigation

Bloods: FBC and blood film. A megaloblastic anemia which is characterized by raised mean corpuscular volume (MCV), hypersegmented neutrophils, and in some instances a pancytopenia. However, neurological features of vitamin B_{12} deficiency may develop in the absence of any hematological abnormalities. Vitamin B_{12} and folate levels: usually low. However, the assay is variable and so in the first instance, a low value should prompt a repeat assay. If the level is still low it may be worthwhile measuring the levels of the mctabolites homocysteine and methylmalonic acid, and/or performing a Schilling test in which an amount of radioactive vitamin B$_{12}$ is given and the amount excreted in the urine over 24 h calculated:

	Pernicious anemia	Malabsorption
Part 1	Abnormal	Abnormal
Part 2 (+ intrinsic factor)	Corrected	Not corrected

Routine biochemistry screen is usually normal. Autoantibody screen can be abnormal: especially important are whether antibodies reactive with intrinsic factor and gastric parietal cells are present, as in cases of pernicious anemia. Neuroimaging: CT/MRI brain is usually normal. Occasionally, a leukoencephalopathy is found. MR spinal cord may show a "longitudinal myelitis" of the posterior columns in SACDOC, especially in the cervical cord. CSF is usually normal. Neurophysiology: EMG/NCS shows sensorimotor neuropathy of axonal, demyelinating, or mixed axonal/demyelinating type; visual evoked potentials may be abnormal (even in absence of visual symptoms, likewise SSEPs, but BSAEPs are rarely abnormal).

Neuropsychology may reveal deficits in memory. Other investigation of hematological and/or gastroenterological features may necessitate specific consults.

Differential diagnosis

- Coeliac disease
- Vitamin E deficiency
- Cerebellar degenerations
- Mitochondrial disease
- Multiple sclerosis
- Neurosarcoidosis

Treatment and prognosis

Once vitamin B$_{12}$ deficiency is diagnosed, a cause should be sought. The mainstay of treatment is vitamin B$_{12}$ replacement: a typical regime for pernicious anemia is 1 mg i.m. on 5 consecutive days, followed by 1 mg every month thereafter. Occasionally neurological symptoms worsen with vitamin B$_{12}$ treatment; folate therapy with vitamin B$_{12}$ deficiency has been said to exacerbate neurological deficits, although this has been questioned. In the early stages, a full clinical and hematological recovery may be expected. All patients make some improvement in the first 3 months of therapy, and it is rare to be left with a severe neurological deficit from pure vitamin B$_{12}$ deficiency, although troubling dysaesthetic symptoms sometimes persist after SACDOC.

References

Larner AJ. Missed diagnosis of vitamin B$_{12}$ deficiency presenting with paraesthetic symptoms. Int J Clin Pract. 2002;56:377–378

Larner AJ. Visual failure caused by vitamin B$_{12}$ deficiency optic neuropathy. Int J Clin Pract. 2004;58:977–978

Larner AJ, Janssen JC, Cipolotti L, Rossor MN. Cognitive profile in dementia associated with vitamin B$_{12}$ deficiency due to pernicious anaemia. J Neurol. 1999;246:317–319

Vitamin deficiencies and the nervous system: overview

Nutritional deficiency of vitamins may have profound adverse effects on nervous system function. These conditions are usually seen in individuals with poor nutritional intake; alcohol abuse may lead to vitamin deficiency. Disorders causing fat malabsorption may also lead to deficiency of fat-soluble vitamins (A, D, E, K).

Clinical features

- Vitamin A (β-carotene): xerophthalmia, nyctalopia (night blindness)
- Vitamin B complex (riboflavin, thiamine): *beriberi*, pellagra; nutritional polyneuropathy; nutritional amblyopia; *Wernicke–Korsakoff syndrome*; ? Strachan's syndrome
- Vitamin B$_6$ (pyridoxine): polyneuropathy
- Vitamin B$_{12}$ (cobalamin): *subacute combined degeneration of the spinal cord* (predominantly posterior column myelopathy + peripheral neuropathy), optic neuropathy, neurobehavioral disorder, reversible cognitive decline (rare), white matter lesions on MR imaging (significance uncertain)
- Vitamin C: scurvy
- Vitamin D (calciferol): rickets, *osteomalacia*, muscle weakness (?myopathy), tetany; deficiency may be induced by prolonged use of antiepileptic medications (especially phenytoin, phenobarbitone)
- Vitamin E (tocopherol): spinocerebellar ataxia (in context of intestinal malabsorption, e.g., cystic fibrosis), although an autosomal recessive condition called *ataxia with vitamin E deficiency (AVED)* due to mutations in the α-tocopherol gene does occur
- Vitamin K: clotting disorders

Investigation

Assay of certain vitamins is possible, but usually the dietary status leads to clinical suspicion strong enough to suggest diagnosis and appropriate treatment.

Treatment and prognosis

Restoration of adequate nutrition +/– vitamin supplements may reverse many neurological features.

Reference

Mancall EL. Nutritional disorders of the nervous system. In: Aminoff MJ, ed. Neurology and General Medicine: The Neurological Aspects of Medical Disorders. 2nd ed. New York: Churhcill Livingstone; 1995:323–339

Vogt–Koyanagi–Harada (VKH) syndrome

Uveoretinal meningoencephalitic syndrome

Vogt–Koyanagi–Harada (VKH) syndrome is an inflammatory disorder, but not a true *vasculitis*, affecting predominantly the eyes and skin, and sometimes cranial nerves and brain parenchyma. There is some evidence for cellular and humoral immune responses to melanocytes.

Clinical features

- Neurological:
  - Aseptic meningitis
  - Sensorineural hearing loss
  - Headache
  - Cranial nerve involvement (especially III, IV, VI)
  - Hemiplegia
  - Transverse myelitis
  - Neuropsychiatric changes
- Ophthalmological:
  - Uveitis: chronic, diffuse, granulomatous panuveitis
  - Retinal hemorrhages
- Dermatological:
  - Depigmentation of eyebrows, eyelashes, and scalp hair (vitiligo, poliosis)

Investigation

Neuroimaging (MRI) may show high-intensity periventricular lesions, choroidal changes. CSF may show lymphocytic pleocytosis, raised protein. Ophthalmic assessment may show an acutely hyperemic disc with retinal hemorrhages and detachments; convalescent pale atrophic disc with orange-red discoloration of the fundus.

Differential diagnosis

Uveoretinal meningoencephalitic syndromes: may be inflammatory, for example, *neurosarcoidosis, systemic lupus erythematosus (SLE)*, vasculitis; infectious, for example, *neurosyphilis*, tuberculosis, herpes viruses (simplex or zoster); or malignant, for example, *lymphoma*, leukemia.

Treatment and prognosis

High-dose intravenous steroids are advocated. For refractory cases other immunosuppressive therapies may be used such as ciclosporin, chlorambucil, cyclophosphamide, azathioprine, or intravenous immunoglobulin. The majority of patients retain moderate-to-good vision.

Reference

Fang W, Yang P. Vogt-Koyanagi-Harada syndrome. Curr Eye Res. 2008;33:517–523

Von Hippel–Lindau (VHL) disease [OMIM#193300]

Cerebello-retinal angiomatosis, Hemangioblastoma of the cerebellum

Von Hippel–Lindau (VHL) disease is an autosomal dominant *neurocutaneous syndrome* characterized by hemangioblastomas of the cerebellum (60%), retina and optic nerve head (60%, often asymptomatic), spinal cord (13–44%), and brain stem (18%), and sometimes associated with renal cell carcinoma and pheochromocytoma. It is usually diagnosed in the third decade. It is caused by mutations in the VHL gene.

Clinical features

- Neurological:
  - Cerebellar signs (gait, limb ataxia)
  - Raised intracranial pressure
  - Cord compression, pain
- Non-neurological:
  - Polycythemia: secondary to renal cell carcinoma
  - Hypertension, orthostatic hypotension: due to pheochromocytoma
  - Abdominal mass (renal cell carcinoma; pancreatic cyst, adenoma)
  - Endolymphatic sac tumor
  - Cystadenoma of the epididymis or broad ligament

Family history of similar conditions.

Investigation

Bloods: polycythemia. Urine: elevated VMA may be found with pheochromocytoma. Neuroimaging (MRI) may show a cerebellar cyst with enhancing nodular lesion on wall; MRA/Angiography shows hypervascular nodule(s) with dilated draining veins; MRI cord may show hemangioblastoma of cord, often multiple, often of posterior columns, causing compression +/– syrinx formation. Other investigations include CT/MRI/ultrasonography of kidneys, adrenals, pancreas; ophthalmology opinion +/– fluorescein angiography. Neurogenetic testing.

Differential diagnosis

Isolated cerebellar or spinal cord tumors. *Wyburn–Mason disease* (retinal angioma).

Treatment and prognosis

Surgical resection of cerebellar/cord lesions may be possible, but ataxia, paraplegia may persist. Laser therapy of retinal lesions may be required. Debulking of renal tumors, partial nephrectomy; renal cell carcinoma is leading cause of death. Appropriate medical management of pheochromocytoma followed by surgical resection. Tumors have a tendency to recur, hence screening of patients as well as at-risk individuals is recommended.

References

Latif F, Tory K, Gnarra J, Yao M, Duh F-M, Orcutt ML. Identification of the von Hippel-Lindau disease tumor suppressor gene. Science. 1993;260:1317–1320
Maher ER, Yates JRW, Harries R, et al. Clinical features and natural history of von Hippel-Lindau disease. Q J Med. 1990;77:1151–1163
Sims KB. Von Hippel-Lindau disease: gene to bedside. Curr Opin Neurol. 2001;14:695–703
Singh AD, Shields CL, Shields JA. Von Hippel-Lindau disease. Survey Ophthalmol. 2001;46:117–142

Von Winiwarter–Buerger's disease

Cerebral thromboangiitis obliterans, Spatz–Lindenberg disease

Von Winiwarter–Buerger's disease is an isolated cerebral form of thromboangiitis obliterans, a noninflammatory occlusive vasculopathy which usually affects peripheral tissues. Cases were described in the late 1930s by Spatz and Lindenberg which, unlike Buerger's disease, occurred in the absence of vascular risk factors (hypertension, smoking). The condition usually presents with dementia and pyramidal signs; there are no specific clinical or histopathological features. Only a handful of cases with pathological verification have been published.

Clinical features

- Dementia; informant interview required
- Pyramidal signs
- Focal and secondarily generalized epileptic seizures

Investigation

No specific abnormalities known in blood, neuroimaging, or CSF, although MRI may show subcortical leukoencephalopathy and brain atrophy. Diagnosis is based on brain biopsy which shows an occlusive arteriopathy affecting both leptomeningeal and intraparenchymal vessels, due to profound intimal thickening, with an intact and reduplicated internal elastic lamina, but no evidence of inflammation or infiltration of blood vessels. Cortex shows nonspecific gliosis.

Differential diagnosis

Other causes of vascular dementia with subcortical leukoencephalopathy, including multi-infarct dementia, Binswanger's disease/encephalopathy, CADASIL, and cerebral vasculitis.

Treatment and prognosis

No specific treatment known; symptomatic control of seizures, spasticity; neurorehabilitation.

References

Larner AJ, Kidd D, Elkington P, Rudge P, Scaravilli F. Spatz-Lindenberg disease: a rare cause of vascular dementia. Stroke. 1999;30:687–689
Zhan S-S, Beyreuther K, Schmitt HP. Vascular dementia in Spatz-Lindenberg disease (SLD): cortical synaptophysin immunoreactivity as compared with dementia of Alzheimer type and non-demented controls. Acta Neuropathol (Berlin). 1993;86: 259–264

W

Wartenberg's neuropathy

Multifocal relapsing sensory neuropathy, Wartenberg's migrant sensory neuritis

Wartenberg's neuropathy is a rare disorder characterized by recurrent attacks of pain followed by sensory loss in the distribution of various cutaneous sensory nerves (hence "migrant"), with resolution of symptoms over a period of weeks. Onset is usually in the fourth or fifth decade. This may be a syndrome produced by more than one underlying condition rather than a single entity. A possible genetic influence is suggested by its coincidence with hereditary *neuralgic amyotrophy*.

Clinical features

- Pain followed by sensory loss in the distribution of a cutaneous nerve; attacks may be precipitated by limb movement or stretching.
- Motor function not affected. Reflexes retained.

Investigation

Neurophysiology: NCS may be able to confirm involvement of cutaneous sensory nerve(s); motor studies normal. Nerve biopsy: may show loss of large myelinated fibers, fibrosis, and axonal regeneration.

Differential diagnosis

Other causes of sensory mononeuropathy, usually compression.

Treatment and prognosis

No specific treatment known. Symptomatic treatment of pain if necessary. Sensory loss usually improves over a few weeks and often returns to normal.

References

Matthews WB, Esiri M. The migrant sensory neuritis of Wartenberg. J Neurol Neurosurg Psychiatry. 1983;46:1–4
Thomas PK, Ormerod IEC. Hereditary neuralgic amyotrophy associated with a relapsing multifocal sensory neuropathy. J Neurol Neurosurg Psychiatry. 1993;56:107–109

Weber–Christian disease

Systemic panniculitis

Weber–Christian disease is an inflammatory condition of fatty tissue (cf. *vasculitis*) usually presenting with red tender nodules in the skin, recurrent or relapsing fevers, with myalgia and arthralgia, and sometimes associated with pancreatic or autoimmune pathology but often idiopathic. Neurological features are rare, but include meningeal xanthogranuloma, with brainstem or cerebellar signs; myopathy; and intramedullary partial myelopathy. Bloods may show raised ESR, CRP, LFTs, ACE, hypergammaglobulinemia, hypocomplementemia (all nonspecific). CSF shows no specific abnormalities but may have oligoclonal bands matched with serum. Neuroimaging (CT/MRI) may show a meningeal mass lesion, or may be remarkably normal. Diagnosis is usually by biopsy of skin lesions showing a non-suppurative lobular panniculitis, with a mononuclear or pleomorphic cellular infiltrate with fat-laden macrophages. Empirical immunosuppressive treatment, with steroids and/or cyclophosphamide, may be attempted.

References

Larner AJ, Marshall B, Ma RCW, Ball JA. Systemic Weber-Christian disease complicated by partial transverse myelopathy. Int J Clin Pract. 2000;54:472–474
Panush RS, Yonker RA, Dlesk A, Longley S, Caldwell JR. Weber-Christian disease. Analysis of 15 cases and review of literature. Medicine. 1985;64:181–191

Wegener's granulomatosis

Wegener's granulomatosis is a granulomatous *vasculitis* predominantly affecting the respiratory tract with destructive cartilaginous change (e.g., saddle nose deformity). Renal disease is usual, ocular disease may occur. Neurological features are predominantly in the peripheral nervous system, and result from spread of granulomata, more frequently than is the case in vasculitis. It may occasionally involve only the CNS often presenting as a single lesion involving the meninges with negative ANCA serology.

Clinical features

Neurological features, affecting either central of peripheral nervous system, are present in about one third of cases:

- Peripheral neuropathy (10–20% of cases): mononeuropathy multiplex, distal symmetrical sensorimotor polyneuropathy.
- Cranial neuropathy, external ophthalmoplegia, *cavernous sinus disease*; involvement of II, V, VI, VII, VIII; ca. 10% of cases: possibly due to granulomatous infiltration of orbit, cavernous sinus.
- Cerebrovascular events.
- Epileptic seizures.
- Raised intracranial pressure (extravascular jugular vein compression).
- Orbital pseudotumor.
- + Respiratory, renal (glomerulonephritis) involvement.

Investigation

Bloods: +ve cANCA is a marker, although this may be persistently negative in the early stages of disease, becoming positive only with disease progression; there may be eosinophilia. Neurophysiology (EMG/NCS) for peripheral neuropathic involvement. Neuroimaging (CT/MRI) may be indicated, especially for cavernous sinus or orbital disease. CSF may show raised protein, lymphocytosis, but may be normal. Nerve biopsy may confirm presence of necrotizing granulomatous vasculitis.

Differential diagnosis

Other intracranial vasculitides.

Treatment and prognosis

Immunosuppression, usually involving a combination of prednisolone and oral cyclophosphamide (reported remission rate of 75%). Methotrexate has also been used. For acute disease, a course of intravenous methylprednisolone is recommended. Limited disease may respond to trimethoprim/ sulphamethoxazole.

References

Nadeau SE. Neurologic manifestations of systemic vasculitis. Neurol Clin. 2002;20: 123–150

Nishino H, Rubino FA, DeRemee R, Swanson JW, Parisi J. Neurological involvement in Wegener's granulomatosis: an analysis of 324 consecutive patients at the Mayo Clinic. Ann Neurol. 1993;33:4–9

Weinberger LM, Cohen ML, Remler BF, et al. Intracranial Wegener's granulomatosis. Neurology. 1993;43:1831–1834

Welander's myopathy

Late adult onset distal myopathy, Swedish type distal myopathy

Weakness in the distal muscles of the upper extremities, usually commencing in the fifth decade, is typical of this condition, with spread to the distal lower extremities but seldom with proximal involvement; reflexes are preserved with the possible exception of ankle jerks. Creatine kinase is normal or slightly elevated; EMG shows myopathic or mixed myopathic–neurogenic features. Muscle biopsy shows a dystrophic pattern with central nuclei, fiber splitting, increased connective tissue, and sometimes rimmed vacuoles. The condition is linked to chromosome 2p13.

Reference

Borg K, Ahlberg G, Borg J, Edström L. Welander's distal myopathy: clinical, neuro-physiological and muscle biopsy observations in young and middle aged adults with early symptoms. J Neurol Neurosurg Psychiatry. 1991;54:494–498

Werdnig–Hoffmann disease [OMOM#253300]

Acute infantile spinal muscular atrophy, Hereditary motor neuropathy type I, Severe spinal muscular atrophy, Spinal muscular atrophy type I

This autosomal recessive *spinal muscular atrophy* has childhood onset (always before 6 months) and generally poor prognosis.

Clinical features

- Hypotonia ("floppy baby"); severe limb weakness worse proximally; "frog's leg" posture; areflexia.
- Tongue fasciculation (50%); facial muscles little affected if at all.
- Bulbar, respiratory (intercostal, not diaphragm) involvement; weak cry.
- Failure to attain developmental motor milestones (i.e., sitting).
- (Decreased fetal movements in pregnancy, in perhaps one third of cases).

Investigation

Bloods: creatine kinase normal (cf. SMA type III, Kugelberg–Welander disease).

Neurophysiology: EMG/NCS shows reduced compound muscle action potential amplitude, acute denervation; sensory studies normal. Muscle biopsy shows types I/II muscle fiber atrophy in fascicles or groups of fascicles, + hypertrophied type I fibers in other fascicles. Neurogenetic testing shows SMN deletions in ca. 95% (exons 7 and 8).

Differential diagnosis

- Infantile hypotonia:
  - Pompe disease
  - Centronuclear myopathy
  - Nemaline myopathy
  - Congenital muscular dystrophy
  - Central core disease
  - Dystrophia myotonica type 1

Treatment and prognosis

No specific treatment; supportive, respiratory care. Most die by age 2 years, from overwhelming respiratory infection; some survive into childhood.

Reference

Le Febvre S, Bürglen L, Frézal J, et al. The role of the SMN gene in proximal spinal muscular atrophy. Hum Mol Genet. 1998;7:1531–1536

Werner syndrome [OMIM#277700]

Werner syndrome is a rare autosomal recessive disorder, also known as "progeria of the adult," first described by Werner in 1904. Development is normal until the third decade when premature aging phenotypes begin, including scleroderma-like thin tight skin, bilateral cataracts, greying and baldness, thin arms and legs. Reported neurological features include transient ischemic attacks due to common carotid artery atherosclerosis, peripheral neuropathy, and possible myelopathy. MR brain imaging may show low normalized brain volume and reduced NAA/Cr ratios. The condition has been associated with mutations in the WRN gene whose protein product has both helicase and exonuclease activities, loss of which leads to abnormal DNA repair, replication, and telomere maintenance.

References

Anderson NE, Haas LF. Neurological complications of Werner's syndrome. J Neurol. 2003;250:1174–1178
Muftuoglu M, Oshima J, von Kobbe C, et al. The clinical characteristics of Werner syndrome: molecular and biochemical diagnosis. Hum Genet. 2008;124:369–377

Wernicke–Korsakoff syndrome (WKS)

A neurological (Wernicke's disease) and neuropsychological (Korsakoff's psychosis) syndrome, the features of which may be seen in isolation or combination, occurring in nutritionally deficient individuals, most usually chronic alcoholics but also following chronic vomiting as in pregnancy (hyperemesis gravidarum). Thiamine deficiency may be of particular pathogenetic significance; thiamine preparations should be given to all patients in whom this diagnosis is suspected.

Clinical features

- Wernicke's disease/encephalopathy:
  - Acute/subacute nystagmus (horizontal and vertical), ophthalmoplegia (horizontal > vertical, e.g., internuclear ophthalmoplegia), cerebellar ataxia of gait, + disturbance of consciousness/mentation: global confusional state, alcohol withdrawal, stupor and coma, amnesic state.
- Korsakoff's psychosis:
  - Amnesic disorder: anterograde and retrograde amnesia. Pathological evidence of thalamic and mammillary body involvement.
  - Confabulation occurs, but is very rare, probably requiring an additional frontal lobe lesion. There is relatively intact immediate memory, attention, and language function.
- Concurrent features in some cases:
  - Peripheral neuropathy
  - Optic neuropathy
  - Impaired olfaction
  - Vestibular paresis (unilateral, bilateral)

Autopsy studies demonstrate a higher incidence of Wernicke–Korsakoff syndrome than recognized in life, isolated delirium without eye signs or ataxia being the most common feature in cases not diagnosed during life. Conditions associated with WKS include alcoholism, prolonged intravenous feeding, hyperemesis gravidarum, anorexia nervosa, prolonged fasting, refeeding after starvation, gastric plication, and bariatric surgery.

Investigation

Bloods: low erythrocyte transketolase level (= index of thiamine deficiency); raised LFTs may indicate chronic alcohol abuse. Neuroimaging (MRI) may show medial thalamic and periaqueductal changes. CSF is usually normal, there may be slightly increased protein. EEG may show diffuse mild to moderate slow activity.

Differential diagnosis

- Encephalopathy: delirium.
- Acute ophthalmoplegia: Miller Fisher syndrome, Bickerstaff's brainstem encephalitis.
- Internuclear ophthalmoplegia: multiple sclerosis, cerebrovascular disease.
- Amnesic disorder: Alzheimer's disease, temporal lobe epilepsy, transient global amnesia, head injury, third ventricular tumor, and herpes simplex encephalitis.

Treatment and prognosis

Thiamine should be given as soon as diagnosis is considered. Features of Wernicke's encephalopathy are promptly reversed; neuropsychological deficits may persist.

Diagnostic criteria

Caine D, Halliday GM, Kril JJ, Harper CG. Operational criteria for the classification of chronic alcoholics: identification of Wernicke's encephalopathy. J Neurol Neurosurg Psychiatry. 1997;62:51–60

References

Galvin R, Brathen G, Ivashynka I, et al. EFNS guidelines for diagnosis, therapy and prevention of Wernicke encephalopathy. Eur J Neurol. 2010;17:1408–1418

Kopelman MD, Thomson AD, Guerrini I, Marshall EJ. The Korsakoff syndrome: clinical aspects, psychology and treatment. Alcohol Alcohol. 2009;44:148–154

Victor M, Adams RD, Collins GH. The Wernicke-Korsakoff Syndrome and Related Neurologic Disorders due to Alcoholism and Malnutrition. 2nd ed. Philadelphia, PA: Davis; 1989

Whipple's disease

Whipple's disease is a multisystem granulomatous disorder caused by the organism *Tropheryma whippelii*. Gastrointestinal and systemic features usually predominate but neurological involvement, sometimes in isolation, occurs in perhaps 10% of cases. Although uncommon, Whipple's disease is treatable and hence the condition often figures in the differential diagnosis of multisystem disease.

Clinical features

- Neurological (in 10% of patients, presenting features in 5%):
  - Dementia (>70%)
  - Ophthalmoplegia (may be supranuclear; >50%)
  - Epileptic seizures (ca. 20%)
  - Cerebellar ataxia (ca. 20%)
  - Pyramidal signs (>30%)
  - Myoclonus
  - Oculo-facial or oculo-masticatory myorhythmia with vergence oscillations: said to be pathognomonic of Whipple's disease
  - Hypothalamic features: somnolence, polydipsia, hypogonadism
  - Eye disease: keratitis, uveitis, papilledema, ptosis
  - Cranial neuropathies
  - Stroke-like episodes
- Systemic:
  - Weight loss, abdominal pain, diarrhea, steatorrhea
  - Fever, malaise
  - Arthropathy
  - Anemia
  - Erythema nodosum, pigmentation
  - Lymphadenopathy

Investigation

Neuroimaging (CT/MRI) may be normal; may sometimes show multiple high signal intensity areas on T_2-weighted images, particularly in region of hypothalamus; enhancing mass lesions are also reported. CSF shows elevated protein, pleocytosis; PAS +ve bacilli may be identified (ca. 30%). Small bowel/

mesenteric lymph node biopsy: periodic acid-Schiff (PAS) positive bacilli; electron microscopy is mandatory (diagnosis may otherwise be overlooked). PCR amplification of *Tropheryma whippelii* DNA in CSF, *in situ* in brain tissue.

Differential diagnosis

Neurosarcoidosis, multiple sclerosis.

Treatment and prognosis

Uniformly fatal without treatment. Responds to antibiotics, e.g., penicillin, streptomycin, and cotrimoxazole. Relapse is not uncommon; PCR for *T. whippelii* may be useful to monitor treatment efficacy.

Diagnostic criteria

Louis ED, Lynch T, Kaufmann P, Fahn S, Odel J. Diagnostic guidelines in central nervous system Whipple's disease. Ann Neurol. 1996;40:561–568

Reference

Panegyres PK. Diagnosis and management of Whipple's disease of the brain. Pract Neurol. 2008;8:311–317

Wilson's disease [OMIM#277900]

Hepatolenticular degeneration, Westphal–Strümpell pseudosclerosis

Wilson's disease is an autosomal recessive disorder of copper metabolism, due to mutations in the ATP7B gene, usually presenting in young adults with hepatic and/or neurological dysfunction, due to accumulation of copper in affected tissues.

Clinical features

- Hepatic (tend to be first features to manifest, in later childhood):
  - Fulminant hepatic failure
  - Chronic active hepatitis
  - Cirrhosis

- Neurological (adolescence, early adulthood):
  - Early:
    - Abnormal behavior, psychiatric symptoms
    - Kayser–Fleischer rings (copper deposition in Descemet's membrane)
    - Akinetic-rigid syndrome: dystonia, rigidity, grimacing, excessive salivation
    - Cerebellar syndrome: ataxia, tremor (flapping, wing-beating), titubation, dysarthria
  - Late:
    - Dystonia.
    - Spasticity
    - Epileptic seizures
    - Dementia
    - Flexion contractures

Investigation

Bloods: elevated copper (although this is nonspecific and may occur in cholestatic liver disease); reduced caeruloplasmin (<20 mg/dL) is more specific. Urine: 24 h copper excretion is high (>100 mg). Slit lamp examination for Kayser–Fleischer rings; sunflower cataracts.

Neuroimaging (CT/MRI) may show low attenuation/signal intensity lesions in basal ganglia.

Liver biopsy: for hepatic copper content; may be required in cases lacking Kayser–Fleischer rings, neurological features and with a normal plasma caeruloplasmin. Neurogenetics: linked to chromosome 13q14.3-q21.1; mutated gene encodes a copper transporting ATPase (ATP7B).

Differential diagnosis

Other early-onset *parkinsonian syndromes*. *Non-Wilsonian hepatocerebral degeneration* is an acquired disorder, occurring as a rare complication of chronic (usually alcoholic) liver disease.

Treatment and prognosis

Early and continued copper chelation therapy is mandatory to prevent the otherwise progressive and irreversible neurological sequelae. Options include:

- D-penicillamine (250–500 mg qds) + prophylactic oral pyridoxine.
- Trientine (triethylene tetramine).
- Tetrathiomolybdate.
- British anti-Lewisite (now rarely used).

- Oral zinc reduces dietary copper absorption (i.e., it is not a chelating agent); its use is favored in asymptomatic patients and during pregnancy.

Liver transplantation cures the condition and may reverse some neurological features Family screening may be required.

References

Lorincz MT. Neurologic Wilson's disease. Ann NY Acad Sci. 2010;1184:173–187
Walshe JM. The conquest of Wilson's disease. Brain. 2009;132:2289–2295
Wilson SAK. Progressive lenticular degeneration: a familial nervous disease associated with cirrhosis of the liver. Brain. 1912;34:295–509

Wolfram syndrome

Diabetes insipidus, Diabetes Mellitus, Optic Atrophy, and Deafness (DIDMOAD) syndrome

Wolfram syndrome is an autosomal recessive neurodegenerative disorder characterized by juvenile-onset diabetes mellitus and optic atrophy, with various other neurological features including diabetes insipidus and deafness, related to brainstem atrophy and dysfunction. Pathogenesis is unknown; mutations in a gene on chromosome 4p (WFS1, wolframin) encoding a transmembrane protein of undetermined function are suspected.

Clinical features

- Juvenile-onset diabetes mellitus and optic atrophy (*sine qua non*)
- Other features:
  - Positive family history
  - Brainstem signs: dysarthria, dysphagia, nystagmus, gaze palsies (Parinaud's syndrome), primary respiratory failure
  - Diabetes insipidus (50%)
  - Sensorineural deafness (50%)
  - Anosmia
  - Seizures/myoclonus
  - Truncal ataxia
  - Axial rigidity
  - Neuropsychiatric/cognitive abnormalities
  - Neurogenic incontinence
  - Hyporeflexia, areflexia
  - Extensor plantar responses
  - Renal tract abnormalities, GI dysmotility, primary gonadal atrophy

Investigation

Neuroimaging (MRI) shows brainstem atrophy, especially involving pons and midbrain. Neurophysiology: NCS/EMG may show mild axonal neuropathy (consistent with diabetes mellitus); EEG may show nonspecific abnormalities, e.g., slowing. Neurogenetics: Mitochondrial DNA analysis has occasionally been reported to show mutations.

Differential diagnosis

The full DIDMOAD syndrome is characteristic, but in partial forms there may be confusion with inflammatory disorders (multiple sclerosis, Behçet's disease) or degenerative conditions.

Treatment and prognosis

No specific treatment known. Appropriate medical treatment of diabetes mellitus, diabetes insipidus. Low vision/hearing aids for visual failure/deafness. Respiratory support may be necessary in cases of primary respiratory failure/central apnea. The median age of death is 30 years.

References

Ganie MA, Bhat D. Current developments in Wolfram syndrome. J Pediatr Endocrinol Metab. 2009;22:3–10
Inoue H, Tanizawa Y, Wasson J, et al. A gene encoding a transmembrane protein is mutated in patients with diabetes mellitus and optic atrophy (Wolfram syndrome). Nat Genet. 1998;20:143–148
Scolding NJ, Kellar-Wood HF, Shaw C, Shneerson JM, Antoun N. Wolfram syndrome: hereditary diabetes mellitus with brainstem and optic atrophy. Ann Neurol. 1996;39:352–360

Writing tremor

Primary writing tremor

Writing tremor is a task-specific *tremor*, evident as a pronation–supination movement of 5–7 Hz on attempting to write. It may be limited to writing or evident in other movements as well; some individuals also have a postural tremor.

The condition is much rarer than writer's cramp, a focal *dystonia* in which tremor may also occur. Whether the two conditions are separate or related remains uncertain; cerebellar activation similar to that seen in *essential tremor* has been reported in PET scan studies of primary writing tremor.

Treatment may be attempted with anticholinergic drugs (as for dystonias), propranolol, primidone, alcohol (as for essential tremor), botulinum toxin injections, and stereotactic thalamotomy.

Reference

Bain PG, Findlay LJ, Britton TC, et al. Primary writing tremor. Brain. 1995;118: 1461–1472

Wyburn-Mason disease

Dechaume–Blanc–Bonnet syndrome

Wyburn-Mason disease is a sporadic *neurocutaneous syndrome* characterized by retinal arteriovenous malformation (AVM), usually unilateral, and independent intracranial AVM, which may extend along the visual pathway to the cerebral peduncle and cerebellar hemisphere. Facial (periorbital) involvement may also occur. Rupture may occur. Onset is usually in adulthood. The retinal AVM may cause proptosis, visual loss (acute or chronic), glaucoma, and optic atrophy. Neurological features may include epileptic seizures, headache, and subarachnoid hemorrhage. Facial angiomas may be unilateral or bilateral. Fluorescein angiography may demonstrate the racemose angioma; MRI may demonstrate intracerebral AVM. The differential diagnosis includes *Von Hippel–Lindau disease* (inherited) and *Sturge–Weber syndrome.* Treatment may require surgical resection, embolization, and radiosurgery.

References

Skorin L, Simmons DK. Wybrun-Mason syndrome. Mayo Clin Proc. 2008;83:135
Wyburn-Mason R. Arteriovenous aneurysm of midbrain and retina, facial naevi and mental changes. Brain. 1943;6:163–189

XYZ

Xeroderma pigmentosum (XP)

De Sanctis–Cacchione syndrome

Xeroderma pigmentosum (XP) is a rare, heterogeneous, group of autosomal recessive disorders characterized by cutaneous lesions in childhood (dermatitis, skin cancer) due to the inability to repair DNA damaged by ultraviolet (UV) radiation (i.e., hypersensitivity to UV radiation). Various mutations underpin the reduced capacity for excision repair of UV-induced DNA damage. The De Sanctis-Cacchione syndrome forms a subgroup of XP in which skin changes are associated with retarded growth and sexual development and neurological complications. In trichothiodystrophy, mental retardation is associated with ichthyosis, brittle hair, and nails. Neurological manifestations are said to occur in about 20% of XP patients.

Clinical features

- Neurological: (not all patients)
  - Motor/mental retardation
  - Microcephaly
  - Sensorineural deafness
  - Cerebellar ataxia
  - Choreoathetosis
  - Axonal polyneuropathy
  - Spastic quadriplegia
- Ocular:
  - Keratitis, conjunctivitis
- Dermatological:
  - Hyperpigmented macules, atrophy, telangiectasia; benign tumors (e.g., keratoma, fibroma, angiomyoma); malignant tumors (basal cell, squamous cell, melanoma).

Investigations

Neurophysiology: EEG shows generalized slowing; focal slow-wave and spike discharges may be seen; EMG/NCS may show axonal polyneuropathy. Neurogenetics: heterogeneous, seven subtypes or complementation groups are recognized, caused by mutations in a number of genes that encode DNA repair proteins.

Treatment and prognosis

Protection from sunlight; skin surveillance; early excision of tumors. Death from disseminated tumors by second to third decade is usual.

Reference

Mimaki T, Itoh N, Abe J, et al. Neurological manifestations in xeroderma pigmentosum. Ann Neurol. 1986;20:70–75

X-linked dystonia-parkinsonism syndrome [OMIM#314250]

DYT3, Lubag

This rare condition, manifest almost exclusively among men originating from the Philippine Islands, usually begins in midlife with axial and lower limb involvement, although upper limb involvement and cranial *dystonia* at onset are also recognized. The majority develop a generalized dystonia within the first few years, others have *parkinsonism*, which is levodopa unresponsive. The patients typically die of their disease after 5–10 years, and at postmortem there is degeneration with a so-called mosaic pattern within the striatum. The condition is linked to the DYT3 locus at Xq13, and results from an insertion into an intron of the TATA-binding protein-associated factor-1 gene.

References

Singleton A, Hague S, Hernandez D. X-linked recessive dystonia-parkinsonism (XDP; Lubag; DYT3). Adv Neurol. 2004;94:139–142
Waters CH, Faust PL, Powers J et al. Neuropathology of lubag (X-linked dystonia parkinsonism). Mov Disord. 1993;8:387–390

X-linked myopathy with excessive autophagy (XMEA)

A rare hereditary myopathy of childhood onset, characterized by a slowly progressive proximal myopathy (especially of the lower limbs), with normal life expectancy. EMG shows polyphasic motor units with high mean amplitude and normal duration; abundant myotonic discharges occur in clinically affected and unaffected muscles. Muscle biopsy shows abundant sarcoplasmic vacuoles, immunopositive for dystrophin and laminin, containing debris and lysosomal enzymes. These features distinguish the condition from other *limb girdle muscular dystrophies*. XMEA is distinct from the X-linked vacuolar myopathy with cardiomyopathy and mental retardation due to deficiency of lysosome-associated membrane protein 2 (LAMP-2), also known as *Danon disease*.

Reference

Kalimo H, Savontaus M-L, Lang H, et al. X-linked myopathy with excessive autophagy: a new hereditary muscle disease. Ann Neurol. 1988;23:258–265

Zinc deficiency

Acrodermatitis enteropathica

There is an autosomal recessive disorder of zinc metabolism and malabsorption, acrodermatitis enteropathica, usually presenting in the first year of life following weaning from breast milk, with a distinctive vesico-bullous skin disorder, especially around orifices (mouth, anus), alopecia, diarrhea, failure to thrive, increased susceptibility to infection, with or without neurobehavioral features (lethargy, irritability, depression). Lifelong oral zinc sulfate supplementation is associated with a normal life expectancy. Untreated, patients progress and succumb to infection.

Whether disordered zinc metabolism may contribute to adult cognitive decline, specifically in the context of *Alzheimer's disease*, remains contentious, with different groups advocating too much or too little zinc as important factors in the pathogenesis of the typical neuropathological lesions of AD. A poor diet will also result in biochemical zinc deficiency, not necessarily accompanied by neurological features.

References

Nachev PC, Larner AJ. Zinc and Alzheimer's disease. Trace Elem Electrolytes 1996;13:55–59
Prasad A. Zinc deficiency. BMJ. 2003;326:409–410